Geriatric Physical Therapy

A Clinical Approach

Carole B. Lewis, PT, GCS, MSG, MPA, PhD
President
Physical Therapy Services of Washington

Adjunct Associate Professor
George Washington University
College of Medicine
School of Health Care Sciences
Washington, DC

Jennifer M. Bottomley, PT, MS
Area Rehabilitation Coordinator
Medicare and Rehabilitation Specialists/Hillhaven Corp.
Norwood, Massachusetts

APPLETON & LANGE
Norwalk, Connecticut

Notice: The authors and the publisher of this volume have taken care to
make certain that the doses of drugs and schedules of treatment are correct
and compatible with the standards generally accepted at the time of
publication. Nevertheless, as new information becomes available, changes in
treatment and in the use of drugs become necessary. The reader is advised to
carefully consult the instruction and information material included in the
package insert of each drug or therapeutic agent before administration.
This advice is especially important when using new or infrequently used drugs.
The publisher disclaims any liability, loss, injury, or damage incurred as
a consequence, directly or indirectly, of the use and application of any of
the contents of this volume.

Prentice Hall International (UK) Limited, *London*
Prentice Hall of Australia Pty. Limited, *Sydney*
Prentice Hall Canada, Inc., *Toronto*
Prentice Hall Hispanoamericana, S.A., *Mexico*
Prentice Hall of India Private Limited, *New Delhi*
Prentice Hall of Japan, Inc., *Tokyo*
Simon & Schuster Asia Pte., Ltd., *Singapore*
Editora Prentice Hall do Brasil Ltda., *Rio de Janeiro*
Prentice Hall, *Englewood Cliffs, New Jersey*

Library of Congress Cataloging-in-Publication Data

Lewis, Carole Bernstein.
    Geriatric physical therapy : a clinical approach / Carole B.
Lewis, Jennifer M. Bottomley.
        p. cm.
    Includes index.
    ISBN 0–8385–8875–1
    1. Physical therapy for the aged.   I. Bottomley, Jennifer M.
II. Title.
    [DNLM: 1. Physical Therapy—in old age.   2. Geriatric Assessment.
3. Aging.   WB 460 L673g 1994]
    RC953.8.P58L479   1994
    615.8'2'0846—dc20
    DNLM/DLC   93–5965
    for Library of Congress   CIP

Acquisitions Editor: Cheryl L. Mehalik
Production Editor: Elizabeth C. Ryan
Designer: Michael J. Kelly

PRINTED IN THE UNITED STATES OF AMERICA

ISBN 0-8385-8875-1

9 780838 588758
90000

Dedication

I dedicate this book to my newly born daughter, Madison Wagner. Even though you won't remember, Madison, you were instrumental in the compilation of this book. In your first month of life, you worked intensely with me on the completion of the final drafts, developing the Pearls, and preparing the chapter outlines. Your adorable little face and your wonderful demeanor gave me the strength and patience to persevere. As I held you in my arms and wrote some of the final passages, your enthusiasm for life was inspirational. I hope that you will have a long, healthy life, full of love and happiness, and that you will enjoy your old age.

With much love, your mother,
Carole

I dedicate this book to the loving memory of my grandparents, Anna Uebele, and Edna and Newton Bottomley, whose influence on my life inspired my professional direction in geriatric physical therapy.

Jennifer Bottomley

About the Cover

Eastern cultures are known for their respectful treatment of the elderly. They are valued members of society. A long and healthy life is desirable, as well as attainable. It is with this image and idea that we selected the symbol that appears on the cover as well as throughout the pages of *Geriatric Physical Therapy*. As you read this book, and learn from it, we hope that respect and care will always be a part of the treatment plan for your geriatric patients.

Contents in Brief

Contents in Detail

Preface

This book was developed based on the need for a geriatric physical therapy text that transcended the classical clinical and academic texts currently available. The profession of geriatric physical therapy has evolved rapidly in the past decade, but the textbooks available have not kept pace with the need for specialized clinical information. With the inauguration of a geriatric specialty exam in physical therapy, the need became more pressing. This book is designed to provide a single, comprehensive source for the advanced applied science of normal and pathological aging, clinical problems, implications for therapeutic interventions, and considerations specific to the elderly.

The main objective of this textbook is to present therapists with a thorough review of advanced clinical information. The target audience for this text is clinicians already exposed to geriatric patients who seek to improve their background and skill level. In addition, advanced master's students seeking specific clinical information will also find relevant material in the text.

At the time this text went into publication, a small group of physical therapists had successfully passed the first geriatric specialty exam. Many of the therapists who sat for this exam had difficulty in locating up-to-date information to prepare for the exam, or a comprehensive source of information. The authors believe this text addresses both of these criteria.

Both of the authors have worked extensively in the field of geriatrics. They have combined their knowledge to provide clinical information that is grounded in the literature and research-based references.

The text is divided into three parts. Part I provides advanced applied gerontological concepts. These chapters contain the most recent background information available and provide a clinically useful basis for a sound foundation for the following two sections.

Part I covers the important areas of demographic trends in the aging population as well as aging theories and their impact on clinical strategies. A thorough description of age-related changes in biology, physiology, and anatomy of all organ systems of the body is provided, as well as a comprehensive examination of pathological manifestations commonly seen in the aged population.

Descriptions of detailed psychological aspects of aging and a presentation of evaluative tools that can be used to evaluate and treat these conditions are provided as useful tools for the clinician. Background information on assessment tools—particularly functional assessment tools—is presented to provide the reader with objective indices for thorough evaluation in a variety of settings.

Part I also incorporates a clear explanation of some of the common nutritional problems and risk factors seen in the older population, as well as a discussion on the components of good nutritional programs. Finally, identification of various drug regimens, adverse drug reactions, and common pathologies seen with inappropriate drug management afford a practical approach to identifying pharmacological aspects of patient intervention.

Part II presents a comprehensive consideration of patient care concepts. This section begins with an overview, "Principles and Practices in Geriatric Rehabilitation," which bridges the gap between the background information presented in Part I and applies it to advanced clinical concepts. The importance of immobility and disuse is emphasized. This section provides an introduction to evaluation and presents treatment suggestions for common problems, including treatment design and rationale.

Orthopedic, neurologic, and cardiopulmonary problems, as well as strategies for evaluating and treating these conditions, contribute invaluable means for comprehensively addressing and intervening in problems commonly seen in an elderly population. Practical suggestions guide the therapist in establishing and implementing health maintenance programs, such as the provision of screening programs as a means of preventive health care and early intervention to avoid the pathological consequences of "hypokinetics."

Part III covers administration and management. Effective communication with the aging population is discussed, as well as the evaluation of personal attitudes toward the elderly, cultural biases, ethnic considerations, and other factors relating to the care of the elderly. A discussion of educational services and objectives for the elderly with a differentiation of various learning theories applied to the older population completes this section.

Practical information is also provided on the identification and description of geriatric physical therapy services. Other practical information includes how to address administrative needs, prepare budgets, and develop marketing proposals for nursing homes and outpatient facilities. The role of the consultant and the development of the consultative tasks for geriatric specialists is presented. A thorough discussion of methods for reviewing research by identifying the various aspects of a research proposal and by examination of research characteristics that make clinical data collection unique for an aging population is also presented. Finally, resources for the aging network available for the older person, including legislative, social and federal programs, are presented in a user-friendly style that afford a one-stop information resource on providing the most appropriate services to an aging population.

It became necessary to condense the large and all-encompassing body of geriatric rehabilitation literature into a manageable textbook size. The authors hope that this book provides a strong clinical foundation for a practicing geriatrician in a clear, concise manner, and will facilitate the provision of optimum care to their elderly patients.

Carole B. Lewis
Jennifer M. Bottomley

Acknowledgments

I would like to acknowledge all of the individuals that have helped to make the compilation of this book possible. I would especially like to thank Janet Jensen for her assistance with the ethics chapter and Amy Ellis for her contributions to the pharmacy chapter. Barbara Woo, Suzanne Stragand, and especially Beth Hoffman and Terry Scanlin provided much hard work and ensured that all the details were in order, especially in organizing and proofing the manuscripts. A special thank you to the staff at Physical Therapy Services of Washington, DC, Inc. and to my family for their patience and understanding in allowing me the time to put together this manuscript. Your on-demand feedback and assistance helped this book get off the ground.

Carole B. Lewis

I would like to acknowledge the forsightedness of Stephanie S. Scott, who was instrumental in the conception and development of this book.

Jennifer M. Bottomley

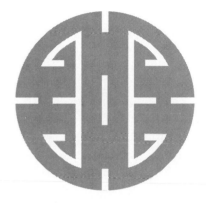

PART I

Applied Gerontological Concepts

CHAPTER ONE

Understanding the Demographics of an Aging Population

Demography is the scientific study of the population. Increasing attention has been paid to the demography of aging as a subfield of general demography that relates in important ways to the concerns of social gerontologists.[1] Demography continues to evolve as a fundamental knowledge base for the study of aging. The study of the "demography of aging" is focused on determining: the state of the older population; changes in the numbers, proportionate size, and composition of this subpopulation; the component forces of fertility, mortality, morbidity, migration, and immigration; and the impact of these demographic changes on issues related to the social, economic, and health status of the elderly in an aging society.[1,2]

Distinct subgroups within the older population, somewhat ignored in the past, have also been receiving increased demographic emphasis in the past few years.[3] This development appears to reflect the societal concerns about the policy challenges of meeting the welfare and health care needs of all components of an aging society.[4]

Gilford[5] has determined that there are serious data gaps that are present in existing demographic information. One such data gap has been identified in the area of the subgroup termed the "oldest-old" (also called the "frail elderly" or the "extremely old"). Because of the special concerns regarding the relatively high rates of illness and disability and the concommitant implications for health care and social service provisions in this age group, they have been presented by demographers as a "geriatric imperative" for future research.[6] This trend toward specialized demographic studies is also apparent in an analysis of a broad range of issues specific to the situations of racial and ethnic minorities[3] and older women. These areas will be dealt with more extensively in the later sections of this chapter.

AN HISTORICAL PERSPECTIVE ON THE STUDY OF POPULATION AGING

The study of population aging has a relatively long history. Attention to population aging emerged in France at the close of the nineteenth century, when the proportion of persons aged 65 years of age and over exceeded 5%. By the 1900s, this proportion increased to 8%.[7] Sweden was another country that experienced considerable population aging in the nineteenth century.[8] Sundbarg[9] was the first to place emphasis on the relative proportions of aged individuals in a society, and the first demographer to note systematic differences in age composition among countries. By implication, he hypothesized that there would be a demographic shift over time toward an aging population structure in all countries.[9]

For most Western countries, the aging of the population has been a twentieth-century phenomenon. In the United States, concerted demographic attention to the aging process can be found as early as the 1920s,[10] and increasing concern was expressed in the 1930s when the declining fertility of the Depression era led demographers to project rapid changes in the age structure of the United States.[11-13] It also led to a growing interest by demographers in capturing the dimensions of this phenomenon. Following World War II, there was a steady increase in the body of literature related to population aging in the United States as well as other Western countries.

There is also an increasing awareness that population aging will be an important issue in underdeveloped countries currently experiencing social and economic development.[14] Population aging is now recognized as a worldwide phenomenon that commands immediate attention if effective societal responses are to be made to changing demographic realities.[1] As a result, many issues have emerged that relate to the rapid growth in the number of older persons (such as the degree to which countries are able to make commitments to social welfare and health care policies in light of other priorities that they face in the allocation of social and economic resources).[15,16]

DEMOGRAPHIC PROCESSES AND AGE STRUCTURE OF POPULATION

Demography views aging as an aggregative process through which the population structure is modified. It is defined in terms of the mean or median age of the population, the size and proportion of various age categories of the population, and the ratios between different age categories.[1] Though these are relatively static concepts, when they are examined over time, demographic patterns and trends begin to develop. In projecting changes in population structure, demographers focus on the rate and timing of events over the entire life course, using chronological age as a reference scale on which to measure important social transitions and to identify demographic trends.

Change in the size of a population over time depends on the rate persons join the population through births or immigration and the rate they leave the population through death or emigration. Persons born in a common year (e.g., classified by common age) are often grouped together as a "birth cohort."[17] Such cohorts can be followed over time to reconstruct population history and to project future population changes.

Traditionally, demographers have used the age of 65 for delineating old age. This facilitates standardized analyses and is grounded in social practices (i.e., retirement, Social Security provisions). In addition, because slightly more males than females are born to humans and the mortality experiences of men and women differ over their lifetimes, demographers typically distinguish the sex of persons when constructing models of population change.[3]

The number of persons who survive to any given age depends on the number of persons born into that cohort, the rate at which they have survived, and the extent to which their numbers have changed because of cumulative differences between immigrants and emigrants. For example, the number of persons reaching the age of 65 in 1990 depended on the number of persons born in 1925, the cumulative probability that they survived each of the next 65 years, and the relative balance between the movement of persons from that age cohort into or out of the United States from 1925 to 1990. The number of persons aged 65 and older in 1990 increased compared to the number of elderly in 1989 because of the addition of this new cohort to the population of older persons was greater than the subtraction of persons who have died in all cohorts aged 65 and older during that year.[3] The population of older persons can thus grow either because the size of the entering birth cohort is much larger than that of previous cohorts or because improvements in survivorship have reduced the number of deaths that might otherwise have occurred among the elderly. Demographers use the "aging pyramid" to graphically depict cohort distribution from year to year. Figure 1–1 pictorially shows the age structure of the US population in 1910.[18] Contrast this pyramid with the age structure of the US population in 1980 that is depicted in Figure 1–2, which is when the 1900–1910 birth cohort reached the 70 years of age and older catagory.[18] A distinction is drawn between "aging at the apex" (e.g., when the proportion of older persons in a population increases) and "aging from the base" (e.g., when the proportion of younger persons in a population decreases).

In studying the elderly population, the absolute number of older persons, the rate of change in the number of older persons, and the proportion of the total population that is old are important components in demography. The aggregate older population is composed of a population that includes persons who range in age over a span of some 45 years.[1] The relative numbers of men and women at each age and the age characteristics of the elderly are also important compositional factors. Explicit attention to the composition of the aged population leads to the recognition of important changes taking place to modify the population structure, such as the high relative increase in the numbers of extremely old persons, declining sex ratios, and shifts in marital status, living arrangements, racial and ethnic status, and health status. In understanding the demographics of an aging population, these aspects of the demography of aging will often be discussed to present a global picture of the characteristics of the population aged 65 and over in any given year.

Historically, fertility is the most important determinant of population growth and the age structure of the population. Demographers view fertility as the demographic process of renewal. When the fertility rate is high, the cohort for each year has more members than the cohorts that preceded it. At moderate to low

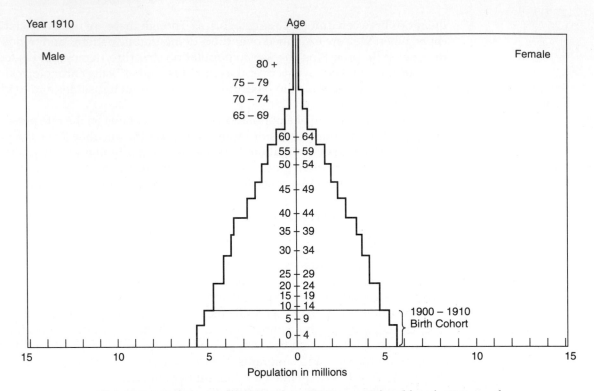

Figure 1–1. Age Structure of the US population: 1910 census. *(Adapted from the US Bureau of the Census, 1970 Census of Population:* United States Summary, General Population Characteristics, PC(1)-B1. *Washington, DC: US Government Printing Office; 1972. Reproduced with permission from Soldo BJ. America's elderly in the 1980's.* Pop Bull. 1980; 35(1):1–48.)

levels of mortality, then, the number of newborns added to the population exceeds the number of older persons who die; the proportion of the population that is young increases, and its median age declines. When the birthrate is low, the proportion of the population that is old increases, and the median age of the population rises.

The effect of a decline in mortality from high to moderate levels, which occurred in the United States in the late nineteenth and early twentieth centuries as infectious diseases were brought under control, paradoxically caused the population to become younger.[19] The reason for this relationship between mortality and age structure is that the most important improvements in survivorship during this period occurred in the age groups of infants and children. Recent improvements in the prevention and treatment of cardiovascular disease, however, have increased the survivorship of older persons. Since 1940, the major reason for the increase in the number of the oldest-old, those aged 85 years and older, has been the improved survivorship of the old.[20] About two-thirds of the 1980 to 1985 increase in the proportion of older persons in the population was caused by a mortality rate decline.[21] The tremendous increase in the projected number of elderly and of the very old during the next 50 years results from the large cohorts born during the post-World War II baby boom that will be reaching old age *and* the improved survivorship in all age cohorts, especially those regarded as the oldest-old.[19]

The growth of the total population is particularly sensitive to declining mortality rates, whereas the growth of the older population, especially in their proportionate size relative to the total population, occurs when the fertility rate declines.[22] In fact, declines in mortality focused at younger ages that are not accompanied by decreases in the fertility rate can lead to an overall younger population. The sustained decrease in mortality that extends into older ages is the main reason for the current population's aging.[21]

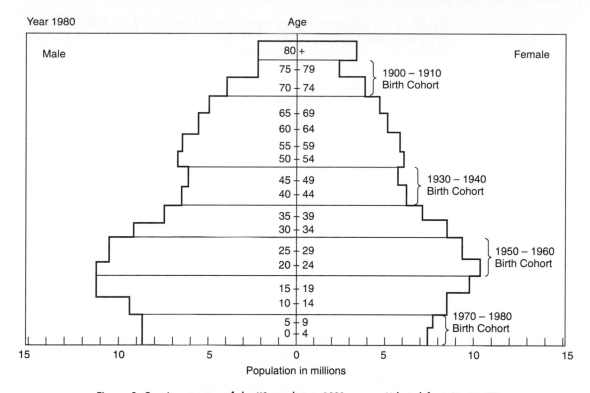

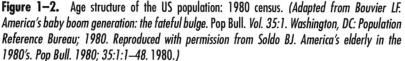

Figure 1–2. Age structure of the US population: 1980 census. *(Adapted from Bouvier LF. America's baby boom generation: the fateful bulge. Pop Bull. Vol. 35:1. Washington, DC: Population Reference Bureau; 1980. Reproduced with permission from Soldo BJ. America's elderly in the 1980's. Pop Bull. 1980; 35:1:1–48. 1980.)*

PROJECTED POPULATION TRENDS IN AN AGING SOCIETY

The major demographic forces that alter the size of a population and its age composition are the levels of fertility and mortality. Measures used by demographers to estimate these two factors are, respectively, the general fertility rate (i.e., the number of live births per 1000 women annually) and the life expectancy at birth. Demographers, in making their projections, typically use low, middle, and high estimates. For the purpose of this chapter, the middle series projections are used unless otherwise indicated.

The projected demographic trends indicate that by the year 2050 there will be 69 million elderly Americans.[19] In 1960, the Census Bureau's statistics indicated that there were 16.6 million persons aged 65 and over, but by 1990, an estimated 31.6 million persons were age 65 and older.[23] Proportionally, the elderly made up 9.2% of the American population in 1960 and increased to 12.6% by 1990. If Census Bureau projections are accurate, it is anticipated that these proportions will climb to 17.7% in 2020 and 22.9% by 2050.

Between the years 1960 and 1990, there was a 2% annual growth in the overall elderly population. This trend is expected to decrease to about 1% by the year 2010 as a result of the small Depression era and World War II age cohorts that will be reaching the age of 65. After 2010, the rate of growth will exceed 2% as the baby boom cohort reaches the age of 65. This trend is anticipated to persist until 2030. Between 2030 to 2050, it is projected that the population of elderly Americans will stabilize to a 1% level of growth annually.[19]

Projected demographic trends reflect an assumption that there will be a sharply declining fertility rate accompanied by a decreasing mortality rate until

TABLE 1–1. LIFE EXPECTANCY OF US POPULATION AT BIRTH, BY RACE AND GENDER: 1900, 1950, AND 1978

Race and Gender	Life Expectancy at Birth		
	1900	1950	1978
White			
Men	47	67	70
Women	49	72	78
Nonwhite			
Men	33	59	65
Women	34	63	74

Reproduced with permission from Soldo BJ. America's elderly in the 1980's. Pop Bull. 1980;35(1):1– 48.

the year 2050.[19] These forecasted changes indicate that there will be a reduction in the growth of the total population to a level of 1% annually.[1] However, even at a level of 1% annual growth, it is anticipated that the total population will double over the next 60 years.[19]

Table 1–1 shows how dramatically the life expectancy of the US population has increased since the early 1900s.[18] Life expectancy at birth is projected to increase from 74.3 years in 1982 to 76.7 years in 2000 and to 81.0 years of age by 2050.[19] Male life expectancy will increase from 70.6 years in 1982 to 72.9 years in the year 2000 and 76.7 years by the year 2050. Females, who can expect to live 78.1 years under current conditions, are projected to attain a life expectancy of 80.5 years in 2000, and 85.2 years by 2050. Other researchers feel that life expectancy will improve even more than the Census Bureau projections assume.[24–26] Life expectancy is, therefore, expected to gain an additional 12.8 years if the current demographic trends persist over the next 60 years.

Female life expectancy has been about 7.5 years higher than male life expectancy since 1970.[19] While there is much disagreement as to whether this differential will narrow or widen, several demographers believe it may narrow by several years.[27–29] Others, however, believe it may widen to 10 or 12 years by the turn of the century.[25,26] Spencer[19] predicts that the sex difference in life expectancy will gradually widen to 8.5 years by 2050.

PROJECTED COMPONENTS OF CHANGE IN AN AGING POPULATION

Fertility Patterns

In the middle series for the overall US population, the number of births is expected to remain above the present level of 3.7 million throughout the early 1990s. The peak number of births (3.9 million) may actually have already occurred in the late 1980s.[19] After the early 1990s, it is anticipated that the birthrate will not surpass 3.7 million because of a decline in the female population of childbearing age. Instead the number of births is projected to fluctuate between 3.4 and 3.7 million.

Mortality Patterns

The first year in which 2 million Americans died was 1983, and it is projected that it is not likely that there will ever be a year again with less than 2 million deaths.[19] Deaths in the next century are expected to steadily increase and reach 2.4 million by the turn of the century and 3.8 million by the year 2040. After that time, the death rate would be between 3.8 and 4.0 million deaths annually.

Because we have already established that the population is getting older, it is not surprising that the proportion of all deaths that happen at older ages would increase in the future. Currently, about 70% of deaths occur at age 65 and older. This proportion is anticipated to increase to 80% by 2030 and remain relatively stable until the end of the twenty-first century. More noteworthy is the likely change in the proportions of deaths that happen at age 85 and over. While 18% of all deaths now occur at such old ages, this percentage is expected to reach 30% by 2010 and increase to more than 43% after 2050.[19]

Immigration and Migration Patterns

A great deal of interest about future levels of net immigration concerns the impact of immigration on the future of US population sizes. This is the only demographic area where projections based on the low, middle, and high estimates from the census data will be covered, because the uncertain immigration rate could profoundly impact the size of the US population. According to Spencer,[19] if there were no net immigration, the US population would grow to 258 million people by the year 2000 and peak at approximately 275 million people around 2030. If future net migration is relatively low (i.e., 250,000 per year), the population would be 264 million in the year 2000 and then level off around 2040 at 294 million. In comparison with the zero migration estimates, this population would be 2.1% or 5.5 million people larger in the year 2000, 6% larger in 2030, and 10% larger by the year 2050. Net immigration at the middle level (i.e., 450,000 per year) has an interesting effect on the population size after 2050. Essentially, there would be a zero-growth population after the year 2050. Therefore, if middle fertility and mortality assumptions are correct, net immigration much below 450,000 eventually produces a stable or declining population.[19] The highest net immigration estimates (i.e., 750,000 per year) show an increase in the population continuously throughout the twenty-first century.

Age Composition of the Aging US Population

It is anticipated that the percentage of the total population that is 65 and over will increase from the current level of 12.6% to 13.0% by the year 2000 and to 21.2% by 2030 (nearly double), when using the middle series Census Bureau estimates.[19]

The population that is 85 years of age and over will grow at a more rapid rate than the entire 65 and over population, assuming that the extremely old will benefit from the improvements in future mortality rates.[23] According to Spencer,[19] there are currently 2.4 million Americans aged 85 and over. This number is expected to double by the beginning of the twenty-first century to approximately 4.9 million, and reach 8.6 million persons over the age of 85 by 2030. Currently, about 1% of the population is aged 85 years and older. By 2050, 5.2% of the population will be that old. Those aged 85 and above compose 9.1% of the present population that is 65 years of age and older.[23] Projections indicate that by the year 2050, those 85 years of age and older will make up one-quarter of the entire elderly population.[25]

For the population of those aged 100 years and over, a substantial growth in the overall numbers is also anticipated. According to the 1990 Census Bureau report,[23] there are about 32,000 centenarians in the population. By the year 2000, this is expected to grow to 108,000, and by 2030 an estimated 492,000 persons will be over the age of 100. Currently, about 30 elderly persons turn 100 every day; by the year 2030, 280 persons each day are expected to be passing their first century of life.[19]

Gender Composition of the Aging US Population

Accompanying the aging of the population is an increasing proportion of females compared to males as age increases. Elderly women outnumber men three to two as a result of sex differentials in mortality that favor females at all ages. For those 85 years of age and older, women outnumber men five to two.[30] In other words, higher proportions of females than males survive to old age. These ratios are expected to increase gradually through the end of this century and then sharply increase through the middle of the twenty-first century as large entry cohorts, in which the sex ratios are higher, enter the 65 years of age and older population.[1]

Marital Status of the Aging US Population

Another demographic characteristic that warrants examination is the marital status of older persons. The importance of this characteristic is its meaning for the elderly individual and its impact on family status, living arrangements, and available support systems.[31] The composition of the aged population with respect to marital status is influenced by complex patterns of family formation and dissolution that vary cross-culturally as well as by the important constraints imposed by differential mortality rates of males and females.[32] The reduced mortality that distinguishes the demographic transitions reportedly occurring, lengthens the duration of marriage as the joint survival of both men and women is extended. However, with the widening gap in survival between the sexes, widowhood becomes more common for women at older ages. For males over the age of 65 years of age, over 75% are currently married, but, for females of the same age, over 65% are widowed.[33]

Marital dissolution through divorce or separation and remarriage in later life are additional factors that need to be considered. In addition, those never married or those cohabitating certainly confound any clean analysis of living arrangements and support systems for the elderly. The proportion of older persons who are divorced is less than 7%. The proportions of never-married males and females are quite high at approximately 12.5%.[1] Remarriage at older ages plays a relatively small role in modifying the marital status distributions.[33]

Projections of marital status in the United States indicate that there will be a slight reduction in the proportions of older males married and widowed in the next century and that there will be proportionately fewer females who are widowed.[34] It is anticipated, however, that cohorts reaching the older ages after 1990 will be more likely to be divorced or separated as a result of the substantially higher proportions of divorced and separated persons in younger cohorts.

Living Arrangements of the Aging US Population

Associated with these marital changes have been pronounced changes in the living arrangements of elderly women. The most notable of these have been the sharp increase in the proportion of women living alone and the sharp decline in the proportion of women living with other family members.[31] There has been relatively little change in the proportion of elderly men living alone or with other family members. As of 1990, about one in seven men live alone and more than four out of five elderly men live with family members.[23] Elderly men are much more likely to be living with a wife than to be widowed or living with other family members.[33]

The increased tendency of older women, including extremely aged women, to live alone is likely to continue. It is expected that by 1995, over 60% of the women 75 years of age and over will be living alone. The proportion of aged men living alone is not expected to change much.[31] The US Census Bureau projections suggest that in 1995, about 52% of the households maintained by persons 75 years and over will be maintained by women living alone or with nonrelatives; the current proportion is about 46%.[35]

The trends toward independent living has come about partly as a result of improvements in the economic and health status of the elderly, partly from a desire not to be dependent on others, and partly, for some, from a simple lack of alternatives.[36]

TABLE 1–2. PREVALENCE OF DISABILITY IN BASIC ADL*^a* AND INSTRUMENTAL ADL*^b* IN ADULTS 65 AND OVER: UNITED STATES

Disability	Age		
	65–74(%)	75–84 (%)	85+ (%)
Needs help in one or more basic ADL	5.3	11.4	34.8
Needs help in one or more instrumental ADL	5.7	14.2	40.0

*^a*Basic ADL: Includes walking, going outside, bathing, dressing, using toilet, getting in and out of a bed, and eating.
*^b*Instrumental ADL: Includes shopping, doing routine household chores, preparing meals, and handling money.
Adapted from Advance Data. *National Center for Health Statistics. Government Document No. 92, September 4, 1982.*
Reproduced from National Center for Health Statistics. *Current Estimates from the National Health Interview Survey: United States, 1981. Washington, DC: US Government Printing Office; 1982. US Dept of Health and Human Services Publication No. 10-141.*

Health Status of the Aging US Population

Clinical measures clearly indicate the decline of health status with age. The elderly are more likely to have chronic conditions that limit their activities, and they experience about twice as many days of restricted activity because of illness compared to the general population.[37] However, to be aged in the United States today is not necessarily to be beset with numerous and complex disabilities. Life after age 65 years is not a period inexorably marked with massive physical deterioration.[38] Nevertheless, the increasing life expectancy of those reaching age 65 years has had an important impact on the prevalence of functional disabilities in the elderly population. The National Health Interview Survey conducted in 1981 by the National Center for Health Statistics provided national estimates of the level of functioning of the noninstitutionalized aged in the United States.[38] Table 1–2 provides a summary of the data collected in that survey. In 1981, about 20% of those community-dwelling elders 65 years of age or older reported some restrictions in their mobility. A similar trend is seen with respect to restrictions in elders' major daily activities. Forty-three percent reported some limitation in their functional activity levels.[38] Viewed as a homogeneous group, the majority of elders are free from disability, and for most, the later years of life are characterized by substantial physical ability.

DEMOGRAPHIC TRENDS AND PROJECTIONS IN THE MINORITY ELDERLY

The aging of the US population will affect every institution and every individual in our society. Projections of the proportion of the population 65 years of age and over is anticipated to dramatically increase over the next 60 years.[3] This phenomena of population aging is of particular importance in minority groups in America. There is a marked differential between majority and minority aging with respects to fertility, mortality, and migration, and it is expected that the racial and ethnic diversity of the aged in the United States will increase rapidly as we enter the twenty-first century. In other words, as the elderly population becomes a larger percentage of the overall population, a greater proportion of the elderly will be minority group members. This shift in the composition of the elderly population will have a great impact on public policy development in the arenas of social welfare and the health care system. This section of the chapter examines the projected demographic trends and the compositional changes in the United States of the minority elderly.

Age is sometimes called "the great equalizer";[3] however, today's elderly are a highly diverse group, and this makes simple analysis difficult. Age, gender, race, and ethnicity determine an individual's status in American society, and as a result, influence life-course experiences. Differences in income, health, and social supports significantly affect the elderly's quality of life, and each of these demographic variables is important to understanding the social, intergenerational family relations, economic status, longevity, and health status of the elderly. The status and resources of many minority elderly reflect social and economic discrimination experienced in earlier life. Many, especially those who migrated to the United States, face cultural and language differences as well. Demographic data provide a sound foundation upon which to examine health status, life expectancy, economic status, family patterns, household structure, and support systems of minority elderly.

Projected Population Trends in the Minority Elderly

Projected demographic trends indicate that by the year 2050 there will be 69 million elderly Americans. Within that group 54 million will be white, 10 million will be black, and 5 million will be composed of other ethnic and racial groups.[39] Eight million of these elderly (of any race) will be of Hispanic origin.[40] If life expectancy improves more rapidly than presently anticipated, these numbers could increase even more dramatically.[30]

Projections of minority elderly population growth are based on the "middle series," intermediate assumptions by the Census Bureau.[19] The growing statistical significance of the elderly population as a whole, and of the minority aged population in particular, is clearly illustrated in the recent rapid growth rates reported by the Census Bureau over the past three decades and the trends extrapolated from that data into the middle of the twenty-first century.[19]

In 1990, 89.9% of America's elderly were white; in fact, the total number of elderly white persons nearly doubled between 1960 and 1990, from 15.4 million to 28.3 million, however, demographic shifts reveal that this situation is changing rapidly. Though it is projected that the white elderly population will double again by the year 2030, it is estimated that the number of minority elderly will grow at a more rapid rate compared with the white elderly over the next 60 years.[3] As a consequence, the percentage of America's elderly that comprise blacks and races other than white would increase from 10.2% in 1990 to 15.3% in 2020 and to 21.3% in 2050. The number of black elderly doubled as well from 1960 to 1990 (1.2 million to 2.6 million) and will nearly triple to 7.8 million in 2030. It is anticipated that the number of black minority group elderly will escalate from 2.6 million blacks in 1990 to 9.6 million by the year 2050. Races other than white or black will increase from 600,000 to 5.0 million. Hispanic elderly of any origin, the fastest-growing population group as a whole in America, will more than double from 1.1 million in 1990 to 2.5 million by 2010, and it will reach 5.6 million by 2030 and 7.9 million in 2050. All nonwhite and nonblack elderly populations have shown a considerable increase from 81,000 in 1960 to 603,000 in 1990. Based on the middle series projections, this number would increase to 1.5 million persons in 2010, doubling again by 2030.[19] From these statistics it appears that although non-Hispanic white elderly will remain the majority group, blacks, Hispanics, and other racial and ethnic groups will grow at a faster rate and become a very large and important component of the aging American populace.

It is also expected that there will be a projected increase in the proportion of elders in each ethnic group. In 1960, 6% of the black population was 65 years of age or older. This percentage is anticipated to increase to 10% by 2010 and be over 17%

by 2030. The other races, including Asian, Native American, Eskimo, and Aleut, could more than double between now and the middle of the next century from 7% elderly to 16.1% in 2030. The Hispanic population would also age considerably. Currently 6% of the Hispanic population is 65 years of age or older. By 2030 this percentage is expected to increase to 13%.[39]

Between the years 1960 and 1990 there was a 2% annual growth in the white elderly population. This is expected to decrease to about 1% from 1990 to the year 2010. This drop is anticipated as the small Depression era and World War II cohorts reach old age. When the baby boom cohort reaches 65 years of age, the rate of growth of elderly whites will exceed 2% per year[19] until 2030. Between 2030 and 2050, projections indicate that there will be no increase in the population of white elderly Americans. Similar growth patterns for the black elderly will also occur, however, it is expected that the rate of increase of black elderly will be substantially greater than for white elderly.[39] On average, the black elderly population will increase at a rate of 1.0 to 1.5% higher than the white elderly each year.[40] For elderly of other races there was a 7% annual increase from 1960 to 1990. It is projected that this group will grow at a rate of 5% per year between 1990 and 2020, and between 2020 and 2050 it will remain relatively constant with a 2% growth rate annually. Hispanic elderly are anticipated to steadily increase 4% per year from 1990 to 2030.[41]

Projected Components of Change in the Minority Elderly

The demographic processes of minority populations in the United States typically vary from the majority population on the demographic dimensions of fertility, mortality, immigration, and migration.[3] For instance, blacks, Native Americans, and Mexican Americans have a higher mortality rate when compared to whites. Conversely, Japanese Americans tend to show a lower mortality rate than whites.[21] In addition, age and gender characteristics seem to influence mortality within a minority group. For example, infants and young men in the black minority have substantially higher mortality rates when compared to other age groups and young women.[3]

Fertility Patterns

The number of births for the population as a whole is projected to fluctuate between 3.4 and 3.7 million from 1990 through the middle of the twenty-first century.[19] The minority population birth statistics are grouped in the census data as "Black-and-Other-Races." The number of black-and-other-races births is already at an all time high of 725,000.[19] If the middle series proves correct, the number of black-and-other-races births would increase to almost 900,000 in 2030 and then stabilize. There is not much of a decline in black-and-other-races births during the 1990s because the number of women of childbearing age in the minority populations will continue to increase.

Mortality Patterns

The pattern of mortality rates in minority elders varies substantially from that seen in the white population as a result of differences in life expectancies and health status.[21] Since declines in the mortality rates for blacks have historically lagged behind white mortality declines, the life expectancy of blacks is not projected to reach white levels until 2080 under all assumptions.[19] Overall life expectancy is projected to decline substantially in the future, and it is not deemed likely that blacks could attain white mortality levels any sooner than 2080. Even with this postponement of convergence, black life expectancy at birth is expected to improve two to four times more rapidly than white life expectancy.[3] There is a good deal of evidence that black and white differences in life expectancy for women are narrowing more quickly than those of men, and this trend is expected to continue.[19] Other than the black population, ethnic subgroups have not been isolated for specific demographic analysis.

Immigration and Migration Patterns of Minority Elders

As a result of high fertility rates and high levels of immigration, Hispanics are a relatively young population. Between 1970 and 1980, the Hispanic population as a whole grew 61%,[40] a surge that makes Hispanics the fastest growing population in the United States. During the first half of the twenty-first century an overall growth and an increased proportion of the aged among Hispanics are expected to occur. Through the separate Hispanic national origin groups (Mexican Americans, Puerto Ricans, Cuban Americans, and Central and South Americans) have not been isolated in demographic projections, examination of the national origins of current older Hispanics reveals the diversity of the elderly Hispanic population.[41] The importance of the history of immigration patterns in the history of this ethnic group is clear.

Fewer than 5% of Hispanics of Mexican American, Puerto Rican, and South and Central American origin were 65 years of age or older in 1989.[3] On the other hand, Cuban Americans aged 65 and over made up approximately 20% of the entire Cuban American population making that subgroup a relatively "old" proportion of Hispanics. Mexican Americans, or Chicanos, constitute 48% of the total Hispanic elderly population, Puerto Ricans constitute 11%, Cuban Americans represent 18%, and Central and South Americans are 8%. One reason for this heterogeneity within the older Hispanic population of the United States is their varied immigration histories.[41] Some Mexican Americans immigrated to the southwestern United States during the colonial times. Others arrived during the "bracero" period when the use of temporary Mexican agricultural labor was encouraged in the United States. Recent documented and undocumented immigrants to the United States from Mexico have further increased the size of the Mexican American population. While the early immigrants of the colonial and "bracero" times are now reaching or have reached the age of 65, the more recent immigrants are relatively young.[41] It is the aging of this latter group that will play a major role in the growth of the Hispanic elderly in the next century.

The current aging of the Cuban subgroup is a result of their immigration to the United States as political refugees of the Castro regime during the 1960s. They came to America as young and middle-aged families, and now they are turning 65 years of age. That is why the Cuban Americans constitute a much larger proportion of the Hispanic elderly compared to the overall Hispanic population.

There is much diversity within the Asian elderly population as well. This population is also growing at a relatively rapid rate and will become an increasingly significant proportion of the US population in the first half of the twenty-first century. In 1980, 6% of the Asian origin population was 65 and older.[42] The Asian population is made up of Chinese, Filipino, Japanese, and, most recently, Vietnamese and Cambodian immigrants. Each of these Asian origin groups comprise about one-quarter of the Asian elderly.[42]

The immigration history of each of these subgroups varies considerably and results from three primary immigration waves. The first wave consisted of those Asians who came to the United States as young persons in the early 1900s; a second wave is made up by the children who were born in the United States to the earliest immigrants from Asia, and the last wave was those middle-aged and elderly persons who came to the United States after the changes in the US immigration laws in the mid-1960s.[42] Many of the Asian elderly today were young when they immigrated to the United States in the early part of this century, or they were the native-born children of these immigrants. In contrast, the Vietnamese and Cambodians came to the United States as political refugees after immigration quotas were lifted in 1965, and they will make up the future wave of Asian elderly.[42]

The elderly Native American population is a truly "statistically invisible" subgroup of the Native American population. Approximately 80,000 Native Americans 65 years of age and over were counted in the 1980 census,[43] which means that elderly persons make up approximately 5% of the total Native American population. It is suggested that due to the low proportions of the Native American population who are aged and the changing patterns of self-identification as Native Americans, that this group of minority elderly is virtually imperceptible within the census.[3] Overall, less than 1% of the minority aged are Native Americans.[19] Between 1970 and 1980, the older Native American population grew at nearly twice the rate of the population of elderly whites or blacks.[39] This apparent increase is credited to a renewed sense of ethnic awareness that developed among Native Americans following the Wounded Knee uprising in 1970.

The population distribution of minority elders is affected by patterns of international immigration and by migration within the United States. Approximately one-fifth (20%) of the black elderly live in rural areas, and over 59% of these are concentrated in the Southeastern states. Of the remainder, most live either in the North Central or Northeast regions of the United States.[44] The vast majority of Hispanic elderly live in four states, each with a different concentration of Hispanic groups. The majority of the Hispanic population in California and Texas are from Mexico and Central America; Florida attracts the Cuban population, while New York receives a large number of immigrants from Puerto Rico and the Caribbean Islands.[41]

The proportion of the Hispanic elderly that live in rural areas is approximately 11%, less than half of the rural white elderly population, which is estimated to be 26%.[44] The 1980 census shows that approximately 10% of Asian Pacific Islander elderly live in rural areas and that over 55% are concentrated in California, Hawaii, and Washington. Of the remainder, most live in the New York and New Jersey metropolitan areas or in Illinois and Texas.[43] About one-quarter of Native American elderly live on American Indian reservations or in Alaskan Native villages. Over half of these are concentrated in the Southwestern states of Oklahoma, California, Arizona, New Mexico, and Texas. Of the remainder, most live along the Canadian border. A far greater proportion (52%) of Native American elderly live in rural areas than any other subgroup of the population.[44] It becomes apparent that the population distribution and migration within the United States creates substantial variations in the age structure of the populations in the various states and regions of the nation. Demographic studies indicate that racial and ethnic minorities are more geographically concentrated than is the majority population.[39]

Race Distribution Trends

The black-and-other-races population as a whole is expected to grow during the next 100 years from the present level of 33.6 million to 45.3 million in the year 2000, 63.2 million in 2030, and 79.1 million by 2080. About two-thirds of the growth is predicted to occur during the next half century, and the rate of growth thereafter will slow relative to any previous time.[19] In contrast, the overall white population is projected to increase from its existing size of 198.5 million, reaching 222.7 million in 2000, peaking at almost 242 million shortly after 2030, and then declining slowly to 231.6 million in 2080.[19]

In the future, projections indicate that the white population will never increase more than about 40% as rapidly as will the black-and-other-races population.[43] The effect of this will be that the proportion of the population that is composed of black-and-other-races will continue to rise. In 1950 this proportion was 10.7%, increasing in 1970 to 12.4%, and then to 14.5% in 1982.[43] It is expected that this proportion will increase about 1.3 percentage points a decade with the black-and-other-races reaching 16.9% in 2000, 20.7% in 2030, and 25.5% by 2080.[39]

Conversely, the fraction of the black-and-other-races population that is black will continue to decline. Blacks constituted 89.7% of the black-and-other-races population in 1970 and 82.5% of this population in 1982.[43] That proportion will be down to 78.9% in 2000, 75.4% in 2030, and 70.4% in 2080. This occurs despite the fact that black fertility is assumed to be considerably above the other races. In large part, the black proportion declines because of the relatively high net immigration of races other than white or black.[19]

Even if there were no growth resulting from net immigration, the proportion of black-and-other-races is projected to increase because of higher future black fertility and the younger age structure of the black-and-other-races population as compared to the white population. In fact, it is expected that the black-and-other-races population will eventually exceed the white population by 20%.[30]

Age Composition of Minority Elderly

The age composition of the minority aged is another important demographic feature, because the elderly population is aging within itself. People of all races are living longer. Blacks 85 years and older increased from 67,000 in 1960 to 251,000 in 1990, and it is expected that the number of the oldest-old blacks will increase to 500,000 by 2010 and 1.8 million by the year 2050.[19] Between 1980 and 1990, the oldest-old Hispanics nearly doubled, increasing from 49,000 to 95,000. It is anticipated that this minority group will number more than 1.5 million by 2050.[41] The very old for all other races increased from 4000 in 1960 to 41,000 in 1990, a remarkable tenfold growth rate.[44]

Projected estimates of minority population growth indicate that the most significant and dramatic changes will occur between 2020 and 2050.[19] Around 62% of the aged in all minority groups currently falls within the 65 to 74 year age range. By 2050, the number in this age group will decrease to about 50% for Hispanics and other races, and about 55% for blacks.[19] Growth is projected to occur in the percentage of those aged 85 years and older. Currently, fewer than one in ten of the minority elderly are in the oldest-old age range, but it is anticipated that this ratio will increase to one in five by the year 2050.[19]

Gender Composition of the Minority Elderly

The gender composition of the minority aged varies considerably from the gender differences in the US elderly population as a whole. In the entire population, elderly women outnumber men by three to two as a result of differences in the life expectancy between males and females. For those 85 years of age and older, women outnumber men five to two.[30] In the minority elderly, both because of the gender imbalances in previous migration patterns and the variations in the extent to which females have better survival rates than males, these ratios have become more equalized.[39] If sex ratio is defined as the number of males per 100 females, the following ratios for elderly minority groups were calculated for 1990[3]: In the young-old group (65 to 74 years old), the sex ratio for non-Hispanic whites was 81:100, for blacks it was 71:100, for Mexican American and Puerto Rican Hispanics the ratio was 100:100, for Hispanics of Cuban and Central and South American origin the ratio was 91:100, and it was 95:100 for Asian Americans. The sex ratio of the young elderly was more balanced among those ethnic groups that had a substantial history of immigration.[39] The less balanced ratio among blacks than whites is credited to the increased mortality rate of black men at every age.[3]

The sex ratio drops among those minority elders 75 years of age and older in all groups with the exception of Asian elderly.[3] For non-Hispanic whites the ratio becomes 59:100, for blacks it is 63:100, for Hispanics the ratio drops to 72:100, and for Asians the ratio actually increases to 124:100. Asian elderly men outnumber females until they reach the oldest-old age group of 85 years of age and over.[42] It is suggested that the more balanced sex ratio among young-old Asian Americans is the result of differences in male migration history. For example, in the early 1900s among the Chinese population, there were 14 males for every female. It is expected that in the future, the relative ratio of Asian men to women will evolve to resemble more closely the ratios of other Asian cohorts that had more sex-balanced immigration patterns (i.e., Asian immigrants since 1965) and the increasing proportion of the Asian American elderly who were born in America.[42]

Marital Status of the Minority Elderly

Among both whites and blacks aged 65 or older, the majority of men are married and the majority of women are widowed,[44] however, among older males, more than twice as many blacks compared to whites are divorced or separated, and the proportion of widowed black men is also higher.[45] The marital status of older black and white women is generally the same, except that the percentage of older black women divorced or separated is slightly higher.[44]

Mirroring the white elderly population, nearly twice as many Hispanic men as women aged 65 and older are married and living with their spouses.[41] Almost twice as many older Hispanic men and women are divorced or separated compared with whites, but the same proportion of Hispanic and white women are widowed.[41]

The majority of Asian men aged 65 and over are married, while the majority of women are widowed. Asian women are much more likely to be married to white partners, and there is a smaller proportion of Asian women who remain single in their later years.[46]

The marital status of Native Americans is comparable to that of the white elderly population. The majority of elderly men are married, and the majority of women are widowed. Like Asian women, Native American elderly women are more likely to be married in their later years than are white women.[44]

Living Arrangements of the Minority Elderly

Household living arrangements of non-Hispanic white, black, Mexican American, Puerto Rican, other Hispanic, and Asian in 1989 reveal some intriguing differences between these groups. One-third of whites and blacks live alone, though generally, the minority aged rarely live alone.[39] This is particularly true of the Asian elderly who tend to live in multigenerational households.[46] With the exception of black elders, living with a spouse is the most common household situation for most elderly groups.[3] It is interesting that the black elderly are less likely to be married than other minority groups, which reflects their higher rates of marital disruption during their life course.[44] In contrast, Puerto Rican and Asian elderly are three times as likely as non-Hispanic whites to live with others, including family members other than their spouse.[45] One-third of black elderly persons live with others, related or unrelated, as do approximately one-fifth of the Mexican Americans and other Hispanics.[21]

While about 94% of all elderly live in the community, a slightly higher proportion (96%) of black elderly do.[44] Since relatively more older blacks compared to whites are widowed, divorced, or separated, a smaller proportion live with their spouses; however, sharing a home with a grown child, usually a daughter, is a common living arrangement for older blacks.[45] Only about 3% of the entire black elderly population are institutionalized, whereas about 5% of the white elderly are. This trend is more apparent among the oldest-old (85 and over) who generally are more likely to be widowed and in need of physical and medical assistance. Among the eldest population, only 12% of blacks live in nursing homes. Twenty-three percent of the white elderly over the age of 85 live in nursing homes.[30]

About 97% of the Hispanic elderly live in households in the community, either alone, with family members (72% of Hispanic elders live with at least one family member), or with nonrelatives. The remaining 3% live in nursing homes.[41] Among elderly Hispanics 85 years of age or older, 10% are in nursing homes compared to 23% of whites.[39]

Among the Asian elderly, 96% live outside of institutions and in the community, while only 19% live alone. The proportion of Asian elderly living in nursing homes is approximately 2%.[42] Only 10% of those elderly Asians aged 85 and over reside in nursing homes.

About 96% of the Native American elderly individuals live in households in the community with only 4% living in institutions. About the same percentage of Native American elderly compared with white elderly live with family members (66% vs 65%), and for both groups, more men than women live with family members.[44] The proportion of Native American elderly living in nursing homes is low (i.e., less than 0.2%), and this trend is most pronounced in the oldest-old who comprise only 13% of the 85 year old and above population.[39]

Income Status of the Minority Elderly

Blacks as well as other minority elderly typically are less likely to work in professions or jobs with high benefits. Also, less education, fewer skilled jobs, lower salaries, and long periods of unemployment mean that blacks are less likely to accumulate income and other assets, benefits, or pensions.[27] As a result, the black elderly, on the average, have less personal postretirement income and are, therefore, more dependent on Social Security benefits for the majority of their retirement funds. The medium income of black elderly Americans is substantially less than that of the white elderly. Black elderly men average an annual income of $4,113, and black elderly women average $2,825, compared to $7,408 for white men and $3,894 for elderly white women.[44] The median personal income of Hispanic men aged 65 years and older is $4,592, or 62% that of white males the same age. Elderly Hispanic women have a median income of $2,873, while white elderly women have a median income of $3,894.[44] The income status of Asians is higher than for blacks or Hispanics, with Asian men aged 65 years or older averaging an annual income of $5,551 and women having a median income of $3,476 per year. Lastly, the median income for elderly Native American men is $4,257, and for women in the age group of 65 years or older it is $3,033.[44]

Poverty Status of the Minority Elderly

With the exception of Asians, a higher proportion of minority group elderly compared with non-Hispanic white elderly live in poverty.[27] Living alone makes the situation even worse for the minority group elderly.[44] Over half of black and Puerto Rican elderly persons report household incomes below the poverty level.[3] A smaller percentage of Asian and non-Hispanic white elderly who live alone are impoverished compared to other racial and Hispanic groups, and it appears that living with a spouse reduces the fraction of elderly in the poverty groups.[44] Yet, married elderly blacks and Hispanics are three times more likely than non-Hispanic whites and Asians to be poor. The 1990 census data indicates that, with the exception of Asians, approximately one minority group member in five who lives with others, lives in poverty.[23]

In urban areas, 32% of black elderly live in poverty (one in three), while 11% of older whites live in poverty (one in nine). In rural areas nearly one out of every two black elderly persons lives in poverty.[44] In rural areas, almost 40% of white women over the age of 75 are poor but over two-thirds (68%) of rural black women live in or near the poverty level.[44]

The percentage of Hispanic elderly with incomes below the poverty level is twice as large (26%) as that among elderly whites (13%). Hispanic poverty rates are higher in rural than in urban areas, and they are higher among Hispanic women as compared to men. Thus, rural women are the most impoverished Hispanic group of all. For example, among the Hispanic elderly, 38% of rural women have a below-poverty income as compared to 21% of rural white women.[41]

The proportion of the Asian elderly living below the poverty level closely resembles that of the white elderly population. Overall, 14% of Asian and 13% of white elderly Americans live below the poverty level. Twenty-six percent of Asians living in rural areas and 37% of Asians in urban areas are poor.[46]

The Native American elderly population is comparable to the black elderly poverty status in that 32% are below the poverty level. In rural areas the proportion is 39% and in urban areas it is 25%.[44]

In light of the demographic trends previously discussed, it appears that there will be a large increase in the number of female-headed households among blacks and Hispanics, and there probably will be an increase in the minority elderly who live alone.[47] Both of these trends portend a substantial increase in the number of minority group elderly who live in poverty.

CONCLUSION

Over the next 60 years, the number of Americans who are 65 years of age or older will increase to nearly 20% of the population, an increase from the present level of just under 12%. As the population ages, increasing levels of functional disability will impact the need for rehabilitative services for home care and nursing home care. Within this older age group, there will be a growing number who will reach "extreme" old age within the proportion of the population that is the 85 years and older. It is this latter group who will have a significant impact on the nation's health care needs and costs.

At present, 22% of those 85 years of age and older are institutionalized and this statistic is not likely to change. The 85 year and older age group is anticipated to increase eightfold, creating an increased demand for home care, nursing home care, and services from all health care providers. Health care providers must begin to plan now for this increase to ensure that as the demand for home care and nursing home care grows, the necessary rehabilitative and restorative services, provisions for nursing care, and financing mechanisms will be available.

Census information and research data are scarce for minority elderly populations. In fact, some researchers have alluded to the "statistical invisibility" of the minority aged.[3] Census data often underrepresent ethnic minorities and do not provide information on their health and disabilities, which are essential indicators of well-being for the elderly.[48] Most of the research surveys available provide data for blacks, whites, and those of Hispanic origin. Very little information is available on other subgroups of the American culture.

Clearly, in the field of gerontology we need to become more conscious of the increasing ethnic diversity of America's aged and to attend seriously to that diversity in the design and execution of research on the elderly. All too often the elderly are seen as a homogeneous group. The elderly in the United States are a melange of different social classes, national origins, and family types, and this diversity will lead to conflicting demands on our social institutions and will require creative policy solutions.

The status of the minority elderly is not likely to improve greatly in the immediate future; however, the importance of projections of the minority aged population—not only in terms of total size but in terms of social characteristics of the older minority populations—should assist in directing effective policy development and implementation to meet their needs. An expanded data base will permit "interactive projections" that will enable analyses to be made of the social and economic implications of demographic developments implicit in the process of majority and minority aging in the United States. This will have an important bearing on the public policy and decision making that are needed for a constructive response to be made to an aging population.

From a demographic prospective, the patterns that surface in the changing size and composition of the aged population modify consumer demands, political constituencies, economic conditions, and social structures. A focus on the aged as a subpopulation emphasizes the needs that arise from the absolute number and differing types of older persons, as well as from their relative proportion to the total population. This is particularly important for public policy development and program implementation, and it calls attention to the need to recognize the differential demands on public and private services and resources that arise from the growth and changing composition of the aged population.

PEARLS

- Consideration of population aging began in Europe in the 1800s but is now a recognized worldwide, twentieth century, phenomenon.

- Change in population size depends on birth, immigration, deaths, and emigration. Growth in the total population is most sensitive to a decline in mortality rates, whereas growth in the older population is due to a decline in fertility rates.

- The elderly made up 12.6% of the US population in 1990, and this figure is expected to climb to 17.7% in 2020.

- The US birthrate will decline or stay below 3.7 million per year, and the death rate will steadily decrease.

- The current ratio of elderly women to elderly men is three to two, and it is five to two over age 85. These ratios are expected gradually to increase through the end of this century and to increase sharply in the middle of the twenty-first century.

- Viewed as a homogeneous group, the majority of elderly are free of disability.

- It is estimated that the number of minority elderly will grow at a more rapid rate compared with the white elderly over the next 60 years.

REFERENCES

1. Myers GC. Demography of aging. In: Binstock RH, George LK, eds. *Handbook of Aging and the Social Sciences.* 3rd ed. San Diego: Academic Press, Inc.; 1990.
2. Zofp PE, Jr. *America's Older Population.* Houston: Cap & Gown Press; 1986.
3. Angel JL, Hogan DP. The demography of minority aging populations. In: *Minority Elders: Longevity, Economics and Health: Building Public Policy Base.* Washington, DC: Gerontological Society of America; 1991.
4. Committee on an Aging Society, Institute of Medicine/National Research Council. In: *Health in an Older Society.* Washington, DC: National Academy Press; 1985.
5. Gilford DM, ed. *The Aging Population in the Twenty-First Century.* Washington, DC: National Academy Press; 1988.
6. Rosenwaike I, Logue B. *The Extreme Aged in America: A Portrait of an Expanding Population.* Westport, CT: Greenwood Press; 1985.
7. United Nations. *The Aging of Populations and Its Economic and Social Implications.* New York: United Nations; 1956. (ST/SOA/SER.A/26).
8. Sundbarg G. *Grunddragen of befolkningslaren.* Stockholm. 1894.
9. Sundbarg G. Sur la repartition de la population par age et sur les taux de mortalite [On the separation of the population by age and the rates of mortality]. *Bul Internat Institute Statistics.* 1900; 12(99):89–94.

10. Dublin LI. *Health and Wealth: A Survey of the Economics of World Health: The Problem of Age*. New York: Harper; 1928; 149–168.
11. Pearl R. The aging of populations. *J Am Statistical Assoc Am*. 1940; 209:277–297.
12. Dublin LI, Lotka AJ. *Length of Life: A Study of the Life Table*. New York: Ronald Press; 1937.
13. Thompson WS, Whelpton PK. *Population Trends in the United States*. New York: McGraw-Hill; 1933.
14. Kinsella K. *Aging in the Third World*. Washington, DC: US Government Printing Office; 1988. US Bureau of the Census, International Population Reports, Series P-95, No. 79.
15. United Nations. *Economic and Social Implications of Population Aging*. New York: United Nations; 1988. (ST/ESA/SER.R/85).
16. Treas J, Logue B. Economic development and the older population. *Pop Dev Rev*. 1987; 12:645–673.
17. Winsborough HH. A demographic approach to the life cycle. In: Back KW, ed. *Life Course Integrative Theories and Exemplary Populations*. Boulder, CO: Westview; 1980. (AAAS Selected Symposium 41).
18. Soldo BJ. America's elderly in the 1980's. *Population Bull*. 1980; 35(4):1–48.
19. Spencer G. *Projections of the Population of the United States by Age, Sex, and Race: 1982 to 2050*. Washington, DC: US Bureau of the Census. Current Population Reports, Series P-25, No. 1007; 1989.
20. Rosenwaike I. A demographic portrait of the oldest-old. *Milbank Memorial Fund Quarterly Health and Society*. 1985; 63:187–205.
21. Preston SH, Himes C, Eggers M. Demographic conditions responsible for population aging. *Demography*. 1989; 26:691–704.
22. Grigsby JS. *The Demographic Components of Population Aging*. University of Michigan and Pomona College; 1988. Working paper.
23. US Bureau of the Census. *Population Estimates by Age, Sex, Race, and Hispanic Origin: 1980 to 1988*. Washington, DC: US Government Printing Office; 1990. Current population reports, series P-25, No. 1045.
24. Bourgeois-Pichat J. *Future Outlook for Mortality Decline in the World*. United Nations, Population Bulletin of the United Nations, 1978. No. 11; 12–41.
25. Crimmins EM. Implications of recent mortality trends for the size and compostition of the population over 65. *Rev Public Data Use*. 1983; 11(1):37–48.
26. Rice DP. Long life to you. *American Demographics*. 1979; 1(9):9–15.
27. Siegel JS, Davidson M. *Demographic and Socioeconomic Aspects of Aging in the United States*. Washington, DC: US Bureau of the Census. Current Population Reports, Series P-23, 1991.
28. Verbrugge LM. Recent trends in sex mortality differentials in the United States. *Women and Health*. 1980; 5(3):17–37.
29. Waldon I. Sex differences in longevity. In: Haynes SG, Feinleib M, eds. *Second Conference on the Epidemiology of Aging*. 1980; 163–186. Washington, DC: NIII Publication No. 80-969.
30. Taeuber C. Diversity: the dramatic reality. In: Bass SA, Kutza EA, Torres-Gil FM, eds. *Diversity in Aging*. Glenview, Ill: Scott, Foresman & Co.; 1990.
31. Soldo BJ, Agree EM. America's elderly. *Population Bull*. 1988; 43(3):1–51.
32. Myers G, Nathanson C. Aging and the family. *World Health Stat Quart*. 1982; 35:225–238.
33. Ryder N. Effects on the family of changes in the age distribution. In: *Economic and Social Implications of Population Aging*. New York: United Nations; 1988; (ST/ESA/SER.R/85, pp. 98–120.
34. Myers GC, Manton KG, Bacellar H. Sociodemographic aspects of future unpaid productive roles. In: *Productive Roles in an Older Society*. Washington, DC: National Academy Press. Committee on an Aging Society, Institute of Medicine and National Research Council; 1986; 110–147.
35. US Bureau of the Census. *Projections of the Number of Households and Families: 1979 to 1995*. Washington, DC: US Government Printing Office; 1989. Current population reports, Series P-25, No. 805.
36. Riley AG. *Aging and Society: Notes on the Development of New Understandings*. Ann Arbor: University of Michigan Press; 1983; 13–17.
37. Jette AM, Branch LG. The Framingham disability study: II. physical disability among the aging. *Am J Public Health*. 1981; 71:1211–1216.
38. National Center for Health Statistics. *Current Estimates from the National Health Interview*

Survey: United States, 1981. Washington, DC: US Government Printing Office; 1982. US Department of Health and Human Services Publication No. 10-141.

39. Taeuber C, Smith D. Minority elderly: an overview of demographic characteristics and 1990 census plans. Presented to the National Council on Aging Symposium; 1988; Washington, DC.

40. Torres-Gil. Hispanics: a special challenge. In: Pifer A, Bronte L, eds. *Our Aging Society: Paradox and Promise.* New York: Norton & Co. 1986; 219–242.

41. Cubillos HL, Prieto MM. *The Hispanic Elderly: A Demographic Profile.* Washington DC: Policy Analysis Center, National Council of La Raza; 1987.

42. Agree E. *Portrait of Asian Elderly.* Washington, DC: American Association of Retired Persons, Minority Affairs Initiative. 1985, Georgetown University Population Research Center; 1985.

43. US Bureau of the Census. *Preliminary Estimates of the Population of the United States by Age, Sex, and Race: 1970 to 1981.* Washington, DC: US Government Printing Office; 1982. Current population reports, series P-25, No. 917.

44. Agree E. *A Portrait of Older Minorities.* Washington, DC: American Association of Retired Persons, Minority Affairs Initiative; 1985. Georgetown University Population Research Center; 1985.

45. Siegel JS, Taeuber CM. Demographic perspectives on the long-live society. *Daedalus.* 1986; 115:77–117.

46. Kim PK. Demography of Asian-pacific elderly: selected problems and implications. In: McNeely RL, Colen JL, eds. *Aging in Minority Groups.* Beverly Hills: Sage Publications; 1983; 29–41.

47. Worobey JL and Angel RJ: Functional capacity and living arrangements of unmarried elderly persons. J Gerontol. 1990; 45(3):95–101.

48. Jette AM, Bottomley JM. The graying of America. *Am J Phys Ther.* 1987; 67(10):1527–1542.

Comparing and Contrasting the Theories of Aging

Historical Perspective	Developmental-Genetic Theories
Fundamental Considerations	Stochastic Theories of Aging
Theories of Aging	Conclusion

The search for the arcanum of that nemesis called "old age" has enticed many scientists to theorize and experiment with possible causes. The study of gerontology is a relatively new discipline, and the excitement of exploring its territory has seduced many scientific minds. Several theories of aging have been proposed, and the most prominent theories will be reviewed and compared in this chapter. This critical look at "current" theories will provide a basic framework for understanding and critically evaluating the following chapters on normal and pathological aging and clinical observations and strategies for managing the care of elderly individuals.

HISTORICAL PERSPECTIVE

The study of aging has a long history. Much of the research in the biology of aging has focused on prolongation studies rather than on the actual mechanisms of aging. In a comprehensive monograph by Freeman,[1] research on aging over the last 2500 years was presented, and the reader is referred to that source for a more in-depth history of the research on aging.

Research on aging began around the turn of the twentieth century.[1] Metchnikoff introduced the concept that aging was caused by the continuous absorption of toxins from intestinal bacteria, and he received the Nobel Prize in 1908 for his contributions to biology and the study of aging. Systematic studies that described the aging phenomena in terms of cell morphology, physiology, and biochemistry began about 1950.[2] There was an improvement in experimental designs that led to accurate definition of valid and reliable hypotheses. Two major groups of aging theories have evolved from those studies. Comfort[2] described the first group of theories about aging as "fundamentalist" or developmental-genetic theories. These theories are based on the premise of "wear and tear,"[3] because aging is attributed to pathological decrements that are tissue-specific (e.g., connective, nervous, vascular, or endocrine tissue). The second group of aging theorists view aging as an epiphenomenon in which environmental insults, such as gravity, toxins, and cosmic rays, result in the aging process. These theories are termed "nongenetic" or stochastic theories of aging. Many additional theories not contained in these two theoretical groups (though they could arguably be forced into one of the two preceding categories) view aging as a continuum with development and morphogenesis,[4] while others relate aging to a cessation of somatic cell growth[5] and energy depletion.[6]

Current modified versions of these theories have been introduced that involve the immune system, the neuroendocrine system, failures in deoxyribonucleic acid (DNA) repair, random mutation in somatic cells, errors in protein synthesis, and random damage from free radicals. These theories, though often presented as separate from each other, are not mutually exclusive. Clearly, there has not been *one* theory that fully identifies all of the causes, mechanisms, or bases of aging. The processes regulating the rate of aging may be different in different cell types and in different tissues, and the combined effects of environmental damage and intrinsic pathologies may further obscure a fundamental mechanism for aging. Clear mechanisms of aging depend on interdependent sets of variables and causes.

From a historical perspective, the concept of aging as a cell-based phenomenon versus organismic aging is comparatively new. Weissman[5] was the first to emphasize the distinction between somatic cells that age and germ cells that do not age. He suggested that the inability of somatic cells to replicate indefinitely was the reason for the limited life span in humans. This theory was under serious questioning because of a flawed series of experiments by Carrel,[7-9] and the study of cellular aging was set back by this historic event in biologic science. In 1912, Carrel and Ebeling[8] began a series of experiments using normal chick embryo fibroblasts cultured in vitro. Based on Carrel's series of experiments, it was thought that fibroblasts could replicate indefinitely and were immortal. The findings were considered to be compelling evidence that individual cells could live forever. This hypothesis dominated gerontology until 1950, and it was an accepted fact that cells did not characteristically age. It was thought that cells were immortal in isolation and that it was the tissues that were involved in aging. Scientists later discovered that the method of preparation of the chick embryo extract by Carrel was contaminated with the continual addition of fresh embryonic cells. The result was erratic miotic activity coinciding with the periodic addition of chick embryo extract.[10] In summary, these cells lived forever because young embryo cells were mixed with the older prepared culture.

In 1961, a landmark study by two then unknown cell biologists, Hayflick and Moorehead,[11] turned the study of senescence of cultured cells completely around. Conclusions from in vitro studies on fetal fibroblast cells (lung, skin, muscle, heart) were that in culture human fibroblasts have a limited life span. Hayflick and Moorehead[11] reported that there was a period of rapid and vigorous cellular proliferation consistently followed by a decline in proliferative activity and characteristic senescent changes (i.e., decreased replication and wasting). They proposed that aging was a cellular as well as an organismic phenomenon. The loss in functional capacity of the aging person reflected the summation of the loss of critical functional capabilities within individual cells. For instance, the loss of type II fibers in the muscle with aging results in atrophy and a decrease in the muscle force production, thereby decreasing functional capacity. The Hayflick and Moorehead experiment altered the direction and interpretation of aging research and cellular biology. In essence, they were among the first scientists to change the philosophy of modern biology and gerontology.

FUNDAMENTAL
CONSIDERATIONS

A discussion of the theories on aging must include a review of the observations and correlations associated with the aging process. A great deal is unknown about the nature of the mechanisms involved in aging; therefore, the study of aging is intrinsically difficult. The myriad of aging scenarios and trajectories that occur in nature, the different combinations of environmental and intrinsic changes, the lack of measurable transition points or biomarkers to define the kinetics of the process of aging, and the lack of a measurable means for aging other than death all serve to obscure any unifying principles. It is even difficult to define "aging," although it is characterized by an increasing vulnerability to environmental changes, and it is known that increasing chronological age increases the probability of death.

There are several underlying assumptions related to "theoretic gerontology." The following fundamental considerations are an important basis upon which to build further knowledge in the studying of aging.

Aging is developmental. This concept is very simple: We do not suddenly age. Our aging time capsules do not ignite at the age of 65. We evolve into mature adults and grow older developmentally, not chronologically. Aging is unique among all developmental stages. A 70-year-old person in chronological age may have the physiologic age of a 50-year-old person. Yet a 50-year-old person with chronic diseases may parallel the physiologic decline of a 90-year-old person.

Old age is a gift of twentieth-century technology and scientific advancement. The gerontologist, James Birren, has penned the notion that the extended life expectancy that we now have is really a gift of modern medicine and technology. Some biologists argue that the "survivorship kinetics" of biological aging may be an artifact of civilization and domestication. In nature, populations of species (including humans) only recently began to live long enough to show the characteristic kinetics of biological aging. Since the discovery of insulin, the development of vaccinations for diseases, improved sanitation, a decline in infant mortality, and the development of modern surgical techniques and advanced treatment modes for formerly fatal diseases, humans now experience longer lives. We are also staying *older* longer (not younger longer) in the twentieth century. The whole phenomenon of aging is new.

The effects of normal aging versus pathologic aging must be differentiated if possible. A confounding problem in understanding aging is the fact that there is a vast spectrum of aging changes. The process of aging is probably multifactorial in its regulation; however, it is virtually impossible to tell which changes are primary to a senescence-regulated event and which are secondary. Often we assume that a functional decline is due to aging. However, disease may often cause functional decline, which is not a normal aging process. For example, if one has adult-onset diabetes, then the probability of cardiovascular disease increases as a result of the effect of the diabetes. It is not "normal" to get diabetes; it is a function of life-style and heredity in North America. A confusion exists between aging, disease, and dying. Aging characteristically brings a loss in homeostasis and with it increased vulnerability to diseases, some of which result in death. Death has been used as the end point measurement of aging; however, death can occur from many causes, some of which are related to the aging process only secondarily, and in some cases they are totally unrelated to the process, as is true of accidents.

There is no universally accepted theory of aging. Aging does not occur in all species or in all organisms of the same species in exactly the same way. While one tissue may be losing functional capacity rapidly, others may be comparatively quite "young" functionally. (A more comprehensive discussion of this is in Chapter 3, Comparing and Contrasting Age Related Changes in Biology, Physiology, and Anatomy.) Although aging is a universal phenomenon, no one really knows what causes it or why we age at different rates. Chronological age is a much less useful and definitive measure of functional capacity than scientists would like.

Amid all these confusing assumptions of aging, there have been a set of aging characteristics that have been identified to be consistent. First, there is an increased mortality with age.[12] Second, consistent changes in the biochemical composition of the body with age have been well documented,[13] including a decrease in lean body mass and an increase in fat. There is also characteristic increases in lipofuscin in certain tissues and an increased cross-linking in matrix molecules such as collagen.[12] Thirdly, a broad spectrum of progressive deteriorative changes have been demonstrated both in cross-sectional and longitudinal studies.[14] (These changes will be discussed in detail in Chapter 3, Comparing and Contrasting Age Related Changes in Biology, Physiology, Anatomy, and Function.) Fourth, there is a reduced ability to respond adaptively to environmental change (perhaps the hallmark of aging). This can be demonstrated at all levels from individual molecule to the complete organism.[15] Thus, the changes of age are not so much the resting pulse rate or the fasting serum glucose, but the ability to return these parameters to normal after a physiological stress. Lastly, there is an increased vulnerability to many diseases with age.[14] The age-associated increase in vulnerability to diseases occurs at the cellular level. Aging is a process that is distinct from disease. The fundamental changes of aging provide the substratum in which the age-associated diseases can flourish.

Aging theories can be divided into two major categories: genetic ("fundamentalist") and nongenetic (environmental). Genetic theories focus on the mechanisms for aging located in the nucleus of the cell, while nongenetic theories focus on areas located elsewhere, such as in organs, tissues, or systems within the body, or extrinsic environmental causes. In order to understand both of these theories of aging, a basic understanding of three somatic cell types is necessary.

Not all somatic cells age at the same rate, nor do they have similar aging characteristics. Somatic cells are divided into three categories: (1) continuously proliferating or mitotic cells, (2) reverting postmitotic cells, and (3) fixed postmitotic cells.[16] Continuously proliferating mitotic cells never cease to replicate themselves, and injury done to these cells is healed through regeneration. Such cells can be found as superficial skin cells, red blood cells, cells of the lining of the intestine, and bone marrow cells. Reverting postmitotic cells have a slower rate of division than the continuously proliferating cells; but when there is injury, the rate of division is speeded up, and regeneration is possible. An example of these are kidney and liver cells. The final type of somatic cells, the fixed postmitotic cells, never replicate once the cells reach maturity.[10,16] Muscle cells and nerve cells are examples of fixed postmitotic cells.

In our adult life, therefore, nerve and muscle cells replicate and repair themselves only if the nucleus is intact. Because the postmitotic cell will not replicate itself, no new vital cells are produced; therefore, the need for residual fixed somatic cells to remain vital is crucial to the well-being and life expectancy of the individual.

THEORIES OF AGING

Historically, one of the major problems in gerontology is the ease and frequency with which new theories have appeared. There is not currently one theory that fully explains the process of aging. Researchers have viewed aging as "an event" that happens, rather than as a period in the life of organisms that begins at maturity (or conception?) and lasts for the rest of the life span. It seems that aging should be considered a developmental process. Numerous primary and secondary changes occur during development and aging. Some changes are programmed and directed within the body, while other changes are caused by the environment.

Understanding aging and formulating coherent, testable hypotheses requires that various aspects of aging be dissected from each other and examined critically. Different authors use different classification systems for the theories of aging. All are useful, and all have inherent difficulties. One effective way to present this information is to group the multiplicity of theories into the two classes of theories based on their fundamental conceptual basis, as described previously, and then describe prominent examples of each of these categories. The reader is reminded that this classification is only operational and that neither the catagories of theories nor the theories themselves are mutually exclusive.

Developmental-Genetic Theories

The developmental-genetic theorists consider the process of aging to be part of a continuum with development genetically controlled and programmed. Opposition to this idea comes from two sources. Some opposing researchers believe that there is a selection for aging mechanisms through evolution. In other words, aging processes are controlled extrinsically by environmental influences. The second source of opposition is the result of an intuitive sense that the diverse scenarios and trajectories of aging are not likely to be controlled by a process whose mechanisms regulate the precise processes of development.[13] That is, aging is not dependent on a single developmental process, but rather it is influenced by multifactoral ascendants.

There is no question that environmental factors can regulate or modify mortality, and in some cases influence the rate of aging (e.g., the aging of the skin is accelerated by exposure to the sun); however, the dimension of aging controlled by genetic processes clearly has some solid foundations. Gerontologists agree that the maximum life span and the rate of aging are regulated intrinsically. The primary evidence of this is the species-specific maximum life span. Variation in life span is far greater among species than within species. Because maximum life span is a species characteristic, it would seem evident that this is genetically determined. Further supporting evidence for the genetic basis of aging and maximal life span comes from the recognition of genetic diseases of precocious aging, such as in genetic progeroid syndromes.[17] The "classic" progeria—Werner syndrome, Hutchinson-Gilford syndrome, and Down syndrome—are among these diseases. The precise mechanism of human aging is not replicated at an accelerated rate in these individuals, however, many of the commonly recognized aging changes occur more rapidly. These diseases are important probes in the study of aging.

Of interest are studies that compare the longevity of monozygotic and dizygotic twins and nontwin siblings. It has been shown that there is a remarkable similarity in longevity between human fibroblast cell cultures in monozygotic twins that is not demonstrated in the other two groups.[17,18] A greater similarity of cell behavior and replicative life span is observed in these twins when compared to nontwin, age-matched controls.[19] One could argue that genetics governs susceptibility to certain diseases but not aging per se. Alternatively, a certain "vigor" could be inherited that protects against the developmental susceptibility to a wide variety of diseases. It clearly is difficult to distinguish between the two mechanisms. Nonetheless, there is circumstantial evidence for genetically controlled mechanisms of aging that potentially operate in a similar way to developmental processes.

Hayflick Limit Theory

Hayflick and Moorehead[11] were able to show that a deterioration in cells (i.e., mitotic and mitochondrial activity) was not dependent on environmental influences, but rather, that cell aging was intrinsic to the cells. They found that there was a limited number of cell population doublings or replications ranging from 40 to 60, the average doubling being 50 per life cycle of the cell. The developmental senescence process of cultured cells includes three phases. Phase I is the beginning stage of cell life, phase II involves a rapid cell proliferation, and the final cessation of cell division occurs in phase III. Hayflick and others have repeatedly shown that phase III is nearly always between 40 and 60 population doublings for embryo cells. Hayflick noted alterations and degeneration occurred within the cells before their growth limit[20] evident in the cell organelles, membranes, and genetic material. Hayflick demonstrated that functional changes within cells are responsible for aging and that the cumulative effect of improper functioning of cells and eventual loss of cells in organs and tissues is probably responsible for the aging phenomenon. Transformation can occur at any point in the life of the cell. Cells acquire a constellation of abnormal characteristics, including chromosomal abnormalities and an indefinite life span (e.g., properties of tumor cells). The generality of the Hayflick phenomenon is that, in the absence of transformations in the cells, senescence always occurs.

Hayflick's limit of cellular life has served as a model to other investigators who have shown that cell replication potential is a function of donor age.[21,22] In other words, an inverse correlation exists between donor age and the population doubling potential[22] and this correlation is directly related to the maximum life span of the species.[23] Evidence of the Hayflick limit has also been seen in cultures taken from individuals with progeria (Hutchinson-Gilford syndrome and Werner syndrome). Inasmuch as progeria is a premature aging syndrome, the decreased life span of the donor's cells shows a lower Hayflick limit, as expected.[16] The length of the longest life span for different species and the number of cell replications are correlated. For example, the Galápagos tortoise has a maximum life span of 175 years with a maximum doubling of 125, whereas the human maximum life span is 110 years with a maximum doubling of 60.[24]

The relationship between the cellular aging phenomenon in cultures and the aging of the individual is not specific to fibroblasts. It has been demonstrated in smooth muscle cells, endothelial cells, glial cells, and lymphocytes. Several changes that occur during in vitro senescence are parallel to those that occur in vivo with advancing age. It is not clear that the observed cellular aging in cultures, however, actually contributes to what we recognize as the in vivo aging phenomenon of the organism. There is no evidence to support that the in vitro replication life span of mesenchymal cells is important in determining the life span of the organism. Contrary to this is that living cells maintain their functional capacity through processes of replacement and repair over long periods of time. So proliferative homeostasis needs to be evaluated with regard to the ability of the organism to respond to environmental stresses. It is also important to keep in mind the aging of proliferating or mitotic cells may be quite different from that of fixed postmitotic or reverting postmitotic cells. The results of the studies cited suggest that, underlying the effects of various proposed "master timekeeping" systems, cells have individual "clocks" that ultimately limit their life span.[24]

Neuroendocrine and Hormonal Theory

This group of theories regard functional decrements in neurons and their associated hormones as central to the aging process. Given the major interactive role of the neuroendocrine system in physiology, this is an attractive approach. D. Donner Denckla, an endocrinologist turned gerontologist, believes that the center of aging is located in the brain.[25] He bases his theory on past studies of hypothyroidism, a disease that mimics mature aging (e.g., a depressed immune system, wrinkling of the skin, gray hair, and a slowed metabolic rate). Hypothyroidism can be fatal if not treated with thyroxine, inasmuch as all the manifestations of aging are evidenced.

Another aspect of the neuroendocrine basis of aging depends on the role of the pituitary hormones.[26,27] The anterior pituitary gland controls the thyroid gland by the thyroid stimulating hormone and thus the secretion of thyroxine. Thyroxine is the master rate-controlling hormone within the body for metabolism and protein synthesis. The focus of this theory is the proposed ability of the anterior pituitary to release a blocking hormone labeled DECO (decreasing oxygen consumption hormone) that blocks the cell membrane from taking up thyroxine as a check-balance in the human system. Denckla has not isolated the antiaging serum, but what Denckla has given us is an alternative philosophic point of view in theoretic gerontology: the in vivo versus the in vitro controversy. Denckla believes that the aging process in vitro is an artifact and unrelated in any meaningful way to true aging. Denckla says,

> "I don't care what happens to cells in tissue culture. What is important is what people die of." He believes that for good evolutionary reasons—to ensure the turnover of generations so that mutations can take place that enable a species to adapt to a changing environment—nature cannot trust to chance (wear and tear). There must, therefore, exist "an absolutely failsafe killing mechanism without which the species would not survive."[25]

Denckla[28] has shown that elderly rats have a lower O_2 consumption and a reduced increase in O_2 consumption in response to the thyroid hormone T_4. This effect is abolished with hypophysectomy and hormone replacement. Denckla concluded that this finding provided evidence for the presence of a previously undescribed pituitary hormone called "decreasing oxygen consumption hormone" (DECO), which probably begins to be produced at puberty under stimulation by the thyroid hormone. DECO is proposed to be responsible for the decreasing oxygen consumption and the reduced effect of thyroid hormone observed in aging.[28]

There have been other theories proposed with regard to functional decline of various aging organs and aging systems. As Hayflick[29] notes, aging changes may simply be the result of more fundamental causes, or the organ system in question may not be universally present in all aging animals.

An important version of Denckla's theory proposes that the hypothalamic, pituitary, and adrenal axis is the master timekeeper for the organism and the primary regulator of the aging process. Functional changes in this system are accompanied by or regulated by decrements throughout the organism. The cascade effect of functional decrements in the hypothalamus, for example, and their potential sequelae have been documented in humans.[30] The neuroendocrine system regulates early development, growth, puberty, the control of the reproductive system, metabolism, and, in part, the activities of all the major organ systems. Support of the neuroendocrine and hormonal theories of aging is evidenced by the decline in reproductive capacity due to a decrease in the release of gonadotropin releasing hormone by the hypothalamus, which appears to be the result of diminished activity of hypothalamic catecholamines.[30] Similarly, it has been shown that the release of pulsatile growth hormone declines with age.[31] These changes would have profound effects on estrogen and progesterone release and subsequently on functional capacity. Wise[31] has suggested that there is a loss of neurons in discrete areas of the brain and a loss of neurotransmitter responsiveness by the remaining neurons.

Satisfactory evidence to relate endocrine function to aging is not present to substantiate a significant contribution of endocrine gland function to the process of aging.[32] In response to stress and trophic hormones, the adrenal cortex and thyroid gland remain intact. For women, menopause is a hormone-mediated event that chronicles but does not regulate aging.[32] The ovary is the sole endocrine gland whose functional capacity predictably declines with normal aging. On the other hand, androgen production by the testis is not as predictable because there are individual differences.

The importance of neuroendocrine research cannot be overemphasized. Critics of these theories, however, point out that the master timekeeper of aging, the neuroendocrine system, lacks universality. Many organisms that age (e.g., higher vertebrates) have no complex neuroendocrine system. It can also be argued that the changes that occur in the neuroendocrine system are fundamental changes and occur in all tissues. Aging of the brain, however, produces additional secondary effects that, although not fundamental to aging, contribute to the development of the overall aging process. What the neuroendocrine system contributes to the aging process is evidenced by the effects of the lack of estrogen with respect to its effects on bone density and vascularity. Its contribution to other aging processes remains to be determined.

The Theory of Intrinsic Mutagenesis

Another theory in the developmental-genetic aging group of theories is referred to as the theory of intrinsic mutagenesis. This idea was first proposed by Burnett[33] and is an attempt to reconcile stochastic theories of aging with the genetic regulation of maximum life span. Burnett suggests that each species is endowed with a specific genetic constitution that "regulates the fidelity of the genetic material and its replication." The degree of fidelity regulates the rate of appearance of mutations or errors, thereby, affecting the life span. Alternatively, we can envision a case in which new "fidelity regulators" appear at different stages in an animal's life. Each successive evolutionary set of regulators could have a decreased capacity allowing an increase in mutational events. Another aspect of intrinsic mutagenesis is concerned with the increase in DNA excision repair associated with maximal life span.[34] There is evidence that the accuracy of DNA polymerase may decrease with age,[35–37] but the research in support of both of these hypotheses is rather controversial.

It has been found that the role of DNA methylation as a regulatory factor may have some implications in light of the intrinsic mutagenesis theory. For example, diploid fibroblasts in culture are unable to maintain a constant level of 5-methylcytosine,[38–40] and in other systems DNA methylation patterns have been linked to X chromosome inactivation-reactivation.[41] These hypotheses are potentially important but need further testing before a reliable and valid body of evidence will emerge.

Immunological Theory

The immunological theory of aging is also categorized as a developmental-genetic theory. This theory was proposed by Walford[42] and has two major observations upon which it is based: (1) that the functional capacity of the immune system declines with age as a result of reduced T-cell function[43] and a reduced resistance to infectious diseases, and (2) that the fidelity of the immune system declines with age as evidenced by the striking age-associated increase in autoimmune diseases. Walford[44] has related these immune system changes to the genes of the major histocompatibility complex genes in rats and mice. Congenic animals that differ only at the major histocompatibility locus appear to have different maximal life spans, suggesting that life span is regulated, at least in part, by this locus. Interestingly, this locus also regulates superoxide dismutase and mixed function oxidase levels, a finding that relates the immunological theory of aging to the free radical theory of aging, which will be discussed subsequently.

As with the neuroendocrine theory, the immunological theory is attractive. The immune system has a primary integrative role and is of major importance in health maintainance. Conversely, life span differences could simply be due to the prevention of diseases. The same argument can be leveled at the immunological theory as at the neuroendocrine theory. It lacks universality, and it is difficult to defend the immune system's role as the primary timekeeper in the biology of all organisms. The inability to distinguish between primary and secondary effects on aging and the possibility that changes in the immune system are no different from changes in other cell types makes interpretation of this theory difficult.

Free Radical Theory

Another example of developmental-genetic theory has to do with free radicals. This theory is attributed to Harman,[45-47] who proposed that aging changes are due to damage caused by free radicals. Basically, free radicals are highly charged ions whose outer orbits contain an unpaired electron. Chemically, they are highly reactive species that are generated commonly in single-electron transfer reactions of metabolism. Free radicals have been shown to damage cell membranes, lysosomes, mitochondria, and nuclear membranes through a chemical reaction called lipid peroxidation. Both membrane damage and cross-linking of biomolecules resulted from free radical chain reactions.[48] The net result of free radical reactions, as summarized by Leibovitz and Siegel,[48a] is a decline in cellular integrity caused by reduced enzyme activities, error-prone nucleic acid metabolism, damaged membrane functions, and accumulation of aging pigments (lipofuscin) in lysosomes.

Free radicals are rapidly destroyed by protective enzyme systems, such as superoxide dismutase. According to this theory, however, some free radicals escape destruction and cause damage that accumulates in important biological structures. This accumulation of damage eventually interferes with function and ultimately causes death. The accumulation of age pigments does not refer to the dark brown spots on one's hands. Age pigments (lipofuscin) are seen at microscopic levels in self-selected tissues of the body, such as nerve and muscle tissue. Lipofuscin is the oxidation product of free radical action on polyunsaturated fatty acids. The rate of accumulation of age pigments is a good index of chronologic age and perhaps one of the few aging phenomena universally demonstrated in mammals. Age pigments as an entity are examples of degenerative change. When accumulated in tissue, they cut off oxygen and nutrient supplies to surrounding areas, causing further degeneration and eventual death of tissue.

There is much support for free radical reactions and their implications in the aging process, as well as their probable pathologic effects as a hypothesized cancer-causing and atherosclerosis-causing agent. This is an appealing theory because it provides a mechanism for aging that does not depend on tissue-specific action but is fundamental to all aerobic tissues. Although this theory has an aspect of random damage, it is not included in the nongenetic stochastic theories because some observations about free radicals are more suggestive of the developmental-genetic theory. For example, Rubner[6] found that the larger the mammal, the lower its metabolic rate. The adaptive significance of this is that as animals get bigger, their surface-to-volume ratio changes. This results in a reduction in the animal's ability to dissipate the heat produced in metabolic reactions. Therefore, a high metabolic rate could cause a hyperthermic effect in a large mammal. Another observation is that life span is a function of body size.[49] Larger animals live longer. This suggests an inverse relationship between metabolic rate and life span. Researchers have speculated that each species is capable of burning a given number of calories in its lifetime.

Metabolic rate is related directly to free radical generation and inversely to life span. It is reasonable to hypothesize that the rate of free radical production is in some way related to life span determination or to senescence. Proponents of this theory suggest that caloric restriction can increase the mean and maximal life span of a species. The notion is that caloric restriction lowers the metabolic rate and, therefore, decreases the free radical production.

The Caloric Restriction Theory

Walford[50] is a staunch proponent of caloric restriction, also known as energy restriction (ER). Dr Walford himself serves as living evidence of the in vivo experiment and that a life-style committed to the high/low diet, with moderate vitamin and mineral supplementation and a regular exercise regimen is beneficial. Caloric restriction and its effects on life span extension is perhaps one of the most promising probes of the mechanisms of aging. Caloric restriction may exert its effectiveness through the neuroendocrine system. Everitt[51] has shown a striking similarity between dietary restriction and hypophysectomy (previously discussed).

This high-nutrient/low-calorie diet is a result of years of animal in vivo experimentation, exploring longevity and maximum life span potential. Dr Walford's experiments have been well received and respected, and other noted theorists, such as Leonard Hayflick, have acknowledged Walford's works.[52]

Walford's caloric restriction program prescribes that an individual gradually lose weight over several years until a point of maximum metabolic efficiency is reached for maximum health and life span.[52] Despite more recent reports associating being a little overweight as "healthier" than being underweight, most recent results from the National Institutes of Health Nutrition Committee and the Centers for Disease Control have concluded that "the weights associated with the greatest longevity are below average weights of the population," as long as such weights are not associated with diseases.[52] The result of the high-quality but low-caloric diet serves to retard aging in the sense that one would be chronologically old but functionally younger.

The calorie restricted diet influences both aging rate and disease susceptibility. It has been said that the immune system is the pacemaker of aging,[32] and caloric restriction has been shown to affect the immune system. For example, it slows down the immune system's decline and inhibits the increased autoimmune reaction.[43] Further, pilot studies in mice provide supportive evidence that caloric restriction may also slow the decline in DNA repair capacity,[53] as well as affect the generation or persistence of free radicals.[54] Recent studies regarding the free radical theory show that lipid peroxidation is lower and that catalase reactions are higher in calorie restricted mice compared with noncalorie restricted controls.[55]

What is the relationship of energy restriction to other aging theories? Caloric restriction influences widely diverse phenomena, particularly those whose mechanistic possibilities include effects on the immune system, cell basal state and proliferation potential, metabolic rate, DNA repair, levels of free radical scavengers, chromatin structure, and protein synthesis and turnover.

As can be seen by other theories discussed in this chapter, aging may be caused by a single factor or by many. Thus, the energy restriction model might be useful in analyzing single-factor theories of aging; it might also clarify the significance of physiologic aging markers that correlate with differences in maximum life spans between species.[50]

A simple extrapolation of the free radical theory of aging leads to the conclusion that active persons would have a shorter life span than nonactive ones. There is no evidence to support this view. Intuitively, the beneficial effects of exercise preclude this logical extrapolation. Paffenberger[56] has shown that greater caloric expenditure is positively correlated with increasing life span and health in humans. A caveat here, as with other statements, is that exercise could have beneficial effects in preventing disease while at the same time accelerating aging through increased free radical generation. On the other hand, disease prevention through exercise could completely obscure the effects of free radicals.

Extensive research has been done regarding the use of antioxidants with free radicals. Vitamin E, vitamin C, selenium, gluthathione peroxidase, and superoxide dismultase have been used as free radical and lipid peroxidase inhibitors.[48] The implication is that there appears to be effective free radical inhibitors that may prevent further cellular degeneration, such as reduced accumulation of lipofuscin.

Stochastic Theories of Aging

The second category of theories is described as stochastic theories. These theories proport that aging is caused by an accumulation of insults from the environment. The result of these insults is that the organism eventually reaches a level incompatible with life.

Error Theory

The error theory, also known as the error catastrophe theory, was first presented by Orgel in 1963.[57] It states that, although random errors in protein synthesis may occur, the error containing protein molecule will be turned over, and the next copy will be error free. If the error containing protein is one that is involved in synthesis of the genetic material or in the protein synthesizing machinery, however, then this molecule could cause further errors. If this is the case, the number of error containing proteins expands to result in an "error crisis" that would be incompatible with proper function and life. The theory specifies that "any accident or error in either the machinery or the process of making proteins would cascade into multiple effects."[58] A decrease in the fidelity or accuracy of protein synthesis was specifically hypothesized to be caused by errors in proper initiation of the pairing of messenger RNA codon with an anticodon of transfer RNA. However, "it may not be possible to distinguish between contributions to cellular aging caused by errors in protein synthesis from those due to accumulation of somatic mutations."[29] It is questionable whether or not accurate protein synthesis is distinguishable from inaccurate DNA synthesis and whether or not the accuracy of both processes are dependent on the fidelity of the other. The interdependence and cumulative effects of errors remain deeply intertwined and somewhat indistinguishable.

Recent experiments contradict Orgel and no longer lend support to the error theory. In human cell cultures fed two amino acids (p-fluorophenylalanine and ethionine) early in their life spans, both the short-term, high-dose cultures and the long-term, low-dose cultures had essentially the same replicative life spans.[59] This result seems irreconcilable with the error theory. It is an appealing theory because of its apparently straightforward testability through the detection of missynthesized proteins. Experiments have shown that not all aged cells accumulate missynthesized protein molecules and that aging is not necessarily accelerated when missynthesized protein molecules are purposely introduced.[29] Despite numerous reports of altered proteins in aging,[60] no direct evidence of age-dependent, malsynthesis has yet been obtained. Altered proteins do occur in aging cells and tissues, however, at present it seems that the accuracy of the protein synthesizing mechanism does not decrease with age. Rather, the capacity of the protein removal machinery in old cells is compromised.[61] It may follow that old cells that contain many modified copies of functionally important proteins could have impaired functional capacity. From a historical viewpoint, the error theory was important to test these hypotheses in order to move toward a more plausible theory.

Redundant DNA Theory

Another dimension of the error theories is the premise that the ability to repair damage to the genetic material is somehow associated with aging or the rate of aging.[62] Medvedev[62] suggests that biologic age changes are a result of errors accumulating in functioning genes. As these errors accumulate reserve, genetic sequences with identical information take over until the system's redundancy is exhausted. This theory is known as the redundant message theory. Medvedev[62] writes that different species' life spans may be a function of the degree of *repeated* genetic sequences. If an error occurred in a nonrepeated gene sequence, the chance of preserving a final intact gene product during evolution or a long life span would be diminished. Hart and Setlow[34] obtained evidence that the ability to repair DNA cells after ultraviolet damage in cell cultures derived from various species of different maximum life spans and was directly correlated to maximum life span potential.

Redundancy seems to protect mammals from losing vital genetic information during the life span.[62] The major criticism of Medvedev's theory is that it fails to explain other possible aging factors, such as radiation-induced aging and quantitative aspects of normal aging. Although the idea that differences in DNA repair provides the basis for the life span differences in species, current experimental support for this theory remains inconclusive.[61] It is probable that if DNA repair is involved in the determination of maximum life span, it is more likely to be site-specific than generalized.[13]

Somatic Mutation Theory

One of the most prominent theories in the stochastic theories category is the somatic mutation theory of aging.[63,64] This theory emerged following World War II as a result of increased research in the area of radiation biology. The theory hypothesizes that mutations or genetic damage result from radiation and that radiomimetic agents accumulate and eventually create functional failure and ultimately the death of the organism. The somatic mutation theory is based on the scientific observation that exposure to ionizing radiation shortens the life span. Szilard[64] showed that exposure to radiation was recessive. It requires two or more "hits" from radiation to inactivate a given locus, and the exposure must occur in a sufficient number of cells for the damage to be manifested. Comparison of chromosomal aberrations in dividing liver cells to mice supports this view.[65] Curtis and Miller[65] found a higher frequency of these chromosomal abnormalities in short-lived as compared to long-lived strains of mice, which supports the somatic mutation theory. There are several arguments against the somatic mutation theory: (1) life span shortening by radiation does not define whether or not the life span mechanism bears any relationship to the normal mechanism of aging.[13] Numerous treatments that would shorten the life span are not related to normal aging (e.g., radiation treatment). (2) Inbred animals would have a longer life span than outbred animals because inbred animals would be homologous at most genetic loci and, therefore, more resistant to random damage. In fact the opposite is true as exemplified in the well-known phenomenon of hybrid vigor. Maynard-Smith[66] showed that inbreeding actually shortened the life span in mice. Some of the most compelling experiments addressing somatic mutation were done on the effects of radiation and life span comparing haploid and diploid animals.[67] Although the haploid animals were much more sensitive to ionizing radiation, both haploids and diploids had the same life span when radiation was withheld. This finding is difficult to reconcile in light of the somatic mutation theory.

Transcription Theory

Other scientists have developed theories focused specifically on stages of genetic processing. One of these processes, transcription, is the first stage in the transfer of information from DNA to protein synthesis. It entails the formation of messenger RNA so that it contains, in the linear sequence of its nucleotides, the genetic information located in the DNA gene from which messenger RNA is transcribed. Hayflick's[29] theory maintains that with increasing age, deleterious changes occur in the metabolism of differentiated postmitotic cells. He also suggests that the alterations are the results of primary events occurring within the nuclear chromatin. A control mechanism responsible for the appearance and the sequence of the primary aging events exists in the nuclear chromatin complex.

Insufficient experimentation to test this hypothesis exists, though Hayflick[29] suggests this should not imply that the hypothesis is wrong. When contemplating these theories thus far, one must ask, why is it that some cells, such as germ cells and some cancer cells, never age or die? Hayflick[29] suggests that "in order to maintain immortality, genetic information is exchanged between these cells in the same way that the genetic cards are reshuffled when egg and sperm fuse." The reshuffling of a fused sperm and egg cell may lead to a fixed life span. In all species, there appears to be a specific time for decrement and eventual death. Hayflick[29] and others refer to this as "mean time to failure." Perhaps species-specific genetic apparatus runs out of correctly programmed material, and some species-related repair systems are better than others because they have a longer life span.

Cross-Linkage Theory

A theory related to the redundant DNA theory is based on cross-linking in macromolecules. In 1942, Johan Bjorksten first related the concept of cross-linkage to developmental aging.[68,69] Prior to the 1940s, cross-linking was used as a method to stabilize macromolecules for individual purposes, such as vulcanizing rubber. Although cross-linking is not restricted to proteins, most experimental research has been on collagen and elastin because these molecules are accessible, do not readily turn over, and show increased cross-linking with age. Bjorksten[68] looked at large reactive protein molecules within the body, such as collagen, elastin, and DNA molecules, and surmised that their cross-linkage was responsible for secondary and tertiary causes of aging. According to Bjorksten

> Crosslinking [sic] reactions result in the union of at least two large molecules. A bridge or link between these is usually formed by a crosslinking agent: a small, motile molecule or free radical with a reactive hook or some other mechanism at both ends, capable of reacting with at least two large molecules. It is also possible for two large molecules to become crosslinked by the action of their own side chains or reactive groups present on one or both of them, or pathologically formed by ionizing radiation.[69]

Matrix molecules constitute more than 20% of mammalian body weight. The vital physiological processes that occur in a bed of matrix molecules will not be able to proceed effectively because cross-linking increases with age. The concepts underlying this theory are probably overly simplistic. Though collagen shows increasing cross-linking with age, is there more to matrix molecule metabolism than simply cross-linking? Some collagen types are replaced by other collagen types in development and aging. Cross-linking is a process of maturation for which increased cross-linking at some sites leads to improved function, but at other sites it impairs function.[70] Further investigation needs to be done to learn more about the matrix molecules.

Bjorksten[68] implies that cross-linking is the primary cause of sclerosis, failure of the immune system, and loss of elasticity. Aging of the skin is perhaps the most obvious example of cross-linking and exposure to solar radiation promotes cross-linkage. Loss of flexibility of the aging body was thought to be due to the cross-linking of tendon, ligament, and muscle tissue. We now see active aging individuals remain more flexible despite constant exposure to cross-linking agents (e.g., unsaturated fats, polyvalent metal ions, such as aluminum, magnesium, zinc, radiation), and few if any researchers view collagen cross-linking as a major underlying cause of aging.

CONCLUSION

Two major categories of scientific theories on aging exist: the genetic-based and the nongenetic (stochastic) theories. Gerontology has evolved into a sophisticated scientific realm enabling us to distinguish between logical, plausible explanations and idealistic searches for the fountain of eternal youth. But the question remains: What causes us to age?

Frolkis, a Soviet gerontologist, was quoted as saying, "the number of hypotheses is generally inversely proportional to the clarity of the problem."[25] This overview of theories should confirm the complicated nature of theoretic gerontology.

It is clear that no single theory adequately explains the entire process of growing old. Aging processes could better be explained if a number of these theories were integrated. For instance, theories on programmed control of aging can readily explain differences in the aging process of different species. The genetic makeup of a species determines the early development of an individual and will determine the rate of growth and metabolism directly affecting aging. Theories that suggest reasons for aging other than genetic makeup are useful in explaining why all members of the same species do not age in an identical manner. It may be that programmed aging directs the similar changes characteristic of all individuals with identical genetic makeup in their earlier years, but eventually bodily changes due to disease, the presence of excessive accumulations of substances in the cells, errors in protein synthesis, and so forth, may alter programmed aging. Because these factors can be expected to vary between individuals it is expected that individual aging will vary, even among members of the same species.

Gerontology is an emerging field that will make it possible for more people everywhere to live healthier and fuller lives and will help us to understand the determining factors in the human life span.

PEARLS

- Aging research began in the early 1900s, and the two major groups of aging theories that have evolved are the developmental-genetic theories and the environmental stochastic theories.

- Hayflick and Moorehead conducted a landmark study that showed that in culture human fibroblasts have a limited life span.

- Theoretic gerontology uses these fundamental considerations: (1) aging is developmental, (2) old age is a gift of modern technology, (3) differentiate normal versus pathological aging, and (4) there is no universally accepted theory of aging.

- Neuroendocrine and hormonal theory regard functional decrements in neurons and their associated hormones as central to the aging process.

- The theory of intrinsic mutagenesis states that successive evolutionary regulations have a decreased capacity allowing an increase in mutations.

- Immunological theory states that the immune system declines with age.

- According to the free radical theory, free radicals accumulate with age and cause destruction to important biological structures.

- Caloric restriction theory prescribes that an individual gradually loses weight until a point of maximum metabolic efficiency is reached for maximum health and life span.

- The error theory specifies that any error in the process of making proteins will cascade into multiple effects.

- Redundant DNA theory states that as errors accumulated, reserve, genetic sequences with identical information take over until the system's redundancy is exhausted.

- Somatic mutation theory hypothesizes that genetic damage will result from radiation and that radiometric agents accumulate and create functional failure and death of the organism.

- Transcription theory relates to deleterious changes that occur in postmitotic cells in the transcriptive phase of protein synthesis.

- In the cross-linkage theory, cross-linkage of macromolecules is responsible for secondary and tertiary aging.

REFERENCES

1. Freeman JT. *Aging, Its History and Literature.* New York: Human Science Press; 1979.
2. Comfort A. *The Biology of Senescence.* 3rd ed. New York: Elsevier; 1979.
3. Pearl R. *The Rate of Living.* New York: Vropfu; 1928.
4. Warthin AS. *Old Age, the Major Revolution: The Philosophy and Pathology of the Aging Process.* New York: Hoeber; 1929.
5. Weissman A. *Uber die dauer des lebens.* Germany: Jena; 1882.
6. Rubner M. *Das problem der lebensdaver und seine beziebungen zum wachstum und ernabrung.* Munich: Oldenbourg; 1908.
7. Carrel A, Burrows MT. On the physiochemical regulation of the growth of tissues. *J of Experimental Med.* 1911; 13:562–569.
8. Carrel A, Ebeling T. On the permanent life of tissues outside the organism. *J of Experimental Med.* 1912; 15:516–522.
9. Carrel A. Present condition of a strain of connective tissue twenty-eight months old. *J of Experimental Med.* 1914; 20:1–13.
10. Hayflick L. Senescence and cultured cells. In: Shock N, ed. *Perspectives in Experimental Gerontology.* Springfield, Ill. Charles C Thomas; 1966.
11. Hayflick L, Moorehead PS. The serial cultivation of human diploid all strains. *Exp Cell Res.* 1961; 25:585–593.
12. Strehler BL. *Time, Cells and Aging.* 2nd ed. New York: Academic Press; 1977.
13. Cristofalo VJ. Overview of biological mechanism of aging. *Annual Review of Gerontology and Geriatrics.* 1991; 6:1–22.
14. Shock NW. Longitudinal studies of aging in human. In: Finch CE, Schneider EL, eds. *Handbook of the Biology of Aging.* New York: Van Nostrand Reinhold; 1985; 721–739.
15. Adelman RC. Hormone interaction during aging. In: Schimke RT, ed. *Biological Mechanisms in Aging.* Washington, DC: US Department of Health and Human Services; 1980.
16. Fries I, Crapo L. *Vitality and Aging.* San Francisco: WH Freeman; 1981.
17. Martin GM, Turker M. Genetics of human disease, longevity and aging. In: Hazzard EG, ed. *Textbook of Genetic Medicine.* New York: McGraw-Hill; 1990.
18. Kallman JF, Jarvik LF. Twin data on genetic variations in resistance to tuberculosis. In: Gedda L, ed. *Genetica Della Tuberculosi e dei tumori.* Rome: Gregorio Mendel; 1957; 15–41.
19. Jarvik LF. Survival trends in a senescent twin population. *Am J of Human Genetics.* 1960; 12:170–181.
20. Hayflick L. The cellular basis for biological aging. In: Finch C, Hayflick L, eds. *The Handbook of the Biology of Aging.* New York: Van Nostrand Reinhold; 1977.
21. Martin GM, Sprague CA, Epstein CJ. Replicative lifespan of cultivated human cells. *Lab Invest.* 1970; 23:26.
22. Schneider EL, Mitsui Y. The relationship between in vitro cellular aging and in vivo human age. *Proceedings of the National Academy of Sciences.* 1976; 73:3584–3597.
23. Rohme D. Evidence for a relationship between longevity of mammalian species and lifespan of normal fibroblasts in vitro and erythrocytes in vivo. *Proceedings of the National Academy of Sciences of the USA.* 1981; 78:3584–3591.
24. Stanley JF, Pye D, MacGregor A. Comparison of doubling numbers attained by cultural animal cells with life span of species. *Nature.* 1975; 255:158.
25. Walford RL. The immunologic theory of aging: current status. *Fed Proc.* 1974; 33:2020.
26. Brody H, Jayashankar N. Anatomical changes in the nervous system. In: Finch CE, Hayflick L, eds. *Handbook of the Biology of Aging.* New York: Van Nostrand Reinhold; 1977.
27. Everitt AV. The hypothalamic pituitary control of aging and age-related pathology. *Experimental Gerontol.* 1973; 8:265–269.
28. Denckla WD. Role of the pituitary and thyroid glands in the decline of minimal O_2 consumption with age. *J of Clin Investigation.* 1974; 53:572–577.
29. Hayflick L. Theories of aging. In: Cape R, Coe R, Rodstein M, eds. *Fundamentals of Geriatric Medicine.* New York: Raven Press; 1983.
30. Finch CE, Landfield PW. Neuroendocrine and autonomic functions in aging mammals. In: Finch CE, Schneider EL, eds. *Handbook of the Biology of Aging.* New York: Van Nostrand Reinhold; 1985: 567–579.
31. Wise PA. Aging of the female reproductive system. *Rev Biol Res Aging.* 1983; I:15–26.

32. Rosenfeld A. Are we programmed to die? *Saturday Rev.* 1976; 10(2):10.
33. Burnett M. *Intrinsic Mutagenesis: A Genetic Approach for Aging.* New York: Wiley; 1974.
34. Hart RW, Setlow RB. Correlation between DNA excision repair and life span in a number of mammalian species. *Proceedings of the National Academy of Sciences of the USA.* 1974; 71:2169–2183.
35. Krauss SW, Linn S. Studies of DNA polymerases alpha and beta from cultured human cells in various replicative states. *J of Cellular Physiol.* 1986; 126:99–107.
36. Linn S. Decreased fidelity of DNA polymerase activity isolated from aging human fibroblasts. *Proceedings of the National Academy of Sciences of the USA.* 1976; 13:2818–2826.
37. Murray V, Holliday R. Increased error frequency of DNA polymerases from senescent human fibroblasts. *J of Mol Biology.* 1981; 146:55–82.
38. Fairweather S. The in vitro lifespan of MRC-5 cells is shortened by 5-azacytidine induced demethylation. *Experimental Cell Research.* 1987; 168:153–158.
39. Holliday R. Strong effects of 5-azacytidine on the in vitro lifespan of human diploid fibroblasts. *Experimental Cell Research.* 1986; 166:543–548.
40. Wilson VL, Jones PA. DNA methylation decreases in aging but not in immortal cells. *Science.* 1983; 220:1054–1071.
41. Wareham VA. Age related reactivation of an X-linked gene. *Nature.* 1987; 327:725–732.
42. Walford RL. Immunopathology of aging. In: Eisdorfer C, ed. *Annual Review of Gerontology and Geriatrics.* New York: Springer Publishing Co.; 1981:2.
43. Walford RL. *The Immunologic Theory of Aging.* Copenhagen: Munksgaard; 1969.
44. Walford RL. Multigene families, histocompatibility system, transformation, meiosis, stem cells and DNA repair. *Mechan Ageing and Develop.* 1979; 9:19–28.
45. Harmon D. Aging: a theory based on free radical and radiation chemistry. *J of Gerontol.* 1956; 11:298–311.
46. Harmon D. Prolongation of life: roles of free radical reactions in aging. *J Am Geriatr Soc.* 1969; 17:721.
47. Harmon D. The aging process. *Proceedings of the National Academy of Sciences of the USA.* 1981; 78:7124–7141.
48. Tappel AL. Lipid peroxidation damage to cell components. *Fed Proc.* 1973; 32:1870.
48a. Leibovitz BE, Siegel B. Aspects of free radical reactions of biological systems: aging. *J Gerontol.* 1980; 35(1):45.
49. Sacher GA, Duffy PH. Genetic relation of life span to metabolic rate for inbred mouse strains and their hybrids. *Federal Proceedings.* 1979; 38:184–198.
50. Walford RL, Harris S, Weindruch R. Dietary restriction and aging: historical phases, mechanisms and current directions. *J Nutr.* 1987;117:1650–1654.
51. Everitt AV. The effects of hypophysectomy and continuous food restriction, begun at ages 70 and 400 days, on collagen aging, proteinuria, incidence of pathology and longevity in the male rat. *Mechan Ageing and Develop.* 1980; 12:161–169.
52. Walford RL. *The 120-Year Diet.* New York: Pocket Books; 1986.
53. Weindruch R, Chia D, Barnett EV, Walford RL. Dietary restriction in mice beginning at 1 year of age: effects in serum immune complex levels. *Age.* 1982; 5:111–112.
54. Harmon D. Free radical theory of aging: role of free radicals in the origination and evaluation of life, aging, and disease processes. In: Johnson JE, Walford RL, Harmon D, Miguel J, eds. *Free Radicals, Aging, and Degenerative Diseases.* New York: Alan Liss; 1986: 3–50.
55. Koizumi A, Weindruch R, Walford RL. Influence of dietary restriction and age on live enzyme activities and lipid peroxidation in mice. *J Nutr.* 1987; 117:361–367.
56. Paffenberger RS. Physical activity, all-cause mortality, and longevity of college alumni. *N Engl J of Med.* 1986; 314:605–609.
57. Orgel LE. The maintenance of the accuracy of protein synthesis and its relevance to aging. *Proceedings of the National Academy of Sciences of the USA.* 1963; 49:517–531.
58. Sonneborn T. The origin, evolution, nature and causes of aging. In: Behnke J, Fince C, Moment G, eds. *The Biology of Aging.* New York: Plenum Press; 1979; 341.
59. Ryan JM, Duda B, Cristofalo VJ. Error accumulation and aging in human diploid cells. *J of Gerontol.* 1974; 29:616–627.
60. Holliday R, Tarrant GM. Altered enzymes in aging human fibroblasts. *Nature.* 1972; 238:26–34.
61. Rothstein M. Age-related changes in enzyme levels and enzyme properties. In: Rothstein M, ed. *Review of Biological Research in Aging.* New York: Alan Liss; 1985; 1:421–444.
62. Medvedev Z. Possible role of repeated nucleotide sequences in DNA in the evolution of life spans of differential cells. *Nature.* 1972; 237–453.

63. Failla G. The aging process and carcinogenesis. *Annuals of the NY Academy of Sciences.* 1958; 71:1124–1130.
64. Szilard L. On the nature of the aging process. *Proceedings of the National Academy of Sciences of the USA.* 1959; 45:30–51.
65. Curtis HF, Miller K. Chromosome aberrations in lower cells of guinea pigs. *J of Gerontol.* 1971; 26:292–299.
66. Maynard-Smith J. Review lecturer on senescence: I. the causes of aging. *Proceedings of the Royal Society of London.* 1962; (B):157:115–124.
67. Clark AM, Rubin MA. The modification of X-irradiation of the life span of haploid and diploid Hagrogracon. *Radiation Research.* 1961; 14:244–251.
68. Bjorksten J. Crosslinkage and the aging process. In: Rockstein M, ed. *Theoretical Aspects of Aging.* New York: Academic Press; 1974: 43.
69. Bjorksten J. The crosslinkage theory of aging: clinical implications. *Compr Ther.* 1976; II:65.
70. Hall DA. *The Aging of Connective Tissue.* New York: Academic Press; 1976.

CHAPTER **3** THREE

Comparing and Contrasting Age Related Changes in Biology, Physiology, and Anatomy

The aging process occurs along the continuum of life. Beginning at conception and terminating in death, certain biological, anatomic, physiological, and functional changes are recognized as transitional markers in the human aging process. Aging is viewed as characteristically decremental in nature and lacking in defined chronological points of transition, though it is linear with time.[1]

The notion of a "maximal achievable life span" is inherent in the concepts of aging.[2-4] Identifying and describing changes in function that are common to all individuals and not produced by pathology is a very difficult task. The use of the term "eugenic" distinguishes changes related to the natural aging process from those related to pathology.[5] The hypothesis of eugenic death is that the decline of function continues linearly to the point where an internal environment compatible with cell life can no longer be maintained.

The changes that a human experiences with the passage of years can be categorized in several ways. For the purpose of this chapter, these age related changes will be discussed in terms of the biological, anatomic, physiological, and functional changes that occur eugenically in various systems in the human body. While the process of aging is very complex and does not uniformly result in decreased functional capacity,[6] this survey of the body's systems will be based on the assumption that the losses associated with the aging process are due to declines in biological cellular functioning. Some changes in function go hand in hand with anatomic or structural changes. In these cases, some functional units are lost, but the remaining units continue to function normally. The kidney is an excellent example of this—function is diminished in proportion to the number of nephrons lost. Skeletal muscle is another example. While muscle mass decreases secondary to the loss of muscle fibers, the remaining muscle mass is capable of oxygenation and consuming metabolic substrates at a constant rate. In some aging processes, there is no anatomic loss but rather a reduced physiological efficiency of each unit. The reduced conduction velocity seen in aging nerve fibers is an example of this. The most obvious aging changes are those in which function is totally lost: The capacity of the female to reproduce is one excellent example, while another would be the loss of the ability to hear sounds above a certain frequency.

Homeostasis is a concept describing the "constancy of the internal environment."[7] This internal constancy enables humans to survive in many environments and to withstand many biological and physiological challenges, thereby expanding the habitable world of the human. Perhaps the single most salient and age related difference is the diminishing ability of the body to respond to physical and emotional stress and return to its prestress level.[8,9] This decrease in homeostatic capacity is seen in all the systems of the body, but it is most marked in neuroendocrine interaction and in the systemic functional alteration in the responsiveness of the nervous and endocrine systems.[7]

The changes associated with aging through adulthood into old age are gradual. During adult life, in the absence of overt pathology, there is a slow decrement in function. Homeostasis can be maintained, albeit at a lower level. Another observation is that the more complex the function, the more decline is seen. Decrements are greater in the functions involving a number of connections between nerve and nerve, nerve and muscle, and nerve and gland. For instance, the decrease in nerve conduction velocity compared to the decrease in maximum breathing capacity. In the former a single system is involved, while in the latter the coordination of a number of nerve and muscle activities is required.

Lastly, it is important to keep in mind that individuals age at different rates. Different tissues and systems within one person demonstrate different aging rates as well. Therefore, while it is useful to discuss the average declines of function, it is important to keep in mind that any one individual may show remarkable variability from his or her peers.

CELLULAR CHANGES IN AGING

General changes in cell growth, division, repair, and regeneration have been found to occur with the aging process. Not all body cells age in the same way or at the same rate; however, in general, the total number of cells in the body decreases with age while remaining cells become less alike in structure and less organized in functions. Within cellular nuclei, nucleoli increase in size and number, loosely coiled fibers of chromatin demonstrate clumping, and the nuclear membrane becomes invaginated. Alterations in the number and shape of mitochondria, distortions of chromosomes, and the fragmentation of the Golgi apparatus have been reported to occur. Though also found in younger cells, there is an increased deposition of an autoflourescent chemically inert substance called lipofuscin. The degree of lipofuscin deposition varies among body tissues but is particularly present in critical tissues like the heart and the brain. The possible correlation between lipofuscin accumulation and system pathology is not yet well established. Though general agreement has been reached regarding the existence of these changes, debates continue over their significance as related to cellular function in normal aging.[10]

Cells can be classified in many different ways. For our purposes, cells will be classified as "mitotic," those that are capable of reproductive division (epithelial cells, hemopoietic stem cells), and as postmitotic cells (neurons, myocardial cells), which are not capable of division. Mitotic cell life is ultimately ended by limited cellular division, while postmitotic cell life (assuming no trauma) is terminated by senescence or death of the organism.

Mitotic cells were previously, and erroneously, believed to have an infinite capacity for division. Instead, Hayflick[11] demonstrated with human fibroblasts that mitotic cells are capable of approximately 50 cell divisions. As a cell ages, the rate of cellular division decreases and becomes more irregular. Eventually, the cell is incapable of further division, and it dies. Hayflick also found that cellular division could be temporarily interrupted for years via an imposed dormancy with ultra cold liquid nitrogen temperatures. Upon thawing, the cells resume their original sequence and rate of division until senescence. This evidence suggests that aging and cell death may be programmed events predetermined by aging genes.[7]

Because enzymes control cellular function, they have been widely studied for age related changes. Though changes have been observed, the amounts of enzymes available are usually adequate if the system is not challenged. In general, the functional effectiveness of many enzymes does not diminish with age while production under stress may be limited.[12]

CARDIOVASCULAR CHANGES WITH AGE

Cellular Changes

Few cellular changes in the aging heart can be attributed to biological changes alone, as evidenced by morphological studies.[13,14] Age can not be accurately determined by pathologic examination of cardiac muscle cells. The only consistent myofibrillar change documented has been lipofuscin accumulation at the poles of the nuclei of cardiac muscle cells.[14] Baker[15] found that cardiac muscle cell diameter and protein production within the nuclear region of the cell were significantly increased with age. A rise in cellular degeneration was also observed with age, and this included an increase in lipofuscin deposition in the muscle cells, lipid deposition, and tubular dilation in the cardiac muscle cells. A marked decline in the total number of pacemaker cells at the sinoatrial node occurs at the approximate age of

60, and by the age of 75 there are less than 10% of pacemaker cells compared to the healthy adult heart.[13-15] It has also been found that there is an increase in interstitial fibrous tissue specifically in the internodal tracts.[14]

Vascular changes with age include a thickening of the supporting membranes of the vessels including capillaries, an elongation of the arteries that becomes tortuous and calcifies, and an increase in amyloidosis (depositing of excess starch-like material in the vessels).[16] The aging process affects each area of the vascular tree differently. Yin[16] reports that changes in the vascular structures are more prominent in the thoracic aorta and less prominent in the renal artery. Changes appear first in the proximal vessels progressing to involve the distal vasculature. It is also noted that the distal vessels undergo the most pronounced changes.[16,17] Changes in the coronary arteries appear first in the left branches, but they do not appear in the right and posterior descending coronary arteries until well into the fifth decade of life.[17]

The endothelial cells of the intima become irregular in size and shape, and the cells lose their parallel orientation to the longitudinal axis of the vessel.[16-18] More giant multinucleated cells are present in the intima with age. Thickening of the subendothelial layer is apparent in aging. There is an increase in the connective tissue content, more thinned, frayed, and fragmented elastic laminae and an increase in lipid deposition and calcification around the internal elastic membrane.[16,19]

In the media, the most prominent age related changes are increased calcification and thickening elastic fragmentation.[16,19,20] The aortic media thickens by approximately 40% (1.21 to 1.67 mm) after the fifth decade of life. The thoracic aorta thickens predominantly secondary to an increase in the elastic laminae.[21] In the abdominal aorta, the thickening is due to smooth muscle proliferation.[21] Ninety-eight percent of human aortas demonstrate significant medial calcification by the fourth decade. Calcium binding to decarboxylic acid-containing amino acids demonstrates a parallel increase with age.[21,22]

Anatomic Changes

The heart shows a slight increase in the thickness of the left ventricular wall with age, though there is no significant change in heart chamber sizes.[13] Pomerance noted that the number of proximal-bundle fascicles connecting the left bundle with the main bundle of the conduction system may be less, and there is a small age related reduction in the density of the distal conduction fibers.[13] Relatively little change appears in the His bundle or AV node. The elastic tissue, fat, and collagen content of the myocardium shows only a slight increase in end stage aging, and small areas of fibrosis in the myocardium show an age related increase. The atrial surface of the atrioventricular and atrial endocardial valves thicken with age. As a result of mechanical stresses induced by repeated contact, nodular thickenings are often noted to form along the line of closure in the atrioventricular valves.

In the vasculature, as previously described, there is an increase in lumen size and thickness in the human aorta.[16] In the renal and carotid arteries there is an increase in the ratio of wall thickness to the radius of the vessel. In the aorta and femoral artery there is a decrease in this ratio.[16] The aorta thickness to radius ratio shows a progressive increase in the peripheral vasculature and vascular tortuosity increases significantly with age.[23]

Physiological Changes

All of these biological and structural changes result in physiological and functional alterations of the cardiovascular system. Generally there is a decrease in cardiac output at rest, a decline in the cardiovascular system's response to stress, an increase in the systolic blood pressure, and a progressive increase in the peripheral vascular resistance to blood flow.

Heart rate, loading conditions, intrinsic muscle performance, and neurohumoral efficiency all affect cardiac output. The maximum heart rate achievable declines linearly with age at peak exercise levels.[24,25] Heart rate response is usually not affected at submaximal exercise levels. Heart rate response has been demonstrated to diminish in response to various physiological stimuli, such as coughing, postural changes, or during Valsalva's maneuver.[26] The rate with which the heart rate peaks also becomes prolonged with increasing age.[24] Cardiac filling and vascular impedance are loading conditions that influence cardiac output. Diastolic filling rate has been shown to decrease with age,[27] and this is attributed to prolonged isometric relaxation, thickening and sclerosis of the mitral valve that impedes ventricular filling, and an age associated decrease in left ventricular compliance.[27] Vascular impedance is affected by the central-aortic stiffness or compliance, peripheral vascular resistance, and the inertial properties of blood.[16] Systolic pressure in the aorta and pulse pressures are increased with age.[14,16] Late systolic pressure exceeds early systolic pressure in the elderly, and the index of elastance (characteristic impedance) and peripheral resistance are increased with age.[28] These changes are indicative of less aortic compliance and a reduced cross-section of the peripheral vasculature, which causes an increase in pulse-wave velocity and in wave reflection. Wei[16,24] hypothesizes that the consequent increase in vascular load could explain the age associated reductions in stroke volume and cardiac output as well as the development of mild left ventricular hypertrophy and prolonged myocardial relaxation in the elderly.

Intrinsic muscle performance is estimated by the mean velocity of circumferential fiber shortening, and this does not change with age.[27] However, isometric relaxation and early diastolic relaxation are prolonged as age increases.[29] Left ventricular wall thickness may result from prolonged relaxation.[27]

Cardiac output is also affected by neurohumoral regulation. In the myocardium and in the peripheral vessels the end-organ responsiveness is decreased to beta-adrenergic stimulation.[16] The autonomic tone is increased based on plasma catecholamine levels.[30] Reflex activity of the cardiovascular system (i.e., Valsalva's maneuver, orthostasis, and cough) are weaker in the aged cardiovascular system, due in part to a decreased baroreceptor sensitivity, and the weaker reflexes are associated with changes in the cardiopulmonary system.[14,26,31]

The ability of the body to maintain a homeostatic blood pressure is a function of the autonomic nervous system, the arterial baroreceptor reflex, circulating neurohumoral factors, local vascular tone, and the extracellular fluid volume. There is an alteration in the homeostatic blood pressure regulatory role as a result of an altered autonomic nervous system with age.[16,31] According to Shimada, an elevation of blood pressure in the elderly can be attributed to an increase in plasma norepinephrine levels, which leads to an increase in the sympathetic responsiveness.[31] The functioning of the arterial baroreceptor reflex is lessened with age.[14,31] Atherosclerosis and the presence of hypertension also decrease the baroreceptor reflex.[31] Catecholamines and circulating neurohumoral factors assist in the maintenance of a homeostatic blood pressure.[32] These factors include renin, aldosterone, vasopressin, atrial natriuretic factor, and angiotensin II. The level of renin in the plasma has been found to remain either unchanged or to decrease in relation to age. It is hypothesized that this is due to a decrease in the concentration of active renin and is not a result of the concentration of renin substrate in the plasma.[32] In proportion to the decreased renin activity in the plasma, there is a related decline in aldosterone and plasma angiotensin II levels with increasing age.[32] Vasopressin remains unchanged or decreases with age. A decrease in vasopressin activity is most often related to blood loss or dehydration.[33] The level of plasma atrial natriuretic factor does not show a change with age. Vascular tone may show a local increase with age, though the constriction of the vessels is not changed in response to norepinephrine with age.[16]

The effect of these changes on the cardiovascular system is seen in changes in cardiac output, stroke volume, and blood pressure at rest and in response to stress. Resting heart rate does not show a consistent age related change in humans.[14] Resting cardiac rate and cardiac output remain relatively unchanged, although peripheral resistance (blood pressure) is increased.[34] With age, myocardial weight tends to increase, and myocardial cells show an increase in lipofuscin deposition. Mitochondria decrease in size and myochondrial cells are less responsive to catacholamine stimulation. A reduction in baroreceptor response and vascular elasticity combines to result in the tendency for older people to experience postural hypotension.[7,35] When sitting at rest, the cardiac output does not show a change with age; however, when supine there is often an age related decrease in cardiac output.[14] There is also a similar position-associated change in stroke volume. This is explained by the changes with age in cardiac compliance and preload conditions.[14,16] Resting blood pressures, both diastolic and systolic, tend to show an increase with age.[24] It is not clear whether this increase in blood pressure is a reflection of eugenic aging or the result of heredity, environmental factors, or both.[14]

In response to stress the cardiovascular system shows a decrease in heart rate acceleration and a decrease in the ejection fraction with physical exertion.[14] Postural changes also affect cardiac output and blood pressure as previously discussed. Following a moderately sized meal, the elderly tend to show a decrease in systemic blood pressure.[14] With increasing levels of exercise, there is a concomitant rise in the systemic blood pressure. This rise is credited to the changes in preload conditions during cardiac filling.[14] In the absence of pathology, the described cardiovascular responses to increased activity levels are consistently seen with increasing age, however, aerobic conditioning exercises may alter this. The effects of exercise on the cardiovascular system are positive and will be discussed in a subsequent chapter.

PULMONARY CHANGES WITH AGE

For the purpose of this chapter, aging changes defined by Butler as those changes that are "universal, intrinsic, progressive and irreversible" within the cardiopulmonary system will be discussed here.[36] The pathologies of the lung will be further discussed in Chapter 5, Pathological Manifestations of Aging.

In the pulmonary system, age changes can be organized according to mechanical properties, changes in flow, changes in volume, alteration in gas exchange, and impairments of lung defense. Decreases in chest wall compliance and lung elastic recoil tendency are two mechanical properties that are altered with age. Increased calcification of the ribs, a decline in intercostal muscle strength, and changes in the spinal curvature all result in a lower compliance and an increased work of breathing.

At normal lung volume airway resistance is not increased, however, normal aging results in a reduction of maximum voluntary ventilation, maximum expiratory flow, and forced expiratory volume in one second (alone and in relation to forced vital capacity). Though tidal volume remains fairly constant throughout life, vital capacity decreases while residual volume increases.

Ventilation, diffusion, and pulmonary circulation are the three major components of the respiratory system that lose efficiency with age. There is an increased thickening of the supporting membranes between the alveoli and the capillaries, a decline in total lung capacity, an increase in residual volume, a reduced vital capacity, and a decrease in the resiliency of the lungs. It is difficult to completely separate pulmonary changes resulting with age from those associated with the pathology of emphysema or chronic bronchitis. Throughout a lifetime, exposure to occupational and environmental inhalants as well as secondary cigarette smoke may result in chronic pulmonary changes and lung pathologies. These disease states closely parallel those of the aging process and also increase in incidence with advancing age.[37] "Normal" pulmonary aging includes a loss of elastic tissue leading to expiratory collapse of the larger airways, difficulty with expiration, and dilatation of the terminal air passages.[38]

There are changes in the diffusion efficiency of the peripheral vascular system with age. Starting with the pulmonary system, impairment of gas exchange is illustrated by a reduced diffusing capacity of carbon monoxide, a lower resting arterial oxygen tension, and an increased alveolar–arterial oxygen gradient. Alveolar surface area and pulmonary capillary blood volume diminish with age. Small changes in red blood cell metabolism produces a decrease in 2,3-diphosphoglycerate (DPG). As a result, the oxygen dissociation curve shifts to the left, which makes oxygen less available at the tissue level.[38]

The ability to provide oxygen to working tissues is altered as normal aging affects the cardiopulmonary system in a variety of ways. In the absence of pathology, the heart and lungs can generally meet the body's needs; however, reserve capacities are diminished. With any challenge, the body's demand for oxygen and perfusion may exceed available supply.

In an older person, normal changes result in an impairment of pulmonary defenses. Cilia are reduced in number, and those that remain become less strong. The "mucus escalator" and alveolar macrophages are less effective in removing inhaled particulate matter. In the absence of physiological challenges, the system maintains fairly adequate defenses. However, an older individual who is chronically exposed to air laden with particles will be at risk for pulmonary dysfunction.[7,39]

The recovery period following physical effort is prolonged in the elderly. Among other factors, this reflects a greater relative work rate, an increase proportion of anaerobic metabolism, a slower heat elimination, and a lower level of physical fitness. As a result, the cool down phase of exercise needs to be lengthened when elderly individuals are exercising to allow for a more gradual return to their baseline vital signs. Abrupt cessation of exercise without considering an adequate recovery period could have negative effects for a person of any age, but it is particularly important in the elderly to provide adequate recovery time.

MUSCULOSKELETAL CHANGES WITH AGE

Cellular Changes

Extracellular and connective tissue changes with age are related to hydration of the tissues and collagen and elastin extensibility. There are many types of connective tissue in the body (loose, adipose, fibrous, etc.). It is "loose" connective tissue that functions to bind organs together while holding tissue fluids and permitting cellular–molecular diffusion. Loose connective tissue is located beneath most layers of epithelium and fills the spaces between muscles (fascia). The most common type of cell in loose connective tissue is called a fibroblast. Fibroblasts work to produce protein fibers called collagen and elastin.[35]

In youth, collagen fibers are strong and flexible, and they are arranged in bundles that criss-cross to form a structure in the body. As a person ages, there is an increased criss-crossing or cross-linkage of the fibers, resulting in denser extracellular matrices. The collagen structure becomes stiffer as it becomes denser. This increased density also impairs molecular movement of nutrients and wastes at the cellular level.[35]

Structurally, elastin fibers also develop increased cross-linkage with age. Water and elasticity are lost. The elastin fibers become more rigid, may tend to fray, and, in some cases, are replaced by collagen completely.[7]

Connective tissue cells develop from the primitive mesenchymal cell. As a result of this common origin, all connective tissue have similar cellular features. All connective tissue cells secrete collagen, elastin, glycoproteins, hyaluronic acid, and contractile proteins.[40] These substances vary in proportion in different tissue types. For example, the predominant secretion in white fibrous tissue is collagen, elastin is the prevalent secretion in yellow elastic tissue, and glycoprotein is the common secretion in cartilage. The pattern of secretion of these substances by connective tissue will be altered under different environmental conditions within the body. In this portion of the chapter, the effects of aging on the production and functional significance of each of these secretions will be considered.

Collagen is the basic protein component in fibrous connective tissue inclusive of bone, tendon, ligament, and cartilage.[41,42] Procollagen, a protein material, is secreted by the ribosomes of connective tissue cells. Individual procollagen molecules bind together to form tropocollagen strands. These strands group together in a spiral fashion to form the mature collagen fiber.[43] The diameter of the collagen fiber is increased by the surface aggregation of additional tropocollagen strands with a resulting characteristic of a compressed and increasingly cross-linked central fiber.[44] Further cross-linkages continue to be added even after the fiber has reached maturity. It has been determined that the diameter of collagen fibers is greater in older subjects when compared to that in younger subjects.[45] Generally, the tensile strength of connective tissue in older persons is greater than that in younger individuals. The increased cross-linkage of collagen fibers is considered a "normal" change related to aging.

The clinical significance of this increased cross-linking is seen in resultant collagenous contractures. Bonds between adjacent collagen strands can produce shortening and distortion of the collagen fibers. This shortening may result in contractures with a progressive restriction in tissue mobility.[42] Collagen fibers are tough and inelastic, and their bonds cannot be broken by mechanical stretching forces. Of interest clinically, however, has been the determination that some of these chemical bonds are temperature sensitive.[46] Lehman and associates[46] found that at temperatures of 42.5°C and above the bonds between collagen fibers become unstable and the tissues can be mobilized. Continuous stretching while heating the tissues followed by 30 minutes of maintained stretching during the cooling period is recommended.[46]

The ribosomes within the connective tissue secrete elastin during the developmental stages.[40] Elastin molecules join together in an end-to-end and branching manner to form a lattice-like network that gives elastin its ability to return to its original length after being stretched.[45] There is a progressive reduction in the amount of elastin in the skin, the walls of the arteries, and the bronchial tree with age.[6,7] If the elastin fibers are overstretched to the point of tearing, scarring occurs, which further decreases the elasticity of the tissues.

The glycoproteins form a group of relatively small molecules of soluble protein material. The presence of glycoproteins in the extracellular area produces the osmotic force that is important in maintaining the fluid content of the tissues.[40] The higher the glycoprotein concentration, the greater the amount of fluid that will be retained in the tissues by osmotic attraction forces. A variety of glycoprotein secretions have been identified, and these vary among tissue types and locations.[47] The production and release of glycoproteins within the connective tissues is reduced with age. As a result, it becomes increasingly difficult for the tissues to maintain a normal fluid balance. Dehydration is commonly found in the tissues of elderly individuals.[40]

Hyaluronic acid helps to regulate the viscosity of tissues, and it is produced by some of the ribosomes in the connective tissue cells, particularly those located in the cartilage. This substance helps to decrease the friction between cellular components during movement. There is a reduction in the amount of hyaluronic acid secreted that is associated with age and, thus, reduced ease of movement (viscosity) of the connective tissues, which results in tissue degradation.[48] The production of hyaluronic acid is enhanced by activity. Thus, exercise becomes particularly important for maintaining the viscosity of tissues in the elderly. Lack of exercise and activity will negatively affect the production of hyaluronic acid producing tissue restrictions and further decreases mobility.

Contractile proteins provide motility within the connective tissues. Their presence provides for the removal of waste products or debris and enhances mobility within the tissue spaces, as well as facilitates the capacity of cellular proteins to cross a capillary or lymphatic wall.[40] During aging, there is a reduction in the secretion and organization of contractile proteins with a resultant decrease in motility.[47] Contractile protein secretion is relatively small in normal fibroblasts. Connective tissue cells that produce abnormally high amounts of contractile protein are called myofibroblasts.[48] Ryan found excessive amounts of contractile protein in chronically restricted tissues, such as the rotator cuff in shoulder-hand syndrome and in Dupuytren's contraction.[48] Again, the importance of activity for the elderly must be stressed to prevent the accumulation of contractile proteins and soft tissue restrictions and contractures.

Fibrinous adhesions have great clinical implications in working with the elderly. Fibrinogen, a soluble plasma protein, is a normal molecular exudate within the capillary, and when this substance passes through the capillary wall into the surrounding tissues, it is converted to strands of insoluble fibrin.[49] Fibrin strands can adhere to tissue structures and restrict movement of these structures. Normally, fibrin is removed as debris by reticuloendothelial cells. With age, as well as with inactivity, the exudation of fibrinogen into the surrounding tissues is increased.[47] With reduced activity levels, complete breakdown of fibrin may not occur leading to the accumulation of this substance, which restricts movement and may possibly result in adhesions. Following an injury (traumatic or surgically induced), fibrinogen also accumulates at the site of tissue damage. If activity is limited, these strands can consolidate and create an adhesion.[40] Activity enhances the removal of fibrinogen and should be resumed as quickly as possible following an injury to prevent irreversible tissue restriction and contractures. The importance of early intervention and mobilization in the elderly is clear.[48]

Changes in Cartilage

Other connective tissues also affected by aging include bone, hyaline cartilage, elastic cartilage, and articular cartilage. Changes in bone will be presented separately.

Hyaline cartilage is found in the nose and the rings of the respiratory passages as well as in the joints. Elastic cartilage is found in parts of the larynx and in the outer ear. Articular cartilage is found between the intervertebral discs, between the bones of the pelvic girdle, and at most articular joint surfaces.[50] With aging, cartilage tends to dehydrate, becomes stiffer, and thins in weight bearing areas.

Cartilage is formed when the primitive mesenchymal cells are subjected to compressive forces in an environment of low oxygen concentration. The predominant secretions of the chondroblast are the glycoprotein, chondroitin sulfate, and hyaluronic acid. Collagen is produced in lesser amounts than these. Cartilage is a unique connective tissue in that it has no direct blood supply. Blood flow in adjacent bones and synovial fluid provide nutrients to the chondroblasts. A strong osmotic force, created by glycoprotein secretions from the chondroblasts passing from the cells into the surrounding matrix, attracts water with dissolved gases, inorganic salts, and organic materials into the matrix, thereby providing the materials necessary for normal metabolism. The concentration of glycoproteins in the matrix determines the amount of fluid drawn into the cartilage. Normal aging is accompanied by a reduction in the amount of chondroitin sulfate produced[51] and results in a decrease in osmotic attraction forces and an impairment in the ability of the matrix to attract and retain fluids.

Nutrients enter the matrix of the cartilage only when compressive forces are absent.[51,52] In a loaded or compressed state fluid and nutrient substances are squeezed out. To provide regular movement of substances in and out of the cartilage, it is necessary that alternating application and release of compressive forces occur. Metabolites remain in the matrix in the absence of compression. The presence of metabolites reduces the oxygen content resulting in a reduction of the secretion of glycoproteins and an increase in the amount of procollagen produced.

With inactivity hyaline cartilage is converted to fibrocartilage.[51,52] Therefore, weight bearing exercises become particularly important in the elderly individual. The movement of nutritional substances in and out of the cartilage with activity could enhance the overall health of the cartilage and preserve the viability of the joints.[51]

In synovial joints the articular surfaces are covered by hyaline cartilage. Lubrication at the interface of the hyaline cartilage is provided by the secretion of hyaluronic acid by the chondroblasts. Hyaluronic acid molecules form a viscous layer covering the hyaline cartilage. Compression facilitates production of hyaluronic acid ensuring continual lubrication of the joint during movement.[52] As previously noted, the secretion of hyaluronic acid decreases with age, thereby reducing the efficiency of the lubrication system of the joint.[51] Degenerative changes of the cartilage are not reversible and rehabilitation efforts need to be directed toward regular compression and release of compression in the aging joint. Normal weight bearing exercises are recommended to maintain cartilaginous health.

The cartilage that normally covers body joints thins and deteriorates with aging. This especially occurs in the weight bearing areas. Because cartilage has no blood supply or nerves, erosion within the joint is often advanced before symptoms of pain, crepitation, and limitation of movement are perceived. Decreased hydration, reduced elasticity, and increased fibrous growth around bony prominences all contribute to increase stiffness and decreased functioning. Advanced stages of cartilage–joint deterioration is commonly known as osteoarthritis.[7,12,53]

Since some types of connective tissue exists almost everywhere in the body, the effects of aging are widespread. Increased rigidity of collagenous and elastin fibers results in a greater amount of energy being needed to produce a given stretch. Skin becomes less elastic and more wrinkled. Lungs lose some recoil tendency, arteries become more rigid and the heart becomes less distensible. Joints become stiffer while decreased hydration in the intravertebral discs results in vertebral compaction and shrinkage of height. Cellular repair, nutrition, and waste removal are impaired.[7,54] Other effects of connective tissue changes will be discussed as various systems are reviewed.

Changes in Body Composition

A brief mention of the changes in body composition and weight needs to be included. The most notable of these changes occurs with the body's fat and water content.[55] While extracellular water remains constant, intracellular water decreases, reflecting either a dehydration of the cell or a decrease of cell mass in the presence of adequate hydration.[55–57] Dehydration is a particularly common consequence of aging, especially during exercise. Adequate fluid intake should be encouraged in the elderly and closely monitored in the exercising aged individual.

In general, there is a decrease in lean muscle tissue while there is an increase in fat concentration. Almost all the organs demonstrate a decrease in weight and mass, an exception being the prostrate, which may actually double in size with age.[57,58]

MUSCLE CHANGES WITH AGE

Cellular Changes

Muscles are composed of postmitotic cells. Intact motor neuron innervation is required for proper functioning and survival. A loss of muscle mass with aging is caused by a reduction in the size and number of muscle fibers.[59] As fewer fibers are lost from the contracting muscles as compared to the opposing muscle mass,[60] the body develops a tendency toward flexion at the joints. Lipofuscin deposition is increased. The density of capillaries per remaining motor unit is decreased, and a reduction in myosin ATP activity has been shown.[61] Neuroconduction of muscle impulse is prolonged and coordination is affected. The sum total of these changes includes a decrease in muscle strength and body stability. Deconditioning and malnutrition often compound the effects of normal age related changes. Though reconditioning will improve muscle function, the speed and degree of potential improvement does decline with age.[62]

Alterations in skeletal muscle with aging resemble those observed with denervation. The classic cross-innervation studies of Buller and associates[63] established the importance of the trophic influence on skeletal muscle function and demonstrated that the metabolic and physiological profile of a muscle fiber (i.e., the fiber type) was primarily determined by the type of neural innervation (phasic or tonic firing pattern and other trophic factors) received. Adult skeletal muscle is composed of three distinct fiber types: type I (slow twitch, high oxidative fiber), type IIA (fast twitch, high oxidative fiber), and type IIB (fast twitch, low oxidative fiber). Based on the histochemical demonstration of myofibrillar ATPase and the mitochondrial enzyme succinic dehydrogenase, this heterogeneous fiber pattern is lost with aging, and fibers become more homogeneous in respect to their physiological and metabolic profile.[60,61,63]

It is well known that decreases in muscle mass occur with old age, with proximal muscles of the lower extremity particularly affected. This decrease in muscle mass is due to a decrease in both fiber number and diameter. No change in the number of motor neural fibers has been found, but the size of the motor unit decreases due to the loss of muscle fibers. The reported decrease in fiber number primarily affects the red oxidative fiber, but the preponderance of evidence based on enzyme histochemistry and physiological properties suggests a greater loss in the fast type II fiber. The decrease occurs in both type IIA and IIB fibers such that the type IIB/IIA fiber ratio is unaltered with increasing age. As a result of this selective loss of type II fibers, the percentage of type I fibers increases from about 40% in 20 to 30 year olds to 55% in 60 to 65 year olds.[64]

Besides atrophy and a decrease in the number of fibers, senile skeletal muscle exhibits a number of ultrastructural changes:

1. Thickening and protrusion of the sarcolemma into the extracellular space.
2. An increase in collagenous material in the extracellular space.
3. Disorganized and disrupted myofilaments at the cell periphery.
4. Proliferation of the tubular T-system, the sarcoplasmic reticulum, and the terminal cisternae.
5. Enlarged mitochondria with vacuolated matrix, short cristae, and loss of dense granules.
6. Accumulation of ribosomes and polysomes in subsarcolemmal region.
7. An increase in lysosomal vesicles and pinocytic activity.

The majority of these age related changes are located at the fiber surface where considerable cell debris associated with proteolytic activity can be observed.

Cellular changes are found in all organs with aging. Among the most visible signs of aging are alterations in skin and the development of movement dysfunction. As we age, strength and coordination decline and movements tend to become slower. Movement dysfunctions are caused by many factors, and some of these factors are peripheral and central synaptic mechanism changes, motivation, skeletal disorders (such as osteoarthritis or structural imbalances caused by tonal changes in cerebral vascular accidents [CVAs] or other neurological syndromes), and muscle changes. Several factors may be occurring simultaneously. Loss of strength, seen as a decrease in muscle hypertrophy and as changes in muscle function, are a result of a complex interaction of factors. For instance, there is a reduced ability of the cardiovascular system to deliver raw materials to working muscles and alterations in the chemical composition of muscle fibers.[64a,65] On a quantitative level, all measurements of muscle, physiological, anatomic, histochemical, or enzymatic, decrease after the age of 40. It is estimated that 20% to 40% of maximal strength is lost by the age of 65 in the nonexercising adult.[66] The general reaction to aging involves a decline in muscular strength accompanied by signs of atrophy. Qualitative measurements of changes in muscle function show loss of lean body mass and primary skeletal muscle. Clinically it is apparent that aging affects certain muscles more than others. For example, flexor muscles of lower extremities show age related changes relatively early compared to other muscle groups.

In the "aging phenomena" there is a decrease in the number of active functional units (motor units or muscle fibers) and a loss in the concentration of specific enzymes or fiber types. The major fiber types show a differential response to aging. Gutmann and Hanzlikova[67] have characterized the essential features of the "senescent motor unit," and these features indicate that age related changes are a distinct biological entity. Changes are similar to changes seen in denervated muscle and immobilized muscle. In aged and denervated muscle there are

- Decreases in the number and size of muscle fibers.
- Proliferation of T tubules and sarcoplasmic reticulum.
- Considerable histochemical evidence of fiber grouping.

Biochemical changes at the cellular level[61] include

- Loss of activity of glycolytic and oxidative enzymes.
- Decreased concentration of adenosine triphosphate (ATP).
- Decreased rate of creatin phosphate resynthesis.
- Changes at the neuromuscular junction altering trophic interactions between muscle and nerve compromising fast synaptic activity (reduced endplate potentials).

Some alterations in aged muscle may be secondary to other age related changes, such as weight loss. Most changes in the senescent motor unit, however, are usually evident before an age associated loss of body weight. It is unlikely that muscle dysfunction is secondary to weight loss in the elderly unless a true state of malnutrition exists.

Pathological causes of strength declines are many including arthritis, cerebral vascular accidents, cardiovascular disease and so on, all of which will be covered more extensively in Chapter 5, Pathological Manifestations of Aging. Functional causes of muscle strength declines can be related to the "use it or lose it" principle. Studies on astronauts in a gravity eliminated environment, as well as research involving immobilization of body parts or the whole body, reveal significant parallels to those muscle changes seen as "normal aging."[7]

Endurance is another factor of muscle function that appears to be affected by aging. Larsson and his colleagues[64] studied the physiological, anatomical, and histochemical effects of aging changes in a cross-sectional study of 55 healthy men 22 to 65 years of age—all sedentary office workers.

To determine whether or not these changes correlated with performance, strength and endurance testing was done using the Cybex.[68] Isometric endurance was measured using the time subjects could maintain 50% of their maximal isometric force and dynamic endurance was measured by having subjects perform 50 maximal isokinetic contractions at 180 degrees/second. The percent of change was determined by dividing the mean torque of the last three contractions by the mean torque of the first three contractions. It was found that at all velocity settings there was an age related decline in isometric force and an age related decrease in the peak isokinetic torque. A decline in maximal knee extension was also noted. There was no age related difference in muscle mass as measured by thigh circumference. Endurance, both dynamic and isometric, was similar in all age groups. With age, force values linearly declined as did the proportion and area of the type II fibers. However, Larsson[68] postulated that, based on multiple regression analysis, type II fiber atrophy could not account for all of the decline in strength measures. Other factors, such as age and activity levels, influenced the results. Combining the factors of increased hydroaldoase dexokinase (HAD) activity, a shift in lactic dehydrogenase (LDH) isoenzyme patterns, an increased proportion of type I fibers, and a decreased age of type II fibers, we see an indication that with aging there is an overall increase in oxidative capacity of the muscle. Another possibly clinically significant finding is the elevated enzyme activities in the older, active group compared with the younger sedentary group. The increased enzyme levels raises the question of how "trainable" the aged motor unit is.[69] Specific measurements of muscles' isometric and isokinetic performances all show deterioration. Interestingly, no change in endurance capacity was correlated with age.

Electromyographic patterns indicate an increasing recruitment of motor units for a given task by skeletal muscle with age. In other words, it takes more to do less.[69] This effect is due to the generalized denervation of muscle fibers requiring a larger number of motor units to produce a given force. These physiological changes in skeletal muscle are associated with the aging process.

Anatomic Changes

Anatomically, a pattern of gross skeletal muscle wasting is seen with aging. On a microscopic level, changes in muscles with aging are similar to those described in myopathy, disuse, and neuropathic atrophy.

The ultrastructure of the sarcoplasm also undergoes some age related changes. The hypertrophy of the sarcoplasmic reticulum is felt to correlate with an increase in the rate of calcium ion transport or absorption by the reticulum. This effect may in turn cause contractile protein dysfunction due to the paucity of calcium ions available for normal contraction. The thickening of the muscle fiber's basement membrane is hypothesized as an explanation of the decreased depolarization sensitivity of aged muscle cell membranes.[70]

Histological Changes

Histopathological changes occur in aging as well as in disuse or denervation. Aging muscles show a general increase in type I muscle fibers. Etiology of this is felt to be twofold: Either there is a selective loss of type II muscle fibers, or there is an reinnervation of denervated type II fiber motor units by type I motor fibers. In the "extremely old" muscle, muscle grouping of fibers of one type occur, a process associated with denervation and subsequent reinnervation. Gutmann[67] found no evidence of disintegration of the terminal axons in senile muscle fibers, but he observed major changes at the neuromuscular junction resulting in muscle atrophy. These changes included an increase in the number and agglutination of presynaptic vesicles, the appearance of neurotubules and neurofilaments in the peripheral axons, the enlargement of primary synaptic clefts, the thickening of the basement membrane, and an increased branching of the junctional folds. These changes produce a slow reduction of synaptic contact in senile muscle and result in a "functional denervation." In addition, the neuromuscular junction in senile muscle shows a reduced frequency of miniature end-plate potentials and a reduced conduction velocity in the presynaptic axons.

The decrease in senile muscle mass is associated with a decrease in total protein and nitrogen concentration and an increase in connective tissue and fat. Intracellular water and potassium are unaltered or decreased, while muscle amino acid concentration increases with aging. Extracellular water, sodium, and chloride are all higher in older adults.

The molecular mechanism of the age related muscle atrophy is not clear, but the process is likely to be linked to the neural and neuromuscular changes already reviewed.

The ability of the muscle to meet energy demands declines linearly with age. It is well known that aging is associated with a progressive decline in physical work capacity. Maximal oxygen uptake (liter/minute $\dot{V}O_2$ maximum) shows a steady decline with age and with disuse or in gravity eliminated situations. The decline in maximal $\dot{V}O_2$ with age is related to cardiovascular, respiratory, and peripheral skeletal muscle changes.

The effect of age on the oxidative rate of heart and skeletal muscle mitochondria appears to be substrate dependent. The cardiovascular system loses some efficiency with age. The consequence of this is that various proteins are not delivered to the muscle tissue in the same quantity as when the muscle was younger. Glycoproteins, the small molecules that produce an osmotic force and are important in maintaining fluid content of tissues, decrease in quantity with aging resulting in the increased difficulty of tissues to retain their normal fluid content.

Chemically, the greatest change is a decrease in the efficiency of muscle cells' selectively permeable membrane.[70] Potassium, magnesium, and phosphate ions are normally in high concentration in the sarcoplasm, but other materials, such as sodium, chloride, and bicarbonate ions, are prevented from entering the cell under resting conditions. A characteristic feature of senescent muscle is a shift from this pattern. In particular, the concentration of potassium is reduced. There is a lack of potassium ions in aging muscle that reduces the maximum force of contraction that the muscle is capable of generating. Often, complaints of tiredness and lethargy in the clinic setting are a result of decreased potassium. Exercise in someone with potassium depletion will only fatigue them more. So it is important to check electrolytes.

SKELETAL CHANGES

The skeletal system functions to support, protect, and shape the body. Additionally, bone has the metabolic functions of blood cell production, the storage of calcium, and a role in the acid–base balance.

The most commonly known age related change involving bone is a calcium related loss of mass and density. This loss ultimately causes the pathological condition of "osteoporosis," in which bone density is lost from within by a process termed "reabsorption." As we grow older, an imbalance occurs between osteoblast activity (bone buildup) and osteoclast activity (breaks down bone). Osteoclast activity proves to be the stronger. As one ages, a decline in circulating levels of activated vitamin D_3 occurs.[71] This causes less calcium to be absorbed from the gut and more calcium to be absorbed from the bones to meet body needs. In postmenopausal women, decreased estrogen levels influence parathormone and calcitonin to increase bone reabsorption, which decreases bone mass. Certain factors, such as immobility, decreased estrogens, steroid therapy, and hyperthyroidism, to name a few, are known to accelerate bone erosion to pathological levels. Easily occurring fractures are the most common result.[7,35]

Osteoporosis is a major bone mineral disorder in the older adult, because it decreases the bone mineral content and, as a result, bone mass and strength decline with age. It is difficult to draw the line between what is normal and what is pathological in osteoporosis. This bone loss appears to be a normal aging process and has been characterized by a decreased bone mineral composition, an enlarged medullary cavity, a normal mineral composition, and biochemical normalities in plasma and urine. The rate of bone loss is about 1% per year for women starting at age 30 to 35 and for men at age 50 to 55. In elderly subjects, regions of devitalized tissue with osteocyte lacunae and haversian canals containing amorphous mineral deposits have been described.[7] These have been identified as micropetrotic regions and are noted to increase in frequency in the skeleton with age. Thus, it is clear that the mineral content of bone qualitatively changes with age.

Qualitatively, osteoporotic bone exhibits a reduction in bone mass with a resulting decrease in bone strength, and there is some evidence that alterations occur in the composition and structure of bone in the aged. Tensile strength of bone in man is related to the number and size of osteons. It has been found that bone from older humans have smaller osteons and fragments and more cement lines than younger bone, and this would account for some of the reduced bone strength of the older bone specimens. The remaining difference in strength results from the geometric structure of the bone in its distribution per unit area as a response to environmental stress placed on the bone. A more comprehensive discussion of osteoporosis is in Chapter 5, Pathological Manifestations of Aging.

Throughout life, red blood cells continue to be replaced after a life span of about 120 days. Some morphological changes do occur with aging. For instance, red cells are slightly smaller and more fragile; however, blood volume is well maintained until approximately 80 years of age. In the absence of pathology, few changes are seen in the white blood cells and in the platelet count. What is lost with aging is the functional reserve to quickly accelerate the production of red blood cells when needed.[7,72]

NEUROMUSCULAR CHANGES WITH AGE

Quantitatively, all muscle measures, including biological, anatomic, and physiological, decline after the age of 40.[73] Many of the changes associated with aging indicate a decrease in the number of active functional units (i.e., motor units or muscle fibers) and a loss in concentration of specific enzymes or fiber types.

CENTRAL NEUROLOGICAL CHANGES

After peaking in the early decades of life, brain mass or weight slowly decreases by as much as 6% to 7% by the time a person ages to 80 years. Though the brain stem appears to be minimally affected by cell loss, widely varied but significant losses occur in the cerebral cortex lobes and cerebellar area. Central nervous system cells are postmitotic. The central neurons that remain continue to decline in number and efficiency of function.

Cell number and composition decrease, and, with aging, the cells of the hippocampus undergo a degeneration caused by numbers of vacuoles surrounding dense central granules. Amyloid plaques develop, and lipofuscin is deposited within many remaining neuronal cells. After age 60, the number of neuronal microtubular structures may decrease and are often replaced by so-called "neurofibrillary tangles." Though plaques and tangles occur with normal aging, they are most commonly associated with the occurrence of senile dementia of the Alzheimer's type (SDAT).

Impulse conduction and cerebral synaptic transmission are both delayed with aging, which affects the transmitter competence of the central nervous system. A particular explanation lies in the general decline of available neurotransmitters. Serotonin, catecholamines, and gamma-aminobutyric acid (GABA) are less prevalent in the older brain. A decrease in the neurotransmitter dopamine is found in normal elderly but it is also associated with the pathology of Parkinson's disease.[74]

Conduction velocity of the central nervous system has been shown to decrease with advancing age. A loss of the myelin sheath and a loss of large myelinated fibers decreases the axons' ability to transmit impulses, especially in the posterior spinal column tracts. These tracts provide for reflex positive-righting responses. Remembering that balance impairment partially results from cerebellar losses (now coupled with central nervous system delays), one can begin to see why an older person has a greater tendency to fall and less ability to quickly correct the center of balance before injury occurs.[75]

INTERSYSTEM HOMEOSTASIS

Thermal Regulation

The role of the hypothalamus in homeostatic regulation is a major factor in age related declines. With increasing age the hypothalamus becomes less sensitive to the physiological feedback and consequently is less able to maintain the stability of the internal environment of the body. Processes such as increased body weight, increased serum cholesterol, and decreased glucose tolerance ensue and subsequently diseases result.[76] The hypothalamic thermostat is the principal control center for regulating the body's response to ambient, locally applied, and internal temperature gradients. Many investigators have attributed the increased rate of heat stroke, hypothermia, and climate related deaths among the aged population to faulty thermoregulation.[77]

Not only the hypothalamic thermostat and basal metabolic rate but also the overall reactivity of the autonomic nervous system decline with age, altering skin hydration and circulation in turn.[78] The vasomotor system is less responsive to warming and cooling, and the normal transient bursts of vasoconstrictor activity are reduced. It is unclear whether or not thermoreceptors in the skin are altered. Because cold receptors are dependent on a good oxygen supply, it may be reasoned that decreased circulatory supply may decrease the perception of cold because of the vulnerability of cold receptors to hypoxia.

Changes in the thermal regulatory response in the elderly have clinical significance in the aged individual's ability to maintain homeostasis with increasing exercise levels, because the cooling time following exercise is often prolonged. In addition, a decrease in the receptiveness of temperature gradients impacts the application of heat and cold modalities in treatment interventions. Consideration of these changes needs to be employed when treating the elderly patient.

Hormonal Balance

Aging is marked by a deterioration not only in the function of individual cells and organs, but also by a failure of mechanisms for the coordination of function between various parts of the body. A weakening of both neural and hormonal controls reduces the ability to adjust to external and internal stresses.[77] Among other responsibilities, the body hormones contribute to (1) the regulation of circulating fluid volumes and cardiovascular performance, (2) the mobilization of fuels for exercise (maintenance of blood glucose, liberation of fat, and breakdown of protein), and (3) the repair of body structures with the synthesis of new protein (anabolism). All of the changes in these functions impact on exercise tolerance and the healing process in the elderly. The aged are slower to reach homeostasis during exercise, and the return to a balanced homeostatic state following exercise is prolonged.[73] In addition, the healing process is slower due to a diminished synthesis of new protein.

In a small number of neurons in the central nervous system the peptide produced within the cell body of the neuron is adrenocorticotropic hormone (ACTH).[74] Liberation of ACTH from the axon terminals of these neurons produces different effects on different groups of postsynaptic cells. ACTH and a number of other peptide transmitter substances that have been identified are substances produced outside the nervous system by cells of the endocrine system. When produced by endocrine cells, these substances are termed hormones.

At neuron-to-neuron connections, the transmitter molecules are produced in moderate amounts and will be released from the presynaptic cell only through the axon terminals. The small amount of transmitter substance liberated from the terminal is rapidly deactivated at the release site. The effect of release of neurotransmitters is limited to a very localized area for only a short period of time.[74]

Movement of molecules between capillaries and extracellular spaces in the central nervous system is more difficult than in other tissues. Nerve cells have become more sensitive than other types of cells to their immediate chemical environment to facilitate a variety of specific transmitter mechanisms.[77]

The capillary wall thickening is achieved partly by a thickening of the basement membrane of the epithelial cells that form the capillary wall and partly as a result of glial cell activity. The glial cells are connective tissue cells responsible for producing the connective tissue packing material for the nerve cells and their fibers. The protein glial membranes that are produced contain finer fibers than those contained in other connective tissues, and the presence of a glial membrane around the small blood vessels and capillaries in the brain produces the so-called blood–brain barrier.[73] While all neuron-to-neuron connections in the brain are protected by the blood–brain barrier, some nerve connections are made with cells outside the nervous system, and these connections form the neuroendocrine system. Connections from the hypothalamus to the posterior lobe of the pituitary gland belong to this system. Normally, the activity of many endocrine glands is finely balanced and highly coordinated, but in the elderly the coordination is increasingly disrupted.[74]

Much of this disruption is the result of the body's reaction to increasing stress. When a person is exposed to stress, whether physical, emotional, or sociological, changes take place in the body as it attempts to deal with the stress. Many of these changes involve a shift away from the normal endocrine balance. Aging can be a period of chronic and increasing stress. As the result of chronic stress the body's defense mechanisms may be unable to cope. This stems from imbalances of the hormonal mechanism.

Circulation

A blood flow rate of approximately 40 mL/min/100 g of brain tissue is regarded as minimal necessary requirement to maintain adequate cerebral perfusion. As compared to the flow rate of 50–60 mL/min/g experienced in youth, an elderly person may have as much as a 20% reduction in cerebral perfusion by the age of 70. Though cerebral perfusion is adequate if the body is not challenged, in the presence of pathology (arteriosclerosis, decreased cardiac output), the older person experiences an increased risk for cerebral damage.[7]

PERIPHERAL NEUROLOGICAL CHANGES

Aging is often characterized by reduced sensibility, coordination, and cognitive abilities, as well as a reduced ability to react to changing circumstances. A general assumption is made that the loss of nerve tissue (i.e., a reduced number of cells) is a predominant feature of aging.[75] In reality, although some loss of nerve cells does take place during the aging process, the extent to which this loss occurs is less than is usually assumed. The lower level of nervous system functioning in the elderly is better explained in terms of biochemical changes that take place in the neurons during aging and senescence.

Granules of lipofuscin accumulate in the cell bodies of neurons as a function of age, changing the cellular composition.[73] Traditionally, this has been regarded as resulting from wear and tear processes in those cells with high oxidative activity. Lipofuscin appears to be formed from lysosomal material within the cell. There is no evidence to support the notion that the presence of lipofuscin granules within the cytoplasm will have a detrimental influence on the normal functioning of the cell. Indeed, one of the heaviest accumulations of lipofuscin occurs in the inferior olivary nucleus, which appears to function normally and from which no neurons are lost in senescence.[73]

Other changes in cellular composition have been reported. Alterations in Golgi's complex, the reduction in ribosome concentration in the endoplasmic reticulum, and the lowered fluid content of the cells are not restricted to nerve cells but are generalized characteristics of degenerating and senescent cells of all types.[73]

In the resting state, the interior of the nerve cell and its processes are rich in potassium ions and low in sodium ions, whereas outside the cell the concentration of these ions is reversed. Because of this unequal distribution of ions, together with the fact that the membrane in its resting state is much more permeable to potassium than sodium ions, the nerve has a resting potential of approximately 70 mV, the outside being electrically positive with respect to the interior.[35,49] A nerve impulse is created by the temporary depolarization of the nerve membrane. Channels in the membrane open up to allow the flow of sodium ions into the cell, with a second set of channels allowing the outward flow of potassium ions from the cell after a slight delay. A wave of depolarization is conducted over the whole surface of the neuron from the point at which it was initially generated. In myelinated nerve fibers, the nerve impulse jumps quickly from one node of Ranvier to the next. The conduction velocity of nerve impulses along myelinated fibers is up to 25 times greater than along unmyelinated fibers of similar diameter. Peripheral nerve conduction velocity shows a progressive decline with aging.[49]

The ionic exchange across the nerve membrane to produce a nerve impulse is a relatively simple mechanism that is altered little during the aging process. In the elderly, there is no significant change in the conduction velocity along a specified portion of a nerve trunk compared to that found in younger adults. In the elderly, as in a younger person, if a reduction in conduction velocity is found, some narrowing of the fiber affecting the integrity of the nerve or some impairment of blood flow to the nerve sheath may be assumed.[70]

SENSORY CHANGES

In the body, information is gathered, interpreted, and transmitted through the integration of the neurosensory system. The "neurosensory system" includes the nervous system and each of the five senses (touch, smell, taste, vision, and hearing). Each of these systems is highly complex, and structural changes are known to occur within them with aging. The sum total of these changes results in a decline of neurosensory function.[79]

Touch

Peripheral receptors are responsible for the sense of touch. As with the other senses, touch also declines with age. Specific receptors for touch, pressure, pain, and temperature are found within the dermis and epidermis of the skin. Receptors can be freestanding or arranged in small corpuscular masses. Meissner's corpuscles (touch–texture receptors), Pacinian's corpuscles (pressure–vibration receptors), and Krause's corpuscles (temperature receptors), as well as peripheral nerve fibers, are noted to decline; therefore, sensitivity to touch, temperature, and vibration frequently declines with age. Though quantitative studies have produced inconclusive results, since freestanding nerve endings remain relatively unchanged, the ability to sense pain should remain intact; however, the elderly person must take special care to avoid injury from concentrated pressures or temperature on the skin[12,50] (e.g., pressures from shoes that are too tight, bathwater that is too hot, and so forth).

The skin is a very important element in touch. In general, skin wrinkles increase with advancing age, but the directional change of epidermal thickness remains controversial. The dermis thins, loses elasticity, and has a diminished vascularity.[79] Loss of tissue support for remaining capillaries results in fragility and easy bruising (senile purpura). Though tanning response diminishes, the appearance of flat pigmented lentigos (age spots) increases with exposure to the sun, and such exposure also increases the risk of neoplastic development from actinic keratosis. The previously reviewed decline in cellular division results in a slower rate and efficiency of tissue repair following any trauma.[58]

Changes in the dermal appendages (i.e., the hair) also occur with age. The degree to which hair becomes gray is largely genetically determined, but in general, a reduction in hair follicles produces a reduction of hair. In contrast, after menopause, facial hair tends to increase in women. Nails grow more slowly, and they develop longitudinal ridges. The number and size of sweat glands is diminished, which results in a reduction of sweat production.[58]

Health care providers need to be sensitive to the fact that some of these changes may effect the self-esteem of an older person. If this is the case, sensitive psychological support must be provided in any interactions.

Vision

Though humans are strongly visual creatures, the eye is vulnerable to many age related changes. Externally, the eyelids show an increased wrinkling and ptosis resulting from losses of elastic tissue and orbital fat, and a decrease in muscle tone.[79] Very often the older person will develop an entropion (a turning inward of the eyelid) or an ectropion (an outward relaxation of the eyelid), which is particularly apparent with the lower lids. Aging results in diminished tear production, and ocular inflammation or infection may occur in some elderly persons if supplementary artificial tears are not provided.[80]

Arcus senilis, a deposition of lipids around the outer edge of the cornea, is a well-known, age related phenomenon that does not interfere with vision.[81] Arcus senilis has been associated with hyperlipidemia in younger people, however, no such association has been shown in the elderly.

In addition to becoming smaller with age, the ocular pupil reacts more slowly to light, and the ability to focus quickly from far-to-near declines. This loss of accommodation is termed "presbyopia."[81] The ability to focus is dependent on the ability of the ocular lens to change shape as needed. Presbyopia is partially caused by a decline in ciliary muscle efficiency, however, as a person ages, the ocular lens continues to grow while becoming more dense and inelastic. With increased stiffness comes decreased flexibility, resulting in a decreased ability to change shapes and focus on desired objects. Far vision is more easily achieved because the ciliary muscles relax and allow the lens to thin.[81] Near vision requires the ciliary muscles to contract to increase the thickness of the lens. This is why older people may require bifocals, which offer a less strong prescription for far vision and a "thicker" one for near. Along with reduced accommodation, older people experience a decreased ability to adapt comfortably and quickly to changes of light and dark. Many older people say they had to give up driving at night because of this age related change.

The older eye demonstrates a tendency toward increased intraocular pressure.[80] As the lens continues to grow into the anterior chamber of the eye, the chamber becomes smaller, and the circulation of aqueous humor is reduced. Though the healthy older eye can tolerate this change, it is possible for a pathological glaucoma to concurrently occur. The increased density of the lens may lead to a form of cataract that can result in a complete loss of useful vision.[81] On a less serious note, the aqueous humor may also develop a yellowish pigmentation creating difficulty in perceiving greens and blues.

An older person may comment to you on the presence of "floaters" in their visual fields. With aging, the vitreous body of the eye loses hydration and tends to demonstrate some clustering of collagen material. This clustering causes shadows or opacities to be projected on the retinal wall. Though the presence of these opacities is normal, an increase in number can be indicative of retinal hemorrhage or detachment.[81]

A decline in visual acuity may ultimately be produced by many age related changes. Even when errors of aged refraction are corrected, a loss of visual receptors in the aging retina or macula will result in a decrease of acuity—with no treatment existing for a cure. Fortunately, with modern technology, the majority of older people are able to maintain a high degree of visual function and independence.[80,81]

Hearing

Though a hearing loss may develop at any age, hearing losses do occur more frequently in later years. A "sensorineural" hearing loss, often called presbycusis, is most common in the elderly. With a sensorineural loss, sound is well conducted through the external and middle ear but age related impairments of the inner ear or auditory nerve prevent the sound transmission to the brain. Age related changes that may contribute to a sensorineural hearing loss include sclerotic changes in the tympanic membrane, cochlear otosclerosis, a loss of hairlike receptors in the organ of Corti, and a degeneration of the auditory nerve.[79]

Presbycusis results in a decreased ability to hear and discriminate speech, particularly at higher and lower frequency levels.[79] Because normal speech contains a broad range of frequencies, the older person may realize that he or she is being spoken to but may not understand all that is being said. Difficulties increase when the speaker talks too quickly or when the hearing impaired individual is unable to observe the speaker's face.

Contrary to common belief, a sensorineural hearing loss does not always preclude the use of a hearing aid. Vision should be corrected so the skill of visual speech conception can be used as much as possible. When speaking with an elder with sensorineural loss, words should be spoken slowly in a medium pitched voice, and face-to-face communication should always be maintained.

Proprioception/Kinesthesia

Proprioception or kinesthetic sense is provided by sensory nerves that give information concerning movements and position of the body. These receptors are located primarily in the muscles, tendons, and the labyrinth system.[7] Though a greater degree of sensory-perceptual loss results from local system changes (i.e., impaired vision from increased lens density), cerebral cortex cell loss may result in less cellular availability for sensory interpretation.[82] This is of great clinical importance in that, as one ages, there may be a concomitant loss of position and movement sense. Coupled with losses in the other sensory systems (e.g., vision), this could significantly impact an elderly individual's awareness of limb or body position and affect safety during transfers and ambulation.

Vestibular System

The vestibular system changes during the aging process. Degeneration occurs in the sensory receptors in both the otoliths and semicircular canals. The function of the vestibular system is to monitor head position and to detect head movements.[82] When an individual is deprived of visual and lower extremity somatosensory information, the vestibular system is left to provide sensation for the control of balance. Healthy young adults are able to balance without meaningful visual or support surface information. Healthy elderly, on the other hand, lose their balance and might even fall when vestibular input is the only spatial orientation information available. All of the major sources of orienting information are compromised during the aging process. Diseases further compound this problem.

Taste and Smell

The senses of taste and smell become less acute with age. As much as 80% of the taste buds may atrophy and perception of taste sensation (i.e., sweet, salty, bitter, acid) becomes less sharp. A reduction of saliva flow occurs as a person ages, and this may aggravate an already dulled sense of taste. The olfactory bulb demonstrates age related cell losses that seem associated with decreased perceptions of various smells. It is proposed that these declines contribute to the appetite decline that is observed in and experienced by the majority of elderly people.[58]

GASTROINTESTINAL CHANGES

The gastrointestinal tract is subject to many changes throughout life. Although normal aging is not responsible for all gastrointestinal changes, it is sometimes difficult to differentiate aging's contributions from those that result from a lifetime of poor habits involving hygiene, food, and substance abuse. Epidemiological studies are beginning to more strongly implicate life-style in relation to some changes in the gut.

Declines in salivation, taste, and smell have already been reviewed, but it is a fallacy to believe that teeth must be lost with aging. Improved dental hygiene and nutrition can prevent common pathologies of tooth loss (dental caries and periodontal disease). With age, the tooth does lose masticating enameled surface area. Intermaxillary spaces decrease, and tooth pulp may atrophy and regress. If teeth are lost, the older person may experience a migration of the normally opposing teeth, with local oral trauma occurring as a result.[83]

The older esophagus demonstrates a reduction of motility and a hesitance of the lower esophageal sphincter to relax with swallowing. To define these changes the term "presbyesophagus" was coined.[84] When eating, the older person may experience an often uncomfortable substernal sense of fullness as food entry into the stomach is delayed. In contrast, the lower esophageal "resting" pressure declines with age. This weakening allows gastric contents to more easily reflux into the lower areas of the esophagus causing heartburn to occur. Hiatal hernias frequently develop in the older person who has a reduced resting pressure of the lower esophageal sphincter.[85]

An age related reduction in motility also affects the stomach, colon, and probably the small intestine. Gastric emptying time often is delayed.[86] Degeneration of gastric mucosa occurs in a small number of elderly and may cause a decrease of intrinsic factor, digestive enzymes, and hydrochloric acid. Usually this "atrophic gastritis" is not the sole cause of B_{12} malabsorption and the resulting pernicious anemia, but gastrointestinal digestion can be reduced. Medications activated by an acid gastric condition may be less effective in the more alkaline environment of an older stomach. A reduced blood supply to the gut and a decrease in the number of absorbing cells can hinder nutrient absorption in the small intestine. Decreased motility in the colon causes the elderly to have a tendency to develop constipation. If the elderly person is particularly immobile or dehydrated, constipation can easily lead into the more serious conditions of fecal impaction and bowel obstruction. Diverticulosis is also common in the elderly. However, its occurrence is probably related more to a diet low in fiber and high in refined, low residue foods than to aging.[7,85,87]

More on the gastrointestinal changes with aging will be covered in Chapter 7, Exploring Nutritional Needs of the Elderly.

RENAL, UROGENITAL, AND HEPATIC CHANGES

It is generally accepted that both liver mass and blood perfusion decline with aging. Metabolism of many drugs is decreased and, following injury, regeneration of hepatic cells occurs more slowly. When compared to those of younger people, no significant differences are found in the serum indicators of liver status of older people. These indicators include the measurement of bilirubin clearance, serum glutamic oxaloacetic transaminase (SGOT), serum glutamic pyruvic transaminase (SGPT), and alkaline phosphatase production. Though total serum protein remains relatively stable, reduced albumin to globulin (A/G) ratios result in a decline of colloidal osmotic pressure. Protein binding of medications may also be decreased. Alterations in protein binding and the prolongation of drug effects within the body are two of the more serious results of normal age changes in the liver.[7,12,88]

When discussing these systems, the gallbladder and pancreas should also be mentioned, because they also demonstrate functional changes with aging. For example, the incidence of biliary stones increases in the elderly, which is probably related to a reduced efficiency of cholesterol stabilization in the body. Controversy exists over the reduction of pancreatic mass with age. A decline in mass may be hidden by an increase in pancreatic fat deposition. Pancreatic cells become less homogeneous, and studies have generally reported a decline in enzyme volume and concentration, though adequate amounts are available for normal digestive functions.[12,58] Another important endocrine age change is the decreased ability of the peripheral tissues to use the available insulin produced by the pancreas.[89] The most important pancreatic age change, however, is the decreased ability of the beta cells to increase insulin production in response to a challenge of increased blood glucose.[12,88]

The aged kidney demonstrates both a loss of parenchymal mass and a reduction of total weight. By the time a person is 85 years old, the amount of remaining functioning nephrons may be decreased by as much as 30% to 40% of what was available in youth. Vascular changes, like a reduction in the number of glomerular capillary loops and an increased tortuosity of arcuate and interlobar arteries, have been reported. Renal perfusion declines by as much as 50% by the later decades of life. The Bowman's capsule basement membrane thickens, glomerular filtration rate declines, and blood urea nitrogen (BUN) tends to rise. The renal tubules show a decline in excretory and reabsorptive capacities, and a loss of urine concentrating abilities occurs. Older kidneys can maintain acid–base homeostasis is an unchallenged environment; however, they are unable to handle increased loads of either acid or base.

The urinary bladder demonstrates an increased number of uninhibited contractions frequently associated with cerebral arteriosclerotic changes. Increases in residual urine and reflux into the ureters provide an ideal environment for bacterial growth. Both asymptomatic and symptomatic bacteria are common in the elderly.[7,90,91]

ENDOCRINE CHANGES

Proper functioning of the endocrine system is essential to maintain the majority of the body's regulatory processes. In some cases (reproductive hormones), age related changes are well known. In other cases, specific information is nonexistent or unclear. Much available information remains highly controversial.

Although age related structural changes in the thyroid do occur, in the absence of pathology its function tends to remain adequate for body needs. A decrease in the basal metabolic rate (BMR) is shown in elderly people, but it seems to be related to the reduction of lean body mass. The elderly are at risk for both hypo- and hyperthyroid problems. However, these problems are unrelated to changes that occur with normal aging.[7,58,92]

Tests of adrenal function show plasma glucocorticoid levels to be similar in both the young and the old. The adrenal cortex response to ACTH remains intact, as does the pituitary's release of ACTH in response to stress; however, circulating levels of aldosterone do decrease with aging.[7]

The pituitary gland demonstrates a reduction in vascularity and an increase in deposition of connective tissue.[7] A reduction in mass is not well established. With aging, nocturnal elevations in growth hormone (GH) disappear. Serum concentrations of ACTH and GH are unchanged with aging,[12] and in most elderly, thyroid-stimulating hormone (TSH) remains normal, although a small percentage develop a slight increase in TSH without obvious symptoms.[93] Postmenopausal women show an increase in the follicle stimulating hormone (FSH) and luteinizing hormone (LH).

Changes in reproductive hormones are most dramatic in the older woman. Following menopause, estrogen and progesterone levels significantly decrease, but serum androgen levels remain relatively unchanged. In the older man, blood levels of testosterone probably decrease, but the controversy over this decline has not yet been resolved.[58]

The uterus, ovaries, and fallopian tubes of the elderly woman become dysfunctional with menopause and decrease in size. A reduction in estrogen causes the vagina to shrink, thin, and lose mucosal protection. The breasts, labia, and clitoris all lose subcutaneous mass, and in advanced years, pubic hair is lost. In contrast, an elderly man will continue to produce sperm throughout his life. However, sperm production and counts are reduced, and spermal abnormalities are increased. The testes may demonstrate very little loss of weight but fibrous tissue deposition increases in the intertubular spaces. With age, the seminiferous tubules' basement membrane thickens. Age changes in the prostate begin around age 40 and continue into the elder years. The most disruptive change involves the replacement of smooth prostatic tissue by dense connective tissue. As the connective tissue accumulates, the resulting prostatic hypertrophy impinges upon the urethra and interferes with smooth release of urine.[7]

SLEEP, MEMORY, AND INTELLIGENCE CHANGES

The phenomenon of sleep is not yet totally understood. Four progressively deeper levels of sleep plus an intermediate level associated with rapid eye movements (REM) are known to exist. Once asleep, a younger person seldom awakens, and the deeper sleep levels of three and four are maintained. In the elderly, consecutive sleep time is decreased, awakenings are more frequent, and less sleep time is spent in levels three and four, though total sleep time is normally only slightly reduced. Because of their possible side effects (such as drowsiness and confusion), the use of sedatives should be discouraged in the aged. In most cases, actual sleep loss is minimal. Other therapeutic supports, such as increased daytime activity and decreased "naps," can be effective in relieving the elderly person's feelings of impaired nocturnal sleep.[12,94]

The process of memory is difficult to separate from the total process of learning. After information is perceived, it is stored in either short- or long-term areas of memory. The elderly typically have more difficulty recalling recently experienced, short-term recall information. In order to be properly perceived, information needs to be presented to an older person at a slower rate and with an increased number of repetitions. If the information is presented in a manner that compensates for age related sensory changes (decreased vision and hearing) and if the information is made to have some personal relevance to the older person, recall of the information is greatly improved.

"Intelligence" may be affected by pathology, but, even in advanced years, it remains unaffected by the physiological changes of normal aging.[7]

The topics of memory and intelligence will be addressed more thoroughly in Chapter 17, Educational Services: Learning, Memory, and Intelligence.

CONCLUSION

Aging as a universal occurrence is regarded as a biological, anatomical, and physiological or "normal" process distinct from pathological processes. As much as aging might be influenced by a predisposition to disease, it is not considered "abnormal." Conceptually, this distinction seems clear enough, but when it is applied to specific cases, the boundaries become blurred. Some degree of decline is noted in all biological, anatomical, physiological, and functional components of the human body with age, but this is not considered pathological. Aging has been excluded from the domain of disease because it is considered normal. Aging is viewed as the result of the accumulation of unrepaired injuries resulting from mostly unavoidable, universal changes. If one defines disease as a "reaction to injury," then is there a distinct aging process? If a steady accumulation of microinjuries causes a linear decline of function, does the presence of redundancy in any system translate into a linear loss of functional capacity, and, is aging an accelerated age-specific failure of each system? The distinction between aging and disease becomes one of arbitrary degree. A variety of degenerative processes are repeatedly termed normal aging until they proceed far enough to cause clinically significant disability. They then become a "disease." In such cases, the distinction between aging and disease is more semantic than biologically, anatomically, physiologically, or functionally normal. The question remains: Is there a normal aging process?

PEARLS

- Individuals age at different rates, and the process of homeostasis helps to keep the internal environmental constant.

- Cardiovascular cellular changes with age are numerous and range from lipofuscin accumulation at the poles of the nuclei of cardiac muscle to increased calcification in the media.

- In the pulmonary system, age changes can be organized according to mechanical properties, changes in flow, gas exchange, and impairment of lung defense.

- Normal weight-bearing exercises are recommended to maintain cartilaginous health.

- The decrease in aging muscle is associated with a decrease in protein and nitrogen and an increase in connective tissue and fat.

- Due to the change in the thermal regulatory response, the aged have a prolonged cooling time following increased activity, as well as a decrease of receptiveness to heat and cold.

- All five senses as well as proprioception/kinesthesia decline with age.

REFERENCES

1. Eveleth PB, Tanner JM. *Worldwide Variation in Human Growth.* Cambridge, England: Cambridge University Press; 1976.
2. Cutler RG. Evolution of longevity in primates. *J Hum Evol.* 1976; 5:169–202.
3. Fries JF. Aging, natural death and the compression of morbidity. *N Engl J Med.* 1968; 303:113–123.
4. Kent S. The evolution of longevity. *Geriatrics.* 1980; 35:98–104.
5. Korenchevksy V. *Physiological and Pathological Aging.* New York: Hafner; 1961.

6. Andres R. Normal aging versus disease in the elderly. In: Andres EL, Bierman EL, Hazard WR, eds. *Principles in Geriatric Medicine*. New York: McGraw-Hill; 1985:38–41.

7. Kenney RA. *Physiology of Aging*. Symposium of the Aging Process Clinics in Geriatric Medicine. Feb 1985; 1(1).

8. Shock NW. Physiological theories of aging. In: Rothstein JL et al., eds. *Theoretical Aspects of Aging*. New York: Academic Press; 1974:119–136.

9. Seyle HA. Stress and aging. *J of Am Geriatrics Society*. 1970; 18(9):669–690.

10. Rowlatt C, Franks LM. Aging in tissues and cells. In: Brocklehurst JC. *Textbook of Geriatric Medicine and Gerontology*. New York: Longman Group Ltd.; 1978.

11. Hayflick L. The cellular basis for biological aging. In: Finch C, Hayflick L (eds). *The Handbook of the Biology of Aging*. New York: Van Nostrand Reinhold; 1977.

12. Goldman R. Decline in organ function with age. In: Rossman I, ed. *Clinical Geriatrics*. 2nd ed. Philadelphia: Lippincott; 1979.

13. Pomerance A. Pathology of the myocardium and valves. In: Caird FI, Dalle JLC, Kennedy RD, eds. *Cardiology in Old Age*. New York: Plenum Press; 1976:11–53.

14. Wei JY. Heart disease in the elderly. *Cardiovasc Med*. 1984; 9:971–982.

15. Baker PB, Arn AR, Unverferth DV. Hypertrophic and degenerative changes in human hearts with aging. *J Coll Cardiol*. 1985; 5:536A.

16. Yin FCP. The aging vasculature and its effects on the heart. In: Weisfeldt ML, ed. *The Aging Heart*. New York: Raven Press; 1980:2.

17. Cotton R, Wartman WB. Endothelial patterns in human arteries, their relation to age, vessel site and atherosclerosis. *Arch Pathol*. 1961;2:15–24.

18. Movat HZ, More RH, Haust MD. The diffuse intimal thickening of the human aorta with aging. *Am J Pathol*. 1958; 34:1023–1030.

19. Milch RA. Matrix properties of the aging arterial wall. *Monogr Surg Sci*. 1965; 2:261–341.

20. Auerbach O, Hammond EC, Garfinkel L. Thickening of wall of arterioles and small arteries in relation to age and smoking habits. *N Engl J Med*. 1968; 278:980–984.

21. Wolinsky H, Glagov S. Structural basis for the static mechanical properties of the aorta media. *Circ Res*. 1964; 14:301–309.

22. Schlatman TJM, Becker AE. Histologic changes in the normal aging aorta: implications for dissecting aortic aneurysm. *Am J Cardiol*. 1977; 39:13–20.

23. Hutchins GM. Structure of the aging heart. In: Weisfeldt ML, ed. *The Aging Heart*. New York; Raven Press; 1980: 269–295.

24. Wei JY. Cardiovascular anatomic and physiologic changes with age. *Topics in Ger Rehab*. 1986; 2(1):10–16.

25. Rodeheffer RJ, Gerstenblith G, Becker LC, et al. Exercise cardiac output is maintained with advancing age in health human subjects: cardiac dilatation and increased stroke volume compensates for diminished heart rate. *Circulation*. 1984; 69:203–213.

26. Shannon RP, Wei JY, Rosa RM, et al. The effect of age and sodium depletion on cardiovascular response to orthostasis. *Hypertension*. 1986; 4:229–242.

27. Gerstenblith G, Frederikson J, Yin FCP, et al. Echocardiographic assessment of a normal adult aging population. *Circulation*. 1977; 56:273–278.

28. Nichols WW, O'Rourke MF, Avolio AP, et al. Effects of age on ventricular-vascular coupling. *Am J Cardiol*. 1985; 55:1179–1184.

29. Miyatake K, Okamoto M, Kinoshita N, et al. Augmentation of atrial contribution to left ventricular inflow with aging as assessed by intracardiac Doppler flowmetry. *Am J Cardiol*. 1984; 53:586–589.

30. Ziegler MG, Lake CR, Kopin IJ. Plasma noradrenalin increase with age. *Nature*. 1976; 261:333–334.

31. Shimada K, Kitazumi T, Sadakne N, et al. Age related changes of baroreflex function, plasma norepinephrine, and blood pressure. *Hypertension*. 1985; 7:113–117.

32. Tsunoda K, Abe K, Goto T, et al. Effect of age on the renin-angiotensin-aldosterone system in normal subjects: simultaneous measurement of active and inactive renin, renin substrate, and aldosterone in plasma. *J Clin Endocrinol Metab*. 1986; 62:384–389.

33. Shannon RP, Minaker KL, Rowe JW. Aging and water balance in humans. *Semin Nephrol*. 1984; 4:346–353.

34. Weisfeldt ML, Gerstenblith G, Lakatta EG. Alterations in circulatory function. In: Andres R., eds. *Principles of Geriatric Medicine*. New York: McGraw-Hill Co.; 1985.

35. Ham RS, Marcy ML. *Normal Aging: A Review of Systems/The Maintenance of Health in Primary Care Geriatrics*. Boston: John Wright, PSG, Inc.; 1983.

36. Butler RN. Current definitions of aging. In: *Epidemiology of Aging.* Bethesda, Md: National Institutes of Health Publication No. 80–969; 1980:7–8.
37. Zadai CC. Cardiopulmonary issues in the geriatric population: implications for rehabilitation. *Topics in Ger Rehab.* 1986: 2(1):1–9.
38. Cummings G, Semple SG. *Disorders of the Respiratory System.* Oxford, England: Blackwell; 1973.
39. Wynne JW. Pulmonary disease in the elderly. In: Rossman I, ed, *Clinical Geriatrics.* 2nd ed. Philadelphia: Lippincott, 1979.
40. Pickles LW. Effects of aging on connective tissues. *Geriatrics.* 1983; 38(1):71–78.
41. Goldberg AL, Goodman HM. Effects of disuse and denervation on amino acid transport by skeletal muscle. *Am J Physiol.* 1975; 216:1116–1119.
42. Hamlin CR, Luschin JH, Kohn RR. Aging of collagen: comparative rates in four mammalian species. *Exp Gerontol.* 1980; 15:393–398.
43. Chapman EA, DeVries HA, Swezey R. Joint stiffness: effects of exercise on young and old men. *J Gerontol.* 1972; 27:218–221.
44. Viidik A. Function properties of collagenous tissue. *Int Rev Conn Tissue Res.* 1982; 6:127–215.
45. Klein FA, Rajan RK. Normal aging: effects on connective tissue metabolism and structure. *J Gerontol.* 1985; 40(5):579–585.
46. Lehman J, Warren C, Scham S. Therapeutic heat and cold. *Clin Orthop.* 1974; 99:207–209.
47. Meyer K. Mucopolysacchrides of costal cartilage. *Science.* 1958; 128:896.
48. Ryan AJ. The role of tissue viscosity in injury prevention. In: Ryan AJ, Allman FL., eds. *Sports Medicine.* New York: Academic Press; 1974.
49. Astrand PO, Rodahl K. *Textbook of Work Physiology.* San Francisco, London: McGraw-Hill; 1970.
50. Hole JW. *Human Anatomy and Physiology.* Wm. C. Brown Co.; 1988.
51. Walker J. Connective tissue plasticity: issues in histological and light microscopy studies of exercise and aging in articular cartilage. *JOSPT.* 1991; 14(5):189–197.
52. Donatelli R, Owens-Burkart H. Effects of immobilization on the extensibility of periarticular connective tissue. *JOSPT.* 1981; 3(2):67–71.
53. Gardner DL. Aging of articular cartilage. In: Brocklehurst JC., eds. *Textbook of Geriatric Medicine and Gerontology.* New York: Longman Group Ltd.; 1978.
54. Akeson WH, Amiel D, Abel MF, et al. Effects of immobilization on joints. *Clin Ortho & Rel Res.* 1987; 219:28–36.
55. Steen, B. Body composition and aging. *Nutr Rev.* 1988; 46:45–51.
56. Borkan GA, Norris AH. Assessment of biological age using a profile of physical parameters. *J Gerontol.* 1980; 35:177–184.
57. Borkan GA, Hults DE, Gerzof SG, et al. Age changes in body composition revealed by computed tomography. *J Gerontol.* 1983; 38:673–677.
58. Jacobs R. Physical changes in the aged. In: O'Hara-Devereaux M, Andrus LH, Scott CD., eds. *Eldercare.* New York: Grune & Stratton; 1981.
59. Brown M, Rose SJ. The effects of aging and exercise on skeletal muscle—clinical considerations. *Top Ger Rehabil.* 1985; 1:20–30.
60. Brown M. Resistance exercise effects on aging skeletal muscle in rats. *Phys Ther.* 1989; 69(1):46–53.
61. Albert NR, Gale HH, Taylor N. The effect of age on contractile protein ATPase activity and the velocity for shortening. In: Tanz RD, Kavaler F, Roberts J., eds. *Factors Influencing Myocardial Contractility.* New York: Academic Press; 1967.
62. Cress ME, Schultz E. Aging muscle: functional, morphologic, biochemical and regenerative capacity. In: Smith EL, ed. *Top Geriatr Rehabil.* 1985; 1(1):11–19.
63. Buller AJ, Eccles JC, Eccles RM. Interaction between motoneurons and muscles in respect of the characteristic speeds of their responses. *J Physiol.* 1960; 150:417–439.
64. Larsson L. Physical training effects on muscle morphology in sedentary males at different ages. *Med Sci Sports Exerc.* 1982; 14:203–206.
64a. Aniansson A, Grimby G, Hedberg M, Krotkiewske M. Muscle morphology, enzyme activity and muscle strength in elderly men and women. *Clin Physiol.* 1981; 1:73–86.
65. Aniansson A, Hedberg M, Henning GB, et al. Muscle morphology, enzyme activity, and muscle strength in elderly men: a follow-up study. *Muscle Nerve.* 1986; 9:585–591.
66. Aniansson A, Sperling L, Rundgren A, et al. Muscle function in 75-year-old men and women: a longitudinal study. *Scand J Rehabil Med.* 1983; 9(suppl):92–102.

67. Gutmann E, Hanzlikova V. Basic mechanisms of aging in the neuromuscular system. *Mech Ageing Dev.* 1972; 1:327–349.
68. Larsson L, Grimby G, Karlsson J. Muscle strength and speed of movement in relation to age and muscle morphology. *J Appl Physiol.* 1979; 46:451–456.
69. Gollnick PD, Armstrong RB, Saltin B, et al. Effect of training on enzyme activity and fiber composition of human skeletal muscle. *J Appl Physiol.* 1973; 34:107–111.
70. Grimby G. Physical activity and muscle training in the elderly. *Acta Med Scand* 1986; 711(suppl):233–237.
71. Bidlack WR, Kirsch A, Meskin MS. Nutritional requirements of the elderly. *Food Technology.* 1988; 40:61–70.
72. Batata M, Spray GH, Bolton FG, Higgins G, Wollner L. Blood and bone marrow changes in elderly patients, with particular reference to folic acid, vitamin B12, iron and ascorbic acid. *Brit Med J.* 1967; 2:667–669.
73. Jokl E. *Physiology of Exercise.* Springfield, Ill: Charles C Thomas Publishers; 1984; 108–112.
74. Burchinsky SG. Neurotransmitter receptors in the central nervous system and aging: pharmacological aspects (review). *Experimental Aging.* 1984; 19:227–239.
75. Bohannon RW, Larkin PA, Cook AC, et al. Decrease in timed balance test scores with aging. *Phys Ther.* 1984; 64:1067–1070.
76. Besdine RW, Harris TB. Alterations in body temperature (hypothermia and hyperthermia). In: Andres R, Bierman EL, and Hazzard WR, eds. *Principles in Geriatric Medicine.* New York: McGraw-Hill; 1985: 209–17.
77. Asmussen E. Aging and exercise. In: Horvath SM, Yousef MK, eds. *Environmental Physiology, Aging, Heat and Altitude.* New York: Elsevier/North Holland; 1981.
78. Ajiduah AO, Paolone AM, Wailgum TD, Irion G, Kendrick ZV. The effect of age on tolerance of thermal stress during exercise. *Med Sci Spts Exerc.* 1983; 15:168. Abstract.
79. Corso JF. Sensory processes and age effects of normal adults. *J Gerontol.* 1971; 26:90–105.
80. Kasper RL. Eye problems of the aged. In: Reichel PE, ed. *Clinical Aspects of Aging.* Baltimore: Williams and Wilkins Co.; 1988.
81. Boyer GG. Vision problems. In: Carnevali P and Patrick B, eds. *Nursing Management for the Elderly.* Philadelphia: Lippincott; 1989.
82. Woollacott MH, Shumway-Cook A, Nasner LM. Aging and posture control: changes in sensory organization and muscular coordination. *Int J Aging Hum Dev.* 1986; 23:97–114.
83. Bennet J, Creamer H, Fontana-Smith DJ. Dentistry. In: O'Hara-Devereaux M, Andrus LH, and Scott CD, eds. *Eldercare.* New York: Grune & Stratton; 1981.
84. Khan TA, Shragge BW, Crispen JS, et al. Esophageal mobility in the elderly. *Am J Digestive Dis.* 1977; 22:1049–1054.
85. Bartol MA, Heitkemper M. Gastrointestinal problems. In: Carnevali P and Patrick B, eds. *Nursing Management for the Elderly.* Philadelphia: Lippincott; 1989.
86. Horowitz M, Maddern GT, Chateron BE, et al. Changes in gastric emptying rates with age. *Clin Sci.* 1984; 67:213–218.
87. Morgan W, Thomas C, Schuster M. Gastrointestinal system. In: O'Hara-Devereaux M, Andrus LH, Scott CD, eds. *Eldercare.* New York: Grune & Stratton; 1981.
88. Hyans DE. The liver and biliary system. In: Brocklehurst JC, ed. *Textbook of Geriatric Medicine and Gerontology.* New York: Longman Group Ltd.; 1978.
89. Fink RL. Mechanisms of insulin resistance in aging. *J Clin Invest.* 1983; 71:1523–1535.
90. Brocklehurst JC. The bladder. In: Brocklehurst JC, ed. *Textbook of Geriatric Medicine and Gerontology.* New York; Longman Group Ltd.; 1978.
91. Sourander LB. The aging kidney. In: Brocklehurst JC, ed. *Textbook of Geriatric Medicine and Gerontology.* New York: Longman Group Ltd.; 1978.
92. Sundwall DN, Ralond J, Thorn GW. Endocrine and metabolic. In: O'Hara-Devereaux M, Andrus LH, Scott CD, eds. *Eldercare.* New York: Grune & Stratton; 1981.
93. Savin CT, Deepak C. The aging thyroid: increased prevalence of elevated serum thyrotrophin levels in the elderly. *JAMA.* 1989; 242(3):247–250.
94. Guilleminault C. Sleep and sleep disorders. In: Cassel S, Walsh B, eds. *Geriatric Medicine.* New York: Springer-Verlag; 1984:II.

Describing Psychosocial Aspects of Aging

Theories of Aging

Full Life Development Theories

Late Life Theories

Cognitive Changes in Late Life

Memory

Intelligence and Learning

Situations Requiring Coping Mechanisms

Depression

Social Isolation

Institutionalization

Anxiety Disorders

Chronic Illness

Death, Dying, Grief, and Multiple Loss

Dementia

Belief Systems Regarding the Aging Process as Fostered by Society

Life-style Adaptation, Stress

Stress Evaluation

Conclusion

The aging process of all aspects of human life is not one dimensional. Besides the obvious physical component, there exists the psychological, emotional, and spiritual components of aging. This chapter will address the psychosocial components. Even though physical health is extremely important, studies and life experience illustrate the effects of cognitive perception on life satisfaction and physical health.[1,2] One study on hip fracture outcomes for older persons showed that the most important variable in successful rehabilitation was the presence or absence of depression[1] This study alone has tremendous implications for physical therapists, because it illustrates that unless the older person's emotional and mental abilities are addressed the physical efforts may have minimal effect.

How does a physical therapist work in the psychosocial realm? Physical therapists are not psychologists and do not receive extensive training in the social and psychological sciences. Nevertheless they can use specific information as an adjunct to daily treatment. For example, examining one's attitudes based on the various psychosocial theories of aging may provide information about a patient's satisfaction or motivation and enhance a therapist's ability to communicate with an older person. In addition, since the goal of physical therapy is to achieve optimal functioning, it is imperative that the therapist be able to recognize situations that require coping mechanisms and provide some assistance in these situations.

This chapter will explore the theories of aging and the cognitive changes in late life. Situations, both normal and pathological, that require coping mechanisms as one ages will be described in detail as well as society's view of aging and the life-style adaptions of older persons.

THEORIES OF AGING

In the last 30 years many psychological theories of aging have been proposed. Prior to this time, however, very few theories existed. The mainstream of thought centered around the theories of Freud and Piaget, then, and these theories place all the emphasis on the psychological development on the child while essentially ignoring the adult. The theories to be discussed in this section are either full life development theories or late life psychological development theories.

Full Life Development Theories

Erikson

Eric Erikson was one of the first psychological theorists to develop a personality theory that extended into old age. Erikson viewed the process of human development as a series of stages that one goes through in order to fully develop one's ego.[3] Erikson describes eight stages in this process. These stages are listed in Table 4–1. Each of these stages represents a choice in the development of the expanding ego. The last two stages are of particular interest to the practitioner working with the older person.

A successful life choice of generativity consists of guiding, parenting, and monitoring the next generation. If an adult person does not experience generativity then stagnation will predominate. Stagnation is evidenced by anger, hurt, and self-absorption. The final stage of Erikson's theory suggests that the older person must accept his or her life with the sense that if "I had to do it all over again, I'd do it pretty much the same."[4] At this stage the person experiences an active concern with life, even in the face of death, and learns to experience his or her own wisdom.

Maslow

Maslow's hierarchy of human needs is not a theory singular to aging, but it is excellent framework for exploring growth, development, and motivation.[5] Maslow's hierarchy of needs is a pyramid of needs, each of which builds upon the other. The lowest level, "biological and physiological integrity," is where the person is trying to feed themselves and keep him- or herself warm and clothed. At the second level,

TABLE 4–1. ERIKSON'S STAGES OF PERSONALITY AND EGO DEVELOPMENT

Period in Life	Erikson's Stage
0–12 months	Trust vs mistrust
2–4 years	Autonomy vs shame
4–5 years	Initiative vs guilt
6–11 years	Industry vs inferiority
12–18 years	Identity vs identity confusion
Young adulthood	Intimacy vs isolation
Adulthood	Generativity vs stagnation
Late life	Integrity vs despair

Reprinted with permission from Erikson EH. Identity, youth and crisis. New York, Norton; 1968.

"safety and security," the person protects him- or herself against the elements and against other people. This cannot be achieved unless the person is first fed and clothed. In the third level, "belonging or love needs," the person begins to seek love from other persons, such as a parent or a significant other. When the person feels the love needs, they can then progress to the next level, "self-esteem," where the person cherishes him- or herself, respects his or her own values and ideas, and feels good about who he or she is. Finally, the level of "self-actualization" is where the person is no longer worried about the lower needs but is now able to give to others and has reached a higher level where they are able to transcend the lower self-esteem needs. They can nurture and feed others, develop their own ideas, and actually live their own values and ideas in the community. According to Maslow very few people in society are self-actualized. Some of our great leaders such as Martin Luther King, Winston Churchill, and Golda Meir were self-actualized people.

One must successfully fill the lower need before ascending to the higher need. When one is in that level one's energies are consumed at that level.[6] One rarely stays at a higher level, but rather the person reverts to lower levels when the lower needs are not met. For example, a recently widowed woman may feel isolated or lonely and be unable to experience the higher levels of self-esteem or self-actualization until her grief has subsided.

This theory is particularly useful in the area of motivation. Since older persons are more likely to have physical decline, their needs will descend to the lower levels of the hierarchy. Therefore, motivation strategies should be aimed at the level of the person's needs. For example, if the person is unstable when walking, then strategies to encourage exercises in this area should appeal to their sense of safety if the person is at that level. If, however, the same person is more concerned about hunger during a treatment session, they will be unable to focus on the exercises.

Maslow believes, however, that it is truly the older person who has the knowledge and experience of life to be able to experience self-actualization, the highest level of the paradigm.[6]

Late Life Theories
Peck

Peck's theory describes tasks that must be accomplished to achieve integrity in old age. In this theory the burden is placed on the older person to redefine the self, dismiss occupational identity, and go beyond self-centeredness. His tasks follow.

1. *Ego differentiation versus work role preoccupation.* In this instance, a retired person must look for new meaning and values beyond their previous work roles.
2. *Body transcendence versus body preoccupation.* Since old age may carry with it ill health, the older person must learn new ways to gain mental, physical, social, and spiritual pleasure that transcend physical discomfort.
3. *Ego transcendence versus ego preoccupation.* This last stage is a way of minimizing the prospect of death by giving to children and making charitable contributions to leave an enduring legacy.[7]

Neugarten

Bernice Neugarten also describes the tasks that must be accomplished in order to be a successfully aging older person. The following are a few of her tasks that directly impact the rehabilitation milieu.

1. Accepting the increasing reality and imminence of death.
2. Coping with physical illness.
3. Coordinating the necessary dependence on support and accurately as-

sessing the independent choices that can still be made to achieve maximum life satisfaction.

4. Giving and obtaining emotional gratification.[8]

Disengagement

The controversial disengagement theory credited to Cummings and Henry in the 1950s postulated that older people and society mutually withdraw. This withdrawal is characterized by a positive change in psychological well-being for the older person.[9] This theory, though not widely accepted at present, has spawned much debate on the subject of late life adaption.

Continuity and Activity

Two well-known theories that developed in response to the disengagement theory are the continuity and activity theories. The continuity theory proposes that activities in old age reflect a continuation of earlier life patterns,[10] while, in contrast, the activity theory states that successful adaption in late life is associated with maintaining as high a level of activity as possible. The older person should find substitutes when a meaningful activity, such as work, must be terminated. The person should develop an active rather than passive role toward their daily life as well as toward biological and social changes that are taking place.[11]

Havighurst

Havighurst's theory on aging relates successful aging to social competence and flexibility in adaption to new roles. He believes in the importance of finding new and meaningful roles in old age, while maintaining comfort with the customs of the time.[12,13] Later, Neugarten and Havighurst noted that successful adaptation to age was related to personality and not age per se. They noted the following four personality types.

1. *Integrated.* Shows a high degree of competence in daily activities and a complex inner life. This type is generally the best adapter.
2. *Passive dependent.* Seeks others to satisfy his or her emotional needs.
3. *Armored.* Attempts to control his or her environment and impulses and tends to be a high achiever.
4. *Unintegrated.* Shows poor emotional control and intellectual competency. This type tends to have the poorest adaptation in late life.[10]

COGNITIVE CHANGES IN LATE LIFE

Several important components of cognition are thought to be affected by age. These are memory, learning, affect, and reasoning. Each of these components of cognition will be discussed in terms of normal aging and pathological mechanisms.

Memory

Memory has been extensively studied for many years, and yet no definitive conclusions have been obtained.[14,15] Some studies show a decrease in memory with age, while others show no change.[14,15] Studies agree that older persons do have poorer techniques for organizing new information into a usable form that will impact information retrieval.[16] In addition, older persons perform better on more familiar memory tasks.[17]

Some problems are inherent in aging research of memory. The population may have an undiagnosed pathology affecting memory. In addition, older persons do not perform as well in unfamiliar laboratories or in paper-and-pencil situations as younger subjects would.[17] Therefore, in the area of normal aging, there is no definitive conclusions as to decline or improvement in memory. A recently defined clinical state, called age-associated memory impairment (AAMI), describes the loss of memory function in healthy persons aged 50 and over, and it is very modest. Nevertheless, AAMI is common enough to be thought to be a feature of aging. Finally, the neurochemical basis of memory loss is currently being explored.[18]

Pathologically, there are several implications of memory loss. First, complaints of memory loss—not actual memory loss—are related to depressive symptomatology.[19,20] Therefore, patient complaints about memory loss should alert the practitioner to check for depression. Actual memory loss is a classic characteristic of dementia or brain syndrome. (See the section on dementia later in this chapter for specifics on brain syndrome and memory loss.)

Treatment techniques for memory loss include the use of classes and educational strategies to assist memory. Classes in self-esteem, accurate record keeping, and the use of mnemonic devices can be helpful. Two additional hints in helping memory are to keep techniques as familiar as possible and to develop some type of reward system. (Refer to Chapter 17, Educational Services: Learning, Memory, and Intelligence.)

Intelligence and Learning

The actual measurement of intelligence is not possible; what is measured is the performance of the person's intelligence. The performance can easily be influenced by health, motivation, and sensory acuity. Even though the word "intelligence" is used, it is not singular. Intelligence can be broken into the "intelligences" of fluid and crystallized.[21]

Crystallized intelligence depends on sociocultural influence and involves the ability to perceive relations, engage in formal reasoning, and understand intellectual and cultural heritage.[22] The growth of crystallized intelligence, even after age 60, can be obtained through self-directed learning and education.[23]

Fluid intelligence depends primarily on the genetic endowment of the individual and the individual's ability to use short-term memory, create concepts, perceive complex relationships, and undertake abstract reasoning. This involves items that are mostly neuropsychologic in nature, and they may decline after age 60.[24]

The implications from this information for the therapist hoping to capitalize on intellectual performance and learning follow.

1. Expect the intellectual ranges in older persons to be varied.
2. Poor performance may not mean poor learning.
3. Emphasize new knowledge that will be consistent with previous learning.[25]
4. Concentrate on one task at a time and be sure that the item is successfully learned before proceeding to the next.[24]
5. Reduce potential for distraction.
6. Space learning experiences sufficiently.
7. Allow for as much self-pacing as possible.
8. Assist older persons in organizing the information to be learned.
9. Present the information in the mode in which it will be used.[26]
10. Make the learning experience as concrete as possible.
11. Use supportive versus neutral instruction.
12. Use as many of the senses as possible to facilitate learning.
13. Provide as much feedback as possible.[27]

These suggestions have come from various studies[21–27] on changes in intelligence and performance and have been suggested as ways of improving performance.

Affect and reasoning appear to remain unchanged as one ages.[23,24] Again, dementia and drug complications are the major cause of decline in these areas.[23,24]

(see section on dementia later in this chapter for specific changes associated with dementia. Also see Chapter 8, Pharmacology, for changes associated with drug interventions.)

SITUATIONS REQUIRING COPING MECHANISMS

Depression

The statistics on the prevalence of depression are varied. Nevertheless, the following quote aptly describes what many medical professionals may see in the health care setting, "Depression has been termed the common cold of the elderly."[28] Many older people cope with the depressive symptoms, and the statistics are quite significant. Depending on the source, cited depressive illness can be found in 5% to 65% of the older population.[29,30] Nevertheless, studies show that it is not aging per se that causes depression but the added variables of cognitive impairment, incontinence, chronic conditions, and disabilities.[31]

The Diagnostic and Statistical Manual of Mental Disorders (DSM-III) describes five categories of depression, all of which have relevance to geriatric patients. They are (1) major depression, (2) organic mood syndrome, (3) adjustment disorder with depression, (4) dysthymic disorder, and (5) dementia with depression.

A listing of these disorders' symptoms is found in Table 4–2.

Major depression is characterized by having at least five of the symptoms listed in Table 4–2 for a period of at least 2 weeks. This type of disorder usually appears very suddenly, and the symptoms are very severe and are likely to end in a suicide attempt.[31] This disorder may occur in one single episode, or it may be recurrent with partial or full remissions between episodes. Mania, or euphoria, can occur between the episodes, but this is more characteristic of bipolar disease, which is much more severe.

Organic mood syndrome is related to a specific organic cause. For example, a patient with a cerebrovascular accident (particularly patients with left hemisphere lesions) may suffer from this type of depression. Endocrinopathies, hypo- or hyperthyroidism, and excessive psychotropic medication are also typical organic factors associated with an organic mood syndrome.[32]

An adjustment disorder with depression is usually the result of a depressive reaction to a psychosocial stressor, such as a physical disability. It is only considered a depressive disorder when the symptoms last longer than 6 months. The major symptom is a depressed mood that impairs physical and social functioning in excess of what one would expect from the physical stressor.

Dysthymic disorders represent the most difficult treatment challenge of all the diagnostic categories. Patients with this type of disorder display at least two of the depressive symptoms listed in Table 4–2 over a period of 2 years. In addition, these

TABLE 4–2. DEPRESSIVE SYMPTOMS

Cognitive	Somatic	Affective
Poor concentration	Fatigue	Sadness
Low self-esteem	Altered sleep	Anxiety
Indecisiveness	Weight change	Irritability
Guilt	Tearful	Fear
Hopelessness	Agitation	Anger
Inability to concentrate	Palpitations	Depersonalization
Suicidal ideations	Weakness	Feels distant

patients have not maintained a normal mood for longer than 2 months. This disorder may be a consequence of a preexisting disorder, such as rheumatoid arthritis.

Dementia with depression is seen in the early stages of the dementing process as the person realizes that he or she is losing cognitive function. This early manifestation of depression may successfully hide the beginning stages of the dementia.

From the description of the different types of depressions, it becomes obvious how important the clinical interview can be. This interview is the first and most important aspect of the evaluation of depression. During the interview the clinician asks about the history of this and previous episodes, the patient's responses to any interventions used in previous episodes, the history of drug or alcohol use, and the patient's social and physical functioning. The next stage is a complete clinical examination including routine laboratory studies. The clinician may also choose to do a mental status examination. (See Chapter 6 for a complete explanation of use and implications of mental status examinations and depression scales.)

The clinician can also choose to conduct biological marker studies for dexamethasone suppression or titrated imipramine binding, as well as optional tests, such as magnetic resonance imaging (MRI). However, it should be noted that these tests are still somewhat controversial as to their usefulness in a differential diagnosis,[31] because they are not definitive for diagnosing other psychological problems. Paper-and-pencil tests and psychological interviews prove just as useful in detecting various dementia and depressions as these more expensive tests. Therefore, physicians may be skeptical when using these to prove a differential diagnosis between dementia and depression.

The treatment of depression involves a four-pronged approach involving psychotherapy, pharmacotherapy, electroconvulsive therapy (ECT), and family therapy. The benefits of insight-oriented psychotherapy have been questioned versus the benefits of behavioral and educationally oriented therapy, which appears to be quite helpful in older depressed patients.[33]

Anyone who talks to the patient in essence is providing psychotherapy. Therefore, the physical therapist should be aware of the treatment plans and goals for the individual patient. In addition, the physical therapist should be aware of some of the themes that emerge when working with the depressed older person. The older depressed person must learn to adjust to new family roles, body image, and a measure of dependency, and they must learn to accept these changes without shame and continue to maintain intimacy with loved ones. In addition, patients must learn healthier coping mechanisms. For example, anticipating future discomfort rather than denying future difficulties is a healthier choice. Using humor, sublimation, and altruism helps the patient focus less on the illness and depression and more on other situations.

Pharmacotherapy primarily involves the use of antidepressants. (For specific information on the use of antidepressants see Chapter 8.) Some general rules on the use of antidepressants are to start the dose at one-third to one-half the adult dose, and the clinician and patient must realize, therefore, that it may take 3 to 4 weeks before a significant response occurs. The clinician also needs to remember that the therapeutic to toxic dose range is a very narrow range with these kinds of drugs. If any side effects are noted, the therapist, patient, or both should consult a pharmacist or physician immediately.

Electroconvulsive shock therapy (ECT) is regaining popularity, and ECT can be very useful in the treatment of severe depressions that are resistant to pharmacological management. It may be especially useful in older patients because of the absence of cardiovascular side effects. The major side effects of ECT are memory loss and confusion, however, these are lessened with unilateral nondominant application.[34]

Family therapy has proven to be a double-edged sword. The family must be helped to cope with the patient's depression, and the family must learn how to effectively help the older patient. Family therapy involves several strategies, such as conflict resolution, problem-solving strategies, and family role assessment. The family can err in several ways, especially by being too helpful, thereby inhibiting the patient's autonomy. They can also deny the problem and display an overly optimistic attitude that overwhelms the older patient.

Social Isolation

Social isolation can be divided into four types.[35,36] One is geographic isolation, and it is a result of territorial restriction. The second, presentation isolation, results from an unacceptable appearance, while the third, behavioral isolation, results from unacceptable actions. Finally, attitudinal isolation arises from cultural or personal bound values. Any one of these types or any combination of them, bars the older person from full acceptance by others. This will cause the person to feel alienated and out of step, and it will effect his or her self-esteem.

Geographic Isolation

Geographic isolation is usually a result of widowhood, urban crowding, rural lifestyle, or institutionalization. In all of these situations the older person may be alienated. For example, in the urban situation the older person may be faced with a fast paced, depersonalized life-style that gives them little opportunity to come in contact with close friends. (Institutionalization will be discussed in the next section.) The intervention techniques for geographic isolation are building upon formal and informal support systems.

Table 4–3 lists formal and informal support systems.[36] In addition, the older person must examine the ramifications of any move they plan for an extended period of time in terms of the significance and size of the social support system they will be leaving behind versus the one they will be gaining.

Presentation Isolation

Unfortunately, in our society many judgments are made on superficial appearance, and as the body ages, its appearance no longer conforms to the Madison Avenue stereotype. On top of this is the disfigurement that accompanies many physical disabilities associated with aging. The physical therapist can help the older person to deal with presentation isolation in several ways:

1. By teaching them to avoid overexposure to individuals with similar image deficiencies, because the older person may capitalize on their weaknesses rather than their strengths.
2. By helping them to establish new relationships with people that can accept them as they are now.

TABLE 4–3. SUPPORT SYSTEMS

Formal	Informal
Involved in social issues for seniors	Neighbors
Senior centers	Nursing home—social corridor
Volunteers	Physician's office
Friends of the Library	Pets
National Retired Teachers Association	Fictional kin—soap operas
Retired Senior Volunteer Program	Psychological withdrawal—dreams, fantasies, hallucinations, daydreams
Foster Grandparents	Beauty salons, restaurants, bars, service personal, shops
Grandparenting	Maids, waitresses in small hotels
	Retirement communities
	Vicarious participation
	Lobby gazers
	Physical therapist

3. By giving lots of positive feedback on present strengths.
4. By asking questions to see what the person really thinks about themselves, and what experience they have had with similar conditions.
5. By teaching them to develop reasonable expectations.[35]

Behavioral Isolation

Behavioral isolation occurs when an older person displays behaviors that are unacceptable. The most likely behaviors to fall into this category are eccentricity, confusion, incontinence, and deviant behavior. The physical therapist can play a role by helping the person to identify the behavior and seek appropriate intervention for alleviating the problem.

Attitudinal Isolation

Attitudinal isolation is strongly entrenched in society's response to the older person. (Society's response will be discussed later in this chapter.) Ageism and the belief that it is acceptable and expected for older persons to be lonely are held by both the older person and the health professional. The intervention for this type of isolation is for both groups to evaluate their prejudices and misconceptions. In addition, the physical therapist must explore whether or not it is, in fact, desirable for the older person to be alone. To do this, the therapist should understand the difference between loneliness and being alone. Loneliness is a state of longing and emptiness, whereas being alone is being apart, solitary, and undisturbed. Figure 4–1

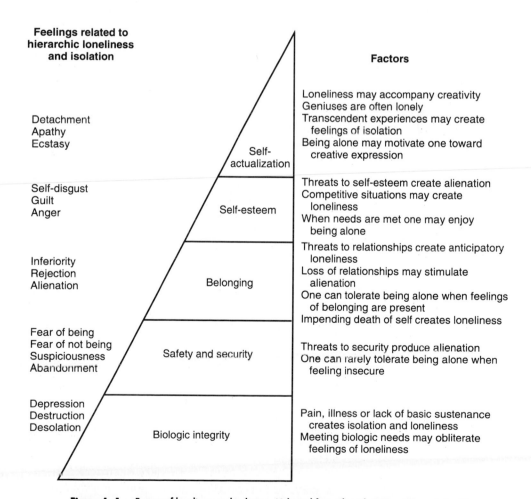

Figure 4–1. Factors of loneliness and isolation. (*Adapted from Ebersole P, Hess P. Towards health aging: human needs and nursing response. St. Louis, Mosby Co.; 1981, with permission.*)

shows Maslow's factors of loneliness and isolation,[36] which may help the physical therapist in this assessment.

Institutionalization

Institutionalization appears to be a bizarre subheading under "situations requiring coping mechanisms." Nevertheless organizational structure can have a profound impact on an individual's behavior. The classic text on the behavioral effects of institutionalization is *Assylums* by Goffman.[37] He identifies five aspects of a total institution (any institution where an individual spends 24 hours a day in residence), and they are

1. A hierarchical authority exists with residents on the lowest rung. This type of authority results in situations where the staff is always right, and the residents are punished or reprimanded.
2. Total institutions take control of personal habits. For example, mealtimes are regulated, as well as urination and defecation. This makes it difficult for the resident to satisfy personal needs in an efficient way.
3. Residents of institutions are often made to feel humiliated, and an example of this is that many residents of institutions are not allowed to close their doors.
4. The setting often makes it impossible for the person to engage in face-saving behaviors. Any defensive behavior a resident may take after being rebuked may then become the focus of a new attack. For example, if a resident becomes angry because the doors must remain open, the staff may then begin to rebuke the resident for inappropriate anger.
5. The person's status within the institution is solely defined by his or her status within the institution and any outside roles are rarely counted. For example, a physical therapist who has worked hard for years to help people in an outside role will be treated the same as a criminal in an institution.

Interventions for helping the older person cope with institutionalization, short of changing the entire system, begin with the individual. The following list gives ways to help personalize the institutional setting.

1. Develop meaningful relationships.
2. Give accurate information.
3. Involve the family.
4. Recognize accomplishments with plaques, posters, and so forth.
5. Recognize and address people by their preferred name.
6. Recognize birthdays on the appropriate day.
7. Provide memorials for residents that have died.
8. Conduct life reviews.
9. Establish contacts with plants, pets, and children.
10. Every person must have some personal items with them.
11. Room sharing should only be done with a compatible resident.
12. Provide legal aide to protect the resident's rights.
13. Provide choices in all matters.[36]

Anxiety Disorders

Anxiety disorders in the older person are frequently underreported and missed.[38] The incidence of anxiety disorders increases with age and is more frequent in women than in men.[39,40] Anxiety disorders either present with symptoms of fear, worry, or nervousness, or as a somatic problem without any physical cause. The DSM-III of the American Psychiatric Association identifies three classes of disor-

TABLE 4–4. THE ANXIETY DISORDERS AND THEIR CENTRAL FEATURES

Disorder	Central Features
Adjustment disorder with anxious mood	Nervousness/anxiety in reaction to identifiable psychosocial stressor
Anxiety states	Persistent or recurrent anxiety not provoked by identifiable stimulus, generally nonsituational
Obsessive–compulsive disorder	Intrusive thoughts and/or repetitive behaviors performed under a sense of pressure
	Attempts to resist increase anxiety
Posttraumatic stress disorder	Acute and delayed reactions to a traumatic event
	Involves "reliving" the experience, emotional numbing, and development of somatic symptoms
Panic disorder	Sudden, unpredictable panic attacks involving intense apprehension and physical symptoms
Generalized anxiety disorder	Generalized, persistent anxiety for more than 1 month
	Includes three of the following: motor tension, autonomic hyperactivity, apprehension, and hypervigilance
Phobic disorders	Persistent, irrational fear or anxiety provoked by stimulus object, activity, or situation
	Avoidance of stimulus
	Fear recognized by patient as irrational or excessive
Agoraphobia	Occurs with or without panic attacks
	Feared stimulus: being alone or in a public place where escape would be difficult or help hard to find
Social phobia	Fear stimulus: social situation involving possible embarrassment or humiliation
Simple phobia	Fear stimulus: situations similar to previous terrifying experience

Adapted and reprinted with permission from Geriatrics. Aug 1985; 40(8):80.

ders that all share the characteristic of anxiety.[41] These three classes are (1) adjustment disorders with anxious mood, (2) anxiety states, and (3) phobic states. Table 4–4 shows the most common anxiety disorders and their central features.

In the assessment of anxiety disorders, the clinician should be aware of the descriptions listed in Table 4–4, as well as some of the frequent symptoms associated with anxiety in the elderly. While the list is quite extensive, several symptoms are seen more frequently by physical therapists,[42] and these include tremor, headaches, chest pain, weakness and fatigue, neck and back pain, dry mouth, dizziness, parasthesias, and nonproductive cough.[42] The presence of these symptoms does not mean that the older person has an anxiety disorder, because there may be physical causes as well as organic causes, such as caffeine, hypoglycemia, or thyroid disease. In addition, therapists should screen for the symptoms of depression already described, as depression may cause some of the symptoms of anxiety disorders.

Finally, the physical therapist should seek additional information. For example, a patient may not tell you that she has a simple phobia; however, when you visit her at home, she may tell you that people are spying on her, listening to her through the walls, and tapping the phone. In further conversations, you discover that this patient had a terrifying experience as a child when she was left alone or when she was harassed and abused by Nazi soldiers. In this instance, the patient has developed a "simple phobic" reaction to always having people around—seen in terms of spying on her—to avoid her deep-seated fear of being alone.

The treatment for anxiety disorders is condensed in Table 4–5. In treating anxiety disorders, the physical therapist can act in several ways. First, the therapist can alert the physician to the problem. Second, the therapist may be able to share addi-

TABLE 4–5. ANXIETY DISORDERS AND THEIR MANAGEMENT

Disorders	Management
Adjustment disorder with anxious mood	Supportive "brief psychotherapies"
	Stress management techniques
	Assertiveness training
	Interventions to eliminate or reduce stressors
Anxiety states	
Obsessive–compulsive disorder	Tricyclic antidepressants
	Avoid use of benzodiazepines
	Psychotherapy
Posttraumatic stress disorder	Crisis intervention techniques
	Supportive brief psychotherapies
Panic disorder	Short-acting benzodiazepines
	Frequent evaluations of medication effects; avoid abrupt withdrawal
	Shield eyes from fluorescent lights
	Stress management techniques
Generalized anxiety disorder	Short-acting benzodiazepines, with frequent evaluations
	Avoid abrupt withdrawal
	Supportive "brief psychotherapies"
	Stress management techniques
Phobic disorders	Avoid use of most benzodiazepines
Agoraphobia	Daily tricyclic antidepressants or MAO inhibitors
	With panic attacks, shield eyes from fluorescent lighting
Social phobia	Behavior therapies
Simple phobia	Behavior therapies

Adapted and reprinted with permission from Geriatrics. Aug 1985; 40(8):80.

tional information collected from the frequent physical therapy sessions. Third, the therapist can play an integral role in any of the behavioral therapies. Finally, the therapist can teach the patient stress management techniques, stress reduction interventions, and assertiveness ideas. These will be discussed in detail at the end of this chapter.

Chronic Illness

As mentioned earlier in this chapter, the importance of coping with chronic illness is imperative for successful aging. In the older population, the percentage of persons with physical illness is staggering. According to Weg, 70% of people over the age of 65 have some type of chronic illness.[43] The three major illnesses for older persons are (1) heart conditions, (2) visual impairments, and (3) arthritis.[43] These types of chronic illnesses can be mild, thereby causing only minimal adaptions or life-style changes, or they can be devastating and cause major life-style modification. Serious illness or a devastating life event can cause profound changes in a person's appreciation of life,[44] and often this will result in a shift in goals, relationships, and values.

Physical therapists can recognize their role in this area by enhancing the older patient's new realizations and thought processes. The following list offers some suggestions to enhance this process.

1. Realize that patients may have a new heightened sense of beauty and of caring relationships.
2. Provide opportunities for the patient to talk about these new changes in values.

3. Encourage the patient in these new realizations, and let them know that these types of thoughts are part of the growth process.
4. Foster communication between the patient and their family, especially in light of the patient's new values.
5. Suggest participating in discussion groups to recovering patients.

Death, Dying, Grief, and Multiple Loss

These final situations that require coping mechanisms fit together well because the insights, manifestations, and mechanisms of coping for each are similar. The legal and ethical aspects of death and dying will be discussed in Chapter 11.

Many people think of aging as a time of loss. In reality, aging represents not just one loss, rather it is a time of multiple losses. Some of the most common losses include the loss of the patient's mobility, productivity, usefulness, body image, time left to live, health, income, and status. These and other losses occur throughout life, however, their frequency increases with old age, and their cumulative effect increases the emotional impact as a person ages. Another very important variable affecting loss is the person's general personality and their ability to tolerate loss. Some people view loss as giving up what one had, while others focus happily on what they had.

The physical therapist constantly works with people who have lost something, whether it is health, mobility, body image, or independence. The therapist's role is extremely important. To evaluate the loss, the therapist must consider if the loss is simple, compound, or symbolic. Losing $10.00 might be simple—if the person is financially healthy. However, if that $10.00 was borrowed with high interest to pay a long standing debt, then it becomes more compound and emotional. In another situation, the $10.00 may be the first money ever received in a business and, therefore, may be symbolic. When evaluating a loss, first check for its type by assessing its significance and by discussing it with the patient and family.

To assist the person, be sure to review the loss with the person and any supportive family and friends. Remember to constantly reorient the person to the reality of the situation. The therapist should not make false promises and set unrealistic goals (see Chapter 14 for treatment suggestions to assist patients with limb loss). Be realistic and set short-term attainable goals. Watch for signs of chronic grief.

Symptoms of a single loss should subside in 6 weeks, however, it may take longer in old age to resolve grief.[45] The symptoms are weakness, tiredness, sighing, and digestive symptoms. The patient may exhibit feelings of anger, deprivation, and guilt, but chronic grief in the older person may be much more subtle. For example, they may not cry, however, they may sigh frequently when talking or complain of constant tiredness. The most useful treatment suggestion for the physical therapist working with a grief-stricken patient is to listen and care. This can help to bridge the isolation. A recommendation for psychological counseling is also imperative.

To some, the death of an older person is viewed as a blessing or the final chapter in a full and rich life. This, unfortunately, does not hold for all older people, because many older people feel they are not ready to die and that they have not fulfilled their lives. According to Kalish, though, the fear of death diminishes as one ages.[46] This may be due to the increased exposure to dying with the aging of family and friends.

Dying has a special significance for the older patient. The following list gives six areas that are different for the older versus the younger patient.

1. Older persons tend to reminisce as a way of integrating their life prior to dying.
2. Older people are less likely to have an advocate. This is especially true for older women, because they tend to outlive their husbands.

3. Older persons are less likely to be communicative than younger patients when dying because of brain syndromes or confusion. This lack of communicative ability makes it more difficult for the health team to provide caring without a reciprocal response.
4. Older people may get less than optimum care because of the belief that they will die soon anyway.
5. The social value of an older person's life is thought to be less than that of a younger person's.[46]

Much has been written about the process of dying. The most well-known author in this area is Dr Kubler-Ross. She is most well known for her stages of dying, which are (1) denial, (2) anger, (3) bargaining, (4) depression, and (5) acceptance.[47] Even though her stages have not been proven to be consistent, they have received great acceptance. In interpreting her stages, it is important to note that not all people go through all of the stages. For example, someone may not experience anger and go straight from denial to bargaining. In addition, there are no time limits on these various stages. Other studies have postulated stages of the dying or grief process. Bowlby and Engel, for example, have similar stages but end their stages with the process of reorganization.[48,49]

The interventions for physical therapists working with the dying patient are to enhance the older person's ability to die with dignity and achieve final growth, and this can be done by recognizing impediments to growth. (These impediments are described in the sections on isolation and institutionalization.)

In addition, the physical therapist can help to fulfill the unmet needs of the dying person. The most common unmet needs are freedom from pain and loneliness, conservation of energy, and maintenance of self-esteem. Physical therapists are well versed in pain management (also see Chapter 14 for more details on pain management), and a full discussion of loneliness was discussed in the isolation section.

Physical therapists can also provide environmental and ergonometric assessment by evaluating an older patient's daily program and provide helpful suggestions to the patient and caregiver to reduce excessive energy expenditure. Finally, there are a few helpful hints for bolstering the self-esteem of an older person who is dying. Be sure that their physical comfort is assured (i.e., cleanliness, personal appearance, and lack of odor). Therapists should use as much sensory feedback as possible in the visual, auditory, and tactile realms. Also, therapists should focus on the immediate future and present opportunities; they should not confuse their values with those of the dying person's. Dying is very individual, and everyone perceives it differently.

The final topic under death, dying, grief, and loss focuses on the health care provider. It is imperative that the provider working with dying patients realizes the extreme amount of stress in this situation. Harper has developed stages that health care providers may experience when working with dying patients for a 1- to 2-year period.[50] They are

1. *Intellectualization* usually occurs in the beginning of employment. The health professional is quite accurate about their job, however, they avoid discussions about death.
2. *Emotional Survival* is characterized by an understanding of the pain and suffering. Here the provider may be unable to face—and may question—his or her own mortality.
3. *Depression* is a stage where the provider accepts the reality of death or quits. Feelings of grief are classic here.
4. *Emotional Arrival* is characterized by a deeper awareness and sensitivity of the dying person.
5. *Deep Compassion* is characterized by full maturity. Here the provider is extremely constructive and has clear emotions on self- and other's issues of death.[50]

DEMENTIA

Millions of older Americans are victims of dementias. Because of this, dementia or cognitive impairment is the major cause of disability in older persons. The statistics are staggering: In the United States the estimated number of people suffering moderate to severe dementia ranges from 1.5 million to 2.3 million.[51,52] One study equates these figures to, "One family in every three will see one of their parents succumb to this disease."[51] The prevalence of dementia also increases as one ages. The estimate for people over 65 is 5%, but for those over 75, it is estimated that 20% will have some degree of cognitive impairment.[53] In addition, in the nursing home setting it is estimated that the prevalence reaches 50%.[53] Besides the amazing emotional burdens, the economic burdens are immense. The care for persons with Alzheimer's disease alone in 1983 was $31 billion.[54]

The categorization of Alzheimer's disease as a cognitive impairment emphasizes the need for precision when describing and categorizing pathologies. The categorization and description of the cognitive impairments of older persons is probably the most important aspect of its assessment and treatment, and yet descriptions and classifications are not always in perfect agreement. This chapter will generally follow a classification scheme derived from the works of Rossman, Eisdorfer, and Cohen.[55,56]

1. *Acute disorders.* These are potentially reversible. Under this subheading is delirium, depression, multiple causes, and accidents.
2. *Chronic disorders.* These are the irreversible cognitive impairments, including Alzheimer's disease, vascular disease, and subcortical disorders.
3. *Presenile dementias.* These diseases tend to be rarer and to occur in younger populations. They are also not reversible.

Acute cognitive disorders have been romanticized in American society. While acute disorders are reversible, their prevalence is not as great as was once reported.[57] In an article entitled "The Reversible Dementias: Do They Reverse?" the results showed only a 3% full resolution and an 8% partial resolution of the dementias.[58]

Despite the less than impressive response rates to treatment, it is still important to understand this aspect of dementia, because it can be reversed. Acute disorders often have multiple causes. Among these causes are drugs, translocation, infection, neoplasm, trauma, malnutrition, toxic states, metabolic imbalances, and depression. According to Clarfield, the most common reversible causes were drugs (28.2%), depression (26.2%), and metabolic changes (15.5%).[58]

The symptoms of this type of cognitive impairment (except for the acute delirium caused by depression) are characterized by a rapidly developing confusion state. The person will often display clouded, fluctuating consciousness accompanied by agitation. In addition the patient will have alterations in the following processes:

1. *Perception.* The person may be hypersensitive to light or sound and suffer from visual, auditory, or tactile hallucinations.
2. *Memory.* This can be significantly impaired more so in the short-term than in the long-term. New information may be difficult to learn possibly because of the delirious patient's decreased attention span.
3. *Thinking.* Delirious patients tend to have illogical and disjointed thoughts. They may have difficulty with problem-solving and word finding. Finally, these patients may also have persecution delusions that they may forget when they recover.
4. *Orientation.* The delirious patient classically is disoriented to time. They may lose orientation to place as the disease progresses, however they rarely lose orientation to person.
5. *Alertness.* The delirious patient may be either hypo- or hyperalert. They may display increased pulse or pressure or decreased alertness.[59]

The manifestation of delirium due to depression differs in several major aspects. The depressed patient will have a slower onset of these symptoms, a longer history of somatic complaints, and a lower self-esteem. The depressed patient will tend to be on the hypo side of alertness. The greatest cognitive decline in the depressed patient will be the ability to process information, and this will be blunted. (For more information on depression in general see the previous section.)

The chronic causes of dementia or cognitive impairment are numerous, with Alzheimer's disease accounting for an estimated 50% of the chronic disorders.[54] Alzheimer's disease results from neuronal degeneration, and it is characterized by neurofibrillary tangles and plaques. While the cause is unknown, some researchers theorize that Alzheimer's is genetically linked, metabolic, or related to a slow virus. The cognitive decline is very slow and gradual, and this type of dementia affects three times as many women as men.

A second category of the chronic dementia is vascular disease or multi-infarct dementia. This type of dementia affects twice as many men as women. The cognitive decline may be due to small cerebral infarcts, arteriosclerotic disease, major cerebrovascular accidents, vertebrobasilar insufficiency, diabetic deterioration of blood vessels, carotid atherosclerosis, and diffuse cerebrovascular ischemia. The cognitive decline is characterized by a stepwise decline.

The third type of chronic dementias are the subcortical disorders. Korsakoff's psychosis is one cause of subcortical disorders, and it is caused by prolonged vitamin B_1 deficiency, which is usually caused by alcoholism. Wernicke's encephalopathy is a more advanced stage of this vitamin B_1 deficiency. Parkinson's disease can also cause irreversible dementia due to the dopamine deficiency. Finally, Huntington's chorea, which is genetically transmitted, can cause profound dementia.

The fourth type of chronic dementias are the presenile dementias. Creutzfeldt-Jakob disease is of particular interest to the geriatrician. Even though this disease can occur as early as the second decade of life, it generally occurs in the fifth to sixth decade. It is a rapidly dementing disease thought to be activated by a slow virus of genetic predisposition. Pick's disease is an extremely rare form of dementia involving the frontal and temporal regions that has symptoms similar to Alzheimer's disease and is often confused with Alzheimer's. It can only be definitively diagnosed at autopsy.

What separates the chronic dementias already noted from the acute dementias is their onset and permanence. All chronic dementias will show signs of cognitive impairment over a course of several months. The family may describe a slow loss of short-term memory with accompanying anxiety or depression. Unlike the acute dementias, the level of consciousness does not fluctuate.

The general characteristics of chronic brain syndrome can be summarized by the following mnemonic device, JAMCO[60]:

J— Judgment. The person may show inappropriate behavior as a result of improper information processing. For example, the patient walks out of his or her room undressed.

A— Affect. The person's affect is more labile, causing them to laugh or cry easily or uncontrollably. An example might be the patient who constantly giggles or weeps.

M— Memory. The person will lose their memory, first the short-term and then long-term. An example might be the patient who evades current questions by relating anecdotes from the past, however, when forced to answer the current questions the patient is unable to do so.

C— Cognition. Cognition will be disjointed and illogical, as well as delusional and hallucinatory. The therapist may be talking to the patient about the patient's exercises and the patient may relate a story about the FBI watching the nursing home.

O— Orientation. The person may, in general, have a very flat level of awareness. The therapist may find that if the patient is left alone to do exercises, they fall asleep or into a daydreaming state.[60]

Alzheimer's disease deserves additional description in terms of manifestations.[61] Hayter has described various stages of Alzheimer's disease. The first stage lasts 2 to 4 years and is characterized by moodiness, hypochondriasis, time disorientation, lack of spontaneity, poor judgment, blaming others, and a sense of helplessness and worthlessness. Generally, the person has difficulty with social adaption and may display catastrophic reactions to stressful events.

The second stage may last several years, and it is characterized by an increase in symptoms. At this point the person is usually in the health care system (i.e., hospital or nursing home) due to unsafe behaviors, such as constant movement, paranoia and hallucinations, and physical abusiveness. At this time the person may display sleep pattern disturbances, as well as incontinence. The third or final stage has no time limit and is characterized by irritability, seizures, disorientation on all spheres, illogical communication, severe anorexia, rigid postures, and explosive sounds and behaviors.

With all the various types and manifestations of dementia, assessment can be very difficult. Assessing orientation (i.e., patient is oriented times three) is not enough and frequently cognitive impairment is missed or dementia and depression are confused. For example, a well-known study found that 64% of the residents of a rehabilitation unit had significant cognitive impairment, yet physicians were unaware of the deficit in 15% of the cases.[62] In addition, Lazarus and associates noted a significant coexistence of depression and dementia in older patients and described methods of differentiating such complications.[63]

What should be in a mental status evaluation and what should be the goals of such an examination? Some suggested goals are to establish a baseline, screen for dementia or depression, determine the patient's ability to follow a rehabilitation program, identify cognitive impairment, and evaluate motor and language skills.[59] The suggested components of a mental status evaluation that can be used by the rehabilitation professional in daily practice are:

1. *Cortical functioning.* Including orientation, attention, concentration, memory, judgment, reasoning, and calculation. Ask questions about the patient's current situation.
2. *Perceptual functioning.* Assess the deficits of the sensory system. Present information with varying intensities of sensory input (i.e., talk loudly and then softly and check the patient's response).
3. *Speech and thought functioning.* Examine appropriateness of questions and statements. Ask questions and note carefully the context appropriateness and complexity of the answer.
4. *Emotional functioning.* Assess affect, mood, and flexibility. Discuss emotionally charged issues, and note the resident's response.
5. *General appearance.* Note posture, dress, hygiene, expressions, motor responses, and general behavior.[59]

The simple and brief tests that meet these goals range from the Blessed Dementia Scale[64] to the Pfieffer Short Portable Mental Status Questionnaire.[65] Nevertheless, one of the most widely used tools for assessing cognitive impairment in the clinical setting is the Mini-Mental State Exam.[66] This can be easily administered in less than a half of an hour, and it meets the criteria already given. (See Chapter 6 for details on administration and scoring of this test.)

Unfortunately, cognitive impairment cannot be assessed by simply administering a simple paper and pencil test. The administration of mental status may be very difficult with a demented patient. Often these patients are resentful or suspicious. In addition, they may have developed evasive skills that may fool the novice evaluator. To minimize these complications, the evaluator should explain clearly and honestly why the test is being administered, and that although some of the items may seem silly, however, it is important that they try to answer them. The therapist should also let the patient know that they will have plenty of time to answer. If the patient appears to avoid questions or to be guessing, the evaluator should repeat the question at a later time, possibly in a different form.

The final aspect of the cognitive impairment evaluation is the recognition of its physiological manifestations. Since the rehabilitation professional is most likely to see the patient on a frequent basis, he or she may notice these abnormalities, which include altered vital signs, such as an increase or a decrease in heart rate, blood pressure, or respiration. The skin may change in color, wetness, and temperature. Finally, the person could also display changes in neurological, cardiorespiratory, gastrointestinal, or urinary functions. It should be noted that all of these manifestations may be a result of an infection, drug complications, or an undetected pathology that can be corrected and may result in a decrease or amelioration of cognitive impaired status.[63]

What is the physical therapist's role in working with the patient with cognitive impairment? A diagnosis of Alzheimer's is often a cause for denial of payment for physical therapy. Many intermediaries cite the inability of Alzheimer's patients to learn as a reason for denial, because rehabilitation is structured around learning, the benefits derived would be minimal. While this argument has its merits, Alzheimer's patients can learn. In addition, therapy is more than learning. A large part of rehabilitation is environmental and physical modification. For example, if a patient with Alzheimer's disease is sent to physical therapy because of muscle weakness in the legs and an increased incidence of falls, then the physical therapist would be judicious in administering a strengthening program on a daily basis to the weakened muscles. Also, an environmental assessment for potential falls might be indicated. Therefore, it is appropriate to design and execute programs for the cognitively impaired elderly with treatable functional decline. In addition, the training and education of the family is crucial to any in-home rehabilitation program.

Some general guidelines for working with the cognitively impaired elderly follow.

1. *Simplify.* That includes simplifying the instructions, programs, and environment.
2. *Explain.* This should be done thoroughly, frequently, constantly, and repetitively, if necessary.
3. *Reorient.* In normal conversation, if possible, remind the patient of the time, place, and activity. Have clocks, calendars, and orienting pictures in view.
4. *Slow down.* Take your time in all aspects. Have a slow, low voice.
5. *Avoid change.* Change should be avoided in the environment, with the personnel, and in all aspects of programming, if possible.
6. *Encourage familiarity.* The environment should have as many familiar objects as possible, exercises should mimic familiar activities, and familiar people should be encouraged to visit.
7. *Touch.* Encourage as much touching as possible. This conveys caring and support to a patient who is going through an uncontrollable change and may desperately need support.
8. *Encourage independence.* This may necessitate simplifying commands and labeling items for ease of recognition.
9. *Respect individual dignity.* Encourage the patient to discuss and demonstrate previous successes and accomplishments. Display pictures of the patient in memorable moments. Respect modesty and dignity.
10. *Educate and support the family.* Be prepared to confront denial in the family and patient. Provide information on additional support services for cognitively impaired patients (see Chapter 21, Aging Network Resources, for listing). Frequently bring up the topic of additional support. (Families frequently refuse initial offerings of help.) Reinforce that the patients behavior is not volitional. Offer helpful suggestions for ways to tell others about the disease when the family is ready.

11. *Listen to the patient.* Even if the patient is not making sense try to listen.
12. *Take care of yourself.* Working with cognitively impaired patients can be emotionally exhausting. If a patient is combative or abusive, tell the patient that this type of behavior upsets you and take time out from the patient.

BELIEF SYSTEMS REGARDING THE AGING PROCESS AS FOSTERED BY SOCIETY

Ageism is the term Butler coined to denote a prejudice against a person or group of persons due to their age.[68] A myth is a belief that a person holds with or without the appropriate facts to gain control of an ambiguous situation. Society holds many of these beliefs. The current belief that is biased toward youth sprung out of the post-depression era. The focus for hope shifted from the older generation to the new, bright-futured baby boomers. The parents who had nothing growing up in the Depression, could now give it all to their children with the hope that they would make a better world. The focus unfortunately shifted from the older population. This shift has combined with the birth of high technology and self-absorption and has led to low self-esteem and negative attitudes for older people.

The Myth of Aging Quiz by Erdman Palmore (Fig. 4–2) is an important tool for assessing bias against older persons.[67] To score this quiz, all the odd-numbered questions are false, and all the even-numbered questions are true. This quiz can be used to test a person's myths, biases, and knowledge.

The problem of ageism or negative attitudes toward older people are particularly pronounced in the health arena. Older patients may be seen as complaining, somatasizing, uninteresting, or helpless. In addition they may not receive the same services as younger persons. In the United States, for example, physicians are often overaggressive with diagnostic tests for older persons but less aggressive in providing rehabilitation services,[69] and physical therapists have been shown to be less aggressive in goal setting for older patients.[70]

The evaluation and treatment of the social misinterpretation of aging is not an easy task. Both the evaluation and the treatment must begin on a personal level. Self-evaluation of myths, belief systems, and the personal evaluation of individual patients must be done daily.

A simple treatment is to show others (by example) healthy and positive ways of working with older persons. The ultimate goal is not to display negative prejudices to other groups in hopes of valuing the older population, but to develop a society with a healthy mixture and respect for all groups. A society to strive for would be one of bright youths, secure middle-aged adults, and wise older persons.

LIFE-STYLE ADAPTION, STRESS

Retirement, illness, and changes in living conditions are all possible life-style adaptations in late life. Are these good or bad situations? Do they cause growth or decline? A simple way of viewing some of these life-style adaptations is through the stress mechanism. Stress, as defined by Hans Selye, is the response of the body to any demand made on it.[71] Stress has both a physical and psychological component.

On the physical level stress has been shown to increase the secretion of adrenalin and cortisol, as well as lower the body's sensitivity to insulin and its tolerance

Facts on Aging Quiz

Please take this short "Facts on Aging Quiz"

T   F   **1.** The majority of old people (past age 65) are senile (i.e., defective memory, disoriented, or demented).

T   F   **2.** All five senses tend to decline in old age.

T   F   **3.** Most old people have no interest in, or capacity for, sexual relations.

T   F   **4.** Lung capacity tends to decline in old age.

T   F   **5.** The majority of old people feel miserable most of the time.

T   F   **6.** Physical strength tends to decline in old age.

T   F   **7.** At least one-tenth of the aged are living in long-stay institutions (i.e. nursing homes, mental hospitals, homes for the aged, etc.)

T   F   **8.** Aged drivers have fewer accidents per person than drivers under age 65.

T   F   **9.** Most older workers cannot work as effectively as younger workers.

T   F   **10.** About 80% of the aged are healthy enough to carry out their normal activities.

T   F   **11.** Most old people are set in their ways and unable to change.

T   F   **12.** Old people usually take longer to learn something new.

T   F   **13.** It is almost impossible for most old people to learn new things.

T   F   **14.** The reaction time of most old people tends to be slower than reaction time of younger people.

T   F   **15.** In general, most old people are pretty much alike.

T   F   **16.** The majority of old people are seldom bored.

T   F   **17.** The majority of old people are socially isolated and lonely.

T   F   **18.** Older workers have fewer accidents than younger workers.

T   F   **19.** Over 15% of the US population are now age 65 or older.

T   F   **20.** Most medical practitioners tend to give low priority to the aged.

T   F   **21.** The majority of older people have incomes below the poverty level (as defined by the Federal Government).

T   F   **22.** The majority of old people are working or would like to have some kind of work to do (including housework and volunteer work).

T   F   **23.** Older people tend to become more religious as they age.

T   F   **24.** The majority of old people are seldom irritated or angry.

T   F   **25.** The health and socioeconomic status of older people (compared to younger people) in the year 2000 will probably be about the same as now.

Figure 4–2. *(Reprinted with permission Palmore E. Facts on aging: a short quiz. Gerontologist. Aug 1977; 17:315–320. © The Gerontological Society of America.)*

to carbohydrates.[72] These physiological changes can cause an increase in blood pressure, as well as a decrease in the body's immune system's ability to combat various diseases. Chronic stress in older people may result in a decreased caloric intake, a lowered body weight, and a lowered lymphocyte count. In addition, older individuals who have experienced this stress response will show an increased systolic pressure and mean arterial pressure, and some degree of left ventricular hypertrophy.[73]

Stress can be both good and bad, and Selye describes both. Eustress is good stress and can be used for growth. A lack of eustress can be exemplified by an older person who sits all day and does nothing, with little initiative or interest. They have no need or desire to adapt or respond to their environment. A possible intervention is placing a hungry, lonely kitten in the same environment. When the older patient begins to take care of this kitten, they will adapt to the new stimulus, and the kitten will give the person something to work for and with. Therefore, the kitten could be considered a eustress.

Bad stress is called distress.[71] The same kitten could be an example of distress if, one month later, it was run over by a truck. The older person would experience loss and a negative need to adapt.

Before evaluating stress, retirement deserves special mention. Retirement is also an example of a life-style adaption that can prove to be good or bad. Retirement presents an emotion-laden change because work fulfills many social needs, and perhaps most importantly, work bestows a status. A physical therapist, for example, knows their status at a social gathering, with patients, and within the medical community. What is the status of a retiree? Work also fixes associations. For example, the physical therapist knows that they will see Bob, the nurse, Jane, the social worker, etc. Who does the in-home retiree see on a regular basis?

Work also regulates activity. The physical therapist knows that she or he works from nine to five, five days a week. The retiree often does not have the same amount of regulated activity. Work also bestows meaningful life experience. A physical therapist helps people to gain independence and to improve the quality of their lives. What is the retiree doing to get meaning in life? These types of questions and issues have spawned the field of preretirement and retirement planning. For a successful retirement, the previously listed attributes of work must continue to be fulfilled. This may mean that the retiree volunteers or participates in strong social programs to meet these needs.[74]

STRESS EVALUATION

Stress can be evaluated in several ways. In Chapter 6, the Life Events Scale and Geriatric Social Readjustment Scale are explained in detail. These two tools provide some information on an older person's stress level. In addition, a complex array of symptoms may indicate stress. For example, on the physiological level an increase in skin temperature, blood pressure, temperature, heart rate, respiration, and autonomic system activity all indicate stress. Impairment in problem-solving ability, social responsiveness, judgment, reality interpretation, and thoughts are all cognitive changes. Motor changes affected by stress are tremor, speech disturbance, and muscle tension. Finally, an older person under stress may display anger, guilt, depression, or anxiety.[73]

The following are the most frequent cues to stress in the elderly: decreased productivity, lack of awareness to the outside environment, decreased interest, rumination, preoccupation, lack of concentration, irritability and angry outbursts, withdrawal, tendency to cry (sobbing without tears), suspiciousness, and critical of self and others.[75]

Stress management or life-style adaption techniques for older adults are different from those suggested for younger persons. Since older persons may have experienced an accumulation of stressors, the intervention itself should impose as few changes as possible. The physical therapist may overload the person's system by suggesting an entire life-style modification for energy conservation, as well as a medication and exercise program. Some additional considerations in planning adaptations for older persons are:

1. If a person is about to experience a high stress situation (a grandchild's wedding, for example) advise them to improve nutrition and increase rest.
2. Respect the individual's time clock. Choose the person's peak performance time to introduce change.
3. Try to encourage continuity of personnel.
4. Explain stress concepts to older persons. Let them know it may take longer to feel the effects of stress management if they are experiencing multiple stress or if they have been experiencing the current stress for a long time.
5. If a person has been experiencing chronic stress, it may be a sign that change is needed (e.g., the kitten and eustress example).

Before suggesting specific stress management techniques, there are several factors that affect coping patterns of older persons. The first is social support. Older persons who believe that they are loved, esteemed, and mutually obligated to a support system have better coping mechanisms.[76] The older person's inner resources have also been found to improve coping responses, and the most important of these are flexibility, past experiences with successful coping, nonavoidance, and resumption of daily activities as soon as possible.[77] Finally, older persons with improved problem-solving ability respond better to stressful events than poor problem solvers.[78]

Stress control techniques range from cognitive to physical. Some examples of cognitive techniques are medication, selective awareness, and systematic desensitization, and a few examples of physical techniques are progressive neuromuscular relaxation, biofeedback, physical activity, and breathing control. (Refer to references 72 and 79 for specific information on these techniques).

The technique that is simplest to learn and most useful for other activities is breathing control. Teaching breathing control for relaxation involves deep diaphragmatic breathing. The older person should breathe in slowly and visualize calmness and relaxation with each inhalation and exhalation. This should be done for 2 to 3 minutes 3 to 4 times a day.

A final note on stress management comes from Hans Selye. Dr Selye was himself an excellent example of a healthy older person. He lived until his 90s, swam and rode his bike daily, and wrote, researched, and lectured until the day he died. Dr Selye's personal recipe for stress was that people should strive to their highest level, but never strive in vain. Second, they should find their minimum daily requirement of stress, because he viewed stress as the spice of life. Finally, he advocated "Altruistic-egoism," which means taking care of oneself by taking care of others.[75]

CONCLUSION

This chapter has reviewed the psychosocial theories of aging, the cognitive changes in late life, as well as multiple situations requiring coping mechanisms. Important problems, such as depression and dementia, were discussed with treatment implications for the physical therapist. Finally, the end of the chapter focused on the aspects of life-style adaption and society's belief system toward aging and older persons.

PEARLS

- Full life development theories, such as Erickson's and Maslow's, discuss accomplishment stages throughout life for successful aging.

- Late life theories, such as those described by Peck, Neugarten, and Havighurst, focus on the state of late life and the older person's role in adapting to this stage of life.

- Memory loss can be assisted by classes and educational interventions.

- Intellectual performance in the aged can be enhanced by the therapist in many ways, including the mode of information presented, pacing, and feedback.

- Depression in its many forms is very common in the elderly and can impact performance. Treatment ranges from behavioral to pharmacological to electroconvulsion shock therapy.

- Social isolation, including geographic, presentation, behavioral, and attitudinal types of isolation, can bar older persons from effectively interacting with their surroundings.

- Institutionalization causes changes in behavior and affects a person's performance. These affects can be countered with recognition of symptoms and behavioral and environmental interventions.

- Anxiety disorders, such as adjustment disorders, anxiety states, and phobic states, are often underreported and missed in the aged.

- Death, dying, grief and multiple loss can be a very different phenomenon in the older person. Recognizing different behavioral interventions can help the older person to die with dignity.

- Dementia affects millions of older persons and can be classified as acute disorders, chronic disorders, and presenile dementias. Assessment and treatment modification for working with these patients is based on behavioral and environmental modification by the therapist.

- Recognizing one's belief systems via the "Myth of Aging Quiz" can help the therapist to work better with the aged.

- Numerous signs, such as a decreased interest in productivity and awareness, may be signs of stress that will respond to rehabilitation interventions, such as life-style adaptations and stress control techniques.

REFERENCES

1. Mossey J, Murtan E, Knott K, et al. Determinants of recovery 12 months after hip fracture: the importance of psychosocial factors. *Am J Public Health*. March 1989; 79:279–286.
2. Magaziner J. Predictions of functional recovery one year following hospital discharge for hip fracture: a prospective study. *J Gerontology*. 1990; 45:101–107.
3. Erikson EH. *Identity, Youth & Crisis*. New York: Norton; 1968.
4. Lewis C. Psychological aspects of aging. In: *Aging: Health Care's Challenge*. Philadelphia: Davis; 1985.
5. Maslow A. *Motivation and Personality*. New York: Harper & Row; 1954.
6. Maslow A. *Toward a Psychology of Being*. Princeton, Van Nostrand Co., Inc.; 1962.
7. Peele B. Psychological developments in the second half of life. In: Neugarten B, ed. *Middle Age and Aging*. Chicago: University of Chicago Press; 1975.
8. Neugarten B. *Middle Age & Aging*. Chicago: University of Chicago Press; 1975.
9. Cummings E, Henry W. *Growing Old: The Process of Disengagement*. New York: Basic Books; 1961.
10. Havighurst R, Neugarten B, Tobin S. Disengagement and patterns of aging. In: Neugarten B, ed. *Middle Age & Aging*. Chicago: University of Chicago Press; 1975.
11. Butler R, Lewis M. Aging and Mental Health. St. Louis: Mosby-Year Book, Inc.; 1982;33–35.

12. Havighurst RJ. Flexibility and the social role of the retired. *Am J Sociol.* 1954; 59:399.

13. Neuhaus R, Neuhaus R. *Successful Aging.* New York: John Wiley & Sons; 1982;9–12.

14. Cockburn J, Smith P. The relative influence of intelligence and age on everyday memory. *J Gerontology.* 1991; 46(1):31–35.

15. Hultoch D, Masson M, Small B. Adult age differences in direct and indirect test of memory. *J Gerontology.* 1991; 46(1):22–30.

16. Craik F, Masani P. Age differences in the temporal integration of language. *Brit J Psychology.* 1967; 58:291–299.

17. Botwinck J. *Aging and Behavior.* 2nd ed. New York: Springer; 1978.

18. McEnte W, Crook T. Age associated memory impairment: a role for catecholamines. *Neurology.* 1990; 40:526–530.

19. Kahn R, Miller N, Zarit S, et al. Memory complaint and impairment in the aged. *Arch Gen Psychiatry.* 1975; 32:1569–1573.

20. Gurland B. The comparative frequency of depression in various adult age groups. *J Gerontology.* 1976; 31:283–292.

21. Labouvie-Vief G. Intelligence and cognition. In: Birren JE, Schaie KW, eds. *Handbook of the Psychology of Aging.* New York: Van Nostrand Reinhold; 1985.

22. Cattell RB. Theory of fluid and crystallized intelligence: a clinical experiment. *J Educ Psychol.* 1963; 54:1.

23. Knox AB. *Adult Development and Learning.* San Francisco: Jossey-Bass; 1977.

24. Botwinick J. *Aging and Behavior: A Comprehensive Integration of Research Findings.* New York: Springer Publishing; 1978.

25. Hayslip B, Kennelly KJ. Cognitive and non-cognitive factors affecting learning among older adults. In: Lumsden BD, ed. *The Older Adult as a Learner.* Washington, DC: Hemisphere Publishing; 1985.

26. Eisdorfer C, Nowlin F, Wilke F. Improvement of learning in the aged by modification of autonomic nervous system activity. *Science.* 1970; 170:1327.

27. Schultz NR, Hoyer WJ. Feedback effects on spacial egocentrism in old age. *J Gerontol.* 1976; 31:72.

28. Bettes S. Depression: the "common cold" of the elderly. *Generations.* Spring 1979; 3:15.

29. Epstein L. Symposium of age differentiation in depressive illness: depression in the elderly. *J Gerontology.* 1976; 31:278.

30. Gurland B. The comparative frequency of depression in various adult age groups. *J Gerontology.* 1976; 31:283–292.

31. Ferucci L, Guralnik J, Marchionni N, et al. Aging and prevalence of depression. *Gerontologist.* October 1990; 30:314A.

32. Starksteen S, Robinson R, Rice T. Comparison of patients with and without major stroke depression matched for size and location of lesion. *Arch Gen Psychiatry.* 1988; 45:247.

33. Nemiroff R, Colarusso C. *The Race Against Time: Psychotherapy and Psychoanalysis in the Second Half of Life.* New York: Plenum Press; 1985.

34. Pettinati H, Bonner K. Cognitive functioning in depressed geriatric patients with a history of ECT. *Am J Psychiatry.* January 1984; 141:1.

35. Goffman E. *Stigma: Notes on the Management of Spoiled Identity.* Englewood Cliffs, NJ: Prentice-Hall, Inc.; 1963.

36. Ebersole P, Hess P. *Towards Healthy Aging: Human Needs and Nursing Response.* St. Louis: Mosby Co.; 1981:382.

37. Goffman E. *Asylums: Essays on the Social Situations of Mental Patients and Other Inmates.* Garden City, NY: Doubleday; 1961.

38. Shader R, Goodman M. Panic disorders: current perspectives. *J Clin Psychopharmacol.* 1982; 2:2–105.

39. Carey G, Gottesman I, Robins E. Prevalence and rates for the neurosis: pitfalls in the evaluation of familiality. *Psychol Med.* 1980; 10:437–443.

40. Kleen D, Robkin J, eds. *Anxiety: New Research and Changing Concepts.* New York: Raven Press; 1981.

41. American Psychiatric Association. *Diagnostic and Statistical Manual of Mental Disorders.* 3rd ed. Washington, DC: American Psychiatric Association; 1980:225–239.

42. Turnball J, Turnball S. Management of specific anxiety disorders in the elderly. *Geriatrics.* August 1985; 40:8, 75–81.

43. Weg R. *The Aged: Who, Where, How Well.* Los Angeles: Ethel Percy Andrus Gerontology Center; 1979.

44. Frankle V. *Man's Search for Meaning.* Boston: Beacon Press; 1959.

45. Ebersole P, Hess P. *Towards Healthy Aging: Human Needs and Nursing Response*. St. Louis: Mosby Co.; 1981; 384.

46. Kalish R. *Death, Grief and Caring Relationships*. Monterey, Calif.: Brooks/Cole; 1981.

47. Kubler-Ross D. *On Death and Dying*. New York: Macmillan; 1969.

48. Bowlby J. Process of mourning. *Int J Psychoanal*. 1961; 42:317.

49. Engel G. Grief and grieving. *Am J Nursing*. 1964; 64:93.

50. Harper B. *Death: The Coping Mechanisms of the Health Professional*. Greenville, NC: Southeastern University Press; 1977.

51. Glenner G. Alzheimer's disease (senile dementia) a research update and critique with recommendations. *J Am Ger Soc*. 1982; 30:59–62.

52. Rocca W, Amaducci LA, Shoenberg BS, et al. Epidemiology of clinically diagnosed Alzheimer's disease. *Ann Neurol*. 1981; 19:415.

53. Gurland B, Cross P. Epidemiology of psychopathology in old age: some implications for clinical services. *Psychiatric Clinics in N Am*. 1982; 5:11–26.

54. Hay J, Ernst R. The economic costs of Alzheimer's disease. *Am J Public Health*. 1987; 77:1169.

55. Rossman J. *Clinical Geriatrics*. 2nd ed. Philadelphia: Lippincott Co.; 1979.

56. Eisdorfer C, Cohen D. The cognitively impaired elderly: differential diagnosis. In: Storandt M, Seigler I, Elias M, eds. *The Clinical Psychology of Aging*. New York: Plenum Publishing Corp.; 1985.

57. Delaney P. Dementia: the search for reversible causes. *South Med Journal*. 1982; 75: 707–709.

58. Clarfield A. The reversible dementias: do they reverse? *Annals of Internal Medicine*. September 1988; 476–486.

59. Teschendorf B. Cognitive impairment in the elderly: delirium, depression, or dementia? *Focus on Geriatric Care and Rehab*. September 1987; 1:4.

60. Lewis C. Psychosocial aspects of aging. In: Lewis C, ed. *Aging: The Health Care Challenge*. Philadelphia: Davis; 1985.

61. Hayter J. Patients who have Alzheimer's disease. *Am J Nurs*. 1974; 74:1460.

62. Luxemborg J, Feigenbaum L. Cognitive impairment on a rehabilitative service. *Arch Phys Med Rehab*. 1986; 67:796–798.

63. Lazarus LW, Newton N, Cohler B, et al. Frequency and presentation of depressive symptoms in patients with primary degenerative dementia. *Am J Psychiatry*. January 1987; 41–45.

64. Blessed G, Tominson BE, Roth M, et al. The association between quantitative measures of dementia and of senile change in the grey matter of elderly subjects. *Br J Psychiatry*. 1968; 114:797.

65. Pfieffer E. A short portable mental status questionnaire for the assessment of brain deficit in elderly patients. *J Am Ger Soc*. 1975; 23:433.

66. Folstein M, Folstein S. Mini-Mental State. A practical method for grading the cognitive state of patients for the clinician. *J Psychiatric Res*. 1975; 189–198.

67. Palomore E. Facts on aging—a short quiz. *Gerontologist*. 1977; 17:4.

68. Butler R. Age-ism: another form of bigotry. *Gerontologist*. 1969; 9:243.

69. Kemp B. The psychosocial context of geriatric rehabilitation. In: Kemp B, Brummel-Smith K, Ramsdell JW, eds. *Geriatric Rehabilitation*. Boston: Little, Brown & Co.; 1990.

70. Kvitek S, Dr Shaver BJ, Blood H, et al. Age bias: physical therapists and older patients. *J Gerontol*. 1986; 41:702.

71. Selye H. *The Stress of Life*. New York: McGraw-Hill; 1959.

72. Allen R, Hyde D. *Investigations in Stress Control*. Minneapolis: Burgess Publishing; 1982.

73. Lakatta E. Hemodynamic adaptions to stress with advancing age. *Acta Med Scand*. 1986; 711(suppl):39–52.

74. Neres M. Coping with stress in nursing. *Am Nurse*. September 15, 1977; 9:4.

75. Selye H. Stress and aging. *J Am Ger Soc*. September 1970; 18:9.

76. Cobb S. Social support as a moderator of life stress. *Psychosom Med*. 1976; 38:300.

77. Henry J, Stephans P. *Stress, Health and the Social Environment*. New York: Springer-Verlag; 1977.

78. Fry P. Mediators of perceptions of stress among community-based elders. *Psychological Reports*. 1989; 65:307–314.

79. Iglarsh. Stress and aging. In: Lewis C, ed. *Aging: Health Care's Challenge*. Philadelphia: Davis Co.; 1990.

Pathological Manifestations of Aging

Aging is considered a normal physiological process because of its universality. As much as the aging process may influence the predisposition to disease, aging in and of itself is not considered to be pathological. This distinction seems conceptually clear, however, the fine line between aging and disease is often blurred when applied to specific cases, and some degree of decreasing biological, physiological, anatomical, and functional capabilities occurs, as one ages. (See Chapter 3, Comparing and Contrasting Age Related Changes in Biology, Physiology, and Anatomy.) Some degree of atrophy is also evident in all tissues of the body. A variety of degenerative processes are called "normal aging" until they proceed far enough to cause clinically significant disability.

The incidence of many diseases is influenced markedly as age advances (Fig. 5–1). The death rates for atherosclerosis, myocardial degeneration, hypertension, and cancer all increase more steeply in older patients than the overall death rate, which arouses the suspicion that aging predisposes an individual either to the development of the condition or to a fatal outcome. With some conditions, such as respiratory infections, the incidence is not increased in the elderly, but the likelihood of the insult being fatal is greater than in younger persons.[1] In a child or young adult, death is most commonly caused by some form of accident (Fig. 5–2); however, in the elderly, the main problems are coronary heart disease, cerebrovascular accidents, respiratory diseases, diabetes, peripheral vascular diseases, and neoplasms.[2]

The purpose of this chapter is to review the pathologies that are commonly manifested in the aged population, but it will not attempt a detailed consideration of every possible geriatric pathology; rather, it will examine some of the more common conditions that afflict the elderly and affect their functional activities and daily living. The format of this chapter follows that of Chapter 3, Comparing and Contrasting Age Related Changes in Biology, Physiology, and Anatomy for easier comparison between "age related" and pathological changes with aging.

AGING AS A DISEASE

There is always the tacit implication that aging, like growth and development, is a normal physiological process lying outside the domain of disease. Though aging may not be considered a disease process, the time dependent loss of structure and

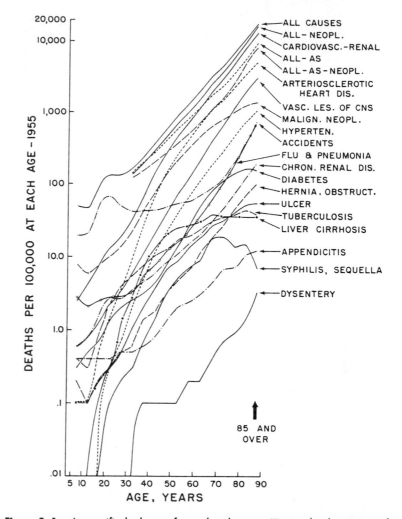

Figure 5–1. Age-specific death rates from selected causes. *(Reprinted with permission from Kohn RR. Principles of Mammalian Aging. 2nd ed. Prentice-Hall, Englewood Cliffs, NJ; 1978.)*[133]

function in all organ systems leads to pathological end states. There is a general decline in the structure, function, and number of many kinds of cells with age. Cellular aging is accompanied by denaturation of extracellular proteins. The collagen and elastin of the skin become irreversibly crystalline and broken. The hyaline cartilage on articular surfaces of joints becomes fibrillar and fragmented, and the beautifully ordered structure of the lens of the eye becomes brittle and chaotic as the lens' proteins are gradually denatured.

The aging process proceeds slowly and ubiquitously over the life course, resulting in a loss of structure and function within every organ or tissue. Countless microtraumas occur and accumulate in small increments as imperceptible injuries. Over a life time, the skin elastin is exposed to microinsults from ultraviolet rays from the sun, repetitive mechanical stresses cause degeneration of articular cartilage, and due to reactions with metabolites the opacity of the lens of the eye diminishes. The most important aging changes occur at the molecular level, as reviewed in Chapter 2, Comparing and Contrasting the Theories of Aging. Small injuries occurring within the cell result in the loss of genetic memory and progressive cross-linking of collagen, the chief structural protein in the body.

Wiley Forbus, a pathologist, defined disease as the reaction to injury.[3] If aging is a gradual accumulation of incompletely repaired injuries due to microtrauma through the life course, it may not be normal, despite its universality. Perhaps "aging" is a pathological process resulting from the tissues' reactions to imperceptible injuries that could have been avoided.

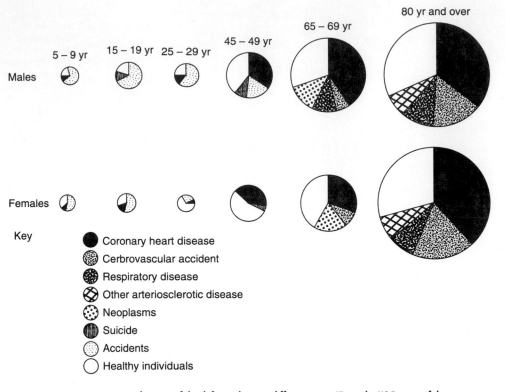

Figure 5–2. Principal causes of death for each sex at different ages. (From the US Bureau of the Census. Statistical Abstract of the United States. 11th ed. Washington, DC; 1990.)

Physical therapists could play a major role in preventing the disabilities that result from these insidious microtraumas. Preventive strengthening and conditioning exercises, positioning, joint and tissue mobilization, and the numerous modalities that could be employed all impact functional capabilities, especially in an aged population. From the authors' clinical perspective, preventing disabilities that can result from pathological processes greatly improves the level of function and the quality of life. There are certainly changes that occur in aging that do not need to be inevitable.

CARDIOVASCULAR MANIFESTATIONS OF AGING

There are no clinically significant effects on heart function that can be solely ascribed to aging. Cardiovascular dysfunction attributed to the aging process closely mimics the decline in cardiac function that is seen with inactivity.[4–6] Arteriosclerosis is a term generally used to describe any form of vascular degeneration associated with a thickening and loss of resilience in the arterial wall.[7] Atherosclerosis is a more specific type of degeneration that is associated with an accumulation of fat in the intimal lining of the vessels and an increase of connective tissue in the underlying subintima.[7] Almost all animal species show some degree of atherosclerosis, and, for this reason, it has been considered an inevitable accompaniment of aging. The pathological consequences of artherosclerosis depend on the site. Weakness in the aorta can cause an aneurysm; ischemic heart disease can result from atherosclerotic changes in the coronary arteries; and cerebrovascular accidents can result from involvement of the cerebral vessels.[8]

Other cardiovascular pathologies increase in incidence with age in addition to ischemic heart disease, and these include cardiomyopathies, conductive system diseases, valvular heart disease, and peripheral vascular disease.[9] The result is that the heart is less effective as a pump and has less reserve to meet increased activity needs. Functional abilities of the individual become more and more restricted as the severity of heart disease increases. Cerebral vascular problems resulting from cardiovascular problems need consideration and are dealt with more extensively in a subsequent section of this chapter on neuromuscular pathologies.

Ischemic Heart Disease

Ischemic heart disease, commonly called coronary artery disease (CAD), results from the blockage of blood flow to cardiac muscle. Some 40% of those aged 65 to 74 years and 50% of those aged 75 years and older have evidence of heart disease.[7] When there is a reversible lack of oxygen in the cardiac muscle in response to an increased activity level or emotional stress, anginal pain results from atherosclerotic changes in the coronary arteries. The effect of ischemia can be reversible, and the muscle cells gradually regain their ability to contract as circulation is restored. A rapid loss of blood flow lasting 30 to 60 minutes can cause death of the myocardial cells.[8] Irreversible damage to a part of the heart muscle from vascular narrowing can result from plaque formation that totally blocks the coronary vessel, such as an embolus or a thrombosis, the consequence of which is a myocardial infarction. Myocardial degeneration can progress with repeated minor episodes of irreversible oxygen depletion in the cardiac muscle. As degeneration progresses, heart muscle functions poorly and congestive heart failure can be the result. Furthermore, muscle deprived of its blood supply becomes prone to chaotic and unregulated contractions that can result in life threatening arrhythmias.

Oxygen extraction in the coronary circulation is relatively complete even at rest.[7] When the work demands are increased on the heart, additional oxygen is required to meet the energy needs of the cardiac muscle cells. This oxygen is obtained through the dilation of the coronary vessels. With rigid, atherosclerotic vessels dilation does not readily occur, and vascular resistance is increased due to the inelastic quality of the vessels and impedence to blood flow by plaque obstruction.

Gross obstruction of the major coronary vessels results in anginal pain typically brought on by vigorous exercise.[10] In the elderly, however, anginal pain is not a consistent symptomatic indicator of ischemia of the cardiac tissue. The elderly more commonly report dyspnea (shortness of breath). Clinically, shortness of breath is a much more reliable indicator of ischemia than anginal pain in the elderly individual.[11] There is a general correlation between ST segment depression on the EKG and the onset of anginal symptoms,[7] though in the elderly, marked ST segment depression occurs with dyspnea without the development of the characteristic anginal pain.[11]

Early intervention in ischemic heart disease takes several forms. The most important is to reduce the "risk factors" that predispose individuals to the development of coronary artery disease, such as cigarette smoking and high blood pressure and serum cholesterol. Secondary prevention of heart attacks, once CAD is established, requires the reduction of risk factors as well as the use of aspirin to prevent platelet aggregation, which may initiate obstruction of a coronary artery, and beta blockers, which appear to limit the extent of muscle injury. Management of symptomatic coronary artery disease is similar in all age groups and consists of medical and surgical interventions. Since the pathophysiology of coronary artery disease is the mismatch between the metabolic demands of the heart muscle and the ability of the coronary arteries to supply blood, interventions are directed at decreasing the metabolic needs of the heart muscle or increasing the ability of the coronary arteries to carry blood. The metabolic demands of the heart muscle can be reduced by lowering the pressure against which the heart has to push, by reducing the rate at which the heart contracts, and by reducing the overall metabolic demands of the body by correcting hyperthyroidism, anemia, low oxygen, or elevated temperature. Calcium channel blocking agents and beta blockers reduce the metabolic demands on heart muscle; and nitroglycerine reduces the pressure against which the heart has to pump by causing dilitation of the coronary vessels. Beta blockers[12] and calcium channel blockers[13] often improve function by reducing myocardial contractility, however, this may leave the elderly individual vulnerable to cardiac failure. It is still debatable how far the effectiveness and toxicity of these drugs is modified by aging.[14]

There are a number of reasons why exercise is helpful to the patient with angina.[7] Development of an enhanced "collateral" flow has not been established.[15] However, the cardiac oxygen demand is decreased by a drop in both heart rate and blood pressure at a given work load. The lengthening of the diastolic phase facilitates coronary perfusion.[7] Though progress is slow in the elderly, dramatic gains of maximum oxygen intake can be achieved if the exercise periods are of sufficient lengths.[7,16] Many activities of daily living can be brought below the anginal threshold by exercise training. Strengthening of the skeletal muscles may help to reduce blood pressure, and, therefore, to reduce the likelihood of developing anginal symptoms during functional activities of daily living.

Surgical intervention is directed at increasing the capacity of the coronary arteries to provide blood to the heart muscle. Critically narrowed sections of arteries can be identified by cardiac catheterization and angiography. Obstructions can be circumvented by grafts or removed by transluminal angioplasty, if the narrowing occurs in larger branches of the coronary arteries. The results of coronary artery bypass graft (CABG) surgery and angioplasty are determined more by the preoperative function of the patient's heart than by the patient's age.[17] In the absence of other severe coexisting disease, the elderly are good candidates for cardiac surgery.

Treatment of acute myocardial infarctions in the aged runs the gamut from infarct reduction (e.g., the use of enzymes such as streptokinase) and emergency angioplasty to comfort measures only. The determination of where in the spectrum of care the individual is most appropriately treated is a decision made jointly by the patient, physician, and family. In this area of medicine, as in few others, the conflict is so stark between the potentially dehumanizing technological imperative of modern treatment and the need to make treatment decisions on the basis of the patient's wishes and preferences. There are appropriate limits to treatment that are often lost in the attempt to apply the latest technology. Further discussion of this important issue is found in Chapter 16, Attitudes and Ethics.

Rehabilitation following myocardial infarction involves an integration of physical and occupational therapy to achieve maximal physical functioning, in addition to nutritional and medical interventions to control the progression of coronary artery disease. Much research has examined the interactions between physical activity and myocardial infarction, however, the general focus has been on middle-aged males even though infarction is more frequent in older age groups.[7,16,18] Two major risk factors, diabetes and hypertension, also become more prevalent with aging.[7]

Some of the postulated mechanisms of infarction (hemorrhage into an atherosclerotic plaque, impaction of an embolus from a fragmented plaque, and development of severe relative oxygen insufficiency) could be induced by vigorous physical activity.[17] However, other pathologies, such as the formation of a thrombus on an ulcerated plaque, seem more likely to occur when an individual is asleep. The histories obtained in nonfatal incidents of myocardial infarction suggest that about 25% were precipitated by physical activity, with exercise increasing the immediate risk by a factor of 6 to 12.[19-21] The potential risk during exercise is outweighed by the benefits of exercise.[16] In older age groups, a smaller proportion of ischemic heart disease deaths occurred suddenly, and, if all age groups are considered, the association between strenuous activity and death is rare.[7,22] A more extensive discussion of exercise intervention following myocardial infarction is provided in Chapter 13, Cardiopulmonary Treatment Considerations.

Cardiomyopathy

Cardiomyopathies are conditions in which the heart muscle hypertrophies and cardiac function is impaired.[8] The muscle of the heart weakens because of poor nutrition, toxins, infections, or genetic factors.[3] This weakening results in dilation of the heart and can lead to congestive heart failure because the heart cannot contract strongly enough to empty a sufficient amount of blood into the peripheral vasculature to meet the body's needs. Hypertrophy of cardiac muscle tissue can be the end results of hypertension, outflow obstruction, or genetic factors.[8] The cardiovascular changes imposed by cardiomyopathies impair function through several pathological mechanisms. The hypertrophied heart is stiff and does not easily fill with blood. As a result, the heart contracts vigorously, but there is little forward circulation to show for the effort, and the body's energy and oxygen needs are not met. In hypertrophic cardiomyopathy, the muscle abnormally contracts, actually creating an obstruction to the outflow of blood from the heart. The more strongly the heart contracts, the greater is the obstruction.

Exercise is often contraindicated in the patient with cardiomyopathy. Medical treatment is directed at correcting or ameliorating the pathophysiology of the underlying cause of the heart failure. Rehabilitative efforts need to be directed toward maintaining the maximal functional capabilities of the elderly individual and preventing the debilitating effects of immobility.

In dilated cardiomyopathies the heart is not strong enough to move blood against the pressure in the blood vessels.[23] As a result, fluid builds up in the pulmonary circulation and causes pulmonary edema, difficulty breathing, low blood oxygen, and further stress on the metabolic needs of the contracting cardiac muscle. Medical intervention is directed toward strengthening the heart's contraction using medications, such as digoxin. More effective emptying of the heart can be achieved if the pressure against which the heart can be achieved if the pressure against which the heart has to move blood is decreased. This is called afterload reduction.[24] Agents that reduce afterload include nitrates, peripheral vasodilators (e.g., prazocin, hydralazine), and other blood pressure lowering agents. Diuretics, which reduce the amount of fluid systemically (termed a preload reduction), also help to reduce pulmonary edema and improve cardiac efficiency.[16] In hypertrophic cardiomyopathy, the problem is the inability of the heart to adequately fill. The rapid, wormy contractions of the hypertrophic heart obstruct the outflow of blood. Dyastolic dysfunction arises when the heart does not adequately fill during its relaxation phase or diastole.[8] Two classes of medication have been found to be effective in improving the efficiency of the cardiac pump. Beta blockers (e.g., propranolol, metoprolol, timolol) and calcium channel blockers (e.g., diltiazem, nifedipine, verapamil) reduce the intensity and speed of cardiac muscle contraction, activating the slow twitch, anaerobic muscle fibers, and thereby improving the strength of muscle contraction. The beta blockers work by blocking the effect of epinephrine on heart muscle, because epinephrine promotes rapid and vigorous contractions. Calcium channel blockers affect the way in which calcium flows into and out of the cardiac muscle. Calcium plays an essential role in regulating the force of contractions.[25]

Conduction System Diseases

Conduction system diseases are those that affect the rate and rhythm of the heart's contractions.[8] The propagation of the electrical wave that results in the coordinated contraction of the heart muscle is initiated in the two pacemaker sites in the heart and is carried initially along specialized pathways, which spread the wave throughout the heart, also known as the conduction system. These pacemakers and pathways can be damaged by many different agents, including those that result in cardiomyopathies and myocardial infarction.[25] The most common consequences of pacemaker dysfunction are extremely rapid (tachycardiac) contractions, poorly coordinated (dysrhythmic) contractions, or extremely slow (bradycardiac) contractions that are less effective in moving blood and result in diminished cardiac output.[7] Low cardiac output can result in confusion, fatigue, poor exercise tolerance, and congestive heart failure. Rapid reductions in cardiac output can cause syncope.

Tachycardias and poorly coordinated rhythms, such as atrial fibrillation, are usually treated with medication to control the rate and convert the rhythm back to normal. Occasionally, electrical cardioversion is required.[8] Bradycardia is usually managed by surgical implantation of an artificial pacemaker, which can be set to trigger a heartbeat at a predetermined rate. Age, per se, is not a contraindication to pacemaker therapy, and the surgery is minor and well tolerated.

Valvular Disease of the Heart

The heart valves, which function to keep the blood flowing in one direction, tend to withstand many microtraumas throughout the life course. Defects of the heart valves are of two types. Stenosis or narrowing of the valve restricts blood flow,[8] and insufficiency or regurgitation results in the backward flow of blood. Both conditions increase the work load on the heart and greatly reduce its efficiency.[7] Two valves are most frequently involved. The mitral valve between the left atrium and ventricle, and the aortic valve, which moves the blood into the systemic circulation.

Rheumatic valve disease, caused by earlier episodes of rheumatic fever, is the most common cause of mitral stenosis and insufficiency in the aged.[25] Congestive heart failure, arrhythmias, and embolization of blood clots from the heart to the brain and other organs are the most common complications of mitral valve disease. These patients require attentive medical management, which includes the use of anticoagulants to prevent emboli, diuretics to control congestive heart failure, and digitalis or other medications to control the heart rate.[8] Nutritional support is often required to assure compliance with a low sodium diet. Because of the potentially serious side effects from too much anticoagulant (bleeding, hemorrhagic stroke) and digoxin (arrhythmias), their narrow range of effective dosages, and the deleterious effect of inadequate dosage, exercise must be gradually implemented and progressed slowly. Protective intervention should focus on skin protection and maintenance of maximal functional capabilities, with close monitoring of the elder's vital signs and subjective responses of perceived tolerance to increasing activity levels.

Surgical intervention to correct mitral stenosis needs to precede the development of fixed pulmonary hypertension and right heart failure.[8] Valve replacement and valvulotomy (where the valve is widened but not replaced) are done through open heart surgery. Transluminal valvulotomy, in which the valve is widened by using catheter-guided balloons, offers significantly lower operative risk in selected patients. Almost all patients continue to require medication for control of heart rate, prevention of emboli, and treatment of congestive heart failure. The response to gradually increasing levels of physical activity following surgery is usually favorable.[8]

Aortic valve disease is common in the aged and results from rheumatic valve disease, increasing damage to a congenitally misformed valve, or the progression of an age related injury to an otherwise normal valve.[25] The latter results from the gradual buildup of scar tissue and calcium on the valve leaflets as part of the normal aging of the valve. The most clinically significant lesion is stenosis of the aortic valve. This results in a progressive increase in the resistance to the flow of blood out of the heart, and, as a result, the heart pumps blood against an increasingly greater afterload.[8] Patients can experience angina even without coronary artery disease, because even normal coronary arteries are unable to deliver sufficient blood to meet the metabolic demands of the overtaxed heart muscle. As the stenosis increases, transient decreases in cardiac output due to arrhythmias or ischemia result in syncope.[7] Finally, when the heart is no longer able to compensate by hypertrophy for the increasing resistance to flow, congestive heart failure supervenes. Unlike previously discussed situations in which congestive heart failure occurs and is amenable to medical intervention, congestive heart failure in aortic stenosis carries a grave prognosis and can be effectively managed only by surgical replacement of the damaged valve.[8] Efforts need to be directed toward maintaining the maximal functional capabilities through exercise programs using activities of daily living as the exercise mode.

Infection of the heart valve, or endocarditis, is a rare but significant illness in the aged.[8] This is due not only to its potential for causing death or severe disability, but also because of its subtle presentation. Lethargy, fatigue, anorexia, failure to thrive, anemia, worsening congestive heart failure, progressive renal failure, low grade fever, embolic stroke or transient ischemic attack, worsening control of diabetes, and development of a new heart murmur are all potentially caused by bacterial endocarditis.[25] Early antibiotic therapy can be lifesaving. Exercise is contraindicated during the acute phase of endocarditis, but gradual resumption of activities of daily living can begin once the infection has been medically controlled.[7]

Hypertension

Hypertension is another common condition affecting the cardiovascular system. It is clear that the aged with systolic blood pressures above 160 mm Hg and diastolic pressures above 95 mm Hg are at increased risk for stroke, congestive heart failure (hypertensive cardiomyopathy), and renal failure. Isolated systolic hypertension carries a similar risk,[8] because much of the cardiovascular morbidity and mortality in the elderly is related to hypertension.[26] This is true for both isolated systolic hypertension and systolic–diastolic blood pressure elevations.[27] In addition to accelerated atherogenesis (myocardial infarction and congestive heart failure), hypertension adversely affects cardiac performance, renal function, and cerebral blood flow; increases aortic aneurysm rupture and dissection; and increases the incidence of cerebrovascular bleeding.[28]

Treatment to lower blood pressure significantly lowers the risk of developing these complications. Medical and dietary management are important in controlling hypertension. In the elderly, most recommendations are for drug treatment for blood pressure in excess of 160/95.[28] There is little evidence whether or not antihypertensive drug therapy alters the course of asymptomatic elderly individuals without evidence of end-organ damage from isolated systolic hypertension.

Nevertheless, isolated systolic hypertension doubles the risk of cardiovascular complications, so that the risk, expense, and inconvenience of drug therapy must be compared with the benefits of systolic blood pressure lowering. Compliance with medication and the early identification and avoidance of drug-induced side effects, such as dizziness, hypokalemia, depression, syncope, and confusion, are major challenges to the health care team. Complications of antihypertensive therapy are more frequent in the elderly individual, both because the diminution of renal function increases the incidence of drug toxicity and because the aged patient with less sensitive baroreceptor responses is more susceptible to the orthostatic complications of volume depletion. Gradually assuming the upright posture may avert dizziness and syncope. Exercise has been shown to have positive effects in reducing high blood pressure and is discussed extensively in Chapter 13, Cardiopulmonary Treatment Considerations. Control of hypertension has the potential to decrease cardiovascular morbidity and mortality.

Myocardial Degeneration

The general decline of cardiac performance with age and inactivity affects the elderly individual's abilities to function at their maximum. The recognized changes in cardiac function include a decrease in right ventricular work rate and a variable change of left ventricular work rate depending on the relative magnitudes of the reduction in maximum cardiac output and the increase of systemic blood pressure.[7,29] While a young person readily accepts a sustained increase of cardiac work rate, in old age an equivalent relative stress may give rise to cardiac failure, particularly if there are other circulatory problems, such as a high systemic blood pressure, a minor disorder of the heart valves, or an excessive intake of fluids. Complaints of shortness of breath in the elderly frequently reflect problems with getting enough oxygen to the working muscle through a failing circulatory system.

The exact reason for a reduction in myocardial function has not been determined. Some authors suggest that it is part of the normal aging process and can be attributed to the wasting of the heart muscle, the loss of elasticity with the slowing of cardiac relaxation,[30] the fibrotic changes in the heart valves, and a modification of catecholamine production or sensitivity.[29] Others suggest that amyloidosis (tissue proteinosis) may precipitate degeneration of cardiac muscle tissue and lead to failure. Pomerance[31] found amyloid material in the hearts of 12% of subjects who died after the age of 80 years from cardiac failure. Other authors have argued that lack of oxygen by numerous repetitive microtraumas to the myocardium leads to myocardial degeneration.[32] They found that cardiac function was well perserved in those with a good myocardial oxygen supply, however, a high proportion of their sample population failed to satisfy that criteria and had chronic oxygen supply problems according to ECG and scintigraphic evidence. On autopsy, most older people showed both atheromatous plaques and small myocardial scars, so ischemic changes over the lifetime could be responsible for impaired cardiac function.[31]

Individuals with a seriously reduced cardiac reserve report a marked need for rest even after mild physical activity.[33] In addition to persistent and undue fatigue, an inadequate cardiac response to exercise usually causes acute shortness of breath (dyspnea), while a restriction of blood flow to the heart itself may produce anginal pain. Inadequate blood flow to the peripheral tissues may give the skin a bluish hue (peripheral cyanosis). The pulse rate typically rises over the day, with a slow and incomplete recovery during rest pauses.[7] Activities of daily living are notably difficult for these elderly individuals. Lying down can induce a sharp reoccurrence or increase of dyspnea and create a "fear of sleeping" that further adds to the severe fatigue experienced on minimal activity by an individual with myocardial degeneration.

The ankle edema of cardiac failure needs to be distinguished from problems of venous drainage. Improper application of modalities, such as a Jobst intermittent compression boot, or elevation of the lower extremities above the horizontal plane could be detrimental to the elderly individual in cardiac failure, whereas they would be quite effective in positively modifying the problems encountered with venous return pathologies. In cardiac failure, a delay in the S_3 sound, a so-called "gallop rhythm," is indicative of a delay in left ventricular filling.[8]

Adverse reactions to exercise in the individual with congestive heart failure (cardiac failure) include an absence of the anticipated rise of systemic blood pressure, an accumulation of a substantial oxygen debt, and a slow recovery of heart rate and ventilation after cessation of the effort.[7] Cardiac stroke volume decreases rather than increases as the intensity of work is augmented. Myocardial contractility is also impaired.

While there is probably merit in persuading subjects with diffuse myocardial disease to preserve existing function through cautiously prescribed effort, the intensity of such activity must be held below the level at which left ventricular failure begins to occur. Once failure has developed, there is little alternative to a combination of traditional medical therapy and rest until the heart is again operating on the favorable (compensated) portion of its pressure/volume reserve.[7] The reduction of muscle mass and decrease of renal function increases the circulatory half-life of digoxin,[34] although the inotropic effect on the heart is diminished with aging.[35] Beta-blocking agents may worsen the tendency to cardiac failure, as may alcohol abuse.[36]

Peripheral Vascular Disease

Peripheral vascular disease is frequently the result of untreated hypertension, cigarette smoking, diabetes mellitus, and elevated serum cholesterol.[25] Atherosclerosis and other forms of peripheral vascular disease can lead to partial or complete obstruction of the main arterial supply to the limbs. The consequences of this are intermittent claudication with walking and skin lesions that may lead to amputation.[7] When early intervention to reduce risk factors is unsuccessful, management is through the modification of diet to reduce weight and cholesterol, medications to enhance blood flow and reduce blood pressure, and behavior modifications to reduce cigarette consumption. Exercise is particularly helpful in treating peripheral vascular disease from a preventative perspective.[7] Buerger-Allen exercises improve the vitality of the peripheral vascular system and impact on back and lower extremity flexibility and strength. They also serve to decrease the debilitating effects of postural hypotension by facilitating adjustment to postural positional changes. Surgical intervention is effective in cases of symptomatic peripheral vascular disease that results in resting pain, claudication, or nonhealing ulcers.[8] As in coronary artery disease, partial obstructions of peripheral arteries, most commonly in the lower extremities, can be treated with bypass grafting or by dilating the obstructed section of the artery using transluminal angioplasty.

Intermittent claudication is muscular pain that, analogous to anginal pain, reflects an acute lack of oxygen to the working muscles. The level of discomfort depends on the level of peripheral vascular obstruction.[37] The condition is seen most often in the elderly, and the subsequent mortality of the claudicant patient is high. A minor orthopedic anomaly, such as a hammer or claw toe, can develop a lesion that can lead to a gangrenous lesion due to the absence of an adequate blood supply in the affected extremity.[37] Immobility created by a gangrenous lesion can lead to depression and renal complications, and death is frequently the result of a coronary thrombosis or hemorrhage.[38]

Amputation is required for the relief of pain and to stop the spread of infection (gangrene) in those patients for whom other surgical procedures are impossible. When an individual has both diabetes and peripheral vascular disease, there is about a 5% incidence of amputations per year.[37] Because the patient's ability to ambulate is greatly affected by the level at which the amputation is performed, the most distal site is preferred. However, the amputation must be performed at a level where there is sufficient blood supply to assure adequate healing. Progressive amputations and a whole lot of immobility is usually required if the amputation is below the area of adequate blood supply and the incision does not heal. The result is that the patient is exposed to the risks of surgery again.

Loss of a limb is a traumatic event. Often the process of grieving must begin before the actual surgery and is helped by contributions from social service, psychiatry, nursing, and rehabilitative services. Depression is a major impediment to the successful rehabilitation of these patients and must be addressed if intensive nursing and physical therapy are to be successful.

PULMONARY MANIFESTATIONS OF AGING

The respiratory system functions to assure the exchange of oxygen and carbon dioxide between the air and the blood within the lungs. This system can be thought of as having several related but separate components: movement of air into and out of the lungs, the exchange of oxygen and carbon dioxide, and the defense of the lung from infection. Changes with age affect every aspect of the respiratory system.

The chest wall becomes a less efficient bellows with age. The anteroposterior diameter of the chest increases and the rib cage becomes more rigid as progressive curviture of the spine, calcification of costal cartilage, and osteoporosis limit the compliance of the chest wall. The chest muscles atrophy with age and also contribute to the gradual decline in the efficiency with which air is moved into and out of the lungs. The collapse of small airways due to the loss of elasticity of lung tissue with age results in increasing resistance to air flow. As a result, the amount of physical effort that must go into breathing increases by 20% between the ages of 20 and 70.[23]

Although the bronchi are not usually affected by normal aging, the surface area of the alveoli decreases by 4% for each decade of life.[18] The aveolar wall is also thinner and contains fewer capillaries for the delivery of blood. The size of the alveoli increases due to the loss of elasticity and recoil. It is the loss of recoil that creates increased susceptibility to airway collapse, the major factor contributing to the altered distribution of air within the lungs.

Ideally, each area of the lung where blood is available for gas exchange would be ventilated, creating a perfect match of ventilation and perfusion. With age, larger areas of the lung are perfused but are not ventilated because of airway collapse and redistribution of blood flow.[7] This results in the return of unoxygenated blood to the general circulation and decreased efficiency of the respiratory system. Pulmonary circulation may also decline with age, further reducing the capacity of the system to respond to the demand for an increased supply of oxygen to tissues.

Changing mechanics within the lung and chest wall also make the lung more susceptible to infection with age. The gag reflex is diminished, thereby increasing the risk of aspiration. Concurrently, the cough reflex is also diminished and the effectiveness of the cough is reduced because of a reduced chest wall compliance and chest muscle strength. Ciliary action, which normally moves secretions up and out of the lungs, also declines, particularly in smokers. These factors combine to compromise the lung's ability to defend against infection. Some drugs play important roles in depressing the respiratory system. Sedative and analgesics, such as alcohol and narcotics, are known to depress respiration and dull the cough and gag reflexes, thus predisposing the elderly person to the risks of hypoxia and aspiration pneumonia.

The two most common types of disease affecting the respiratory system are pneumonias, which compromise gas exchange and serve as a source of sepsis, and diseases that affect the amount of air flow in the lungs, such as chronic obstructive lung disease (COPD) and emphysema.

Pneumonia

Pneumonia is the most common infectious cause of death in the elderly[39] and the most common infection requiring hospitalization. It is often the cause of death for patients with other serious conditions, such as diabetes, cancer, stroke, congestive heart failure, dementia, and renal failure. The increased incidence of pneumonia with aging is due in part to the weakening of the local pulmonary defenses; however, the high mortality of pneumonia is largely due to its more subtle presentation in the elderly. Typical symptoms, such as a productive cough, fever, and pleuritic chest pain, are frequently absent, but subtler symptoms, such as confusion, alteration of sleep–wake cycles, increased congestive heart failure, anorexia, and failure to thrive, are more common. Misdiagnosis and late diagnosis are common and contribute to the high mortality of pneumonia in the aged.[39]

Successful treatment of pneumonia requires early recognition and institution of proper antibiotic therapy. The identification of the causative bacteria in the examination of a sputum sample is the single most important diagnostic test for determining initial antibiotic therapy. Unfortunately, such samples are often difficult to obtain in a dehydrated and confused elderly patient, and, as a result, therapy is often empirical and not as specifically directed or as effective as possible. Hydration, nutritional support, chest physical therapy, and treatment of complicating illnesses are often required in addition to antibiotics.

Obstructive Lung Disease

Conditions that cause obstruction to airflow within the lungs are called obstructive airway diseases. They share the common characteristic of increased resistance to airflow within the airways.[23] Asthma is a reversible obstructive airway disease characterized by episodic increases in airway resistance due to spasms and narrowing of airways in response to infection, allergic reactions, and environmental conditions. Chronic obstructive pulmonary disease (COPD) denotes conditions of increased airway resistance that are irreversible because of permanent structural damage resulting from cigarette smoking, infections, toxic exposures, or any combination of these.

Emphysema is a term used to describe the permanent destruction of aveoli with the resulting expansion of the remaining aveoli. A consequence of emphysema is the reduction of the area in which gas exchange can occur, which results in perfusion/ventilation mismatch and hypoxia. Emphysema is associated with increased airway resistance due to the collapse of small airways.

Chronic bronchitis is a different disease process in which there is chronic inflammation of the small airways with resulting increased mucus, airway plugging, and destruction of small airways.[39] As a consequence, airflow is reduced because of the permanent narrowing of the small airways. There is often a reversible component of the airway obstruction superimposed on the chronic changes. Cigarette smoking is the leading cause of chronic bronchitis and multiplies the deleterious effects of other environmental agents, such as asbestos, silica, coal dust, and fibers. Frequently, emphysema and chronic bronchitis coexist.

Patients with obstructive airway diseases usually manifest disabilities that result either from hypoxia, hypercapnia, or dyspnea. Both hypoxia and hypercapnia can cause confusion, fatigue, and worsening heart failure. Breathlessness, or dyspnea, is usually the most limiting symptom of COPD. Functional impairment due to COPD can be severe, and COPD is often fatal. Over half of the patients die within 2 years of their first episode of respiratory failure.[40,41] These patients require extensive therapeutic and supportive interventions.

The treatment goal of individuals with COPD is to prevent smoking and maintain optimum functioning for as long as possible. This usually involves chest physical therapy, medication, oxygen therapy, and environmental changes designed to reduce exertion. The depression that accompanies chronic illness of all types can be particularly significant in COPD patients, many of whom feel that they have brought it on themselves by smoking. Because of its complexity, COPD is an excellent example of a health problem that requires an interdisciplinary approach.

MUSCULAR MANIFESTATIONS OF AGING

The musculoskeletal system is composed of muscles, tendons, the fascia, the bony skeleton, and joints (including ligaments and cartilage). The individual experiences a gradual decrease in strength, control, and mobility as the components of this system age.

Muscle Changes with Aging

Muscle alterations are complex and poorly understood, because the composition of muscles changes over time with the replacement of myofibrils by fat, collagen, and scar tissue. Individual muscle fibrils also change in their permeability to water, sodium, and chloride, which increases with age.[7] Blood flow to muscles decreases with age, thereby reducing the amount of nutrients and energy available to the muscle, and muscle strength declines.[42] This process begins early in life and accelerates rapidly after the fifth decade, especially when it is overshadowed by inactivity. By age 60, the total loss in lean muscle mass represents 10% to 20% of the maximum muscle power attained at age 30.[7]

Myopathy and Myositis

Muscle dysfunction in the aged is usually the result of toxic or metabolic factors acting on muscle, rather than to any intrinsic disease of the muscle.[43] Symptoms suggesting myopathy include weakness in the hip girdle muscles, made apparent by the person's increasing difficulty rising from a chair, and the development of a waddling gait or shoulder girdle weakness, manifested by an inability to lift objects above shoulder level. Muscle soreness is not a usual finding with myopathy and is more common with myositis, where there is infiltration of muscles by inflammation.[44] Polymyositis can be ideopathic or related to the presence of an underlying carcinoma. Myositis usually responds to steroids or other anti-inflammatory agents.

Muscle weakness can result from several correctable causes, including hyperthyroidism, alcoholism, adrenocortical steroid excess (Cushing's disease or administration of steroids), and hypokalemia (from diarrhea or diuretic use). Correction of the underlying cause usually results in the resolution of the weakness.[42]

SKELETAL MANIFESTATIONS OF AGING

Aging brings about many complex and poorly understood changes in bone structure. Until about the age of 45, bone mass increases in both men and women, but over the next 25 years both sexes show a progressive decline in bone mass, with women losing about 25% and men approximately 12%.[45] Although bone growth continues into old age, resorption of the interior of the long and flat bones (trabecular bones) increases until resorption occurs at a greater rate than the formation of new bone. As a result bone strength and stability decline. This is particularly true of trabecular bone, which is found in the highest proportions in vertebral bodies, wrists, and hips. This correlates with the clinical observation of increased incidence of fractures of these bones with age.[46]

Osteoporosis and Osteomalacia

Osteoporosis is a heterogeneous condition characterized by an absolute decrease in the amount of normal bone (i.e., loss of bone). Osteoporosis results when the production of new bone mass is exceeded by the resorption of old bone, in other words, osteoporosis is the failure of bone formation to keep pace with bone resorption. This is termed coupling. The result is that the bone becomes structurally weakened. Osteoporosis is due neither to a lack of dietary calcium nor to defective bone mineralization,[45] rather it is caused by endosteal resorption, which is greater than the formation of new osteons or bone units.[47] Age related trabecular bone loss starts at age 35, and cortical bone loss starts at about age 40. The loss proceeds at about 0.5% per year; but, at female menopause, the accelerated rate is 2.0% to 8.0% due directly or indirectly to lowered estrogen production.[45] The greater the bone mass attained at the time resorption exceeds the creation of new bone, the more time is needed before significant structural changes result. This, in part, accounts for the higher incidence of clinically significant osteoporosis in women than in men because men have greater bone mass.

The reasons for the differential rates of demineralization of bone between men and women are not understood, but there are several factors that appear to have a role in the process. For example, estrogen deficiency occurring with menopause leads to an accelerated bone loss and is partially reversed by replacing estrogen.[45] Other factors contributing to skeletal weakness include malabsorption of calcium leading to poor bone mineralization (osteomalacia) that affects both sexes. A negative calcium balance can result from many factors, such as calcium deficiency in the diet, malabsorption, and accelerated loss. Impaired absorption of calcium from the intestine can be due to insufficient vitamin D because of diet, or renal or hepatic disease. Calcium absorption can be affected as part of intestinal malabsorption syndromes, such as sprue and regional enteritis.[48] Endocrine disorders affecting calcium balance include hyperthyroidism; excess corticosteroids, as in Cushing's disease or steroid administration; and hyperparathyroidism leading to excess bone resorption as well as hypoparathyroidism resulting in poor calcium absorption. Immobility for any reason and at any age can lead to marked negative calcium balance. When a limb is immobilized, localized osteoporosis occurs.[6]

Thus, for the elderly, decreased mobility for any reason adds to the already abundant factors present for the development of osteoporosis. The presence of osteoporosis requires a thorough review of potentially treatable causes. Treatment is a judicious balance of exercise, medication, and dietary manipulation.

Calcium supplementation does nothing to prevent postmenopausal bone loss in women undergoing menopause or who have undergone menopause within 5 years prior to treatment. In women who are postmenopausal by 6 or more years, calcium citrate malate can significantly reduce bone loss at a dosage of 800 mg/day.[46] Riis and associates[49] suggest that calcium supplementation may have a minor effect on the loss of cortical bone, but it does not effect on trabecular bone.

The importance of osteoporosis relates to the incidence of bone fracture in postmenopausal females. Women are postmenopausal for 40% of their lives. Symptomatic osteoporosis affects one in three of the older female population and results in more than 175,000 femur fractures and 500,000 vertebral fractures per year in American women.[50] Fracture of the femur is a major contributor to mortality in the elderly. Activity (particularly weight bearing activity), calcitonin, sodium fluoride, a calcium intake of 1500 mg/day, and vitamin D 400–600 IU/day may possibly retard further bone loss.[50] Boron supplementation may reduce the urinary excretion of calcium and magnesium and elevate the concentration of 17 β-estradiol,[51] thus, inhibiting the normal bone losses of aging. Calcium supplementation is thought to inhibit immunoreactive and parathyroid hormone (PTH) secretion as levels of PTH increase with age in response to diminished levels of extracellular fluid calcium. Estrogen replacement therapy may retard the normal bone loss of aging, but the protective effect may last no longer than 2 to 3 years after termination of treatment.[52]

Although the entire skeleton loses mass with aging, the distribution of bone loss is not uniform. Those areas of the skeleton with the highest content of trabecular bone, such as vertebral bodies and bones of the wrists and hips, will lose the greatest amount of mass.[47]

Joint Changes with Aging

Degenerative changes in joints begin as early as the second or third decade, and after age 40 progress more rapidly.[53] These changes occur mainly in weight bearing joints, such as ankles, knees, hips, and lumbar spine. Cartilage forms the weight bearing surfaces of these joints. By age 30, it begins to crack, shred, and fray. Over time, deep vertical fissures appear, and the cartilage producing cells die or become less effective. Ultimately, the cartilage layers are eroded, exposing the bone beneath to direct contact with the opposing bone.[54] This contact causes pain and produces the physical sign of crepitus, or grinding, when the joint is moved. New bone formation is stimulated, but the bone growth is irregular. Often, it interferes with joint mobility as the resulting osteophytes enlarge. Synovial membranes, which surround and protect joints, also exhibit changes due to age. With age, the synovial lining thickens and the synovial fluid becomes more viscous. Other changes include the shrinkage of the intervertebral discs in the lumbar spine due to loss of water content in the discs.[54] Coupled with vertebral body collapse, disc shrinkage can produce a significant loss of height. The aging changes associated with bone, cartilage, and synovial membranes are dealt with extensively in Chapter 3.

Degenerative Arthritis/Osteoarthritis

Arthritis is an inflammation within the joint space that causes pain, loss of mobility, and deformity of the joint. There are several different types of arthritis, but all lead to a common final pathway known as degenerative joint disease (DJD) or osteoarthritis.[55] Recurrent joint trauma leads to intra-articular damage, resulting in the release of proteolytic enzymes that often cause bleeding. A cycle is set up with increased cartilage damage, bleeding, and the release of potentially destructive enzymes. Over time, cartilage is eroded, new bone growth stimulated, and the joint gradually loses its ability to respond to trauma, making it even more susceptible to additional trauma and damage.[54] Pain develops from irritation of the periosteum, joint capsule, and fibrotic changes of the periarticular muscles. Unlike rheumatoid arthritis, the synovial membrane in osteoarthritis is not the primary site of involvement. However, over time it can become fibrotic as a result of the primary degenerative process.[55]

The joints most often affected by DJD are the hands, knees, hips, lumbar, and cervical spine. It is manifested clinically by stiffness and pain that increases with use. Impaired mobility makes it difficult to accomplish routine activities of daily living (ADLs).[56]

The development of effective anti-inflammatory medications and the improvement of surgical interventions in joint disease has changed the current management of end stage DJD. Joint replacement can be very effective in restoring function and limiting pain, and joint fusion and anti-inflammatory medications are often effective in pain control.

Rheumatoid Arthritis

Rheumatoid arthritis can occur at any age and is characterized by the abrupt onset of symmetrical joint swelling, erythema, and pain. Inflammation of the synovial membrane results in the release of proteolytic enzymes that perpetuate inflammation and joint damage.[54] Morning stiffness is more pronounced and of longer duration than in DJD. The involved joints tend to be the small joints of the hands and feet, the wrists, shoulders, elbows, hips, knees, and ankles. Essentially every joint is involved in this autoimmune, systemic condition. Eventually deformities occur affecting mobility and basic ADLs. Rheumatoid arthritis is a systemic disease, therefore, other signs and symptoms are often present, including: fever, fatigue, malaise, poor appetite, weight loss, nutritional deficiencies, weakness, anemia, enlarged spleen, and lymphadenopathy (disease of the lymph nodes).[55] Response to therapy is usually quite good. Given the ease with which the aged develop muscle atrophy with disuse, aggressive physical therapy is essential to maintain strength and joint mobility during phases of remission. During exacerbation, physical therapy should be directed toward pain management through decreasing swelling in the joint (ice, electrical stimulation), maintaining joint mobility, and decreasing discomfort (oscillation joint mobility techniques, active motion), and encouraging participation in functional ADLs.

Gout

Gout is a form of arthritis that usually affects only a few joints. Needle-like crystals of uric acid are deposited in joints, tendons, and bursae, and they incite a rapidly progressive inflammatory reaction. The result is the abrupt onset of severe pain and the development of an acutely tender and inflamed joint that can incapacitate the individual very rapidly. In middle age, gout is episodic, but, in later years it tends to occur with greater frequency and in more joints.[23] Gout tends to affect men more than women. It occurs spontaneously or as a result of other illnesses or treatments. Some diuretics used to treat congestive heart failure or hypertension may cause gout because they interfere with the secretion of uric acid from the kidney, thereby causing an elevated uric acid level. Other causes of gout include rapid tissue turnover, such as seen in lymphoma, leukemia, thalassemia, psoriasis, and pernicious anemia. Acidosis of any cause, such as diabetes, alcohol, or renal failure, can also precipitate gout. Treatment is medical, and the prognosis for preventing permanent joint deformity is good if treatment is undertaken early in the course of chronic gout.[53]

Temporal Arteritis/Polymyalgia Rheumatica

Inflammation of small- and medium-sized arteries that are derived from the aortic arch give rise to a condition called giant cell arteritis or temporal arteritis (TA). It is part of a spectrum of conditions that include the entity of polymyalgia rheumatica (PMR), which is only seen in individuals over the age of 50.[23] Neck and hip girdle stiffness and pain, an elevated sedimentation rate, low grade anemia, fever, weight loss, elevated globulins, and rapid response to steroids are the characteristics of polymyalgia rheumatica. Of the greatest clinical significance is the high incidence of sudden monoccular blindness that can occur from the obliteration of the ophthalmic artery by the arteritis.[57] This potential outcome requires early and aggressive evaluation and treatment of anyone suspected of having PMR/TA. Diagnosis is established by biopsy of the temporal artery looking for evidence of arteritis. The biopsy is positive in approximately 50% of cases;[9] however, a negative result on biopsy does not exclude the presence of PMR/TA. It is a relapsing, systemic disease that usually responds to steroids and resolves over 1 to 2 years. It is one of the most common preventable causes of blindness in the aged.

NEUROMUSCULAR MANIFESTATIONS OF AGING

Central Nervous System

Central nervous system (CNS) impairment is a leading cause of functional disability in the aged.[25] The normal process of aging results in the gradual diminution of size and number of cells in all locations within the CNS.[9] The size and weight of the brain declines with age as demonstrated by autopsy and computed axial tomography (CAT) scan results.[50] Metabolic activity declines as measured by oxygen consumption and blood flow, and the conduction rate of peripheral nerves declines steadily.[7] Of great interest, however, is the observation that the changes of normal aging do not result in significant neurological impairment.[25] Although there is a steady diminution of the components of the CNS over time, there is no associated neurological deficit that can be ascribed solely to aging.

Unimpaired, normal aging occurs in the majority of elderly persons. The development of chronic, severe cognitive impairment, however, occurs in nearly 30% of individuals over the age of 80.[25] The functional impairments resulting from CNS dysfunction can be severe. It is useful to think of them as resulting from changes in cognition (such as judgment, comprehension, memory), changes in sensory input (blindness, deafness, neuropathy), and changes in ability to execute actions (paralysis, gait disorders, loss of coordination, incontinence, aphasia). Alterations of capacity in any of these spheres can result from and cause alterations in psychiatric performance as well.

The final common pathways of neurological dysfunction are the transcortical tracts. They involve cognitive functioning, movement, sensation, and sensory integration of movement. A multiplicity of specific diseases and conditions result in dysfunction within these realms. Some are preventable, and early medical intervention is essential. Others are relentlessly progressive and do not respond to disease-specific interventions. In these conditions, interventions are directed at achieving the individual's maximal functional level. The following sections are a brief and greatly simplified survey of the more common types of neurological diseases in the aged.

Confusion/Delirium

Cognitive disorders of all types account for nearly two thirds of nursing home admissions and a significant majority of those elderly persons who are incapacitated by illness.[59] Severe cognitive dysfunction may not impair an individual's longevity, especially with meticulous attention to treatable complicating illnesses. As a result, the aged with cognitive dysfunction make up the largest group of functionally disabled individuals.

Those conditions resulting in alterations in cognitive function can be divided into several groups on the basis of reversibility and chronicity. Acute cognitive dysfunction of rapid onset without underlying damage to brain tissue carries the best prognosis for recovery. This usually results from toxic or metabolic derangements that affect the normal functioning of the brain or from a psychiatric illness, such as depression, that also has a metabolic basis. The term delirium is used to describe these acute confusional states. Susceptibility to toxic/metabolic delirium (toxic encephalopathy) is not limited to the elderly; however, the more limited metabolic reserve of the aging brain makes the elderly person more sensitive than a younger person to minor stresses.

Confusion, restlessness, agitation, poor attention span, reversal of sleep–wake cycles, hallucinations, and paranoia can all be manifestations of delirium. Subtle changes resulting from correctable toxic/metabolic abnormalities can persist for extended periods before they are recognized as resulting from potentially reversible causes. Appropriate interventions are frequently delayed. It is particularly important for these reversible conditions to be identified by the health care team because failure to intervene in a timely manner can cause permanent cognitive dysfunction. Equally important is the risk that inappropriate treatment will result in further functional impairment or a greatly increased risk of injury. Pathological brain dysfunction resulting from toxic/metabolic causes usually has a good recovery prognosis when the underlying abnormality is corrected. Table 5–1 lists the more common causes of toxic confusion/delirium in the elderly.

Interventions are directed at identifying and correcting the underlying metabolic abnormality. Although the prognosis for a return to baseline CNS function is usually good with correction of the abnormality, the patient's overall prognosis is often determined by the underlying disease that caused the metabolic abnormality rather than the degree of brain dysfunction. During a confusional state, however,

TABLE 5–1. COMMON CAUSES OF TOXIC/METABOLIC CONFUSION/DELIRIUM IN THE ELDERLY

Drugs	Metabolic Abnormalities
Alcohol	Hypoglycemia
Psychotropics (tranquilizers, antipsychotics, antidepressants)	Hyponatremia
Over-the-counter sleep, cold, and allergy medications	Hypocalcemia
Analgesics	Hypothermia
Antihypertensives	Hypothyroidism
Beta-blockers (propranolol)	Hypoxia
Antiparkinsonian medications	Vitamin B_{12} deficiency
Anticonvulsants (phenobarital, phenylantoin, carbamazepine)	Cortisol deficiency
Digoxin	Hepatic failure (elevated ammonia)
H_2 blockers (cimetadine)	Renal failure (elevated BUN, creatine)
Amphetamines	Elevated cortisol
	Pulmonary failure (elevated carbon dioxide)

the individual is more prone to accidental injury, complications such as aspiration pneumonia, and further cognitive dysfunction due to inappropriate use of sedatives that may aggravate rather than relieve the agitation. The occurrence of any of these complications may worsen the overall prognosis for recovery. Acute toxic/metabolic delirium may coexist with chronic progressive forms of brain dysfunction, such as Alzheimer's disease.

Dementias

Dementias are characterized by the slow onset of increasing intellectual impairment, including disorientation, memory loss, diminished ability to reason and make sound judgments, loss of social skills, and the development of regressed or antisocial behavior.[60] Frequently, depression is superimposed on dementia as a reaction to the perceived loss of intellectual skills and leads to further cognitive impairment.[61]

Alzheimer's disease and multi-infarct dementia are the two most common forms of irreversible dementia. Each has a fairly characteristic pattern of onset and findings. Alzheimer's disease is usually slowly progressive and begins insidiously. It is not associated with focal neurological deficits or abrupt changes in severity. Patients typically begin with short-term memory deficits and progress to severely regressed behavior, an inability to learn or remember new tasks, and a loss of ability to perform ADLs.[62] Multi-infarct dementia is usually of more rapid onset, occurs in younger individuals, and progresses in a step-wise fashion with abrupt worsening and subsequent plateaus of function. Frequently, there are focal neurological deficits, such as paresis and parethesias.[63] Often, the individual is hypertensive, diabetic, or both. He or she may also show evidence of generalized atherosclerosis.[64]

It is important to distinguish between Alzheimer's and multi-infarct dementias. The prevention of recurrent cerebral infarction may arrest the progression of multi-infarct dementia, which has as its pathophysiological basis irreversible brain damage resulting from repetitive ischemic injury caused by emboli or bleeding. Normalization of blood pressure is the most effective intervention known. Other types of reversible dementia, such as those resulting from hypothyroidism, vitamin B_{12} deficiency, and normal pressure hydrocephalus, can become "fixed" and unresponsive to treatment unless identified and treated at an early stage. Early identification of these correctable dementias is essential. Unfortunately, no such therapeutic imperative exists for Alzheimer's disease, which is of unclear etiology and without treatment at this time.

Regardless of the etiology of dementia, once reversible causes have been ruled out, the main tasks of the clinical team are to minister to the patient's emotional needs, assist in the act of grieving for lost function, alter the environment so that the patient's remaining skills can be used, augment the patient's capacity to successfully undertake ADLs, educate the family, provide emotional and physical support for the family and caretakers, and provide the patient and family with a realistic prognosis. Any superimposed illness can cause a rapid and prolonged decline in mental status, which may totally resolve as the underlying illness is treated.

Cerebrovascular Diseases

In contrast to the dementing illnesses that result in "global" brain dysfunction, cerebrovascular diseases more commonly result in focal brain dysfunction.[64] There are several different types of cerebrovascular disease, each with a different pathophysiological mechanism, prognosis, and treatment. The mechanisms include the rupture of small blood vessels from hypertension, abrupt blockage of vessels by emboli from the heart or atheramatous plaques in the large arteries leading to the brain, and spontaneous formation of blood clots within the blood vessels due to local increases in coagulability. The pathophysiology of cerebrovascular disease is the interruption of blood flow to brain tissue with resultant cell damage or death from ischemia.[7] Decreases in the heart's ability to pump blood can lead to ischemia, as can blockage of the blood vessels to or within the brain from atheromatous plaque, emboli, or inflammation of the lining of the blood vessels. Uncontrolled hypertension, diabetes mellitus, smoking, and elevated cholesterol contribute to cerebrovascular disease directly by affecting the entire circulatory system.

Preventive interventions must be specifically directed at the underlying pathophysiology. Hypertension can be controlled by medication, diet, and exercise. The prevention of emboli usually requires the use of anticoagulants, such as aspirin, dipyridamole, and warfarin. The risk of bleeding, both into the brain and into other organs, increases with the use of these agents and often limits their use in certain patients. If emboli result from cardiac arrhythmias, prevention results from a return to normal sinus rhythm through the use of electrical cardioversion or antiarrhythmics, such as quinidine, procainamide, and digoxin.[25] Because of the heightened risk of intracerebral bleeding, anticoagulants are avoided in the presence of hypertension and in cerebral vascular accidents that result from bleeding into brain tissue.

Recurrent, small cerebral vascular accidents can result in multi-infarct dementia. More commonly, however, limited areas of the brain are damaged and result in more focal disabilities, including the loss of motor or sensory function over the right or left side of the body and alterations in vision, speech, and the ability to interpret sensory inputs. The extent of the deficit following a stroke depends on the location and function of the injured part of the brain, the degree of damage, and the availability of unaffected regions of the brain that can assume the lost function. Residual effects can be so subtle as to be functionally negligible or so extensive that only the most basic brain functions, such as the control of respiration and blood pressure, are preserved.

Parkinson's Disease

Parkinson's disease is a progressive degenerative disease of unknown cause resulting in the loss of melanin containing brain cells in the substantia nigra and locus ceruleus and a decrease of dopamine in the caudate nucleus and putamen. The term Parkinson's disease is reserved for those cases of unknown etiology.[65]

Parkinson's syndrome is used to describe the same constellation of anatomical, motor, and intellectual deficits that result from specific agents. These include postencephalitic (von Economo's disease), post-traumatic (boxer's parkinsonism), and toxin induced (Haldol). Similar movement disorders often result from the use of neuroleptics or reserpine but are not associated with any anatomical changes.

Parkinsonism is a commonly occurring syndrome in the aged.[65] When fully developed, there is characteristic increased limb rigidity, stooped posture, shuffling gait, decreased mental acuity, difficulty initiating movement, and tremor that is usually symmetrical, rhythmic, and abolished by intentional movement. Early in its course, however, parkinsonism may give an asymmetrical tremor, a slight increase in muscle tone with associated decrease in spontaneous movement, a masking of the face with loss of spontaneous expression, and a generalized rigidity in muscle tone. As these restrictions on voluntary movement progress, they result in significant functional impairment. Associated incontinence and constipation further complicate the management of these individuals.

Benign familial tremor is often mistaken for Parkinson's disease early in its course. Characteristically, the tremor is more rapid (7 to 9 per second) and increases with movement. As a result, patients complain of an inability to lift a spoon or cup without spilling its contents. There is no associated hypokinesia or gait disorder. Alcohol, sedatives, and beta-blockers (such as propranolol) effectively reduce the amplitude of the tremor.[66]

In parkinsonism, drug treatment and intensive physical therapy are frequently helpful, however, these interventions do not change the relentless progression of functional impairments. Drug therapy is directed at the amelioration of symptoms at the lowest effective dose. Drugs are of three general classes: (1) those that are anticholinergic, (2) those that mimic the effects of dopamine (such as bromocriptine), and (3) those that replete dopamine (L-dopa). Physical therapy to maintain strength, improve posture, prevent contractures, and maintain the maximal functional capabilities of the individual with parkinsonism is crucial. Despite the progressive nature of this illness, many patients can maintain full function for several decades with a combination of physical therapy and drug intervention.[67]

Normal Pressure Hydrocephalus

Normal pressure hydrocephalus is common in the elderly.[25] It presents with the clinical triad of dementia, slow, shuffling gait, and urinary incontinence. Dilation of the ventricles with hydrocephalus is thought to affect the function of the surrounding brain tissue that controls lower extremity movement and bladder function. CAT scan of the head can establish the presence of ventricular enlargement but cannot determine whether it is due to atrophy of brain tissue or the enlargement of the ventricles. However, in selected cases that have shown clinical improvement after repeated removal of cerebrospinal fluid, placement of a surgical shunt occasionally results in resolution of the dementia, incontinence, and gait disorder.[23]

Cervical Spondylosis

Cervical spondylosis is caused by the impingement upon the cervical spinal cord of bony spurs resulting from severe degenerative arthritis.[23] Patients usually develop a clumsy, spastic, and stiff gait, incontinence, and diminished sensation in the lower extremities. Cervical CAT scanning, myelograms, and magnetic resonance imaging (MRI) can establish the location and extent of spinal cord impingement. Surgical decompression of the spinal cord may be necessary to interrupt the progression of this condition and its associated severe disabilities.[25]

Peripheral Nervous Systems

With aging, the number and size of peripheral nerve fibers diminish with a concomitant decrease in conduction velocity.[68] There is often a clinically insignificant decrease in touch and vibration sense. The peripheral nerves, however, are easily affected by nutritional deficiencies, toxins, and endocrine disorders.[25] The resulting neuropathies can cause marked loss of position sense, resulting in instability, falls, chronic pain, and dysesthesia (a painful and persistent sensation induced by a gentle touch of the skin).

The common nutritional deficiencies that lead to neuropathy are folic acid (caused by poor diet or folic acid antagonists, such as diphenylhydantoin and sulfonamides), vitamin B_{12} (caused by pernicious anemia due to malabsorption of B_{12}), and alcohol related deficiencies of thiamine, pyridoxine, and other B vitamins.[23,69] Toxic neuropathies can result from heavy metal exposure (such as lead and arsenic), medications (such as nitrofurantoin, disulfiram, diphenylhydantoin), or from uremia. Replacement of the deficiency and removal of the toxin are the cornerstones of therapy. Prognosis is good for resolution.[70]

Diabetic neuropathy can take several forms. There is a distal sensory polyneuropathy that affects the hands and feet with diminished sensation and burning pain; a proximal motor neuropathy resulting in proximal muscle wasting and weakness; and a diffuse autonomic neuropathy resulting in orthostatic hypotension, neurogenic bladder, obstipation (intractable constipation), and bowel immotility.[71] In addition to these diffuse forms of neuropathy, single nerves can be affected. The resulting mononeuropathies can cause loss of ocular muscle function and painful nerve root and branch dysfunction wherever an involved nerve travels.[72] Treatment is symptomatic and may involve analgesics, certain physical therapy, and possible splinting. Relief from painful dysesthesias may be obtained in some cases with the use of diphenylhydantoin, amitriptyline, or carbamazepine. Tight control of the blood sugar appears neither to prevent nor lessen diabetic neuropathy.[73] Rarely, another endocrine disease, hypothyroidism, can present with neuropathy. It responds to thyroid hormone replacement. Other causes of neuropathy in the aged include paraneoplastic syndromes (located in the lung, ovary, multiple myeloma) and amyloid.[74]

NEUROSENSORY MANIFESTATIONS OF AGING

Skin Pathologies

The skin is the largest organ of the body and functions to protect the interior of the body from the effects of pathogens, toxins, environmental extremes, trauma, and ultraviolet irradiation. With age, and often as the result of the accumulated effects of repeated injury, the skin changes. It grows and heals more slowly, becomes more sensitive to most toxins, and is less able to resist injury.[75] It becomes less effective as a barrier to infections. The specialized appendages, such as sweat and sebum glands, pressure and touch sensors, and hair follicles, atrophy. This results in dryness, a lowered ability to alter body temperature through sweating, and the loss of hair. The small blood vessels in the skin diminish with age: A change that contributes to the skin's lessened effectiveness as a barrier to infection, diminished reserve for repair, and altered ability to assist in thermoregulation.[76]

There are several skin diseases that are common in the aged and that have significant effects on function. These include malignant tumors, herpes zoster, and decubitus ulcers. A great deal of data have accumulated to demonstrate an association between cutaneous aging and the development of skin cancers, infections, and ulcers.[75] Many of the factors that appear to predispose individuals to the development of pathological manifestations in old age are similarly operative in the development of skin problems.[77] These include cumulative exposure to carcinogens, diminished DNA repair capacity, and decreased immunosurveillance. In addition, the reduced epidermal density in the skin that is seen with senescence is likely to play a role in the development of skin lesions, infections, and ulcerations.

Malignant Tumors

Skin cancer is the most common malignancy known to the human race.[77] As with most malignant disease, its incidence increases exponentially with age, however, there are few cancers that are as age dependent as cutaneous malignant disease. The three most important malignant tumors of the skin in the aged are basal cell carcinoma, squamous cell carcinoma, and malignant melanoma.

Basal cell carcinomas arise in areas of sun exposed skin and increase with the intensity and duration of sun exposure as well as genetic background. These types of nonmelanoma skin cancers account for approximately 50% of all cancers reported each year in the United States,[78] and 80% of all skin cancers fall into the category of basal cell carcinomas.[79] Though basal cell carcinomas occur in all races, the prevalence increases with fair skin and decreases with more intensely pigmented skin. The most common sites are the face, tops of the ears, neck, anterior chest, arms, and hands. Treatment is virtually always successful in eradicating the tumor unless there has been extensive local invasion of muscle and bone. These tumors rarely ever metastasize but can be locally invasive and deforming if not treated early. Fortunately, they are slow growing and seldom get large enough to be more than a cosmetic problem.

Squamous cell carcinomas arise from chronically irritated skin. Sun damage is the most common cause but other irritants include tobacco (lip and mouth), snuff (nose), coal tar, soot, and x-rays. Chronically traumatized scars following burns or surgery are other sites of predilection.[77] These cancers are locally invasive and frequently metastasize to regional lymph nodes, brain, and lung and, therefore, carry a higher mortality rate than basal cell carcinomas. Early detection and excision result in higher cure rates. Extensive surgery with excision of all regional lymph nodes and radiation therapy are frequently employed to cure these tumors. They are poorly responsive to chemotherapy.[80]

Malignant melanoma is also the result of sun damage.[81] It is estimated that approximately 17,700 people develop a new primary malignant melanoma each year.[78] This means that approximately 1 in every 185 individuals living an average life span will develop malignant melanoma in this country.[82] Furthermore, the incidence of this disease is doubling every 10 to 15 years.[82] Despite constantly improving cure rates over the years, the death rate is over 5500 per year and increasing.[78] Although malignant melanoma affects all age groups, the highest age specific incidence rates occur in the population over the age of 60 years of age.[83] In the elderly, lentigo maligna melanomas and acral-lentiginous melanomas (occurring on the plantar surface of the foot, most commonly on the weight bearing areas of the heel and forefoot[84]) occur disproportionately in the geriatric population. Both present as flat areas of increased, multicolored (brown, black, red, and blue) pigmentation. Occasionally, white areas are also present within the lesion, presumably related to foci of spontaneous regression of the tumor. Because the prognosis for survival with melanoma is related to the depth of skin invasion at the time of excision, these melanomas have a good prognosis if removed early. Nonetheless, deaths occur from lentigo maligna melanoma at the same rate as other melanomas when matched for similar anatomic site and thickness.[85] Other forms of melanoma are also found in the elderly and require early detection and excision to avoid the increasingly poor prognosis with lesion depth. As time goes on, particularly if the tumor becomes invasive, nodularity may develop at the surface of the lesion and ulceration may occur. The nodular melanoma, which is more aggressive in nature, comprises approximately 20% of malignant melanomas.[78] Melanomas metastasize early and extensively to brain, lung, liver, and bone tissue.

Skin cancer is a major concern in geriatric populations. Both cumulative exposure to carcinogens and age related factors contribute to the high prevalence of cutaneous malignancy in the elderly. Although mortality rates from skin cancer are relatively low, morbidity can be significant, particularly if lesions are neglected. Physical therapists could have a major impact on the early detection of skin cancers by assessing skin status during the physical evaluation, not only for obvious ulcerations or lesions, but for the more subtle presentations of skin changes as well.

Herpes Zoster

Zoster results from the reactivation of a dormant varicella virus (chickenpox) that had been sequestered for a long time in a sensory nerve root. The result is an intensely painful and pruritic eruption over the area innervated by that sensory nerve root. Immunocompromised hosts, such as those on steroids, or those with chronic diseases that alter the immune response, such as cancer and renal failure, have a greater incidence of herpes zoster.[86] Normal individuals also get herpes zoster. However, the reasons for its reactivation are obscure.

Two types of disability result from this infection. First, the eruption itself requires local care to prevent superinfection by bacteria, and the associated pain inhibits mobility, appetite, and sleep. Second, there is a high incidence of postherpetic neuralgia in the aged.[74] A severe, burning pain can persist for months—long after the local eruption has resolved. Although there are some medications that can lessen the severity of the initial pain, the patient with postherpetic neuralgia usually requires narcotics for relief. Rehabilitative efforts with herpes zoster are important in maintaining mobility through functional exercise and ambulation. In an elderly individual, pain-imposed restriction of activity can lead rapidly to the devastating effects of bed rest, especially when a neuralgia exists.

Decubitus Ulcers

Decubitus ulcers result from prolonged pressure and damage to the skin induced by shear force. Usually occurring over bony prominences, pressure and shear forces impair circulation to the area, resulting in ischemic changes in the tissue and ulcer formation.[87] They are most common in situations in which there is forced immobility due to illness or injury, diminished response to pain because of altered sensorium or inability to move, and altered nutritional status, usually as the result of some other illness or injury. Chronic weight loss leads to a decrease in subcutaneous fat, fragile epidermis, decreased blood flow to the dermal vessels, and a depressed immune function. Although aging skin has altered healing properties, decubitus ulcers are the result of other illnesses and are not simply the result of aging. They are rarely seen in otherwise healthy elderly persons.

Decubitus ulcers are potentially serious in the frail elderly who are chronically ill. The patients most susceptible are those who are among the most debilitated and are confined to a bed or chair.

It takes less than an hour of unrelieved pressure exceeding that of the capillary blood flow to induce pressure necrosis.[87] Bony prominences, such as over the coxa, lateral hips, heels, ankles, elbows, and scapulae, are frequently subjected to pressure high enough to cause ischemic injury. Malnutrition and diminished cutaneous blood flow contribute to the genesis and the perpetuation of these ulcers. Once the skin has broken down, irritation due to incontinence, exposure to bacterial contaminants, and compromised blood flow will contribute to further skin, subcutaneous fat, and muscle breakdown.[88]

Decubitus ulcers are easier to prevent than they are to cure. Prevention requires meticulous attention to potential pressure areas and the development of treatment strategies to assure that pressure is distributed evenly and no spot has pressure applied for too long. Once a pressure sore develops, it must be kept free from any further pressure in order to heal.

Treatment also includes debridement of any dead skin, either surgically or through dressing changes designed to remove necrotic tissue. In order for the ulcer to heal, the base of the ulcer must be free of necrotic debris and bacteria and it must provide a suitable environment for the growth of new skin. It must also be kept pressure free. Furthermore, the patient must receive adequate nutrition, including trace elements and vitamins such as zinc and vitamin C. Restoration of nutritional status is essential to healing decubitus ulcers. Achieving nitrogen balance by providing sufficient protein to make new tissue (with adequate levels of calories to protect the protein from being used for energy) is a primary goal. Surgical closure is sometimes required. Given the intensity and duration of the required treatment to cure an established decubitus ulcer, every effort should be made to prevent their occurrence through careful positioning and turning, air and water mattresses to distribute pressure, and attention to nutrition.

Physical therapy intervention includes low intensity current or nonthermal ultrasound.[89] Debridement can be accomplished using the whirlpool, though prolonged immersion in water in the dependent position should be avoided from these author's perspective. Functional activity and therapeutic exercise should be employed to maintain physical condition and capabilities so as to avoid the prolonged pressure of bed rest.

Disturbances of Touch

Touching provides one with important information about one's environment. It is also an important method of communication. The aging process often leads to a general decline in tactile sensitivity,[75] but the degree of loss is very variable. Some cases are more profound than others due to underlying pathological conditions, declining circulation, or injury. A loss or decline in tactile acuity will effect the aged person's ability to localize and properly identify stimuli. This reduces the patient's response time or his or her reactions that are based on the speed and intensity with which the stimuli were perceived.

The skin is a very important element in the ability to sense touch. The dermis thins, loses elasticity, and has a diminished vascularity with age.[77] Loss of tissue support for the remaining capillaries results in fragility and easy bruising (senile purpura).

The most common appearance of aging skin is dryness, scaling, and an atrophic appearance.[75] These changes may be related to systemic disease or to functional problems, but they are considered to be part of the normal process of aging. Hair loss occurs and is related to vascular insufficiency.[25] These changes are associated with a diminished sebaceous activity, a decrease in hydration of the horny layers, alterations in the metabolic and nutritional components associated with skin production and repair, and a dysfunction in keratin formation.[77] The skin loses its elasticity. The associated involvement of the peripheral arterial and venous systems produce pigment changes and an increased deposit of hemosiderin in the soft tissues, adding to the disturbed keratin formation. In general, the skin appears dry and yellowish with a wrinkled, inelastic, and parchment-like appearance. The decline in cellular division with age results in a slower rate and efficiency of tissue repair following any trauma.[77]

As with the other senses, touch acuity declines with age. Peripheral receptors provide the neurosensory input for the sense of touch, and these receptors for touch, pressure, pain, and temperature are found within the dermis and epidermis of the skin. Receptors can be freestanding or arranged in small corpuscular masses. Meissner's corpuscles (touch-texture receptors), Pacini's corpuscles (pressure-vibration receptors), and Krause's corpuscles (temperature receptors), as well as peripheral nerve fibers are noted to decline in transmission, but the ability to sense pain remains intact because there are few age related changes that occur in the free nerve endings. Sensitivity to touch, temperature, and vibration, however, frequently declines with age, therefore the elderly person must take special care to avoid injury from concentrated pressures or excessive temperature on the skin.[89]

Vibratory sensitivity loss is sometimes related to certain nervous system disorders. Reliable data exist, however, to indicate that there is a clear decline in vibratory sense that may begin as early as age 50 and that has no underlying pathology.[75] The decline appears to be greater in the lower extremities and is thought to be the result of undetected microchanges in the circulation in the legs or lower spinal cord.

Stereognosis is the ability to recognize an object by touching and manipulating it. A decline in this area is not thought to be related to aging but rather to an impairment of the central neurological processes, such as that seen in cerebral vascular accidents.

Ocular Pathologies with Age

Vision is the sense that human beings depend on the most, because our society depends heavily on visual cues. Much of our communication is via visual images and nonverbal communications, such as the written word, facial expressions and body language, billboards, and television. Identification of much that is in one's environment occurs through vision. It is a major tool for environmental safety, independence, and mobility.

With aging, several structural changes occur in the eye that evolve into pathologies, all of which result in a decline in visual acuity. Many of these changes begin at an early age and progress steadily, though slowly, over time. The slowness of this process allows for the patient to gradually accommodate the changes and to continue functioning. At some point, however, the cumulative effects of the process will result in some loss of independence and mobility.

The lens ages early so that by the age of 50 most people will exhibit some signs of aging there.[57] With age, the cytoplasm of transparent crystalline cells that form the lens throughout life become discolored, opaque, and rigid. Additionally, certain ligaments and muscles weaken, thereby limiting the ability of the anterior–posterior diameter of the lens to expand.[90] Gradually, the lens becomes set in size and flat. This condition, known as presbyopia, leads to a decline in both visual acuity and field. As the lens ages, thickens, and becomes yellow and somewhat opaque, the risk of cataracts also increases.[57] Because the lens is clouded, light rays entering through the lens scatter as they move through the visual system. This is the primary cause of the glare that can be so disorienting for the aged person. Also, as the lens thickens, the chamber becomes more shallow. The major danger in this case is the onset of acute angle glaucoma. With increasing age, less light reaches the retina because the pupil becomes smaller.[90] There is a linear decrease in the amount of light reaching the retina from the age of 20 to the age of 60.[57] This results in the need for increasing available light in order to see, and an increase in the time needed to adapt to sudden changes from bright to diminished light or darkness. Further, it should be noted that the eye requires approximately double the illumination for every 13 years of adult life.[57] Thus, the final level of vision in diminished lighting, after time allowed for accommodation, is less for the aged person than for the younger.

Color vision is also affected by age. While the mechanism is still not entirely understood, it is believed that the discoloration of the lens leads to color filtering and a decline in color intensity, especially with greens and blues.[57] It is thought that as the lens yellows, the shorter light waves of the greens and blues are filtered out, while the longer waves of the other half of the color spectrum retain the capacity to pass through the lens to the retina. Yellows, oranges, and reds have been found to stimulate the sympathetic nervous system responses in the elderly.[91] It is not necessarily profound that elderly individuals tend to develop a "taste" for brighter colored clothes.

Over time there is atrophy of orbital fat, which occurs with the pattern of general wasting.[57] This leads to the loss of the normal fat cushion behind the globe and may produce some recession of the eye and the characteristic sunken eye appearance known as enophthalmos. Enophthalmos is often accompanied by a deepening of the upper lid fold and a slight obstruction of the peripheral visual fields. The skin of the upper lid also tends to relax causing the upper lid to drop onto the lashes resulting in some restriction of the lid and leading to an upper lid ptosis. When severe, such a condition will limit vision for objects above eye level, such as traffic lights and stop signs.

The production of tears also declines with age.[57] If there has been sufficient relaxation of the lid, the direction of the tear ducts (the lacrimal puncta) will also change. Normally, the direction is inward, toward the eye itself, but with relaxation the direction is changed so that it is focused away from the eye and is thus exposed to the air. This leads to excessive tearing. This condition, if pronounced enough, leads to senile ectropion, a physical state in which the lower lid is physically unable to cover the lower portion of the eye.[90] This leaves no opportunity for the palpebral conjunctiva to be bathed in tears. This causes chronic dryness of the eye and will lead to metaplasia and keratinization of the epithelial layer. The opposite situation or senile entropion may also occur. This is a turning inward of the lower lid that leads to the irritation of the cornea and lower conjunctiva by the lashes. Severe cases of either ectropion or entropion will require plastic surgery.

The vitreous body also undergoes changes with aging. The gel-like substance undergoes some amount of shrinkage after the age of 60.[90] The primary role of the vitreous is to support the retina, and this becomes compromised as the amount of available fluid decreases. By the age of 70 or 80, most people develop some degree of detachment of the vitreous body from the posterior aspect of the globe. This occurrence is often heralded by transient flashes of light or by a small number of dark, floating opacities. These flashes are noted most often when turning in bed, not when sitting quietly. A sudden shower of dark spots or floating opacities is strongly suggestive of a retinal break and should be treated as an emergency to decrease the possibility of actual retinal detachment. Frequently, surgery will be suggested prophylactically for the uninvolved eye.[57]

Hearing Pathologies with Age

Changes in the morphological structures in the ear with age can lead to pathological changes. Briefly, these changes are atrophy and degeneration of hair cells and supporting cells in the basal coil of the cochlea leading to sensory presbyacusis; loss of auditory neurons causing neural presbyacusis; atrophy of the stria vascularis in the scala media with corresponding deficiencies in bioelectric and biochemical properties of the endolymphatic fluids, known as metabolic presbyacusis; atrophic changes in structures associated with vibration of the cochlear partition, known as cochlear conductive presbyacusis; loss of minute vessels that supply the spiral ligament, stria vascularis, and tympanic lip, which causes vascular presbyacusis; and a loss of neurons from the cochlear nucleus leading to central presbycusis.[92] While each of these entities have been separately identified and studied, it is important to note that they seldom happen independently of each other.

The hearing losses that occur with presbyacusis affects the higher, pure tone frequencies.[92] This leads to a decrease in the ability to understand speech because parts of words or whole words are lost because of higher tones as well as the interference of background noise. The use of hearing aids and surgical implants have provided relief for some, but the process of presbyacusis is such that these steps can only blunt the effects of the problem. Because most cases of presbyacusis are of mixed etiology, as has already been noted, intervention will not completely correct the loss. Thus, the clinical focus should be on improving and maintaining as much of the hearing capability as possible and assisting the aged person, and the family, to adapt to the limitations necessitated by substituting other forms of communication and environmental stimuli to compensate for the hearing loss that remains.[93]

The clinician needs to be very mindful of the effects of hearing loss on all aspects of the aged person's life. Failure to consider the effects of hearing loss when evaluating such problems as depression, confusion, possible attention span deficits, and a variety of other clinical problems may lead to less than adequate clinical intervention.

Tinnitus is the diagnosis given to a variety of "ear noise" disorders. A small percentage of the elderly suffer from this condition to varying degrees,[92] and it is a very annoying problem. Patients often report constant or intermittent noises, such as buzzing, ringing, or hissing, that result in a distortion of accurate reception of environmental sounds and voices. If patients complain of tinnitus, considerations for a quiet treatment environment should be made to decrease the bombardment of external noises superimposed on the internal sources.

Proprioceptive/Vestibular Dysfunction

Proprioception or kinesthesia are affected by changes in the neurosensory mechanisms. Though a greater degree of sensory or perceptual loss results from local system changes (i.e., impaired vision from increased lens density), cerebral cortex cell loss may result in less cellular availability for sensory interpretation. This is important when evaluating an elderly individual's gait pattern and balance. Peripheral vascular disease and diabetes may affect proprioceptive input. Vibratory sense is diminished or lost in the early stages of type II diabetes.

There is scant research on proprioception in the aged population. Skinner and co-workers[94] reported that the ability to replicate passive knee motion and the ability to detect motion diminished with increasing age. Older subjects detect motion less well at low frequencies of movement, though they still accurately report joint motion sensation.[95] Compared to younger individuals, people over the age of 50 required passive movement thresholds of perception that were twice as high in the lower extremities, but there was no difference in the upper extremities.[96] Impairment of proprioception rarely occurred in a neurological screening of a sample of subjects ranging in age from 67 to 87.[97] On the other hand, perception of passive knee movement in individuals 65 years of age and older showed an age related decline in position sense.[98] Perhaps proprioceptive loss is joint specific. Clinically, it appears to decline in the lower extremities with advancing age and is an important consideration when working with the elderly. Loss of proprioception is usually an irreversible deficit and contributes to a great many falls in the elderly. Barrett and associates[98] found that proprioception was improved by almost 40% when an Ace bandage was applied around the knee. The current authors have had clinical success with the use of light cuff weights (i.e., 1 pound) around the ankles for facilitating increased proprioceptive awareness when pathologies manifest in proprioceptive loss. Though the prospect of reversing proprioceptive deficits is low, the elderly individual can be taught to compensate for a decrease in position sense by visual input.

Degeneration occurs in the sensory receptors in both the otoliths and semicircular canals affecting the vestibular system. The function of this system is to monitor head position and detect head movements. When an individual is deprived of visual and lower extremity somatosensory information, the vestibular system is left to control balance. Healthy young adults are able to balance without meaningful visual or support surface information, but healthy elderly adults with normal amounts of vestibular degeneration lose their balance and are at risk for falls when vestibular input is the only spatial orientation information available. Diseases of the neuromuscular system further compound this problem. Balance problems or the "fear of falling" may severely compromise ambulatory capabilities in the elderly. Patients with vestibular lesions can be potentially treated with specific exercises to improve vestibular function or can be taught compensatory techniques using vision.[99,100]

Sensory Changes in Smell

There is a close association between the sense of smell and human behavior. The olfactory memory is a very powerful one, and it can elicit strong emotions. The sense of smell is also a key to recognizing what is occurring in the environment. The effects of aging alone on the ability to smell are minimal, and any decline in the sense of smell is probably related to an underlying pathology. Research has shown that there is a wide variation among elderly individuals' abilities to smell.[93] There does appear to be a decline in fibers in the olfactory bulb, and by the age of 80, almost three-fourths of the fibers are lost.[101] It is recognized that women have greater olfactory acuity than men;[101] however, postmenopausal women have a decreased ability to smell, which is thought to be the result of a decline in estrogen levels following menopause. Eating is perhaps the most directly affected activity when olfactory acuity is involved. In order to detect the flavor of food, one must be able to smell it. Thus, the aged person with a loss of smell may complain that food is tasteless. For the person with olfactory loss, hot foods are more easily perceived than cold foods. As with all of the senses, smell serves as an environmental safety factor. The inability to smell will raise certain safety concerns that can be resolved using alternative methods, such as ensuring that there are smoke detectors in the house to compensate for the loss of ability to smell smoke.

Sensory Changes in Taste

The sense of taste is closely associated with the senses of smell and vision. How food looks and smells enhances or detracts from its taste. There are four basic sensations in taste perceived by the taste buds; bitter, salty, sweet, and sour. Taste buds located in different areas of the tongue are responsible for perceiving the different sensations. Thus, any pathology affecting the tongue will also affect the ability to perceive the sensation for that area. Research indicates that there is a decline in taste sensitivity with age.[93,102] While it is not fully understood, there is a clear decline in the number of taste buds. Taste buds have the ability to rapidly regenerate, but the speed with which they do so declines with age. Eventually, the rate of loss exceeds the rate of replacement. There is some research that indicates that cigarette and pipe smoking is a factor in this decline.[101] While there are other age related changes, such as the decline in the flow of saliva, these changes are not considered significant until they are very advanced. It is unlikely that age related changes will affect the ability to taste prior to the age of 70. When these changes do occur, the aged person seems to have an increased sensitivity to bitterness and a decreased sensitivity to sweetness and saltiness.

Compensation for these losses revolves around recognizing how to enhance the involved senses. It is beneficial to make food visually more appealing, to serve hot foods hot, to increase the use of herbs and spices, to create an enjoyable social and physical environment, and to aggressively maintain good oral hygiene.

GASTROINTESTINAL PATHOLOGIES IN AGING

Age related changes in function are apparent in the gastrointestinal system, and these changes, combined with poor nutrition, can lead to pathological states.[86] This is important to physical therapy, because without an adequate energy source, the functional capabilities of any individual become restrained and limited. For example, the loss of dentition and diminution of salivary gland activity with age impairs mastication and deglutition, thereby affecting the overall function of the system. There are no significant changes in bowel function that can be ascribed solely to aging;[103] however, the aging gastrointestinal system is more susceptible to cancer, vascular insufficiency, and chronic degenerative conditions. Common gastrointestinal problems encountered in the aged include dysphagia; ulcer disease; pernicious anemia; cancer of the pancreas, stomach, and large intestine; constipation; and cholelithiasis. Gastrointestinal complaints are extremely common in the aged, and gastrointestinal disease accounts for over a quarter of hospital admissions.[104]

Dysphagia

Dysphagia is difficulty in swallowing. It commonly results from neuromuscular disorders, such as a cerebral vascular accident, Parkinson's disease, diabetes, or other neuropathies. Malnutrition results from decreased intake; and aspiration of oral contents is a common accompaniment that frequently leads to pneumonia. Siebens and co-workers[105] have identified a fairly high incidence of swallowing problems involving the mouth, pharynx, and upper esophageal sphincter in the elderly population. It is common to classify dysphagia according to the lesions causing the abnormal movement of food through the mouth, pharynx, and upper espohageal sphincter as oropharyngeal dysphagia. Those abnormalities producing difficulty with the passage of ingested material through the smooth muscle portion of the esophagus are classified as esophageal dysphagia.[106] Oropharyngeal dysphagia is characterized clinically by difficulty initiating the process of swallowing and physically by impaired ability to transfer food from the mouth into the upper portion of the esophagus. This process involves a closely coordinated central mechanism between the sensory nerves from afferent receptors (cranial nerves V, IX, and X) and the efferent nerves (V, VII, IX, X, and XII), supplying the muscles in this area. Many lesions of the central nervous system and muscle apparatus of the mouth and upper esophageal sphincter can produce oropharyngeal dysphagia. Cerebrovascular accidents and Parkinson's disease frequently result in dysphagia. Pathologies that affect the motor end plates, such as myasthenia gravis, can inhibit proper muscle functioning. Muscle problems, such as those seen in metabolic myopathy (e.g., thyroid disease, steroid therapy), primary myositis, or amyloidosis, can create swallowing difficulties.[103] Tumors or surgical scarring can cause local obstruction to the passage of food, and motility disorders like abnormal upper esophageal sphincter relaxation or pharyngeal/upper esophageal sphincter incoordination can cause oropharyngeal dysphagia.

True esophageal dysphagia, where the transport of the ingested material down the esophagus is impaired, is common in the elderly.[106] Carcinoma of the esophagus, which occurs with increasing frequency in the elderly, usually presents with dysphagia. The most common symptom is the sensation of food "hanging up" in the esophagus. It has a poor prognosis for cure and usually requires extensive palliative treatment. Hiatus hernia, another cause of dysphagia, is also increasingly common in the aged. Few, however, are symptomatic, and medical management with antacids and H_2 blockers is effective.[104] It is important to understand that achalasia can initially present in the elderly, and that other motility disorders, such as diffuse esophageal spasm and scleroderma, do occur in these individuals.[106] Another cause of esophageal dysphagia that is unique to the elderly population is dysphagia aortica, in which the transport of material down the esophagus is impaired by a markedly tortuous and enlarged aorta, heart, or both.[103]

The role of the physical therapist in treating dysphagia is to coordinate the team efforts of speech pathology, occupational dietary therapy, and nursing to provide a comprehensive positioning and feeding program. The physical therapist is involved in evaluating and treating the patient's head and trunk control; neck range of motion; neck weakness; sitting balance; any abnormal postural reflex activity that interferes with head control, sitting balance, or both; gross facial muscle test; ability to handle secretions; voluntary deep breathing ability; breath control and voluntary cough; and gross motor upper extremity ability. Specific emphasis needs to be placed on wheelchair and bed positioning and respiratory status.

Ulcer Disease

Ulcer disease is common in the elderly, and the presentation is often atypical,[103] because the complications of obstruction, bleeding, and perforation are more common in the aged than in younger individuals. Emergency surgical treatment for bleeding in the elderly carries up to a 20% mortality.[86] Medical management is effective in uncomplicated cases and rests on the use of antacids, avoidance of salicylates, and other nonsteroidal and steroidal anti-inflammatory agents and H_2 blockers, such as cimetadine. Cimetadine induced confusion is a common complication in the aged, and a reduced dose will prevent it.

The difficulties encountered in rehabilitation of the aged with ulcer disease are centered around their poor nutritional status and the decline in their level of activity. Focus needs to be on the maintenance of maximal functional capabilities and adequate nutrition.

Pernicious Anemia

Pernicious anemia results from a common age related decline in the absorption of vitamin B_{12}. This usually occurs in the setting of chronic inflammation of the lining of the stomach called atrophic gastritis.[103] Not only can impaired B_{12} absorption cause significant disease (e.g., dementia, neuropathy, and anemia), but it is associated with a higher incidence of carcinoma of the stomach. Replacement of vitamin B_{12} through monthly injections, in addition to monitoring B_{12} intake through dietary means, effectively prevents or corrects the deficiency. The most clinically significant findings in patients with pernicious anemia are low energy levels, confusion, and peripheral neuropathies that result in proprioceptive problems.

Cancer

Gastrointestinal malignancies account for the second largest number of cancer deaths behind lung cancer.[86] The esophagus, stomach, pancreas, and large intestine are the most common sites. Cancer of the stomach is more common with advancing age, has its peak incidence in the eighth and ninth decades, and has a poor 5-year survival rate. Cancer of the pancreas has a similar 5-year survival rate, but its peak incidence is in the sixth decade.[103] Late diagnosis due to atypical, vague, or misleading symptoms, such as depression or altered mental status, is the rule. Cancer of the colon accounts for half of all gastrointestinal malignancies. Because they are not usually "clinically silent," as with the other malignancies, intervention is usually earlier and more successful. Rectal bleeding, anemia, weight loss, and altered bowel habits are the common presenting complaints. However, weakness, depression, fatigue, anorexia, and decreased functional competence are also early nonspecific clues to colon cancer. Unless the elderly person's condition makes it likely that they will soon die from other causes, surgery is often required to cure the patient and to prevent intestinal obstruction. Colon cancer's 5-year survival rate varies widely depending on the extent of the tumor at the time of initial treatment, but complete cures and long remissions are common.

Constipation

Constipation is increasingly common with advancing age. Although bowel transit times are normal in otherwise healthy adults, many other age related factors can contribute to having fewer than three stools per week. Inactivity, inadequate dietary fiber, inadequate fluids, drug side effects (e.g., narcotics, iron, sedatives, and anticholinergics), over-sedation, confusion, and prior laxative abuse can all contribute to constipation. Alterations in the intestine due to local disease, such as hemorrhoids, strictures, diverticulitis, and cancer, can also contribute to constipation. Correction of contributory factors, use of regular, periodic laxatives, and patient education are usually effective. For those patients who are too confused to respond to the urge to stool, regular disimpaction is important.

Biliary Tract Disease

Cholelithiasis increases with age and occurs in nearly one third of those over the age of 70.[103] Although most gallstones are "silent," infection and biliary obstruction due to stones are common in the elderly. Emergency surgery for cholecystitis in the elderly carries a 25% mortality. This has spurred some to advocate "prophylactic" cholecystectomy in those elderly with multiple small stones because they are at highest risk for passing a stone and causing an obstruction. Nonoperative techniques are being developed, such as endoscopic papillotomy in which the bile duct is widened from within the intestine by use of an endoscope, which avoids anesthesia and surgery. This technique is useful for some elderly who would not otherwise tolerate surgery.

Renal Disease

The kidneys are the major modulators of the amount of water, sodium, and potassium found in the extracellular fluid of the body. They also are a major route of drug excretion and are important in maintaining an appropriate blood pressure.[102] Alterations in renal function can have profound effects on all of these essential functions.

With age, the amount of blood that can be filtered by the kidneys declines steadily.[103] This is due in part to a decline in the amount of blood that arrives at the kidney because of heart disease or the narrowing of the blood vessels. It is also caused in large part by the decrease in the number and size of the glomeruli, which are the areas of the kidney that filter plasma. The ability of the kidney to reabsorb water and solutes from the filtered plasma also declines.[107] Although these reabsorptive capacities remain, they are at a significantly lower level in the aged and help to account for the decreased capability of the aged person to excrete an excessive amount of water or to prevent the loss of water in the face of dehydration.

There are eight commonly encountered problems in the aged to which altered renal function contributes: too much or too little water, too much or too little sodium, too much potassium, drug intoxication, and acute and chronic renal failure.[108] All of these disruptions of body homeostasis can result in an altered mental status and can be life threatening.

Sodium and Water Balance

The aging kidney has a diminished capacity for excreting a water load because of its inability to excrete a very diluted urine.[109] The water excess that results leads to a dilution of serum sodium, which in turn results in fatigue, lethargy, nonspecific weakness, and confusion. In extreme cases, seizures and coma can result. Excess water frequently is retained from the use of hypotonic solutions during intravenous therapy. It may also result from the syndrome of inappropriate antidiuretic hormone secretion (SIADH), which causes the kidneys to excrete a concentrated urine. Head trauma, stroke, pneumonia, and certain drugs can cause SIADH. Several commonly used medications can also induce hyponatremia, including aspirin, haloperidol, chlorpropamide, acetaminophen, barbituates, and amitriptyline.[110]

Regardless of the mechanism, the results of low serum sodium can be life threatening, and they require immediate intervention to reverse the sodium decline. Since the problem is usually one of excess water rather than decreased sodium, treatment consists of restricting free water or promoting the excretion of dilute urine. The addition of sodium through the use of hypertonic solutions is reserved for the most severe cases.[111]

At the other extreme of water balance is dehydration, in which the aging kidney has a diminished capacity to conserve water by making a more concentrated urine. The consequence of this deficit is that the aged individual is much more susceptible to dehydration in the presence of fever. Because of the resulting changes in mental status, the effect of fever and mild dehydration may be enough to initiate a vicious cycle in which the aged person become progressively dehydrated because of the resulting confusion and loss of thirst mechanism.[111,112] Significant dehydration is often an associated finding in elderly persons presenting with other illnesses, such as pneumonia, urinary tract infections, and strokes. The inability to maintain adequate hydration is often the deciding factor that precipitates admission to the hospital in the elderly person.

Intravenous fluid replacement is often required to regain fluid balance. Frequently the mental status changes resulting from dehydration and elevated serum sodium last long after the fluid imbalance has been corrected.

Increasing the amount of sodium presented to the aging kidney results in retention of sodium because the excess load cannot be as effectively excreted as it is in younger individuals.[109] Because the retention of water occurs with the retention of sodium, the result of an increase sodium load is an expansion of the total extracellular fluid. This results in congestive heart failure, edema, and elevated blood pressure.[110]

Alternatively, the aging kidney cannot correct for a decrease in the amount of sodium presented to the kidneys. The aging kidney loses sodium and, therefore, is less able to maintain homeostasis with a limited sodium load. What results is a steady decline in the total extracellular fluid and associated hypotension, dizziness, weakness, and falling. The lessened functional reserve of the aging kidney makes it less able to correct for alterations of water and salt that would not stress the younger individual.[108] The resulting abnormalities of sodium and water accompany other illnesses and increase both morbidity and mortality in the aged.

Potassium

Excess potassium, or hyperkalemia, can cause fatal cardiac arrhythmias.[113] It is more common in the aged because of several age related changes in renal function. Aldosterone is the hormone responsible for maintaining potassium balance, and it effects the kidney by causing potassium to be exchanged for sodium in the urine. The net result is that potassium is excreted and sodium is retained. With age, the amount of aldosterone diminishes, as does the kidney's capacity to excrete potassium.[111] The presence of potassium-sparing drugs or diabetes amplifies these effects. In the setting of dehydration, when there is both decreased renal blood flow and acidosis, there is a marked decrease in the excretion of potassium and a significant shift of potassium from within the cells into the extracellular space. The resulting severe hyperkalemia can cause life threatening arrhythmias.

Drug Intoxication

The kidneys are one of the major routes of drug detoxification and excretion,[108] and a progressive decline in renal function results in lower clearances for many different types of drugs. Higher serum levels are reached and maintained longer in the elderly than in younger individuals by using the same amount of drug.[110] For many compounds this means that standard adult dosages result in toxic blood levels in the elderly. Among the most important drugs that are retained are digitalis, several types of antibiotics, and oral diabetic agents. As a consequence, drug dosages need to be adjusted downward in the elderly.

Acute and Chronic Renal Failure

Acute cessation of renal function can occur at any age, but the diminished blood supply of the aging kidney renders it more susceptible to injury.[108] Hypotension is the usual precipitating cause and can result from dehydration, over-medication, surgery, or sepsis. Acute injury from certain antibiotics or from contrast dye used in radiology can also result in acute renal failure.

Acute renal failure is associated with the rapid buildup of toxic waste products and drugs, fluid overload, and elevation of serum potassium. Any of these complications can be fatal if not managed correctly. In addition, the immune system is impaired, and patients with acute renal failure frequently die from infections.[109]

Chronic renal failure is marked by the slow deterioration of renal function and is usually detected when the presence of another illness stresses the renal system and elevated blood urea nitrogen (BUN), hyponatremia, or increased fluid retention leads to an evaluation of renal function.[111] The functional side effects of chronic renal failure result primarily from anemia and congestive heart failure. Patients with renal disease severe enough to cause significant chronic mental status changes have a poor prognosis and often require dialysis or transplantation—a very touchy subject in light of possible rationing of health care imposed by health care reforms.

The clinical implications of problems in the kidney in relation to exercise and activity tolerance center around the electrolyte balance and the potential inability of the kidney to facilitate homeostasis. Increasing energy expenditure through exercise is positively correlated with an improvement in mortality and morbidity through a number of mechanisms.[114] Despite these benefits, there has been some reluctance, especially with the elderly with renal failure, to recommend fitness programs because of the fear that exercising too intensely will provoke cardiac arrhythmias, myocardial infarction, or increased blood pressure.[115] Regular eccentric training can increase protein turnover (37% higher muscle catabolism) in older people and can require a higher protein intake.[116]

Combined with a calorie-appropriate diet, regular exercise maintains a reasonable body weight, delays the loss of lean muscle mass, and promotes good physical performance. Activity level is also a predictor of survival for people aged 60 to 90 years.[117,118]

ENDOCRINE DISEASES

The endocrine system encompasses a diverse group of organs and specialized glands that produce hormones. Hormones are chemical messengers that instruct those cells with complementary receptors to perform a specific metabolic act.[119] The thyroid gland elaborates thyroxine, which in turn modulates the overall metabolic rate of cells within the organism. Parathyroid glands elaborate parathyroid hormone, which is central to regulation of calcium metabolism. The islet cells of the pancreas produce insulin, which helps regulate glucose metabolism. Three hormones help modulate the fluid and electrolyte balance of the body: the posterior pituitary gland makes antidiuretic hormone (ADH), the kidneys produce renin, and the adrenal glands produce aldosterone.[120]

Although many other hormones exist, excess and deficiency of the previously listed hormones account for most of the clinically significant endocrine diseases encountered in the aged. With aging, there appears to be a reduction in the sensitivity of the target cells to the hormone messenger.[121] This is due, in some cases, to a lessening of the number of hormone receptors found on the target cells.

Thyroid Disease

Clinically, significant disease can result from either an excess or a deficiency of thyroid hormone. In both hyper- and hypothyroidism, the presentation of the syndrome can be very different in the aged than it is in younger patients. As is the rule with most illnesses in the aged, the presentation is usually more subtle, and the symptoms and signs less specific.[121] With advancing age, there is no change in the circulating levels of total thyroxine or triiodothyronine or the free hormone values.[119] However, there is a decreased production of thyroid hormones with aging that is counterbalanced by a decrease in thyroid hormone degradation. In addition, there is a tendency for diminished feedback of thyroid hormones, leading to a mild increase in thyrotropin levels, particularly in women. In older men, there is an increased prevalence of failure for thyroid-stimulating hormone (TSH) to respond to thyrotropin-releasing hormone (TRH).

Hypothyroidism is common in the aged and results from the failure of the thyroid gland to elaborate sufficient thyroid hormone despite maximum stimulation of the gland by TSH. The incidence of hypothyroidism increases from approximately 1% below the age of 60 to 4% to 7% after the age of 60.[122] Vague symptoms abound: dry skin, chronic muscle and joint pains, lethargy, confusion, weight gain, edema, depression, apathy, sensitivity to sedatives, and cold intolerance. Patients with severe hypoglycemia, develop hypothermia and have cognitive dysfunction resembling dementia. These hypofunctions are seen most commonly in the hospitalized elderly patient who experiences the stress of surgery or other acute illness.[123] More subtle abnormalities, such as pseudodementia, depression, and lethargy, are more common in ambulatory patients.

Untreated hypothyroidism places the individual at increased risk of death from concurrent illness. Treatment involves the gradual replacement of thyroid hormone on a daily basis until the TSH value becomes normal. This usually requires monthly dosage adjustments for several months.

In the aged, hyperthyroidism results most commonly from an excess of thyroid hormone released from a multinodular goiter. Between 7% and 12% of patients with hyperthyroidism are over the age of 60.[119] Although many symptoms of hyperthyroidism in the aged are similar to those in the younger patient, they are usually more subtle. Common manifestations include the development of glucose intolerance (diabetes mellitus), congestive heart failure, atrial fibrillation, muscle weakness, weight loss, diarrhea, and agitation. However, there is a small group of the aged with "apathetic hyperthyroidism" in which the presentation of disease is diametrically different from the usual.[124] These individuals show depression, apathy, failure to thrive, and constipation. Although their symptoms are similar to patients with hypothyroidism, correction of the elevated thyroid hormone level abolishes the symptoms.

Surgical ablation of the thyroid gland is rarely done and is usually reserved for situations in which the enlarged gland compromises the patient's airway. The use of radioactive iodine, which is selectively concentrated in the gland, produces the most lasting reduction in hormone levels.[121] It is so effective that virtually all patients treated with this modality develop hypothyroidism requiring hormone replacement. Medications, such as propylthiouracil, that block the production of thyroid hormone are effective alternatives to radioactive iodine. Their use is complicated by the development of bone marrow suppression and a significant relapse rate when the medication is withdrawn. In the majority of cases, however, both types of treatment produce excellent results.

Glucose Metabolism

The number of insulin receptors found on cell membranes decreases with age.[125] Reflecting this change, the incidence of glucose intolerance increases with age and reaches nearly 25% by age 80.[126] In the aged, it is important to identify glucose intolerance, not only to prevent the complications of untreated diabetes (i.e., neuropathy, retinopathy, nephropathy, and accelerated atherosclerosis) but, even more so, to identify those individuals at risk for nonketotic hyperosmolar coma or severe hyperglycemia, which can be precipitated by infection, dehydration, or other physiological stress.

Nonketotic hyperosmolar coma is exclusively a disease of aged diabetics.[125] It is characterized by extremely high blood sugars and osmolarity (hyperosmolar).

Patients present with mental status changes that range from lethargy to coma. They are severely dehydrated and frequently hypotensive. It is often easy to overlook the precipitating event (e.g., pneumonia, urinary tract infection, or myocardial infarction) because the severity of the neurological changes suggest a primary neurological event.

Dehydration and hypotension are more significant clinical problems than hyperglycemia. Treatment consists of fluid replacement and very low dose insulin therapy to slowly bring down the elevated blood sugar.[127] Prevention of this syndrome involves the early identification of diabetic patients who are slipping into the cycle of infection, decreased oral intake, dehydration, increased blood sugar, and the resulting acceleration of dehydration because of the forced excretion of water when the kidneys cannot reabsorb all of the glucose presented to it and glucose is lost in the urine. Rehydration and treatment of the primary illness will usually prevent the development of nonketotic hyperosmolar coma.

Antidiuretic Hormone

Antidiuretic hormone (ADH) increases the reabsorption of water from the kidney, and its release is stimulated by a decrease in circulating fluid volume or an increase in osmolarity. It is an important part of the endocrine system, which maintains fluid balance.[119] Under certain circumstances, the pituitary makes excessive amounts of ADH, which results in SIADH. Several intracranial processes, such as stroke, meningitis, and subdural hematoma, and intrathoracic conditions, such as pneumonia, tuberculosis, and bronchiectasis, can cause SIADH. Recurring episodes of SIADH precipitated by acute viral illness have been reported as well. This syndrome results in excess water retention, which in turn causes a severe dilution of serum sodium.[121] This results in lethargy, confusion, and seizures. It usually responds to restricting free water and correcting the precipitating factors, and it can be intermittent or chronic.

Parathyroid Disease

Parathyroid hormone maintains calcium balance by stimulating the absorption of calcium from the intestine, reabsorption from the urine, and mobilization from bone.[121] The amount of circulating parathyroid hormone increases with age because of age related decreases in the amount of calcium absorbed from the intestine. Part of this decrease results from lower levels of calcium and vitamin D (essential for absorption of calcium) in the diet and less sunlight mediated conversion of vitamin D to more active forms.[128]

A decrease in the circulating levels of ionized calcium triggers the release of parathyroid hormone. In situations such as renal failure, serum calcium levels decrease because of binding with retained phosphates normally excreted in the urine. The resulting decrease in calcium triggers the release of parathyroid hormone and often raises its level out of the normal range. This is called secondary hyperparathyroidism.[121] Parathyroid hormone levels usually return to normal when the stimulus for lowering calcium is removed. Occasionally, however, the parathyroid glands continue to overproduce the hormone even after the stimulus is removed. The result is an autonomous, hyperfunctioning parathyroid gland that raises the serum calcium level and results in a clinically apparent hyperparathyroidism. A more common cause of hyperparathyroidism is the development of a single parathyroid adenoma that produces excess hormone.[120,121] In either situation, the elevated calcium level causes profound mental status changes, including confusion, lethargy, and coma. Elevated calcium is a reversible cause of altered mental status in the aged. Osteomalacia, renal stones, and peptic ulcer disease are also associated with hyperparathyroidism. However, in the aged, they are less common than mental status changes.

Parathyroid surgery is an effective treatment. Conservative management using high sodium diets, phosphate supplements, and diuretics, such as furosemide, is also effective in patients who cannot tolerate surgery.[129] Hypoparathyroidism can result from surgery, or it can develop spontaneously. It is rare, and the main symptom, tetany, can usually be prevented by calcium supplements and agents, such as hydrochlorothiazide, that retard calcium loss by the kidneys.

METABOLIC PATHOLOGIES IN AGING

Diabetes Mellitus

Diabetes mellitus is a chronic disease that affects approximately 12 million people in the United States.[130] Insulin is needed for glucose to be transferred from the blood to the muscle and fat cells.[71] People who suffer from diabetes cannot produce enough insulin (type I) or cannot properly use the insulin they do produce (type II), causing hyperglycemia.[131]

The complex nature of diabetes creates a broad spectrum of physical complications and reactions that can make the condition extremely dangerous. Diabetes is the leading cause of blindness, and it can cause glaucoma and cataracts. Diabetics are twice as likely to have heart attacks and strokes, five times more prone to foot ulceration with the development of gangrene, and seventeen times more prone to kidney disease when compared to the general population.[71] Complications of diabetes also affect the mouth; the reproductive, muscular, nervous, and vascular systems; and the skin. They also reduce an individual's defense mechanism in the presence of infection.

Symptoms of diabetes include increased urination, thirst, hunger, fatigue, and lethargy; weight loss; and numbness or tingling in the feet and hands. Though no clear understanding of the cause of diabetes has been found and there is no cure, the disease has been found to be controllable by achieving and maintaining normal blood glucose levels.[72] This requires a carefully balanced use of four critical components: diet, exercise, education for self-monitoring, and drug therapy.

By its very nature, diabetes is a condition in which food is improperly metabolized, thereby producing too much glucose. Therefore, diet control is critical to diabetes control, especially in type II diabetes.[72] Patients with diabetes should be encouraged to eat less, to consume fewer calories, and to eat less fat and simple sugars.

The second area of control is exercise. Exercise improves blood glucose control and circulation, reduces cardiovascular risk, and keeps the patient fit.[132,133] Daily exercise increases the tissue sensitivity to insulin for 2 to 3 days, thereby decreasing the need for insulin injection.[133] Exercise and the diabetic will be dealt with more extensively in Chapter 13, Cardiopulmonary Treatment Considerations.

Patients with diabetes should receive be thoroughly educated about the disease, its complications, and the specific steps that must be taken to control it. Self-monitoring involves a routine check of glucose levels, either by checking the urine or the blood. Blood glucose monitoring is the method of choice since it is a more accurate measurement of glucose levels. In addition, self-monitoring of skin condition, especially in the lower extremities, is a vital component of diabetic education.

Drug therapy for diabetes consists of oral agents (type II only) and insulin. Insulin is obtained from animal sources, such as cows and pigs, or from a biosynthesis process that results in insulin products that are the same as human insulin.[131] The synthesized insulin has gained popularity in recent years because it causes the formation of fewer insulin antibodies and is less likely to cause allergic reactions. Insulin requirements may change in patients who become ill, especially with vomiting or fever.

Signs of hyperglycemia may be caused by a missed insulin dose, overeating, not following the diabetic diet, or a fever or infection. These signs include excessive thirst, urination, or both; dry mouth, drowsiness, flushed dry skin, fruitlike breath odor, stomachache, nausea, vomiting, and a difficulty breathing.

Signs of hypoglycemia may be caused by too much insulin, missing a snack or meal, sickness, too much exercise, drinking alcoholic beverages, or taking medications that contain alcohol. Symptoms of this include anxiety, chills, cold sweats, cool pale skin, confusion, drowsiness, excessive hunger, headache, nausea, nervousness, shakiness, vision changes, and unusual tiredness or fatigue. If these symptoms occur, the consumption of a sugar-containing food (e.g., orange juice or honey) should reverse the symptoms.

CONCLUSION

The incidence of disease increases as one ages. Disease states seem to be the result of microinsults over one's lifetime that are universal in all systems of the body, though the end state pathology may be different and the progression may evolve at varying speeds. The question arises: Are these small, cumulative injuries avoidable? Free radicals are unavoidable by-products of our own metabolism. Background radiation is a universal fact of life (about one-third of it comes from our own intracellular potassium).[3] A temperature of 37°C is hot as far as molecular stability is concerned, and no chemical bond is immune from rupture by thermal perturbations.[3] In this context, aging, like the microinsults that cause it, may also be ubiquitous and inevitable and lead to pathological problems.

PEARLS

- The death rate for certain diseases increases more steeply than the overall death rate, which arouses the suspicion that aging predisposes one to the development of the condition or a fatal outcome.

- There are no clinically significant effects on heart function that can solely be ascribed to aging. Therefore, the numerous pathologies seen in the cardiovascular system (i.e., ischemic heart disease, cardiomyopathy, conductive system disease, valvular disease, hypertension, myocardial degeneration, and peripheral vascular disease) account more for the decrements in the function of the system.

- The two most common types of diseases affecting the respiratory system are pneumonias, which compromise gas exchange and serve as a source for sepsis, and chronic obstructive lung disease and emphysema, which affect the amount of airflow in the lungs.

- Muscle dysfunction in the aged is usually the result of toxic or metabolic factors acting on the muscle rather than any intrinsic disease of the muscle.

- Disease of the neuromuscular system (i.e., CNS and peripheral nervous system dysfunction, confusion, dementia and delirium, cerebrovascular disease, Parkinson's disease, normal pressure hydrocephalus, and cervical spondylosis), like those of the cardiovascular system, are much more responsible for the decrements seen in aging than the effects of aging.

- Diseases of the sensory system affect all of the body's function involving the skin (the largest organ in the body) proprioception, and pain, and thermal and vibratory sensation.

REFERENCES

1. Kohm RR. Human aging and disease. *J Chron Dis.* 1963; 16:5–21.
2. Timiras PS. Developmental Psychology and Aging, Chapter 28. New York: Macmillan; 1972.
3. Johnson HA. Is aging physiological or pathological? In: Johnson HA, ed. *Relations Between Normal Aging and Disease.* Aging Series Vol. 28. New York: Raven Press; 1985:239–247.

4. Dietrick JE, Whedon GD, Shorr E. Effects of immobilization upon various metabolic and physiologic functions of normal men. *Am J Med.* 1948; 4:3–9.
5. Lamb LE, Stevens PM, Johnson RL. Hypokinesia secondary to chair rest from 4 to 10 days. *Aerospace Med.* 1965; 36:755.
6. Miller PB, Johnson RL, Lamb LE. Effects of four weeks of absolute bed rest on circulatory functions in man. *Aerospace Med.* 1964; 35:1194.
7. Shepard RJ. *Physical Activity and Aging.* 2nd ed. Gaithersburg, Md: Aspen Publishers, Inc.; 1987.
8. Ragen PB, Mitchell J. The effects of aging on the cardiovascular response to dynamic and static exercise. In: Weisfelt ML, ed. *The Aging Heart.* New York: Raven Press; 1980:269–296.
9. Ham RJ, Marcy ML, Holtzman JM. The aging process: biological and social aspects. In: Wright J, ed. *Primary Care Geriatrics.* Boston: PSG, Inc.; 1983.
10. Ellestad MH. Stress testing—principles and practice. 2nd ed. Philadelphia: Davis; 1985.
11. Ewing DJ, Campbell IN, Clarke BF: Heart-rate response to standing as a test for automatic neuropathy. *Br Med J.* 1978; 1(6128):1700.
12. Thadani U, Davidson C, Singleton W, Taylor SH. Comparison of the immediate effects of five beta-adrenoceptor blocking drugs with different ancillary properties in angina pectoris. *N Engl J Med.* 1989; 300:750–755.
13. Cairns JA. Current management of unstable angina. *Can Med Assoc J.* 1988; 119:477–480.
14. Gerstenblith G, Weisfeldt ML, Lakatta EG. Disorders of the heart. In: Andres R, Bierman EL, Hazzard WR, eds. *Principles of Geriatric Medicine.* New York: McGraw-Hill; 1985; 515–526.
15. Kattus A, Grollman J. Patterns of coronary collateral circulation in angina pectoris: relation to exercise training. In: Russek HI, Zohman BL, eds. *Changing Concepts of Cardiovascular Disease.* Baltimore, Md: Williams and Wilkins; 1972; 352–376.
16. Larson EB, Bruce RA. Health benefits of exercise in an aging society. *Arch Intern Med.* 1987; 147:353.
17. Astrand PO. Exercise physiology and its role in disease prevention and in rehabilitation. *Arch Phys Med Rehabil.* 1987; 68:305.
18. Kohl HW, Moorefield DL, Blair SN. Is cardiorespiratory fitness associated with general chronic fatigue in apparently healthy men and women? *Med Sci Sports Exerc.* 1987; 19(S6).
19. Shepard RJ. Sudden death—a significant hazard of exercise. *Brit J Spts Med.* 1974; 8:101–110.
20. Shepard RJ. Do risks of exercise justify costly caution? *Phys Sports Med.* 1977; 5(2):58–65.
21. Shepard RJ. *Ischemic Heart Disease and Exercise.* Chicago: Croom Helm, London and Year Book Medical Publishers, 1981.
22. Romo M. Factors related to sudden death in acute ischemic heart disease. A community study in Helsinki. *Acta Med Scand.* 1972; 547(suppl):7–92.
23. Kenney RA. *Physiology of Aging: A Synopsis.* Chicago: Year Book Medical Publishers, Inc.; 1982.
24. Baker PB, Arn AR, Unverferth DV: Hypertrophic and degenerative changes in human hearts with aging. *J Coll Cardiol.* 1985; 5:536A.
25. Schneider EL, Reed JD. Modulations of aging processes. In: Finch CE, Schneider EL, eds. *Handbook of the Biology of Aging.* New York: Academic Press; 1985.
26. US Bureau of the Census. *Statistical Abstract of the United States.* ed 110. Washington, DC: US Government Printing Office; 1990.
27. NIH. *National High Blood Pressure Education Program Coordinating Committee, 1989: Statement on Hypertension in the Elderly.* Bethesda, Md: National Institutes of Health; 1989.
28. Abrams WB. Pathophysiology of hypertension in older patients. *Am J Med.* 1988; 85(suppl 3b):7–13.
29. Toscani A. Physiology of muscular work in the aged. In: Huet JA, ed. *Work and Aging.* Second international course in social gerontology. International Centre of Social Gerontology, Paris, 1971.
30. Harrington TR, Dixon K, Russell RO, et al. The relation of age to the duration of contraction, ejection and relaxation of the normal human heart. *Amer Heart J.* 1984; 67:189–199.
31. Pomerance A. Pathology of the heart with and without failure in the aged. *Brit Heart J.* 1965; 27:697–710.
32. Weisfeldt ML, Gerstenblith ML, Lakatta EG. Alterations in circulatory function. In: Andres R, Bierman EL, Hazzard WR, eds. *Principles of Geriatric Medicine.* New York: McGraw-Hill; 1985:248–279.

33. Bruce RA. Evaluation of functional capacity in patients with cardiovascular disease. *Geriatrics.* 1957; 12:317–328.
34. Triggs EJ, Nation RL. Pharmacokinetics in the aged: a review. *J Pharm Biopharmacol.* 1975; 3:387.
35. Gerstenblith G, Spurgeon HA, Froelich JP, et al. Diminished inotropic responsiveness to ouabain in aged rat myocardium. *Circ Res.* 1979; 44:517–523.
36. Reeves WC, Nanda NC, Gramiak R. Echocardiography in chronic alcoholics following prolonged periods of abstinence. *Amer Heart J.* 1978; 95:578–583.
37. Thiele BL, Strandness DE. Disorders of the vascular system: peripheral vascular disease. In: Andres R, Bierman EL, Hazzard WR, eds. *Principles of Geriatric Medicine.* New York: McGraw-Hill; 1985:527–535.
38. Berman ND. *Geriatric Cardiology.* Lexington, Ky: Collamore Press; 1982:1–244.
39. Gladman JRF, Barer D, Venkatesan P, et al. The outcome of pneumonia in the elderly: a hospital survey. *Clin Rehab.* 1991; 5:201–204.
40. Cummings G, Semple SG. *Disorders of the Respiratory System.* Oxford, England: Blackwell; 1973.
41. Wynne JW. Pulmonary disease in the elderly. In: Rossman I, ed. *Clinical Geriatrics.* 2nd ed. Philadelphia: Lippincott Co.; 1979.
42. Grimby G, Saltin B. The aging muscle. *Clin Physiol.* 1983; 3:209–218.
43. Cress ME, Schultz E. Aging muscle: functional, morphologic, biochemical, and regenerative capacity. *Top Geriatric Rehab.* 1985; 1(1):11–19.
44. Mense S. Physiology of nociception in muscles. Advances in pain research and therapy. In: Friction JR, Awad EA, eds. *Myofascial Pain and Fibromyalgia.* New York: Raven Press; 1990; 17.
45. Dowd T. The female climacteric. *Nat OB-GYN Group.* 1990; 6(1):32–54.
46. Dawson-Huges B, Dallal G, Krall E. A controlled trial of the effect of calcium supplement on bone density in postmenopausal women. *NEJM.* 1990; 329(13):878–883.
47. Giansiracusa DF, Kantrowitz FG. Metabolic bone disease. In: Keiber JB. *Manual of Orthopaedic Diagnosis and Intervention.* Baltimore: Williams and Wilkins Co.: 1978.
48. Fujiswawa Y, Kida K, Matsuda H. Role of change in vitamin D metabolism with age in calcium and phosphorous metabolism in normal subjects. *J Clin Endocrinol Metab.* 1984; 59:719–726.
49. Riis B, Thomsen K, Christiansen C. Does calcium supplementation prevent postmenopausal bone loss? *N Engl J Med.* 1987; 316(4):173–177.
50. Harrington TR. Preventing osteoporosis in menopausal women. *J MSSK Med.* June 1990.
51. Nielson F, Hunt C, Mullen L, Hunt J. Effect of dietary boron on mineral, estrogen, and testosterone metabolism in postmenopausal women. *J FASEB.* 1987; 1:394–397.
52. Pogrund H, Bloom R, Menczel J. Preventing osteoporosis: current practices and problems. *Geriatrics.* 1986; 41(5):55–71.
53. Chesworth B, Vandervoort A. Age and passive ankle stiffness in healthy women. *Phys Ther.* 1989; 69(3):217–224.
54. Walker J. Connective tissue plasticity: issues in histological and light microscopy studies of exercise and aging in articular cartilage. *JOSPT.* 1991; 14(5):189–197.
55. Klein FA, Rajan RK. Normal aging: effects on connective tissue metabolism and structure. *J Gerontol.* 1985; 40(5):579–585.
56. Donatelli R, Owens-Burkart H. Effects of immobilization on the extensibility of periarticular connective tissue. *JOSPT.* 1981; 3(2):67–71.
57. Boyer GG. Vision problems. In: Carnevali E, Patrick C, eds. *Nursing Management for the Elderly.* Philadelphia: Lippincott Co.; 1989.
58. Payton OD, Poland JL. Aging Process: Implications for clinical practice. *Phys Ther.* 1983; 63(1):41–48.
59. Wedgewood, J. The place of rehabilitation in geriatric medicine: an overview. *Int Rehabil Med.* 1985; 7:107.
60. Molsa PK, Paljarvi L, Rinne JO, et al. Validity of clinical diagnosis in dementia: a prospective clinicopathologic study. *J Neurol Neurosurg Psychiatry.* 1985; 48:1085–1090.
61. Alexopoulos GS, Abrams RC, Young RC, Shamoian CA. Cornell scale for depression in dementia. *Biol Psychiatry.* 1988; 23:271–284.
62. Hughes CP, Berg L, Danziger WL, et al. A new clinical scale for the staging of dementia. *Br J Psychiatry.* 1982; 140:566–572.
63. Cummings JL, Miller B, Hill MA, Neshkes R. Neuropsychiatric aspects of multi-infarct dementia and dementia of the Alzheimer type. *Arch Neurol.* 1987; 44:389–393.

64. Hachinski VC, Illiff LD, Zilhka E, et al. Cerebral blood flow in dementia. *Arch Neurol.* 1975; 32:632–637.

65. Schoenberg BS. Epidemiology of movement disorders. In: Marsden CD, Fahn S, eds. *Movement Disorders.* London: Butterworth; 1987:17–32.

66. Quinn NP, Rossor MN, Marsden CD. Dementia and Parkinson's disease—pathological and neurochemical considerations. *Br Med Bulletin.* 1986; 42:86–92.

67. Hornykiewicz O. Brain neurotransmitter changes in Parkinson's disease. In: Marsden CD, Fahn S, eds. *Movement Disorders.* London: Butterworth; 1987:41–58.

68. Baloh RW. Neurology of aging: vestibular system. In: Albert ML, ed. *Clinical Neurology of Aging.* New York: Oxford University Press; 1984.

69. Batata M, Spray GH, Bolton FG, et al. Blood and bone marrow changes in elderly patients, with particular reference to frolic acid, vitamin B_{12}, iron and ascorbic acid. *Brit Med J.* 1967; 2:667–669.

70. Burchinsky SG. Neurotransmitter receptors in the central nervous system and aging: pharmacological aspects (review). *Experimental Aging.* 1984; 19:227–239.

71. Gambert SR. *Diabetes Mellitus in the Elderly: A Practical Guide.* New York: Raven Press; 1990.

72. Bergman M. *Principles of Diabetes Management.* New York: Medical Examination Publishing Co.; 1987.

73. Riddle MC. Diabetic neuropathies in the elderly: management update. *Geriatrics.* 1990; 45(9):32–36.

74. Gutmann E, Hanzlikova V. Basic mechanisms of aging in the neuromuscular system. *Mech Ageing Dev* 1972; 1:327–349.

75. Gilchrest BA. *Skin and Aging Processes.* Boca Raton, Fla: CRC Press, Inc.; 1984; 67–81.

76. Silverberg N, Silverberg L. Aging and the skin. *Postgrad Med.* 1989; 86:131–136.

77. Pollack SV. Skin cancer in the elderly. In: Cohen HJ, ed. Cancer II: Specific Neoplasms. *Clin Geriatr Med.* 1987; 3(4):715–728.

78. Silverberg E. Cancer statistics, 1984. *CA.* 1984; 34:7–23.

79. Scotto J, Fears TR, Fraumeni JF, Jr. Incidence of nonmelanoma skin cancer in the United States. US Department of Health and Human Services Pub. No. (NIH) 82–2433, Washington, DC: US Government Printing Office; 1981.

80. Albright SD III. Treatment of skin cancer using multiple modalities. *J Am Acad Dermatol.* 1982; 7:143–171.

81. Kopf AW. Malignant melanoma in humans. In: *Causes and Effects of Changes in Stratospheric Ozone: Update 1983.* National Research Council, National Academy of Sciences. Washington, DC: National Academy Press; 1984.

82. Kopf AW. Prevention of malignant melanoma. *Dermatol Clin.* 1985; 3:351–360.

83. McLeod GR, Davis NC, Little JH. Melanoma: experience of the Queensland Melanoma Project. In: Balch CM, Milton GW, eds. *Cutaneous Melanoma.* Philadelphia: Lippincott; 1985.

84. Feldman DE, Stoll H, Maize JC. Melanomas of the palm, sole, and nail bed: a clinico-pathological study. *Cancer.* 1980; 46:2492–2504.

85. Koh HK, Michalik E, Sober AJ. Lentigo maligna melanoma has no better prognosis than other types of melanoma. J Clin Oncol. 1984; 2:994–1001.

86. Andres R. Normal aging versus disease in the elderly. In: Andres EL, Bierman EL, Hazzard WR, eds. *Principles in Geriatric Medicine.* New York: McGraw-Hill; 1985:38–41m.

87. Bennett L, Lee B. Pressure versus shear in pressure sore causation. In: Lee B, ed. *Chronic Ulcers of the Skin.* New York: McGraw-Hill; 1985:39–56.

88. Kosiak M. Prevention and rehabilitation of ischemic ulcers. In: Kottke F, Stillwell G, Lehman J, eds. *Krusen's Handbook of Physical Medicine and Rehabilitation.* 3rd ed. Philadelphia: Saunders; 1982:881–888.

89. McCulloch J, Hovde J. Treatment of wounds due to vascular problems. In: Kloth L, McCulloch J, Feedar J, eds. *Wound Healing: Alternatives in Management.* Philadelphia: Davis; 1990:177–195.

90. Kasper RL. Eye problems of the aged. In: Reichel RJ, ed. *Clinical Aspects of Aging.* Baltimore, Md: Williams and Wilkins; 1988.

91. Andreasen MK. Making a safe environment by design. *J Gerontol Nurs.* 1985; 11(6):18–22.

92. Zegeer LJ. The effects of sensory changes in older persons. *J Neuroscience Nurs.* 1986; 18:325–332.

93. Christenson MA. Designing for the older person by addressing the environmental attributes. *Phys Occup Ther Geriatrics.* 1990; 8:31–48.

94. Skinner HB, Barrack RL, Cook SD. Age-related decline in proprioception. *Clin Orthop.* 1984; Apr(184):208–211.
95. Kokmen E, Bossemeyer RW, Williams WJ. Quantitative evaluation of joint motion perception in an aging population. *J Gerontol.* 1978; 33:62.
96. Laidlaw RW, Hamilton MA. A study of thresholds in perception of passive movement among normal control subjects. *Bull Neurol Inst.* 1937; 6:268–340.
97. Benassi G, D'Alessandro R, Gallassi R, et al. Neurological examination in subjects over 65 years: an epidemiological survey. *Neuroepidemiology.* 1990; 9:27–38.
98. Barrett DS, Cobb AG, Bently G. Joint proprioception in normal, osteoarthritic and replaced knees. *J Bone Joint Surg.* 1991; 73B:53–56.
99. Herdman SJ. Exercise strategies in vestibular disorders. *Ear Nose Throat J.* 1989; 68:961–964.
100. Herdman SJ. Assessment and treatment of balance disorders in the vestibular deficient patient. In: Duncan P, ed. *Balance.* Proceedings of the American Physical Therapy Association Forum. Alexandria, Va: APTA Publications; 1990:87–94.
101. Hayter J. Modifying the environment to help older persons. *Nurs Health Care.* 1983; 4:265–269.
102. Maloney CC. Identifying and treating the client with sensory loss. *Phys Occup Ther Geriatrics.* 1987; 5:31–46.
103. Bartol MA, Heitkemper M. Gastrointestinal problems. In: Carnevali, P and Patrick, B eds. *Nursing Management for the Elderly.* Philadelphia: Lippincott Co.; 1989.
104. Bidlack WR, Kirsch A, Meskin MS. Nutritional requirements of the elderly. *Food Technology.* 1988; 40:61–70.
105. Siebens H, Trupe E, Siebens A, et al. Correlates and consequences of eating dependency in Institutionalized elderly. *J Am Geriatr Soc.* 1986; 34(3):192–198.
106. Castell DO. Dysphagia in the elderly. *J Amer Ger Soc.* 1986; 34(3):248–249.
107. Goldman R. Decline in organ function with age. In: Rossman I, ed. *Clinical Geriatrics.* 2nd ed. Philadelphia: Lippincott Co.; 1979.
108. Goyal VK. Changes with age in the human kidney. *Exp Gerontol.* 1982; 17:321–331.
109. Lindeman RD, Goldman R. Anatomic and physiologic age changes in the kidney. *Exp Gerontol.* 1986; 21:379–406.
110. Lindeman RD, Tobin JD, Shock NW. Longitudinal studies on the rate of decline in renal function with age. *J Amer Ger Soc.* 1985; 33:278–285.
111. Fine LG. Preventing the progression of human renal disease: have rational therapeutic principles emerged? *Kidney Int.* 1988; 33:116–128.
112. Phillips PA, Rolls BJ, Ledingham JJG: Reduced thirst after water deprivation in healthy elderly men. *N Engl J Med.* 1984; 311:753–759.
113. Lindeman RD. Hypokalemia: causes, consequences, and correction. *Am J Med Sci.* 1976; 272:5–17.
114. Nieman DC. *The Sports Medicine Fitness Course.* Palo Alto, Calif.: Bull Publishing Co.; 1986.
115. Drinkwater BL: *The Role of Nutrition and Exercise in Health. Continuing Dental Education.* Seattle: University of Washington; 1985.
116. Suominen H, Heikkinen E, Liesen H. Effect of 8 weeks endurance training on skeletal muscle metabolism in 56–70 year old men. *Eur J Appl Physiol.* 1987; 37:173–180.
117. Kaplin GA, Seemah TE, Cohen RD. Mortality among the elderly in the Alameda County study: behavioral and demographic risk factors. *Am J Public Health.* 1987; 77(3):307–312.
118. Stones MJ, Dornan B, Kozma A. The prediction of mortality in elderly institution residents. *J Gerontol Psychol Sci.* 1989; 44(3):72–79.
119. Mooradian AD, Morley JE, Korenman SG. Endocrinology in aging. *Dis Mon.* 1988; 34:395–461.
120. Greenblatt RB. *Geriatric Endocrinology.* Aging Series Vol. 5, New York: Raven Press; 1978.
121. Morley JE. Geriatric endocrinology. In: Mendelsohn G, ed. *Diagnosis and Pathology of Endocrine Disease.* Philadelphia: Lippincott Co.; 1988.
122. Robuschi G, Safran M, Braverman LE. Hypothyroidism in the elderly. *Endocr Rev.* 1987; 8:142–153.
123. Morley JE, Slag MF, Elson MK, et al. The interpretation of thyroid function tests in hospitalized patients. *JAMA.* 1983; 249:2377–2379.
124. Morley JE. The aging endocrine system. *Postgrad Med.* 1983; 73:107–120.
125. Lipson LG. Diabetes in the elderly: diagnosis, pathogenesis and therapy. *Am J Med.* 1986; 80(suppl 5A):10–21.

126. Morley JE, Mooradian AD, Rosenthal MJ, et al. Diabetes mellitus in elderly patients: is it different? *Am J Med.* 1987; 83:533–544.

127. Rosenthal MJ, Hartnell JM, Morley JE, et al. UCLA geriatric grand rounds: diabetes in the elderly. *J Am Geriatr Soc.* 1987; 35:435–447.

128. Chapuy MC, Chapuy P, Meunier PJ. Calcium and vitamin D supplements: effects of calcium metabolism in elderly people. *Am J Clin Nutr.* 1987; 46:324–328.

129. Chernoff R. *Geriatric Nutrition: The Health Professional's Handbook.* Gaithersburg, Md: Aspen Publishers, Inc.; 1991.

130. American Diabetes Association. Position statement: office guide to diagnosis and classification of diabetes mellitus and other categories of glucose intolerance. *Diabetes Care.* 1992; 15(suppl 2):4.

131. Jackson RA. Mechanisms of age-related glucose intolerance. *Diabetes Care.* 1990; 13(suppl 2):9–19.

132. Jette DU. Physiological effects of exercise in the diabetic. *Phys Ther.* 1984; 64(3):339–342.

133. Kohl HW, Villegas JA, Gordon NF, Blair SN. Cardiorespiratory fitness, glycemic status, and mortality risk in men. *Diabetes Care.* 1992; 15(2):184–192.

134. Kohn RR. *Principles of Mammalian Aging.* 2nd ed. Englewood Cliffs, NJ: Prentice-Hall; 1978.

CHAPTER **6** SIX

Assessment Instruments

The demands in health care for cost-effective care are pushing rehabilitation and medical professionals to prove the efficacy and efficiency of the care provided. The obvious place for caregivers to begin this process is in the area of assessment. The evolution of medicine and rehabilitation has been a mixture of science, philosophy, sociology, and intuition. Some of the finest practitioners may be some of the worst scientists. However, they may have an extraordinary intuitive sense. Because of this fine mixture, it is difficult to quantify assessments, treatments, and outcomes. Nevertheless, this needs to be done. The work in health care assessment has grown exponentially in the last 20 years, and more tools are being developed and more scrutiny is being applied to treatment interventions and outcomes.

In the area of aging, these efforts are extremely timely. As was noted in Chapter 1, the number of older persons is growing dramatically. In addition, the National Long-Term Care Survey noted 3.0 million older persons with impairment in one or more daily activities.[1] The Supplement on Aging portion of the National Interview Survey showed 6.0 million impaired elderly,[2] and the *Journal of Gerontology: Medical Sciences* noted recently that the "quality of life is judged more by the level of functioning and ability to remain independent than by specific diseases diagnosed by the physician."[3]

The implications of improved, appropriate, and standard measures also impact the clinician by improving communication among practitioners, fostering consistency, and reaffirming knowledge and skill.

This chapter will discuss three important components of the physical therapist's assessment of the elderly. The first section will discuss mental status measures for older persons; the second will discuss the most common functional assessment tools for the elderly; and third will discuss the modifications needed when assessing the older person using accepted physical measures, such as goniometry, manual muscle tests, and nerve conduction velocity.

MENTAL STATUS MEASURES

Mini-Mental State Examination

The Mini-Mental State Examination (MMSE) was published in 1975 by Dr Folstein and co-workers,[4] and it has been widely used since then to assess cognitive changes in older patients. The MMSE was developed to assess patients who have deficits in memory, language, or both. These deficits correlate to intellectual impairment that may indicate Alzheimer's disease. The test indicates impairment, though it does not make a diagnosis.[5] The MMSE correlates with Wechsler Intelligence Scales and the Wechsler Memory Test, as well as to cerebral lesions detected by CAT scan.[4,5]

The test is relatively easy to administer and takes between 5 and 10 minutes. The test and its instructions for administration can be found in Figure 6–1.

The maximum score possible on this test is 30. A score below 24 indicates cognitive impairment and is not considered normal for older persons. A score of 21 to 24 is considered mild intellectual impairment, a score of 16 to 20 reflects moderate impairment, and a score below 15 is considered severely impaired.[4] The MMSE also relates to depression, and is indicative of depression at a score of 19. Patients show improvement on the MMSE scores as the depression is ameliorated.[6]

The Mental Status Questionnaire

The Mental Status Questionnaire (MSQ) is composed of ten questions and, therefore, is quick and easy to administer. Because of its ease of use and its validity and reliability, it has been used extensively for the past three decades.[7] This test does show a correlation between low scores and impaired cognition.

Despite the test's convenience and research strength, however, it does have several clinical weaknesses. It lacks sensitivity and may show false positives because it does not pick up impairment until the scores are in the high range. It also omits several important domains of cognitive functioning, including reasoning, visual–spatial relationships, and many aspects of language. Table 6–1 shows the MSQ.[7] The MSQ has also been criticized for a lack of relevancy of its questions to institutional residents.[6]

Depression Scales

Despite the high prevalence of depression in the older population, the diagnosis of depression may be missed.[8] However, when screening instruments are used, the recognition of depression is increased.[9]

The Zung Self-Rating Scale

The Zung Self-Rating Depression Scale is widely used for screening for depression. However, this scale may not be the best choice for older persons. The validity on

Mini-Mental State Exam

Orientation:	Maximum Score	Score	Instructions
What is the (year) (season) (date) (day) (month)?	5	_____	Ask for the date. Then proceed to ask other parts of the question. One point for each correct segment of the question.
Where are we: (state) (county) (town) (hospital) (floor)?	5	_____	Ask for the facility then proceed to parts of the question. One point for each correct segment of the question.

Registration:			
Name three objects (bed, apple, shoe). Ask the patient to repeat them.	3	_____	Name the objects slowly, one second for each. Ask him to repeat. Score by the number he is able to recall. Take time here for him to learn the series of objects, up to 6 trials, to use later for the memory test.

Attention and Calculation:			
Count backwards by 7s. Start with 100. Stop after 5 calculations.	5	_____	Score the total number correct. (93, 86, 79, 72, 65)

Alternate question:			
Spell the word "world" backwards.	5	_____	Score the number of letters in correct order. (dlrow = 5. dlorw = 3)

Recall:	Maximum Score	Score	Instructions
Ask for the three objects used in question 2 to be repeated.	3	_____	Score one point for each correct answer. (bed, apple, shoe)

Language:			
1. Naming: Name this object. (watch, pencil)	2	_____	Hold the object. Ask patient to name it. Score one point for each correct answer.
2. Repetition: Repeat the following— "No ifs, ands or buts."	1	_____	Allow one trial only. Score one point for correct answer.
3. Follow a 3-stage command: "Take the paper in your right hand, fold it in half, and put it on the floor."	3	_____	Use a blank sheet of paper. Score one point for each part correctly executed.
4. Reading: Read and obey the following: Close your eyes.	1	_____	Instruction should be printed on a page. Allow patient to read it. Score by a correct response.
5. Writing: Write a sentence.	1	_____	Provide paper and pencil. Allow patient to write any sentence. It must contain a noun, verb, and be sensible.
6. Copying: Copy this design.	1	_____	All 10 angles must be present. Figures must intersect. Tremor and rotation are ignored.
	Total Score	_____	(Max. 30) Test is not timed.

Figure 6-1. *(Reprinted with permission from Folstein MF, Folstein SE, McHugh PR. Mini mental state. A practical method for grading the cognitive state of patients for the clinician. J Psychiatr Res. 1975; 12:189-198.)*

TABLE 6–1. MENTAL STATUS QUESTIONNAIRE (MSQ)

The patient gets a point for every error when asked the following questions, and the scores show the severity of brain syndrome as follows:

0–2 = none or minimal
3–8 = moderate
9–10 = severe

1. What is this place?
2. Where is this place located?
3. What day of the month is it today?
4. What day of the week is it?
5. What year is it?
6. How old are you?
7. When is your birthday?
8. In what year were you born?
9. What is the name of the president?
10. Who was the president before this one?

Reprinted with permission from Kahn RL, et al. Brief objective measures for the determination of mental status in the aged. Am J Psychiatry. 1960; 117:326.

this test was tested on a university outpatient population,[10] and elderly persons scored higher on it. Because of this, the elderly may be considered "borderline" even when they are not depressed.[11]

The test is composed of ten negative and ten positive statements, with the respondent giving an answer that correlates with a one to four rating. The scores can be expressed as a percentage of 80, with 80 being the highest score and most indicative of severe depression.[12] (Fig. 6–2).

Popoff Index of Depression

The Popoff Index of Depression may be more applicable to the older patient who is seen in the community. This test allows for more covert responses, which can help to identify persons who are not ready to make obvious statements about their depression. It is slightly more sensitive to patients who are somatisizing as well.[13] The test consists of 15 groups of statements. Each group has a covert, overt, and healthy response. If the respondent chooses either the covert or the overt response, he or she will get a point. A score higher than 10 is indicative of depression. This test, as well as the Zung test, has been shown to have sensitivity and reliability when compared to other tests and population studies (Fig. 6–3).[14]

Beck Depression Inventory

The Beck Depression Inventory (Fig. 6–4) is another very popular instrument for depression screening. The test was initially administered by interview, but it is also adaptable for self-administration.[15] The original form has 21 sets of statements with a scoring mechanism from zero to three. In a primary care setting, a cutoff score of 13 was indicative of depression with a high sensitivity and specificity.[16] In elderly patients, it was found that using a cutoff score of 10 only missed 3% of the depressed patients.[17]

The short form of the Beck's Depression Inventory correlates as well as the long version and only takes the patient 5 minutes to complete. The 13 questions for the short version are taken from Figure 6–4[18] as follows: A,B,C,D,E,G,I,L, M,N,O,Q,R. In addition, in the short version the responses are reversed so that the patient reads the most negative response first.[16]

The Zung Self-Rating Depression Scale

1. (–) I feel down-hearted and blue.
2. (+) Morning is when I feel the best.
3. (–) I have crying spells or feel like it.
4. (–) I have trouble sleeping at night.
5. (+) I eat as much as I used to.
6. (+) I still enjoy sex.
7. (–) I notice that I am losing weight.
8. (–) I have trouble with constipation.
9. (–) My heart beats faster than usual.
10. (–) I get tired for no reason.
11. (+) My mind is as clear as it used to be.
12. (+) I find it easy to do the things I used to.
13. (–) I am restless and can't keep still.
14. (+) I feel hopeful about the future.
15. (–) I am more irritable than usual.
16. (+) I find it easy to make decisions.
17. (+) I feel that I am useful and needed.
18. (+) My life is pretty full.
19. (–) I feel that others would be better off if I were dead.
20. (+) I still enjoy the things I used to do.

Statements are answered "a little of the time," "some of the time," "a good part of the time," or "most of the time." The responses are given a score of 1 to 4, arranged so that the higher the score, the greater the depressioin: the statements designated with (+) are given "1" for response "most of time," while those with (–) are given a "4" for "most of the time."

Figure 6–2. *(Adapted and reprinted with permission from Arch Gen Psych. 1965; 12:63–70.)*

The Geriatric Depression Scale

The final tool to be described for assessing depression is the Geriatric Depression Scale. This 30 item, yes-or-no questionnaire determines that a score of over 8 has a 90% sensitivity and an 80% specificity in detecting depression in the older population.[19] There is also a short version consisting of the following 15 questions: 1–4, 7, 9, 10, 12, 14, 15, 17, and 21–23. A score of over 5 on this form may indicate depression.[20] The test and the method of scoring is shown in Figure 6–5.[20]

Stress Measures

A final area of pyschosocial assessment is stress.

The Holmes and Rahe Life Events Scale

The most widely used tool for evaluating stress is the Holmes and Rahe Life Events Scale.[21] This scale is shown in Figure 6–6. In administering this tool, the patient is asked to circle the events that have occurred in the last year or will occur in the coming year. The therapist adds up the scores, and the total score is compared to the following scale. A score of below 180 points indicates mild stress or less than a 40% chance of a serious illness in the next year; a score of 180 to 300 indicates moderate stress or a 40% chance of developing a serious illness in the next year; and a

Popoff Index of Depression

1. **O.** Everything is an effort.
   H. I have a lot of energy.
   C. Maybe I'm just getting older.

2. **H.** I've got a lot of pep.
   C. I tire easily.
   O. I'm tired all the time.

3. **C.** I'm in a rut.
   O. Things are not going well.
   H. I'm pleased with the way things are going.

4. **O.** I don't have much to look forward to.
   H. I look forward to the future.
   C. I go along as best I can.

5. **H.** I enjoy getting up in the morning.
   C. I push myself to get going in the morning.
   O. I find it hard to face the day.

6. **C.** I don't feel rested after sleeping.
   O. I've been having trouble sleeping lately.
   H. I sleep fine and feel rested.

7. **O.** I haven't been eating as well lately.
   H. I enjoy eating.
   C. Food doesn't taste as good as it used to.

8. **H.** Sex is pleasurable to me.
   C. Sometimes I'm too tired for sex.
   O. I've lost some interest in sex lately.

9. **C.** I force myself to do my work.
   O. I don't have much ambition.
   H. I am ambitious.

10. **O.** I don't feel like doing much lately.
    H. I enjoy doing lots of things.
    C. I don't go out much beacuse I am too tired.

11. **H.** Things are going good.
    C. Sometimes everything goes wrong.
    O. I can't cope with things very well lately.

12. **C.** I'd do better if I felt better.
    O. Sometimes I can't do anything right.
    H. Things are running smoothly.

13. **O.** I'm depressed.
    H. I'm happy.
    C. I don't let myself get depressed.

14. **H.** I'm happy with the way I'm doing things.
    C. Everybody feels they could do better.
    O. I'm not doing things as well as I used to.

15. **O.** Sometimes I feel like giving up.
    H. I'm enjoying my life.
    C. I fight it when I feel discouraged.

In the questionnaire, "C" indicates a "covert" response, "O" an overt response, and "H" a healthy response.

Figure 6–3. *(Adapted and reprinted with permission from Clinical Medicine. Philadelphia: Lippincott Co. 1969; 76:26.)*

score above 300 indicates severe stress or an 80% chance of a serious illness in the next year.[21]

FUNCTIONAL ASSESSMENT

The word function is repeated 88 times in the current Health Care Financing (HCFA) regulations on rehabilitation.[22] This fact should encourage rehabilitation professionals to think about and use functional measures, because HCFA uses these regulations as requirements for payment.

Functional measurement is also important because it differs from the current methods physical therapists and occupational therapists use to assess patient status, and they may not truly reflect a patient's functional level. These measures, such as range of motion, strength, and other musculoskeletal parameters, may be important to assessment, but they do not always relate to function. If rehabilitation professionals are to show efficacy in what they do, it is important that they assess function in conjunction with musculoskeletal parameters. Combining these two assessments will make a truly comprehensive rehabilitation evaluation possible.

A recent study by Mary Tinetti scrutinizes the use of musculoskeletal measures.[23] Her study showed very little relationship between musculoskeletal measures and functional outcomes of older patients.[23]

The Beck Depression Inventory

A Mood

0 I do not feel sad.
1 I feel blue or sad.
2a I am blue or sad all the time and I can't snap out of it.
2b I am so sad or unhappy that it is very painful.
3 I am so sad or unhappy that I can't stand it.

B (Pessimism)

0 I am not particularly pessimistic or discouraged about the future.
1 I feel discouraged about the future.
2a I feel I have nothing to look forward to.
2b I feel that I won't ever get over my troubles.
3 I feel that the future is hopeless and that things cannot improve.

C (Sense of Failure)

0 I do not feel like a failure.
1 I feel I have failed more than the average person.
2a I feel I have accomplished very little that is worthwhile or that means anything.
2b As I look back on my life all I can see is a lot of failures.
3 I feel I am a complete failure as a person (parent, husband, wife).

D (Lack of Satisfaction)

0 I am not particularly dissatisfied.
1a I feel bored most of the time.
1b I don't enjoy things the way I used to.
2 I don't get satisfaction out of anything any more.
3 I am dissatisfied with everything.

E (Guilty Feelings)

0 I don't feel particularly guilty.
1 I feel bad or unworthy a good part of the time.
2a I feel quite guilty.
2b I feel bad or unworthy practically all the time now.
3 I feel as though I am very bad or worthless.

F (Sense of Punishment)

0 I don't feel I am being punished.
1 I have a feeling that something bad may happen to me.

2 I feel I am being punished or will be punished.
3a I feel I deserve to be punished.
3b I want to be punished.

G (Self Hate)

0 I don't feel disappointed in myself.
1a I am disappointed in myself.
1b I don't like myself.
2 I am disgusted with myself.
3 I hate myself.

H (Self Accusations)

0 I don't feel I am any worse than anybody else.
1 I am very critical of myself for my weaknesses or mistakes.
2a I blame myself for everything that goes wrong.
2b I feel I have many bad faults.

I (Self-punitive Wishes)

0 I don't have any thought of harming myself.
1 I have thoughts of harming myself, but I would not carry them out.
2a I feel I would be better off dead.
2b I have definite plans about committing suicide.
2c I feel my family would be better off if I were dead.
3 I would kill myself if I could.

J (Crying Spells)

0 I don't cry any more than usual.
1 I cry more now than I used to.
2 I cry all the time now. I can't stop it.
3 I used to be able to cry but now I can't cry at all even though I want to.

K (Irritability)

0 I am no more irritated now than I ever am.
1 I get annoyed or irritated more easily than I used to.
2 I feel irritated all the time.
3 I don't get irritated at all at the things that used to irritate me.

L (Social Withdrawal)

0 I have not lost interest in other people.
1 I am less interested in other people now than I used to be.

—— *Continued* ——

─── *Continued from previous page* ───

2   I have lost most of my interest in other people and have little feeling for them.
3   I have lost all my interest in other people and don't care about them at all.

M (Indecisiveness)
0   I make desicions about as well as ever.
1   I am less sure of myself now and try to put off making decisions.
2   I can't make decisions any more without help.
3   I can't make any decisions at all any more.

N (Body Image)
0   I don't feel I look any worse than I used to.
1   I am worried that I am looking old or un-attractive.
2   I feel that there are permanent changes in my appearance and they make me look unattractive.
3   I feel that I am ugly or repulsive looking.

O (Work Inhibition)
0   I can work about as well as before.
1a It takes extra effort to get started at doing something.
1b I don't work as well as I used to.
2   I have to push myself very hard to do anything.
3   I can't do any work at all.

P (Sleep Disturbance)
0   I can sleep as well as usual.
1   I wake up more tired in the morning than I used to.
2   I wake up 1 to 2 hours earlier than usual and find it hard to get back to sleep.
3   I wake up early every day and can't get more than 5 hours sleep.

Q (Fatigability)
0   I don't get any more tired than usual.
1   I get tired more easily than I used to.
2   I get tired from doing anything.
3   I get too tired to do anything.

R (Loss of Apopetite)
0   My appetite is no worse than usual.
1   My appetite is not as good as it used to be.
2   My appetite is much worse now.
3   I have no appetite at all anymore.

S (Weight Loss)
0   I haven't lost much weight, if any, lately.
1   I have lost more than 5 pounds.
2   I have lost more than 10 pounds.
3   I have lost more than 15 pounds

T (Somatic Preoccupation)
0   I am no more concerned about my health than usual.
1   I am concerned about aches and pains or upset stomach or constipation or other un-pleasant feelings in my body.
2   I am so concerned with how I feel or what I feel that it's hard to think of much else.
3   I am completely absorbed in what I feel.

U (Loss of Libido)
0   I have not noticed any recent change in my interest in sex.
1   I am less interested in sex than I used to be.
2   I am much less interested in sex now.
3   I have lost interest in sex completely.

Items with "a" or "b" are scored the same as the corresponding number.

Figure 6–4. *(Reprinted with permission from Inventory for measuring depression. Arch Gen Psych. 1961; 4:561–571.)*

Geriatric Depression Scale

1. Are you basically satisfied with your life? (no)

2. Have you dropped many of your activities and interests? (yes)

3. Do you feel that your life is empty? (yes)

4. Do you often get bored? (yes)

5. Are you hopeful about the future? (no)

6. Are you bothered by thoughts that you just cannot get out of your head? (yes)

7. Are you in good spirits most of the time? (no)

8. Are you afraid that something bad is going to happen to you? (yes)

9. Do you feel happy most of the time? (no)

10. Do you often feel helpless? (yes)

11. Do you often get restless and fidgety? (yes)

12. Do you prefer to stay home at night, rather than go out and do new things? (yes)

13. Do you frequently worry about the future? (yes)

14. Do you feel that you have more problems with memory than most? (yes)

15. Do you think it is wonderful to be alive now? (no)

16. Do you often feel downhearted and blue? (yes)

17. Do you feel pretty worthless the way you are now? (yes)

18. Do you worry a lot about the past? (yes)

19. Do you find life very exciting? (no)

20. Is it hard for you to get started on new projects? (yes)

21. Do you feel full of energy? (no)

22. Do you feel that your situation is hopeless? (yes)

23. Do you think that most persons are better off than you are? (yes)

24. Do you frequently get upset over little things? (yes)

25. Do you frequently feel like crying? (yes)

26. Do you have trouble concentrating? (yes)

27. Do you enjoy getting up in the morning? (no)

28. Do you prefer to avoid social gatherings? (yes)

29. Is it easy for you to make decisions? (no)

30. Is your mind as clear as it used to be? (no)

Score one point for each response that matches the yes or no answer after the question.

Figure 6–5. *(Adapted and reprinted with permission from Yesavage JA, Brink TI Development and validation of a geriatric depression screening scale: A preliminary report. J Psych Res. 1983; 17:41.)*

The Holmes and Rahe Social Adjustment Scale

Rank	Life Event	Mean Value
1	Death of spouse	100
2	Divorce	73
3	Marital separation	65
4	Jail term	63
5	Death of close family member	63
6	Personal injury or illness	53
7	Marriage	50
8	Fired at work	47
9	Marital reconciliation	45
10	Retirement	45
11	Change in health of family member	44
12	Pregnancy	40
13	Sex difficulties	39
14	Gain of new family member	39
15	Business readjustment	39
16	Change in financial state	38
17	Death of close friend	37
18	Change to different line of work	36
19	Change in number of arguments with spouse	35
20	Mortgage over $10,000	31
21	Foreclosure of mortgage or loan	30
22	Change in responsibilities at work	29
23	Son or daughter leaving home	29
24	Trouble with in-laws	29
25	Outstanding personal achievement	28
26	Wife begin or stop work	26
27	Begin or end school	26
28	Change in living conditions	25
29	Revision of personal habits	24
30	Trouble with boss	23
31	Change in work hours or conditions	20
32	Change in residence	20
33	Change in schools	20
34	Change in recreation	19
35	Change in church activities	19
36	Change in social activities	18
37	Mortgage or loan less than $10,000	17
38	Change in sleeping habits	16
39	Change in number of family get-togethers	15
40	Change in eating habits	15
41	Vacation	13
42	Christmas	12
43	Minor violations of the law	11

Figure 6–6. *(Reprinted with permission from Holmes T, Rahe R. The social readjustment rating scale. J Psych Res. 1967; 11:213–218.)*

A third factor contributing to the importance of functional evaluation is the ability to give a beginning and end point based on a functional outcome, as well as a relationship of this outcome to a patient's independence. For example, the Barthel Index (see Fig. 6–7) can rate a patient's difficulty with bathing or walking. The patient's ability to perform these tasks is assigned a level that is indicated by a number. As the person progresses with treatment, they are moved to higher levels. If they regress, they are ranked at a lower level. In addition, the total scoring on this index indicates to the assessor when the patient is able to go home or is in need of assistance.

These numbers translate to a patient's specific ability to function and can be very helpful in making decisions related to disposition and the need for continued care. On the other hand, a muscle strength measure indicating normal (5/5) muscle strength means nothing if the person cannot get in and out of a tub or eat independently. The combination of strength and function measures are extremely helpful, however, when assessing cause and outcome.

The purpose of this section is to encourage the health professional to avoid doing unnecessary and time-consuming tests. Many of these functional tests can be done by the patient with paper and pencil prior to the treatment program and on discharge without unnecessarily monopolizing the health professional's time.

A final justification of functional evaluation comes from an article written by Robert Kane, Dean of the School of Public Health at the University of Minnesota.[24] Dr Kane is a well-respected researcher in gerontology and health care and an advocate for functional assessment for geriatricians. In his article, he states that a specialty is not truly a specialty until it has its own instrument. He gave radiology as an example. This discipline would not have its current credibility or base if it were not for x-rays. Also, cardiology would not have evolved into a specialty if it were not for heart catheterization. He then asserts that geriatrics will truly not be accepted as a specialty until the professionals in that area have a similar tool. He believes that the tool for geriatrics is functional assessment.[24]

By extrapolating on his thoughts, it can be seen that rehabilitation is an area where functional assessment is a tool, especially for rehabilitation professionals in the area of geriatrics. The following sections follow this argument and advocate functional assessment for rehabilitation professionals, particularly for those working in geriatrics.

What is Functional Assessment?

Functional assessment differs from traditional assessment in several ways. For example, it targets specific behaviors and tasks a patient wishes to accomplish. If a therapist were to ask a patient, "What do you want from physical therapy?," the patient would not say, "I want my muscles to test normal or 5/5." Rather, they would answer, "I want to increase the strength in my legs," or "I want to run 10 miles pain free." These responses are rarely indicated in rehabilitation notes or incorporated into work goals. Instead, many notes state that the goal of treatment is to increase strength or function. This is not enough. A goal stated in a slightly more specific functional terms is, "Increase strength so that the patient is able to run a marathon without pain," or "the patient is able to walk from bed to bathroom unassisted, without falling or losing balance." An even better functional statement would be a quantified response, such as, "The patient scores 80 on the Barthel and can return home independently."

Richard Bohannon, in an article in the *International Journal of Rehabilitation Research*, showed that the number one priority when rehabilitating stroke patients is the patient walking independently.[25] Physical therapists may forget this when implementing various measures and techniques. Therefore, if the focus is on function, therapists will not lose sight of patients' needs.

The goal of rehabilitation is to assist people in achieving their highest level of function, but confusion often interferes with this. Instead of focusing on the goal, therapists focus on the signs and symptoms. When measuring and treating range of motion, strength, or endurance, the goal of function must be maintained. The second area of confusion and poor implementation of function is the use of function to mean different things (for example, the function of a knee or a hip). Instead, function must be examined in terms of the whole individual[26] and, more specifically, how that person functions versus how his or her shoulder functions.

If function is defined as the normal or characteristic performance of the individual,[27] the individual is the unit of analysis rather than the body part or organ system. It is not just a shoulder or a kidney that is being studied, it is a whole person. Can the patient reach up into the cabinet even if they have a rotator cuff tear, and do they need to? Is there some modification that they should be taught to adapt to their environment?

Understanding function includes more than understanding physical function, because there are four components of function.[28] The first is physical function, which is the component that physical therapists work with the most. This subsection of function includes sensory motor performance, walking, climbing stairs, and other activities of daily living. The second component is mental function, including intelligence, cognitive ability, and memory. The third is emotional function defined as coping with life's stressors, anxieties, and satisfactions. The fourth is social function. This area looks at a person's interaction with family members and the community, and any economic considerations. A good reference for functional assessment tools in older persons is Kane and Kane's *Assessing the Elderly*.[26] The next section will examine examples of different functional tools; the majority will be dedicated to physical scales, but some will be multidimensional.

Functional Assessment Tools

The Barthel Index

The Barthel Index is one of the most widely known and well-established physical functional parameters assessment tools.[29] It measures toileting, bathing, and ambulation (Fig. 6–7).[29] On the Barthel Index, the best score is 100 and the worst is 0. Tasks 1 through 9 have a possible score of 53, and tasks 10 through 15 have a possible score of 47, for a total possible score of 100.

Exploring a few items on this index will demonstrate how it is scored. If a patient can drink from a cup independently, they get 4 points. If, however, they need someone's help or they cannot do it at all, they get 0. The reason this scoring mechanism seems strange is because it is a weighted scale. Weighted scales were developed to correlate with other measures. In a weighted scale, the accomplishment of one item may be more important to a specific measure and is, therefore, scored higher than others. Because of this weighing, it is imperative to use the numbers shown on the tool.

To administer this test, give a patient the form without the numbers, and allow the patient to check the appropriate column. Later, the scorer can add up the numbers. This test is most reliable, however, if a health professional assesses and grades each task as the patient performs it.[29]

What do the numbers mean? The test reflects the patient's ability to perform activities of daily living (ADLs) without an attendant.[29] It correlates well with clinical judgment and mortality, as well as with discharge to a less restrictive environment.[29] A score of 60 or above means that a person can be discharged home but will require at least 2 hours of assistance in ADLs. If they score 80 or above, it means that the person can be discharged home but will require assistance of up to 2 hours in self-care. When working with a patient that has been assessed as independent in self-care and scores a 50 on the Barthel Index, this would indicate the contrary.

Barthel Index

The following presents the items or tasks scored in the Barthel Index with the corresponding values for independent performance of the tasks:

	"Can do by myself"	"Can do with help of someone else"	"Cannot do at all"
Self-Care Index			
1. Drinking from a cup	4	0	0
2. Eating	6	0	0
3. Dressing upper body	5	4	0
4. Dressing lower body	7	4	0
5. Putting on brace or artificial limb	0	2	0 (Not applicable)
6. Grooming	5	0	0
7. Washing or bathing	6	0	0
8. Controlling urination	10	5 (Accidents)	0 (Incontinent)
9. Controlling bowel movements	10	5 (Accidents)	0 (Incontinent)
Mobility Index			
10. Getting in and out of chair	15	7	0
11. Getting on and off toilet	6	3	0
12. Getting in and out of tub or shower	1	0	0
13. Walking 50 yards on the level	15	10	0
14. Walking up/down 1 flight of stairs	10	5	0
15. If not walking: propelling or pushing wheelchair	5	0	0 (Not applicable)

Barthel Total: Best score is 100; worst score is 0.

NOTE: Tasks 1–9, the Self-Care Index (including control of bladder and bowel sphincters), have a total possible score of 53. Tasks 10–15, the Mobility Index, have a total possible score of 47. The 2 groups of tasks combined make up the total Barthel Index with a total possible score of 100.

Figure 6–7. *(Reprinted with permission from Mahoney FI, Barthel DW. Functional evaluation: the Barthel Index. Maryland State Med J. 1965; 14(2):61–65.)*

The Katz ADL Index

The Katz ADL Index was one of the first attempts at standardizing functional assessment. This tool includes six major areas of ADLs: bathing, feeding, dressing, toileting, transferring, and continence. The index is show in Figure 6–8, and it can be scored in two ways. The first way that is shown uses letter ratings from A to G on a Guttman type scale. The rater chooses the most accurate assessment of the individual's performance. There is also a Likert-type of rating for this scale. Here, each activity is given a score from 0 to 3, where 0 is complete independence, 1 is a use of a device, 2 is the use of human assistance, and 3 is complete dependence. The scores are added up and averaged. This index has been used in various settings, from institutional to community.[30,31] The reliability in the Guttman version ranges from 0.948 to 0.976, there are no reliability measures for the Likert version.

Kenny Self-Care Index

The Kenny Self-Care Index reports professional judgment of six major ADLs (see items listed in the scale shown in Fig. 6–9). The professional rates the patient on all items on a 5 point scale as follows: 0 = complete dependence, 1 = uses extensive assistance, 2 = moderate assistance, 3 = minimal assistance, 4 = total independence. The scores are added and averaged for each category and all are summed for a basic physical function score. This index can be used to show improvement as evidenced by a higher score. There are no studies on reliability or validity as of yet.[32]

Instruments of Daily Living

The instruments described so far have assessed basic ADLs. Instrumental ADLs are also important to independent living, but they are more complex. Examples of these types of activities are using the telephone, shopping, and managing money. The Instruments of Activities of Daily Living (IADL) identifies seven items and then provides the rater with rankings for independence (see instrument Table 6–2 for items and rankings).[33] Despite the lack of reliability and validity measures for this scale, it can be useful in indicating what services may be needed by the patient. For example, deficits in an area will dictate if a person needs transportation assistance or meal preparation.

PULSES

The PULSES Profile is an acronym for six multidimensional areas of function. These areas are P = physical condition, U = upper limb function, L = lower limb function, S = sensory components, E = excretory function, and S = support factors. The PULSES Profile is shown in Table 6–3. Each of the six items is rated according to the description listed below each item. The PULSES has not been shown to be reliable. However, it has been shown to correlate to other functional measures.[34,35] This tool has been used with a variety of patient settings and patient groups, and it is probably best used in a situation where a significant degree of change is expected.[36]

Functional Independence Measure

The next measure is the Functional Independence Measure (FIM). The Functional Independence Measure is copyrighted and is available from the Research Foundation, State University of New York (SUNY).[36] It is an extensive work containing several scales on transferring, feeding, dressing, bowel and bladder control, communication, and so forth. The whole package together makes up the FIM.

One of FIM's scales measures locomotion scale. The numbers to the left (1 through 7) indicate the need for assistance. For example, number 7 on the scale would be complete independence defined as a patient that "walks a minimum of

Katz ADL Index

The Index of Independence in Activities of Daily Living is based on an evaluation of the functional independence or dependence of patients in bathing, dressing, going to the toilet, transferring, continence, and feeding. Specific definitions of functional independence and dependence appear below the index.

A   Indpendent in feeding, continence, transferring, going to toilet, dressing, and bathing.

B   Independent in all but one of these functions.

C   Independent in all but bathing and one additional function.

D   Independent in all but bathing, dressing, and one additional function.

E   Independent in all but bathing, dressing, going to toilet, and one additional function.

F   Independent in all but bathing, dressing, going to toilet, transferring, and one additonal function.

G   Dependent in all six functions.

Other   Dependent in at least two functions, but not classifiable as C, D, E, or F.

Independence means without supervision, direction, or active personal assistance, except as specifically noted below. This is based on actual status and not on ability. A patient who refuses to perform a function is considered as not performing the function, even though he is deemed able.

Bathing (sponge, shower, or tub)
  Independent: assistance only in bathing a single part (as back or disabled extremity) or bathes self completely.
  Dependent: assistance in bathing more than one part of body; assistance in getting in or out of tub or does not bathe self.

Dressing
  Independent: gets clothes from closets and drawers, puts on clothes, outer garments, braces, manages fasteners, act of tying shoes is excluded.
  Dependent: does not dress self or remains partly undressed.

Going to toilet
  Independent: gets to toilet, gets on and off toilet, arranges clothes, cleans organs of excretion (may manage own bedpan used at night only and may or may not be using mechanical supports).
  Dependent: uses bedpan or commode or receives assistance getting to and using toilet.

Transfer
  Independent: moves in and out of bed independently and moves in and out of chair independently (may or may not be using mechanical supports).
  Dependent: assistance in moving in or out of bed and/or chair, does not perform one or more transfers.

Continence
  Independent: urination and defecation entirely self-controlled.
  Dependent: partial or total incontinence in urination or defecation, partial or total control by enemas, catheters, or regulated use of urinals and/or bedpans.

Feeding
  Independent: gets food from plate or its equivalent into mouth (precutting of meat and preparation of food, as buttering bread, are excluded from evaluation).
  Dependent: assistance in act of feeding (see above), does not eat at all or parenteral feeding.

Figure 6–8. (Reprinted with permission from Katz S, et al. Studies of illness in the aged. The Index of ADL: a standardized measure of biological and psychosocial function. JAMA. 1963; 185:914–919.)

List of Items in the Kenny Self-Care Index

1. Bed
   a. Move in bed
   b. Rise and sit
2. Transfers
   a. Sitting
   b. Standing
   c. Toilet
3. Locomotion
   a. Walking
   b. Stairs
   c. Wheelchair

4. Dressing
   a. Upper trunk and arms
   b. Lower trunk and legs
   c. Feet
5. Personal hygiene
   a. Face, hair, arms
   b. Trunk, perineum
   c. Lower extremities
   d. Bowel program
   e. Bladder program
6. Feeding

Figure 6–9. *(Reprinted with permission from Schoening H, Anderegg L, Bergstrom D, et al. Numerical scoring of self-care status of patients. Arch Phys Med Rehab. Oct 1965; 46:689.)*

TABLE 6–2. INSTRUMENTAL ACTIVITIES OF DAILY LIVING[33]

1. Telephone:
   I: Able to look up numbers, dial, receive, and make calls without help.
   A: Able to answer phone or dial operator in an emergency, but needs special phone or help in getting number or dialing.
   D: Unable to use the telephone.
2. Traveling:
   I: Able to drive own car or travel alone on bus or taxi.
   A: Able to travel but not alone.
   D: Unable to travel.
3. Shopping:
   I: Able to take care of all shopping with transportation provided.
   A: Able to shop but not alone.
   D: Unable to shop.
4. Preparing meals:
   I: Able to plan and cook full meals.
   A: Able to prepare light foods but unable to cook full meals alone.
   D: Unable to prepare any meals.
5. Housework:
   I: Able to do heavy housework (e.g., scrub floors).
   A: Able to do light housework, but needs help with heavy tasks.
   D: Unable to do any housework.
6. Medication:
   I: Able to take medications in the right dose at the right time.
   A: Able to take medications, but needs reminding or someone to prepare it.
   D: Unable to take medications.
7. Money:
   I: Able to manage buying needs, writes checks, pays bills.
   A: Able to manage daily buying needs, but needs help managing checkbook, paying bills.
   D: Unable to manage money.

I, Independent; **A**, assistance; **D**, dependent.
Reprinted with permission and adapted from Multidimensional Functional Assessment Questionnaire. ed 2. Duke University: Duke University Center for the Study of Aging and Human Development; 1978; 169–170.

TABLE 6–3. MODIFIED PULSES PROFILE

P— *Physical condition:* Includes diseases of the viscera (cardiovascular, gastrointestinal, urologic, and endocrine) and neurologic disorders:
  1. Medical problems sufficiently stable that medical or nursing monitoring is not required more often than 3 month intervals.
  2. Medical or nurse monitoring is needed more often than 3 month intervals but not each week.
  3. Medical problems are sufficiently unstable as to require regular medical and/or nursing attention at least weekly.
  4. Medical problems require intensive medical and/or nursing attention at least daily (excluding personal care assistance only).

U— *Upper limb functions:* Self-care activities (drink/feed, dress upper/lower, brace/prothesis, groom, wash, perineal care) dependent mainly on upper limb function:
  1. Independent in self-care without impairment of upper limbs.
  2. Independent in self-care with some impairment of upper limbs.
  3. Dependent on assistance or supervision in self-care with or without impairment of upper limbs.
  4. Dependent totally in self-care with marked impairment of upper limbs.

L— *Lower limb functions:* Mobility (transfer chair/toilet/tub or shower, walk, stairs, wheelchair) dependent mainly on lower limb function:
  1. Independent in mobility without impairment of lower limbs.
  2. Independent in mobility with some impairment in lower limbs, such as needing ambulatory aids, a brace or prosthesis, or else fully independent in a wheelchair without significant architectural or environmental barriers.
  3. Dependent on assistance or supervision in mobility with or without impairment of lower limbs, or partly independent in a wheelchair, or there are significant architectural or environmental barriers.
  4. Dependent totally in mobility with marked impairment of lower limbs.

S— *Sensory components:* Relating to communication (speech and hearing) and vision:
  1. Independent in communication and vision without impairment.
  2. Independent in communication and vision with some impairment, such as mild dysarthria, mild aphasia, or need for eyeglasses or hearing aid, or needing regular eye medication.
  3. Dependent on assistance, an interpreter, or supervision in communication or vision.
  4. Dependent totally in communication or vision.

E— *Excretory functions* (bladder and bowel):
  1. Complete voluntary control of bladder and bowel sphincters.
  2. Control of sphincters allows normal social activities despite urgency or need for catheter, appliance, suppositories, etc. Able to care for needs without assistance.
  3. Dependent on assistance in sphincter management or else has accidents occasionally.
  4. Frequent wetting or soiling from incontinence of bladder or bowel sphincters.

S— *Support factors:* Consider intellectual and emotional adaptability, support from family unit and financial ability:
  1. Able to fulfill usual roles and perform customary tasks.
  2. Must make some modification in usual roles and performance of customary tasks.
  3. Dependent on assistance, supervision, encouragement, or assistance from a public or private agency due to any of the above considerations.
  4. Dependent on long-term institutional care (chronic hospitalization, nursing home, etc.) excluding time-limited hospital for specific evaluation, treatment, or active rehabilitation.

Reprinted with permission from Granger C, Albrecht G, Hamilton B. Outcome of comprehensive medical rehabilitation: measurement by PULSES Profile and the Barthel Index. Arch Phys Med Rehab. 1979; 60:145.

150 feet without assistance/assistive device and does not use a wheelchair and performs it safely." Scores of 6 and 7 are considered no help required. Scores of 5 and below mean that the person does require a helper.

Please remember that insurance reviewers may not feel that a helper is someone who is a skilled care helper, like a physical therapist, and this must be taken into consideration when filling out the form. For example, when treating a patient who scores a 5, it is not obvious that the skilled care of a physical therapist is necessary. Interpret numbers of 4 and 5 to be in questionable need of skilled care, unless the therapist is providing specific skilled services. The rating of 4 and 5 is not enough to justify care. In contrast, a score of 1, 2 and 3 may justify need of care.

This particular test is good for showing a person's improvement through percentages of assistance required. As the patient improves, grade them on this scale accordingly. The therapist can also establish goals based on this scale. A patient may score a 2 initially, but may achieve a 5 later on. Simply state, "on the FIM that the patient has gone from level 2 to level 5." This lends credibility to the treatment application.

Again, this is just one part of a larger tool encompassing many physical and social parameters. It is a huge battery of tests, and it is available for a minimal amount of money from SUNY[37] (Fig. 6–10).

Functional Status Index

The next tool is the Functional Status Index (Table 6–4). This differs from previous tools because it looks at pain—an important component of many patient programs. The Functional Status Index measures the degree of independence, the degree of difficulty, and the amount of pain experienced when performing ADLs.[37] This test was originally developed for patients with arthritis and is, therefore, particularly good for evaluating those patients. The test evaluates gross mobility, hand activities, personal care, and home chores. The best way to administer this test is for the evaluator to ask the patient the questions and give the respondent a list of responses.[38]

The evaluator will say, "Take a look at your assistance sheet and assess your ability when walking outside." The person would look at the assistance list and may say, "My son always has to help me, but I do not use a cane. I guess I am a 3." The evaluator would then say, "Thinking about how you walk inside, would you say that it is extremely easy, somewhat easy . . . ," thus going through the difficulty list. Then finally, the evaluator repeats the same procedure with the pain list (Fig. 6–11). This is very time consuming for the health care professional, but with some sacrifice of validity, a patient can fill out the form by themselves. The advantage of this test is its inclusion of pain. Many older patients may be able to perform most activities, but they experience pain while they are doing them. In many cases, this could be the justification for treatment. None of the previous measures assesses pain, which makes this test a useful tool.[38]

Functional Status Questionnaire

The final functional tool to be discussed here is the Functional Status Questionnaire (FSQ). This tool has been shown to have reliability and construct validity,[38] and it provides a comprehensive assessment of physical, psychological, and social functions. The clinician can use the report to screen and monitor a patient's status. Figure 6–12 is an example of one of the subscales. This form is quite easy for the older person to fill out. The scoring of the scale is extremely complicated, but it provides a visual analog scale of the patient's functioning in terms of maximum function and a warning zone for delineation of functional disability. This information is easily generated from the software package.[39]

Functional Assessment Scales and Indices

Unfortunately, there is not enough room in this chapter to discuss all the available functional assessment tools, though Table 6–5 provides information and references for additional tools that are available.[39] This section is meant to provide an overview of the available tools. After the therapist reviews the separate tools, three im-

---

Functional Independence Measure (FIM)

Locomotion   Includes walking, once in a standing position, or using a wheelchair, once in a seated position, on a level surface.

Check most frequent mode of locomotion. If both are about equal, check W *and* C. If initiating a rehabilitation program, check the mode for which training is intended.

(   ) W = <u>w</u>alking   (   ) C = wheel<u>c</u>hair

No Helper

7. Complete Independence–*Walks* a minimum of *150* feet without assistive devices. Dose not use a wheelchair. Performs safely.

6. Modified Independence—*Walks* a miniumum of *150* feet but uses a brace (orthosis) or prosthesis on leg, special adaptive shoes, cane, crutches, or walkerette; takes more than reasonable time or there are safety considerations.

   If not walking, operates manual or electric wheelchair independently for a minimum of 150 feet; turns around; maneuvers the chair to a table, bed, toilet; negotiates at least a 3 percent grade; maneuvers on rugs and over door sills.

5. Exception (Household Ambulation)—Walks only short distances (a minimum of 50 feet) with or without a device. Could take more than reasonable time, or there are safety considerations, or operates a manual or electric wheelchair independently only short distances (a minimum of 50 feet).

Helper

5. Supervision—*If walking,* requires standby supervision, cuing, or coaxing to go a minimum of *150* feet.

   If not walking, requires standby supervision, cuing, or coaxing to go a minimum of *150* feet in wheelchair.

4. Minimal Contact Assistance—Subject performs 75% or more of locomotion effort to go a minimum of *150* feet.

3. Moderate Assistance—Performs 50% to 74% of locomotion effort to go a minimum of *150* feet.

2. Maximal Assistance—Performs 25% to 49% of locomotion effort to go a minimum of *50* feet. Requires assistance of one person only.

1. Total Assistance—Performs less than 25% of effort, or requires assistance of two people, or does not walk or wheel a minimum of *50* feet.

Figure 6–10. *(Reprinted with permission from Uniform Data System for Medical Rehabilitation. Research Foundation of the State University of New York, Buffalo, NY.)*

TABLE 6–4. FUNCTIONAL STATUS INDEX

Suggested Response Lists		
List I	List II	List III
1. No help	1. Extremely easy	1. No pain
2. Use equipment	2. Somewhat easy	2. Mild pain
3. Use human assist	3. Neither easy nor difficult	3. Moderate pain
4. Use human assist & equipment	4. Somewhat difficult	4. Severe pain
5. Unable to do	5. Extremely difficult	

Reprinted with permission from Jette AM. Functional status index: Reliability of a chronic disease evaluation instrument. Arch Phys Med Rehab. September 1980; 61(9):395–401.

portant points must be made about functional assessment. They are

1. Why is it so important?
2. What are the differences in the tools?
3. When should these tools be used?

In addition, measures of ADLs have been shown to correlate with the following:

1. Admission to a nursing home.[40]
2. Use of physician services.[41]
3. Insurance coverage.[42]
4. Living arrangements.[40]
5. Use of hospital services.[43]
6. Use of paid home care.[44]

As mentioned earlier, therapists must begin to correlate standard measurements, such as a goniometry, to functional assessment for productive values of these parameters.

The biggest problem in functional tools and surveys is that, depending on what is measured, the outcomes can vary greatly.[45] Wiener showed in one comparison a 60% difference in ADL problem identification from one study to another.[46] The reasons stated for this were

1. Methods used to collect data.
2. Age comparison.
3. How the ADLs were classified in terms of difficulty, length of problem, and type of assistance.
4. Which ADLs were used.
5. Sampling method.[46]

Table 6–6 is a list of surveys studied by Wiener and information reviewed on ADLs.[46]

Applegate has also done an excellent comparison of some of the more widely used functional tools[46] (see Table 6–7).

The final question to be answered is when should these tools be used. The most efficient way to use these tools is to have a goal in mind for its use, such as to establish a baseline to show improvement, to screen for problems, to set rehabilitation goals, or to monitor the patient's progress.[47]

The medical community in general is developing a keen interest in functional assessment. Lachs and Williams, in the *Annals of Internal Medicine,* urge general practitioners to use functional assessments.[47,48] In addition, this article specifically delineates physical therapy as an appropriate referral once functional deficits are noted. Table 6–8 is a procedural chart on functional assessment from Lachs and Williams' work.[48]

Physical therapists in geriatrics must get involved in functionally assessing patients not only for the efficacious assessment potential, but also for continuity of care from medical peers.

Functional Status Index

Activity	Assistance	Pain	Difficulty	Comment
Mobility				
Walking inside	☐	☐	☐	_____
Climbing up stairs	☐	☐	☐	_____
Transferring to & from toilet	☐	☐	☐	_____
Getting in & out of bed	☐	☐	☐	_____
Personal Care				
Combing hair	☐	☐	☐	_____
Putting on pants	☐	☐	☐	_____
Buttoning clothes	☐	☐	☐	_____
Washing all parts of the body	☐	☐	☐	_____
Putting on shoes/slippers	☐	☐	☐	_____
Home chores				
Vacuuming a rug	☐	☐	☐	_____
Reaching into high cupboards	☐	☐	☐	_____
Doing laundry	☐	☐	☐	_____
Washing windows	☐	☐	☐	_____
Doing yardwork	☐	☐	☐	_____
Hand activities				
Writing	☐	☐	☐	_____
Opening containers	☐	☐	☐	_____
Turning faucets	☐	☐	☐	_____
Cutting food	☐	☐	☐	_____
Vocational				
Performing all job responsibilities	☐	☐	☐	_____
Avocational				
Performing hobbies requiring hand work	☐	☐	☐	_____
Attending church	☐	☐	☐	_____
Socializing with friends & relatives	☐	☐	☐	_____

Figure 6–11.   *(Reprinted with permission from Jette AM. Functional status index: Reliability of a chronic disease evaluation instrument. Arch Phys Med Rehab. Sept 1980; 61(9):395–401.)*

Daily Activities

This group of questions refers to many types of physical and social activities. We would like to know how **difficult** it was for you to do each of these activities, on the average, **during the past month**. By difficult, we mean how hard it was or how much physical effort it took to do the activity **because of your health**. Circle the number:

> 4   if you usually had **no difficulty** doing it;
> 3   if you usually had **some difficulty** doing it;
> 2   if you usually had **much difficulty** doing it;
> 1   if you usually **did not do the activity because of your health**; or
> 0   if you usually **did not do the activity for other reasons**.

During the Past Month, How Much Physical Difficulty Did You have . . .	Usually Did With No Difficulty	Usually Did With Some Difficulty	Usually Did With Much Difficulty	Usually Did Not Do Because of Health	Usually Did Not Do For Other Reasons
1. Taking care of yourself, that is, eating, dressing, or bathing?	4	3	2	1	0
2. Moving in and out of a bed or chair?	4	3	2	1	0
3. Walking *several* blocks?	4	3	2	1	0
4. Walking *one* block or climbing *one* flight of stairs?	4	3	2	1	0
5. Walking indoors, such as around your home?	4	3	2	1	0
6. Doing work around the house such as cleaning, light yard work, home maintenance?	4	3	2	1	0
7. Doing errands, such as grocery shopping?	4	3	2	1	0
8. Driving a car or using public transportation?	4	3	2	1	0
9. Visiting with relatives or friends?	4	3	2	1	0
10. Participating in community activities, such as religious services, social activities, or volunteer work?	4	3	2	1	0
11. Taking care of other people such as family members?	4	3	2	1	0
12. Doing vigorous activities such as running, lifting heavy objects or participating in strenuous sports?	4	3	2	1	0

Figure 6–12. *(Reprinted with permission from Jette A, Davies A, Cleary P, et al. Functional status questionnaire reliability and validity when used in primary care. J Gen Intern Med. May/June 1986; 1:143–149.)*

TABLE 6–5. FUNCTIONAL ASSESSMENT SCALES AND INDICES

Scale Index	Domain	Assessor	Mode	Rel/Val[a]
Katz ADL	Eating Bathing Dressing Transfer Continence Toileting	Professional	Performance self-report	X X
Modified ADL Scale	Eating Ambulation Bathing Dressing Transfer Personal grooming Continence Toileting	Lay	Self, proxy, performance	X X
PULSES	Physical condition Upper limbs Lower limbs Sensory Excretory Social function	Lay	Performance	X
Kenny Self-Care	Bed activities Transfers Locomotion Continence Dressing Feeding	Professional	Performance	X
Philadelphia Geriatric Center Scale (PGC)	Toileting Feeding Dressing Grooming Ambulation Bathing	Lay	Self, proxy	X X
Philadelphia Geriatric Center Scale II (PGCII)	Telephone Shopping Food Preparation Housekeeping Laundry Public Transport Medications Finances	Both	Self, proxy	X X
Functional Health Scale	Heavy work Current illness Limitation in activities Walk 1/2 mile Climb stairs Socialize	Lay	Self, proxy	
PACE II	Telephone Finances Shopping Housekeeping Meal preparation	Both	Self, proxy	

(continued)

TABLE 6–5. FUNCTIONAL ASSESSMENT SCALES AND INDICES (CONT.)

Scale Index	Domain	Assessor	Mode	Rel/Val[a]
OARS II	Telephone Shopping Transportation Meal preparation Medication Finance	Both	Self	X
PACE II	7 ADL 17 range of motion 8 strength Balance Coordination	Both	Self, proxy, performance	
OARS	Eating Dressing Grooming Walking Transfer Bathing Continence Toileting	Both	Self, proxy	X
Functional Health of the Institutionalized Elderly	Transfer Eating Walking Bathing Dressing Toileting	Professional	Self, performance	X X
Functioning for Independent Living	Vision Hearing Speech Continence Behavior Orientation Communication Wandering	Professional	Self, proxy, performance	X
Performance Activities of Daily Living (PADL)	Shave Wipe nose Drink from cup Comb hair File nails Eat with spoon Turn faucet Switch lights Button on and off Slippers on and off Brush teeth Telephone Sign name Turn key Tell time Stand and sit	Professional	Performance	X X

[a]Rel/Val: Reliability and validity.

TABLE 6–6. TYPE OF INFORMATION ON ADL ITEMS IN NATIONAL SURVEYS

Survey	Population	Number of ADLs[a]	Minimum Duration of Disability	Needs Assistance	Receives Human Assistance	Uses Special Equipment	Receives Standby Help	Level of Difficulty
National Long-Term Care Survey (1982)	Noninstitutionalized, functionally impaired elderly	9	Yes	Yes	Yes	Yes	Yes	No
New Beneficiary Survey (1982)	New Social Security beneficiaries (between mid-1980 and mid-1981)	4	No	No	Yes	No	No	Yes
National Health and Nutrition Examination Survey I Followup (1982–1984)	Persons aged 25–74 (between 1971–1974 and 1974–1975) examined in NHANES I	6	No	No	Yes	Yes	No	Yes
National Long-Term Care Survey (1984)	Functionally impaired elderly, age 65+	9	Yes	Yes	Yes	Yes	Yes	No
National Health Interview Survey Supplement on Aging (1984)	Elderly persons, age 55+	9	No	No	Yes	Yes	No	Yes
Survey of Income and Program Participation—Disability Module (1984)	Noninstitutionalized population	4	No	Yes	Yes	No	No	No
Longitudinal Study of Aging (1984–1986)	Noninstitutionalized persons aged 70+ in 1984	9	No	No	Yes	Yes	No	Yes
National Nursing Home Survey (1985)	Current residents of nursing homes	6	No	No	Yes	Yes	No	No
National Mortality Followback Survey (1986)	Persons aged 25 and over who died in 1986	5	No	No	Yes	Yes	No	No
National Medical Expenditure Survey-Household (1987)	Noninstitutionalized population	7	Yes	No	Yes	Yes	No	No
National Medical Expenditure Survey-Institutional (1987)	Persons in nursing homes and personal care facilities	6	No	No	Yes	Yes	No	No

[a]Some surveys have a different number of ADLs on the instrument that screens for disability than on the detailed survey. Where that occurs, the larger of the two numbers is reported.

Reprinted with permission from Weiner J, Hanley N, Clark R, Van Nostrand J. Measuring the activities of daily living: Comparisons across national surveys. Journal of Gerontol Social Services. *1990; 45(6)229–237. © The Gerontological Society of America.*

TABLE 6–7. COMPARISON OF WIDELY USED FUNCTIONAL TOOLS

Instrument	Function Assessed	Range or Sensitivity	Administration	Strengths	Weaknesses
Katz ADL Scale	Basic self-care	Limited to basic activities; not sensitive to small changes	By patient or interviewer; based on judgments	Simple assessment of basic skills; useful in rehabilitative setting	Limited range of activities assessed; ratings subjective
Barthel Index	Self-care and ambulation	Slightly broader range than Katz ADL Scale; includes stair climbing, wheelchair use	By interviewer; based on judgment or observation	Range of activities useful in rehabilitational setting	Range not useful for small impairments; ratings subjective
Kenny Self-Care Scale	Self-care and ambulation	Similar to Barthel Index	By interviewer; based on judgment or observation	Range useful in rehabilitational setting	Range narrow for small impairments; ratings subjective
Instrumental ADL Scale	More complex activities: food preparation, shopping, housekeeping	Higher range of performance than Katz ADL Scale; not sensitive to small changes	By interviewer or patient; based on judgment	Assesses functions important for independent living	Ratings subjective
Timed Manual Performance	Timed assessment of performance of structured manual tasks	Broad range, from signing name to lifting latches	By interviewer; based on observation; requires special props	Assesses actual performance; sensitive to small changes[7]	Difficult to use in patients who are seriously ill or cognitively impaired
Performance Test of ADL	Self-care, mobility, and transfers	Ranges from ADL and instrumental ADL to mobility and transfers	By professional or trained interviewer; requires observation of patient performing specific activities; requires props	Direct observation of range of functions; useful in variety of clinical settings	Time consuming; difficult to use in seriously ill patients
Framingham Disability Scale	Self-care and physical activities	Broad range of activities, from self-care to lifting objects; not sensitive to small changes	By interviewer	Assesses broad range of activities; detects persons with less serious disabilities	Complex scoring; summary scores may hide important problems observed in individual tasks

Reprinted with permission from Applegate W, Blass J, Williams F. Instruments for the functional assessment of older patients. N Eng J Med. April 26, 1990; 322(17):1207–1214.

MODIFIED PHYSICAL THERAPY MEASURES

Musculoskeletal Parameters

Strength

It is widely accepted that strength decreases with age. However, no studies exist to date that show a difference in the strength decline with age using simple manual muscle test techniques. This makes it difficult for a practitioner to use the current knowledge of age's strength changes in the clinical setting.

In the realm of dynamometer and muscle hypertrophy, some clinically useful information has been generated. The best sources on muscle hypertrophy are Tomanek and Wool, and Goldspink and Howells.[49,50] Basically, these resources contend that older muscle does hypertrophy but not to the same extent.

TABLE 6–8. PROCEDURE FOR FUNCTIONAL ASSESSMENT SCREENING IN THE ELDERLY

Target Area	Assessment Procedure	Abnormal Result	Suggested Intervention
Vision	Test each eye with Jaeger card while patient wears corrective lenses (if applicable)	Inability to read greater than 20/40	Refer to ophthalmologist
Hearing	Whisper a short, easily answered question, such as "What is your name?" in each ear while the examiner's face is out of direct view	Inability to answer question	Examine auditory canals for cerumen and clean if necessary. Repeat test; if still abnormal in either ear, refer for audiometry and possible prosthesis
Arm	Proximal: "Touch the back of your head with both hands" Distal: "Pick up the spoon"	Inability to do task	Examine the arm fully (muscle, joint, and nerve), paying attention to pain, weakness, limited range of motion. Consider referral for physical therapy
Leg	Observe the patient after asking: "Rise from your chair, walk ten feet, return, sit down"	Inability to walk or transfer out of chair	Do full neurologic and musculoskeletal evaluation, paying attention to strength, pain, range of motion, balance, and traditional assessment of gait. Consider referral for physical therapy
Urinary incontinence	Ask: "Do you ever lose your urine and get wet?"	Yes	Ascertain frequency and amount. Search for remediable causes including local irritations, polyuric states, and medications. Consider urologic referral
Nutrition	Weigh the patient. Measure height	Weight is below acceptable range for height	Do appropriate medical evaluation
Mental status	Instruct: "I am going to name three objects (pencil, truck, book). I will ask you to repeat their names now and then again a few minutes from now." [See text discussion.]	Inability to recall all three objects after 1 minute	Administer Folstein Mini-Mental Status Examination. If score is <24, search for causes of cognitive impairment. Ascertain onset, duration, and fluctuation of overt symptoms. Review medications. Assess consciousness and affect. Do appropriate laboratory tests
Depression	Ask: "Do you often feel sad or depressed?"	Yes	Administer Geriatric Depression Scale. If positive (normal score, 0 to 10), check for antihypertensive, psychotropic, or other pertinent medications. Consider appropriate pharmaceutical or psychiatric treatment
ADL-IADL[a]	Ask: "Can you get out of bed yourself?"; "Can you dress yourself?"; "Can you make your own meals?"; "Can you do your own shopping?"	No to any question	Corroborate responses with patient's appearance; question family members if accuracy is uncertain. Determine reasons for the inability (motivation compared with physical limitation). Institute appropriate medical, social, or environmental interventions
Home environment	Ask: "Do you have trouble with stairs inside or outside of your home?"; ask about potential hazards inside the home with bathtubs, rugs, or lighting	Yes	Evaluate home safety and institute appropriate countermeasures
Social support	Ask: "Who would be able to help you in case of illness or emergency?"	...	List identified persons in the medical record. Become familiar with available resources for the elderly in the community

[a]ADL-IADL: activities of daily living-instrumental activities of daily living.
Reproduced with permission from Lachs M, Feinstein A, Cooney L, et al. A simple procedure for general screening for functional disability in elderly patients. Ann Intern Med. 1990; 112:699–704.

Figure 6–13 contains some formulas for assessing hypertrophy and charts illustrating the comparison in muscle hypertrophy.[51]

It is apparent from these formulas that the calculation for the difference in muscle hypertrophy is rather cumbersome and not easily applicable in the clinic. The authors suggest being wary of using muscle hypertrophy measures (i.e., girth) as the only criteria for assessing muscle strength increases with age.

Dynanomomter testing of strength can be replicated in the clinic. Rice carried out a simple assessment of numerous joints' strength using a modified sphygmomanometer.[52] Table 6–9 is his chart of absolute strength measures.[53]

Borges and associates also showed the torque changes with age in the knee using the Cybex dynamometer (see Table 6–10).[53]

Finally, Vandervoort and Hayes found a 71% decrease in plantarflexor muscle isometric strength in the elderly as compared with the young.[54] This study was done on both young and old healthy women.[55] Their findings revealed strength development for the young of 0.16 nm per second and 0.09 nm per second in the elderly group.

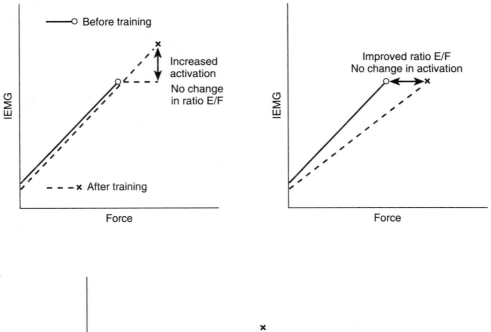

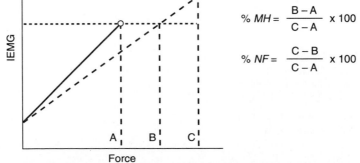

Figure 6–13. Hypertrophy in older men. **A.** Strength gain due to neural factors. **B.** Strength gain due to hypertrophy. **C.** Evaluation of percentage contributions of neural factors (NF) vs. hypertrophy (MH). *(Reprinted with permission from Moritani T, Devries HA. Potential for gross muscle hypertrophy in older men. J Gerontology. 1980; 35(5):673.)*

TABLE 6–9. ABSOLUTE AND RELATIVE STRENGTH MEASUREMENTS

Muscle groups	Men Strength (kg)	Men Strength/ Body Weight (kg/kg)	n	Women Strength (kg)	Women Strength/ Body Weight (kg/kg)	n
Shoulder abductors	12.4 ± 5.0[a]	0.17 ± 0.07	37	9.3 ± 3.3	0.15 ± 0.05	81
Shoulder flexors	12.7 ± 5.0[a]	0.17 ± 0.07	37	9.3 ± 3.4	0.14 ± 0.05	81
Elbow extensors	14.9 ± 4.6[a]	0.20 ± 0.06	37	11.2 ± 3.3	0.19 ± 0.06	81
Elbow flexors	15.2 ± 5.1[a]	0.21 ± 0.07	37	10.9 ± 3.9	0.18 ± 0.06	81
Hip extensors	14.4 ± 5.8[a]	0.19 ± 0.08	31 (2)	11.6 ± 4.0	0.19 ± 0.06	69 (1)
Hip flexors	16.2 ± 6.7[a]	0.23 ± 0.09	31 (2)	10.8 ± 3.3	0.18 ± 0.06	74 (1)
Knee extensors	19.1 ± 5.7[a]	0.27 ± 0.09	31 (5)	16.7 ± 4.8	0.28 ± 0.08	77 (2)
Dorsiflexors	15.1 ± 4.5[a]	0.21 ± 0.07	37	12.6 ± 4.1	0.21 ± 0.06	79
MS grip	23.2 ± 4.4	0.33 ± 0.08	20 (17)	20.1 ± 5.7	0.31 ± 0.09	74 (7)
Dynamometer grip	30.8 ± 6.6[a]	0.43 ± 0.1[a]	37	21.6 ± 6.1	0.36 ± 0.08	64

Values are means ± SD, 1 kg = 9.806 newtons. MS = modified sphygmomanometer. Parentheses indicate the number of measurements that exceeded the upper limit of the MS.
[a]Indicates significant difference (p ≤ 0.05) between men and women for absolute or relative strength measurements.
Reprinted with permission from Rice C. Strength in an elderly population. Arch Phys Med Rehab. May 1989; 70:391–397.

In conclusion, the clinical implications of the information noted in the area of strength changes with age are

1. Be wary of girth measures as a means of reflecting strength gains.
2. Compare outcomes to the norms noted. For example, compare knee extension torques to Borge's measures versus measures of torque on younger persons.
3. Compare strength measures to Rice's norms versus the classic manual muscle test for more comparable findings.

Range of Motion

The literature on range of motion norms is still somewhat controversial. For example, Walker showed no significant differences in range of motion in 28 joints of young and old subjects[55] (Table 6–11).

Frekany and Leslie showed that even if an older group did have motion limitation, it could be normalized with appropriate stretching exercises.[56] James and Parker give probably the most comprehensive and recent reference on joint range of motion norms of the lower extremity[57] (Fig. 6–14).

Information also exists on upper extremity and spinal norms for range of motion. These are listed in chart form in Tables 6–12 through 6–15. These findings,

TABLE 6–10. KNEE EXTENSION TORQUE AT 90 DEGREES PER SECOND

	Age (Years)	Torque
MEN	20	122
	70	78
WOMEN	20	68
	70	38

Reprinted with permission from Borges O. Isometric and isokinetic knee extension & flexion torque in men and women aged 20–70. Scand J Rehab Med. 1989; 21:45–53.

TABLE 6–11. UPPER AND LOWER LIMB RANGE OF MOTION MEAN VALUES AND STANDARD DEVIATIONS FOR AGE GROUPS COMBINED BY SEX AND FOR SEXES COMBINED[a] (AGES 60–84)

Upper Limb Motion	Men (age groups combined)		Women (age groups combined)		Diff. Between M/W	Sexes Combined		
	$\bar{X}$	s	$\bar{X}$	s		p^b	$\bar{X}$	s
Shoulder abduction	155	22	175	16	−20[c]	<0.001	165	21
flexion	160	11	169	9	−9	<0.001	165	11
extension	38	11	49	13	−11[c]	<0.001	44	13
medial rotation	59	16	66	13	−7	NS	62	15
lateral rotation	76	13	85	16	−9	0.02	81	15
Elbow beginning flexion	6	5[d]	1	3	−5[d]	<0.001	4	5
flexion	139	14	148	5	−9	0.002	143	11
Radioulnar pronation	68	9	73	12	−5	NS	71	11
supination	83	11	65	11	+18	<0.001	74	14
Wrist flexion	62	12	65	8	−3	NS	64	10
extension	61	6	65	10	−4	0.05	63	9
radial deviation	20	6	17	6	+3	NS	19	6
ulnar deviation	28	7	23	7	+5	0.01	26	7
Hip beginning flexion	11	3	11	5	0	NS	11	4
flexion	110	11	111	12	−1	NS	111	11
abduction	23	9	24	6	−1	NS	23	7
adduction	18	4	11	4	+7	<0.001	14	5
medial rotation	22	6	36	7	−14[c]	<0.001	29	10
lateral rotation	32	6	30	7	+2	NS	31	7
Knee beginning flexion	2	2	0	1	+2	<0.001	1	2
flexion	131	4	135	7	−4	0.01	133	6
Ankle plantar flexion	29	7	40	6	−11[c]	<0.001	34	8
dorsiflexion	9	5	10	5	−1	NS	10	5
Subtalar inversion	31	11	29	10	+2	NS	30	10
eversion	13	6	12	5	+1	NS	12	6
First metatarsophalangeal beginning flexion	3	7	1	4	+2	NS	2	5
extension	62	17	59	8	+3	NS	61	17
flexion	5	7	8	16	−3	NS	6	8

[a]All values reported in integers.

[b]Univariate t tests, df = 1, 58 (t values can be obtained from any statistical text with table of critical values for t distribution).

[c]Difference > intertester error.

[d]One man deleted because of the presence of pathologically restricted ROM, n = 29.

Reprinted with permission from Walker J, Sue D, Miles-Elkousy N, Ford G, Trevelyan H: Active mobility of extremities in older subjects. Phys Ther. June 1984; 64(6):919–923. Reprinted with permission of the American Physical Therapy Association.

even though controversial, can assist the therapist to set more appropriate goals. If, for example, as was stated in Bassey's chart, the norms for shoulder flexion are 129, then a goal of 170 is inappropriate. Keeping these charts for review can help to design appropriate programs.

Postural Changes with Age

Posture changes with age. Perfect posture demonstrates a plumb line that bisects the ear, just anterior to the acromion process, through the greater trochanter, just posterior to the patella and just anterior to the lateral malleolus (see Fig. 6–15).[58]

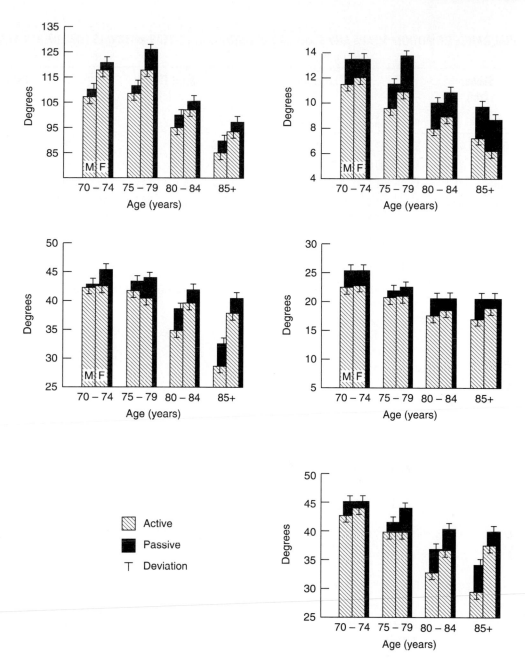

Figure 6–14. Lower extremity range of motion. **A.** Knee flexion. **B.** Ankle dorsiflexion (knee extended). **C.** Ankle plantar flexion (knee extended). **D.** Ankle dorsiflexion (knee flexed). **E.** Ankle plantar flexion (knee flexed). *(Reprinted with permission from James B, Parker A. Lower extremity range of motion. Am J Phys Med Rehabil. 1989; 68(4):162–167.)*

Changes in posture with age include[58]

1. Forward head.
2. Rounded shoulders.
3. Change in lordotic curve (either flatter or more curved).
4. Increased hip flexion.
5. Increased knee flexion.

Standard means of assessing posture are acceptable for older persons. The clinician must be sure to align the plumb line from the malleoli and up, otherwise a false alignment will be noted.

A good tool for rating and screening posture is the REEDCO Posture Score

TABLE 6–12. SPINAL RANGE OF MOTION: MEANS AND STANDARD DEVIATIONS IN 10-YEAR INTERVALS FOR LUMBAR RANGE OF MOTION[80]

Age (yr)	Shöber (cm) $\bar{X}$	s	CV	n[a]	Extension (°) $\bar{X}$	s	CV	n	R Lat Flexion (°) $\bar{X}$	s	CV	n	L Lat Flexion (°) $\bar{X}$	s	CV	n
20–29	3.7	0.72	19.5	31	41.2	9.6	23.3	31	37.8	5.8	15.4	31	38.7	5.7	14.7	31
30–39	3.9	1.00	25.6	42	40.0	8.8	22.0	44	35.3	6.5	18.4	44	36.5	6.0	16.4	44
40–49	3.1	0.81	26.1	16	31.1	8.9	28.6	16	27.1	6.5	24.0	16	28.5	5.2	18.2	16
50–59	3.0	1.10	36.7	43	27.4	8.0	29.2	43	25.3	6.2	24.5	44	26.8	6.4	23.9	44
60–69	2.4	0.74	30.8	26	17.4	7.5	43.1	27	20.2	4.8	23.8	27	20.3	5.3	26.1	27
70–79	2.2	0.69	31.4	9	16.6	8.8	53.0	10	18.0	4.7	26.1	10	18.9	6.0	31.7	10

[a]Different "n's" appear in some age groups because of the difficulty in measuring patients with various medical conditions (e.g., rash).
Reprinted with permission from Fitzgerald GK, Wynveen KJ, Rheault W, Rothschild B. Objective assessment with establishment of normal values for lumbar spinal range of motion. Phys Ther. Nov 1983; 63(11):1778. Reprinted with permission of the American Physical Therapy Association.

TABLE 16–13. SPINAL/NECK RANGE OF MOTION[81]

	Age 10	30	80
Flexion	35°	30°	27°
Lateral Flexion	63°	50°	30°
Extension	60°	50°	35°
Rotation	165°	150°	130°

Reprinted with permission from Lind B, et al. Normal range of motion of the cervical spine. Arch Phys Med Rehab. Sept 1989; 70:692–695.

TABLE 6–14. SHOULDER FLEXION RANGE OF MOTION[82]

Age	Male	Female
65–74 years old	129°	124°
75+ years old	121°	114°

Reprinted with permission from Bassey E, et al. Flexibility of the shoulder joint measured as range of abduction in a large representative sample of men and women over 65 years of age. Eur J Appl Physiology. 1989; 58:353–360.

TABLE 6–15. SHOULDER RANGE OF MOTION[83]

60–74 years old
Flexion: 159°
Abduction: 159°

75+ years old
Flexion: 150°
Abduction: 154°

Reprinted with permission from Boyle S. Geriatric shoulder range of motion. Master's thesis. Philadelphia: University of Pennsylvania, February 1989.

Sheet (see Fig. 6–16). This evaluation tool is self-explanatory, and it is not singular to older persons. It can be used on young and old to provide a quantitative approach to posture analysis. Since posture can be an important variable in movement, balance, and gait of older persons, it is imperative that the clinician assess it as objectively as possible.[59]

Gait Assessment

Gait changes with age are as variable as many of the other characteristics listed in this section are. What will be given here are norms or averages.

To begin the examination of the gait cycle, motion will be discussed. The first place that a change is noted in the old versus the young is in the preswing phase. Older persons show 5° less motion in plantarflexion when compared to young (i.e., 15° as compared to 20°).[60] The knee range of motion shows no difference. However, the hip exhibits 5° more flexion (i.e., 35° versus 30° in the younger population).[61] Gait velocity is also less in older persons. Average velocity in the young is 82.6 m/min, and it is 78.6 m/min in the 60 to 87 age range.[62] Stride length is also shorter in the older population. Healthy older persons have a stride length of 1.39 m and younger persons have an average stride length of 1.5 m.[63]

All of the changes noted are the only significant differences noted in *healthy* older persons. If other pathological factors are taken into consideration, then other gait abnormalities will be noted. (For further information on gait changes noted with pathology see Chapter 13.)

Functional Ambulation Profile

Two tools are particularly good for assessing gait in older persons. The first tool is the Functional Ambulation Profile (FAP) by Dr Arthur Nelson (Fig. 6–17).[64] This tool is particularly useful for older patients who have suffered from a stroke. To use this assessment tool, enter the date and the patient's bilateral time; that is, how long the person can stand on both feet. Some patients cannot stand for 30 seconds without dizziness or support. The longest anyone needs to be timed is 2 minutes. The next entry on the FAP is unilateral time: how long the person can stand on the left leg. Repeat for the right leg. Next, conduct the test with patient's eyes closed, and add the score code for this variation. According to Bohannon, the norms for persons over 70 years old are that they can stand with the eyes open for 14.2 seconds and with the eyes closed for 4.3 seconds.[65]

Begin the notes for the basic ambulation section of this tool by entering the distance needed for functional independence. It may be the distance from bed to bathroom, for example this may measure 50 feet. Count the steps as the patient walks, however. The distance of 12 feet shown on the form is arbitrary; whatever distance is used must be used each time the measurement is recorded in order for it to be consistent and reliable.

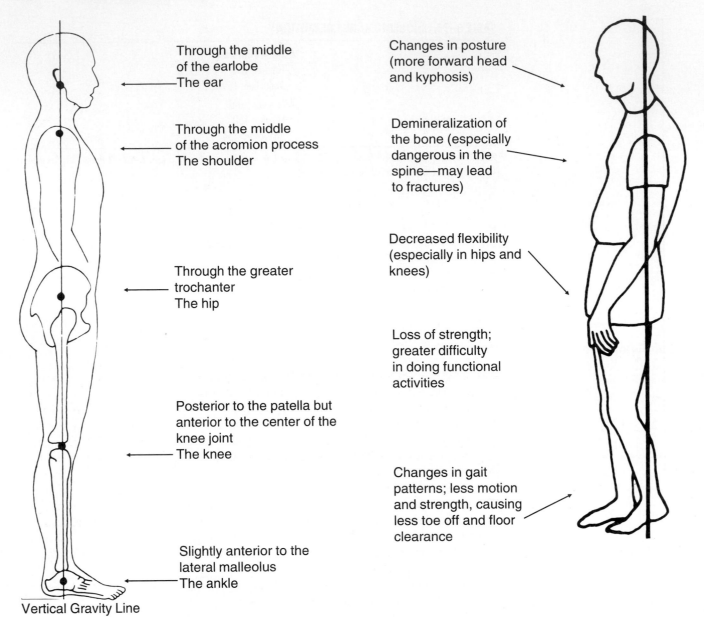

Through the middle
of the earlobe
—The ear

Through the middle
of the acromion process
The shoulder

Through the greater
trochanter
The hip

Posterior to the patella but
anterior to the center of the
knee joint
—The knee

Slightly anterior to the
lateral malleolus
—The ankle

Vertical Gravity Line

Changes in posture
(more forward head
and kyphosis)

Demineralization of
the bone (especially
dangerous in the
spine—may lead
to fractures)

Decreased flexibility
(especially in hips and
knees)

Loss of strength;
greater difficulty
in doing functional
activities

Changes in gait
patterns; less motion
and strength, causing
less toe off and floor
clearance

Figure 6–15. *Posture changes with age. (Reprinted with permission from Lewis C, Bottomley J. Musculoskeletal changes with age. In: Lewis C, ed. Aging: The Health Care Challenge. Philadelphia: F.A. Davis; 1990.)*

A watch will also be needed with a second hand to administer this test. To modify this test for someone using an assistive device, just note the use of the device in the comments. Also note pain with a star or other code.

Gait Abnormality Scale

Another excellent tool is the Gait Abnormality Rating Scale (GARS) by Wolfson and associates.[66] This tool was developed to detect fallers. It is, however, an excellent tool for quantifying aspects of gait patterns for older persons (see Table 6–16).

The GARS is quite easy to score. The patient is given the corresponding numerical value to each item listed, and the scores are added to get the individual's GARS score. Wolfson and co-workers found that persons scoring higher than 18 were more likely to fall. Not only is this a good tool for assessing gait, it also can be used to predict patients who are more vulnerable to falling.[66]

POSTURE SCORE SHEET	Name _____			SCORING DATES			
	GOOD - 10	FAIR - 5	POOR - 0				
HEAD LEFT RIGHT	HEAD ERECT GRAVITY LINE PASSES DIRECTLY THROUGH CENTER	HEAD TWISTED OR TURNED TO ONE SIDE SLIGHTLY	HEAD TWISTED OR TURNED TO ONE SIDE MARKEDLY				
SHOULDERS LEFT RIGHT	SHOULDERS LEVEL (HORIZONTALLY)	ONE SHOULDER SLIGHTLY HIGHER THAN OTHER	ONE SHOULDER MARKEDLY HIGHER THAN OTHER				
SPINE LEFT RIGHT	SPINE STRAIGHT	SPINE SLIGHTLY CURVED LATERALLY	SPINE MARKEDLY CURVED LATERALLY				
HIPS LEFT RIGHT	HIPS LEVEL (HORIZONTALLY)	ONE HIP SLIGHTLY HIGHER	ONE HIP MARKEDLY HIGHER				
ANKLES	FEET POINTED STRAIGHT AHEAD	FEET POINTED OUT	FEET POINTED OUT MARKEDLY ANKLES SAG IN(PRONATION)				
NECK	NECK ERECT, CHIN IN, HEAD IN BALANCE DIRECTLY ABOVE SHOULDERS	NECK SLIGHTLY FORWARD, CHIN SLIGHTLY OUT	NECK MARKEDLY FORWARD, CHIN MARKEDLY OUT				
UPPER BACK	UPPER BACK NORMALLY ROUNDED	UPPER BACK SLIGHTLY MORE ROUNDED	UPPER BACK MARKEDLY ROUNDED				
TRUNK	TRUNK ERECT	TRUNK INCLINED TO REAR SLIGHTLY	TRUNK INCLINED TO REAR MARKEDLY				
ABDOMEN	ABDOMEN FLAT	ABDOMEN PROTRUDING	ABDOMEN PROTRUDING AND SAGGING				
LOWER BACK	LOWER BACK NORMALLY CURVED	LOWER BACK SLIGHTLY HOLLOW	LOWER BACK MARKEDLY HOLLOW				
		TOTAL SCORES					

Figure 6–16. Posture score sheet. (From REEDCO, Auburn, NY. Copyright 1974. Reprinted with permission.)

Modified Functional Ambulation Profile

Patient: _____

STATIC WEIGHT-BEARING CAPACITY

Date   ____ ____ ____ ____ ____ ____ ____ ____ ____

Bilateral Time   ____ ____ ____ ____ ____ ____ ____ ____ ____

Left Unilat. Time   ____ ____ ____ ____ ____ ____ ____ ____ ____

  with eyes closed   ____ ____ ____ ____ ____ ____ ____ ____ ____

Right Unilat. Time   ____ ____ ____ ____ ____ ____ ____ ____ ____

  with eyes closed   ____ ____ ____ ____ ____ ____ ____ ____ ____

DYNAMIC (in place) WEIGHT TRANSFER RATE

Date   ____ ____ ____ ____ ____ ____ ____ ____ ____

Time to complete   ____ ____ ____ ____ ____ ____ ____ ____ ____

4 transfers (8 steps)   ____ ____ ____ ____ ____ ____ ____ ____ ____

BASIC AMBULATION EFFICIENCY

Date   ____ ____ ____ ____ ____ ____ ____ ____ ____

Through//bars
holding on time/steps   ____ ____ ____ ____ ____ ____ ____ ____ ____

Twelve foot distance
outside//bars time/steps   ____ ____ ____ ____ ____ ____ ____ ____ ____

COMMENTS

Figure 6–17.   *(Reprinted with permission from Nelson AJ. Function ambulation profile.* Physical Ther. *1974; 54:1059–1065.)*

TABLE 6–16. COMPONENTS OF THE GAIT ASSESSMENT RATING SCORE (GARS)

A. General Categories
 1. Variability—a measure of inconsistency and arrhythmicity in stepping and arm movements.
  0 = fluid and predictably paced limb movements.
  1 = occasional interruptions (changes in velocity), approximately <25% of time.
  2 = unpredictability of rhythm approximately 25–27% of time.
  3 = random timing of limb movements.
 2. Guardedness—hesitancy, slowness, diminished propulsion and lack of commitment in stepping and arm swing.
  0 = good forward momentum and lack of apprehension in propulsion.
  1 = center of gravity of head, arms, and trunk (HAT) projects only slightly in front of push-off, but still good arm-leg coordination.
  2 = HAT held over anterior aspect of foot, and some moderate loss of smooth reciprocation.
  3 = HAT held over rear aspect of stance-phase foot, and great tentativity in stepping.
 3. Weaving—an irregular and wavering line of progression.
  0 = straight line of progression on frontal viewing.
  1 = a single deviation from straight (line of best fit) line of progression.
  2 = two to three deviations from line of progression.
  3 = four or more deviations from line of progression.
 4. Waddling—a broad-based gait characterized by excessive truncal crossing of the midline and side-bending.
  0 = narrow base of support and body held nearly vertically over feet.
  1 = slight separation of medial aspects of feet and just perceptible lateral movement of head and trunk.
  2 = 3–4″ separation feet and obvious bending of trunk to side so that cog of head lies well over ipsilateral stance foot.
  3 = extreme pendular deviations of head and trunk (head passes lateral to ipsilateral stance foot), and further widening of base of support.
 5. Staggering—sudden and unexpected laterally directed partial losses of balance.
  0 = no losses of balance to side.
  1 = a single lurch to side.
  2 = two lurches to side.
  3 = three or more lurches to side.

B. Lower Extremity Categories
 1. % Time in Swing—a loss in the percentage of the gait cycle constituted by the swing phase.
  0 = approximately 3:2 ratio of duration of stance to swing phase.
  1 = a 1:1 or slightly less ratio of stance to swing.
  2 = markedly prolonged stance phase but with some obvious swing time remaining.
  3 = barely perceptible portion of cycle spent in swing.
 2. Foot Contact—the degree to which heel strikes the ground before the forefoot.
  0 = very obvious angle of impact of heel on ground.
  1 = barely visible contact of heel before forefoot.
  2. = entire foot lands flat on ground.
  3 = anterior aspect of foot strikes ground before heel.
 3. Hip ROM—the degree of loss of hip range of motion seen during a gait cycle.
  0 = obvious angulation of thigh backwards during double support (10°).
  1 = just barely visible angulation backwards from vertical.
  2 = thigh in line with vertical projection from ground.
  3 = thigh angled forward from vertical at maximum posterior excursion.
 4. Knee Range of Motion—the degree of loss of knee range of motion seen during a gait cycle.
  0 = knee moves from complete extension at heel-strike (and late-stance) to almost 90° (@ 70°) during swing phase.
  1 = slight bend in knee seen at heel-strike and late-stance and maximal flexion at midswing is closer to 45° than 90°.
  2 = knee flexion at late stance more obvious than at heel-strike, very little clearance seen for toe during swing.
  3 = toe appears to touch ground during swing, knee flexion appears constant during stance, and knee angle during stance, and knee angle during swing appears 45° or less

(continued)

TABLE 6–16. COMPONENTS OF THE GAIT ASSESSEMENT RATING SCORE (GARS) (CONT.)

C. Trunk, Head, and Upper Extremity Categories

1. Elbow Extension—a measure of the decrease of elbow range of motion.
   0 = large peak-to-peak excursion of forearm (approximately 20°), with distinct maximal flexion at end of anterior trajectory.
   1 = 25% decrement of extension during maximal posterior excursion of upper extremity.
   2 = almost no change in elbow angle.
   3 = no apparent change in elbow angle (held in flexion).

2. Shoulder Extension—a measure of the decrease of shoulder range of motion.
   0 = clearly seen movement of upper arm anterior (15°) and posterior (20°) to vertical axis of trunk.
   1 = shoulder flexes slightly anterior to vertical axis.
   2 = shoulder comes only to vertical axis or slightly posterior to it during flexion
   3 = shoulder stays well behind vertical axis during entire excursion.

3. Shoulder Abduction—a measure of pathological increase in shoulder range of motion laterally.
   0 = shoulders held almost parallel to trunk.
   1 = shoulders held 5–10° to side.
   2 = shoulders held 10–20° to side.
   3 = shoulders held greater than 20° to side.

4. Arm-Heel strike Synchrony—the extent to which the contralateral movements of an arm and leg are out of phase.
   0 = good temporal conjunction of arm and contralateral leg at apex of shoulder and hip excursions all of the time.
   1 = arm and leg slightly out of phase 25% of the time.
   2 = arm and leg moderately out of phase 25–50% of time.
   3 = little or no temporal coherence of arm and leg.

5. Head Held Forward—a measure of the pathological forward projection of the head relative to the trunk.
   0 = earlobe vertically aligned with shoulder tip.
   1 = earlobe vertical projection falls 1″ anterior to shoulder tip.
   2 = earlobe vertical projection falls 2″ anterior to shoulder tip.
   3 = earlobe vertical projection falls 3″ or more anterior to shoulder tip.

6. Shoulders Held Elevated—the degree to which the scapular girdle is held higher than normal.
   0 = tip of shoulder (acromion) markedly below level of chin (1–2″).
   1 = tip of shoulder slightly below level of chin.
   2 = tip of shoulder at level of chin.
   3 = tip of shoulder above level of chin.

7. Upper Trunk Flexed Forward—a measure of kyphotic involvement of the trunk.
   0 = very gentle thoracic convexity, cervical spine flat, or almost flat.
   1 = emerging cervical curve, more distant thoracic convexity.
   2 = anterior concavity at mid-chest level apparent.
   3 = anterior concavity at mid-chest level very obvious.

Reprinted with permission from Wolfson L, Whipple R, Amerman P. Gait assessment in the elderly. A gait abnormality rating scale and its relation to falls. J Gerontology. 1990; 45(1):M14. © The Gerontological Society of America.

In addition, the classic methods of assessing gait, such as the evaluation of shoe wear and standard gait analysis, are still applicable to the older population. The tools that have just been presented are extra ways of assessing gait that are specific to the older population.

Cardiopulmonary Tests

Chapters 3 and 4 provided background information on the complex array of physiological changes in the cardiopulmonary system with age. This section will discuss modifications in the assessment parameters that will be needed to account for

Parameter		Change with Increased Age	
Vital capacity (VC)	Decreased		
Functional residual capacity (FRC)	Increased		
Residual volume (RV)	Increased	Change dependent on size and sex	
Forced expiratory volume ($FEV_{1.0}$ liter)	Decreased		
Forced expiratory flow ($FEF_{25-75\%}$ liter/sec)	Decreased		
		Standard Values/Age-related change	
Partial pressure of arterial oxygen (PaO_2)	Decreased	80–100 mmHG: 104–0.42 × age	
Partial pressure of arterial carbon dioxide ($PaCO_2$)	Unchanged	35–45 mmHG	
pH	Unchanged	7.35–7.45	

CARDIAC RESERVE: EFFECTS OF AGE AND DISEASE

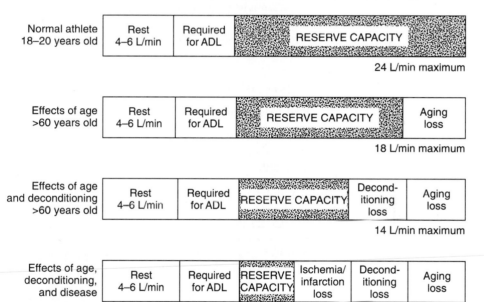

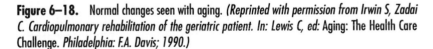

Figure 6–18. *Normal changes seen with aging. (Reprinted with permission from Irwin S, Zadai C. Cardiopulmonary rehabilitation of the geriatric patient. In: Lewis C, ed: Aging: The Health Care Challenge. Philadelphia: F.A. Davis; 1990.)*

these changes. The chart of normal changes found in Figure 6–18 offers an explanation for the parametric change seen in a typical cardiopulmonary assessment.[67] Table 6–17 is an outline of the typical assessment process for a patient interview and physical examination.[67]

In these assessments several changes can be noted for the average older person. These are

1. There may be an increase in the anterior–posterior diameter of the chest with age. This should be very slight. If it is excessive, then it may indicate pathology (i.e., emphysema).
2. There may be a slight use of accessory muscles for breathing. Again, a slight use of these muscles is acceptable, however, as noted previously, more than that is indicative of pathology.

TABLE 6–17. ASSESSMENT PROCESS FOR PATIENT INTERVIEW AND PHYSICAL EXAMINATION

Patient Interview

Patient perception of problem/disease process
  Specific didactic knowledge
  Emotional reaction
    embarrassment
    anxiety
    preoccupation
    denial
  Family perception of problem/disease process
  Patient description of disease progress and physical
    performance ability
  Patient history of dyspnea/orthopnea

Chart Review

Medical history
  Previous admissions and diagnosis
  Present medical problems: active/inactive
    present medications
    admitting diagnosis/objectives/care plan
Laboratory studies
  pulmonary function tests/ABGs
  metabolic studies/blood work
  recent EKG
  significant radiographic findings

Work/Social History

Present and past jobs/working environment
Present and past living locations
Social habits
  smoking
  alcohol
  physical activity

Observation

Patient position
  use of upper extremities
  use of musculature
Thoracic cage
  symmetry
  ratio of AP to Lat diameter
Breathing
  rate and depth
  rhythm
  pattern

Palpation

  subcostal angle/AP to Lat diameter
  localized expansion/symmetry
  excursion/mobility
  locate painful areas

Auscultation

  Normal breath sounds
  Abnormal breath sounds
  Adventitious breath sounds

Reprinted with permission from Irwin S, Zadai C. Cardiopulmonary rehabilitation of the geriatric patient. In: Lewis C, ed. Aging: The Health Care Challenge. Philadelphia: F.A. Davis; 1990.

3. Note that the following are signs of abnormal pathology or deconditioning: an elevated heart rate over 84 BPM prior to start of the exam,[68] a rise of over 20 BPM with the initial evaluation,[68] orthostatic hypotension, anxiety, arrhythmias, or fatigue during or later in the day.[68]

Exercising testing of the cardiovascular system was developed for younger populations, however, the tests can be modified for older persons. Table 6–18 lists four of the more common exercising-testing protocols.

The tests, even with modification and slowing for the older person, may be too vigorous. Table 6–19 gives low-level functional protocol.[67]

One more exercise test protocol was developed by Everett Smith.[69] This test is useful for the very low-level patient that is either unable to get out of a chair or performs better in a chair. This is the Chair Step Test shown in Figure 6–19. This test was developed by Smith and attempts to tax the cardiovascular system while controlling for those patients who may be unsafe on other cardiopulmonary exercise tests.[69] To perform this test, the patient sits in a chair and extends to touch, with alternating feet, boxes of various heights (as listed in Fig. 6–19). Each stage lasts 5 minutes, with the last stage involving alternately raising the arms on the same side

TABLE 6–18. EXERCISE TESTING PROTOCOLS

12-Minute Walk[a]	Level walking for 12 min distance recorded.	No equipment necessary yet correlates well with study results of more complex tests; can be used for patients who cannot accomplish either treadmill walking or bike riding because of dyspnea.
Low Level Functional	See Table 6–19.	Intermittent walk test for use with moderate to severely impaired patients. Allows flexibility of workload assignment and establishes an accurate baseline.
Balke Test[b]	Treadmill: speed constant at 3.0 mph; grade initially 0% increased by 3.5% every 2 min.	Slight increase in speed for patient with less impairment allows pulmonary and cardiovascular stress to come before leg fatigue.
Bruce[b]	Treadmill: speed initially 1.7 mph; grade initially 10%; both are increased every 3 min in a specified manner.	Can be used with relatively fit individuals to stress accurately all systems' response to exercise. Good to assess exercise-induced bronchospasm in fit individuals.
Bicycle Test[c]	Specific workload (i.e., watts or Kg/min) patient rides for a preset time, next workload determined by patient response.	Intermittent subjective test based on patient response. Requires lower extremity strength and endurance to reach high metabolic response level.

[a]McGavin CR, Cupta SP, McHardy GJR. Twelve-minute walking test for assessing disability in chronic bronchitis. Br Med J. 1976; 1:822.
[b]From Physician's handbook for evaluation of cardiovascular and physical fitness, Tennessee Heart Association, 1972.
[c]Ellestad NH. Stress Testing: Principles and Practice. Philadelphia: F.A. Davis, 1979.
Reprinted with permission from Irwin S, Zadai C. Cardiopulmonary rehabilitation of the geriatric patient. In: Lewis C, ed. Aging: The Health Care Challenge. Philadelphia: F.A. Davis; 1990.

of the body to shoulder level. The therapist monitors the patient at 2 minutes and 5 minutes. This test progresses the patient from 2.3 to 3.9 metabolic equivalents (METS).[68]

As noted in the previous sections, classic measures of cardiopulmonary functions are still appropriate for the older person. However, the clinician must be aware of changes that will affect those tests and choose to use more age-suitable ones.

Nerve Conduction Velocity

This section will discuss the manifestation of these systems in terms of nerve conduction velocities. (Again Chapters 3 and 4 describe the normal and pathological changes in the nervous system with age.) In all of the extremities, sensory nerve action potentials proprograte at a slower velocity and decrease in amplitude.[75] This decrement begins in the third decade and progresses in to the eighth decade.[70] The amplitude of sensory potentials drops from 43 to 21 μv, and sensory velocity in digital nerves steadily declines from 57 to 48 m/sec.[71] Despite these changes, the refractory period is relatively unaffected in the older person.[70] Conduction velocity in the dorsal column shows little change before the age of 60; however, it declines sharply after 60 at a rate of ±0.78 m/sec each year.[72] Tables 6–20 and 6–21 compare young and old conduction velocities.[72]

TABLE 6–19. LOW-LEVEL FUNCTIONAL PROTOCOL

Collect resting data supine and sitting	ECG, BP, RR, HR, O_2sat, PFTs
Stage I	Objective assessment of dyspnea/1.5–2 mph, 0% grade Walk 6 min = 4 min stabilization + 2 min gas collection Rest: Patient returns to baseline HR, RR, and O_2sat
Stage II	Functional ambulation assessment/treadmill set at speed and incline equal to functional work capacity based on physiologic and symptomatic response to Stage I Walk 6 min = 4 min stabilization + 2 min gas collection Rest: Patient returns to baseline HR, RR, and ABGs
Stage III	Maximum exercise tolerance/treadmill set to produce HR of 70–85% max or predicted ventilatory max ($35 \times FeV_1$) Walk 6 min = 4 min stabilization + 2 min gas collection Rest: Patient returns to baseline HR, RR, and ABGs
Criteria to terminate test	85% predicted or HR_{max}, desaturation to 85% or lower SaO_2, reaching a ventilatory maximum ($35 \times FEV_1$), development of significant cardiac arrhythmias, or development of significant symptoms

Reprinted with permission from Irwin S, Zadai C. Cardiopulmonary rehabilitation of the geriatric patient. In: Lewis C, ed. Aging: The Health Care Challenge. *Philadelphia: F.A. Davis; 1990.*

Motor conduction velocities slow at an even greater rate as do sensory nerves. The rate of decline of these nerves is 1 m/sec per decade after 15 to 24 years of age.[70] Several tables (see Tables 6–20 through 6–23) show the motor nerve conduction velocity changes with age.[72] Nerve conduction velocity can only be assessed by a therapist or physician specifically trained in this area. Nevertheless, all clinicians should be aware of changes with age that will affect the results of those tests.

Chair Step Test

		HR/BP	HR/BP	HR/BP
6″	2 min	_____	_____	_____
12″	2 min	_____	_____	_____
18″	2 min	_____	_____	_____
18″	2 min	_____	_____	_____

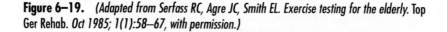

Figure 6–19. *(Adapted from Serfass RC, Agre JC, Smith EL. Exercise testing for the elderly.* Top Ger Rehab. *Oct 1985; 1(1):58–67, with permission.)*

TABLE 6–20. ELECTROPHYSIOLOGIC MEASUREMENTS IN THE YOUNG AND OLD SUBGROUPS AND IN THE COMBINED NORMAL CONTROL POPULATION. FIGURES REPRESENT MEAN ± 1 SD

	Unit	Young Adults	Old Adults	Combined Population
Number of measurements		30	30	60
Age	years	31.6 ± 14.1	74.1 ± 7.5	52.8 ± 24.2
Height	cm	171.4 ± 9.2	163.4 ± 9.9	167.4 ± 10.3
Median motor CV	m/sec	59.4 ± 2.6	52.6 ± 4.0	56.0 ± 4.8
Median sensory CV	m/sec	64.3 ± 3.2	56.9 ± 5.0	60.6 ± 5.6
Median F-wave latency (F)	msec	26.7 ± 2.0	28.4 ± 2.3	27.5 ± 2.3
Tibial F-wave latency (F)	msec	48.5 ± 4.2	55.8 ± 6.7	52.1 ± 6.4
Median SEP latency (SEP)	msec	16.0 ± 1.4	16.2 ± 1.1	16.1 ± 1.3
Tibial SEP latency (SEP)	msec	34.4 ± 4.2	38.2 ± 3.8	36.3 ± 3.8
Spinal conduction (CV)	m/sec	55.8 ± 12.1	42.4 ± 13.1	48.4 ± 12.4

Reprinted with permission from Dorfman L, Bosley T. Age-related changes in peripheral and central nerve conduction in man. Neurology. Jan 1979; 29:40.

Assessing Ethnicity

This final section on assessment deals with the concept of assessing ethnicity.[73] Rempusheski makes a strong plea to health professionals to recognize bias and differences in ethnic views of health care providers and recipients. Table 6–24 is a copy of her assessment categories.[74] These categories can be used by the practitioner interested in evaluating and planning programs most relevant and acceptable to the older person.

TABLE 6–21. CONDUCTION VELOCITY AND LATENCY (NORMALIZED BY HEIGHT) CHANGES WITH AGE CORRESPONDING TO THE LINEAR REGRESSION EQUATION $y = a \times AGE + b$[11]

Variable	Change with age (a)	y Intercept (b)	SD[a] y/x γ	SD[b] y/x₁₉ x₂ γ
Median motor CV	−0.15 m/sec/yr	63.9 m/sec		
Median sensory CV	−0.16 m/sec/yr	69.2 m/sec		
Spinal conduction (CV)	−0.24 m/sec/yr	60.8 m/sec		
Median F-wave latency (F)	+0.04 msec/m/yr	14.4 msec/m	0.056	0.054
Tibial F-wave latency (F)	+0.12 msec/m/yr	24.9 msec/m	0.076	0.067
Median SEP latency (SEP)	+0.015 msec/m/yr	8.8 msec/m	0.050	0.045
Tibial SEP latency (SEP)	+0.08 msec/m/yr	17.6 msec/m	0.078	0.071

[a]Normalized average standard error of y corrected for x in the single linear regression analysis $y = ax + b$.
[b]Normalized average standard error of y corrected for x_1 and x_2 in the multiple linear regression analysis. $y - a_1 x_1 + a_2 x_2 + a_3 x_1 x_2 = b$. ($x_1$ = age, x_2 = height.)
Reprinted with permission from Dorfman L, Bosley T. Age-related changes in peripheral and central nerve conduction in man. Neurology. Jan 1979; 29:40.

TABLE 6–22. MAXIMUM SENSORY CONDUCTION VELOCITY IN DISTAL AND PROXIMAL SEGMENTS OF SUPERFICIAL PERONEAL, SURAL, AND POSTERIOR TIBIAL NERVE IN 34 SUBJECTS 15 TO 33 YEARS OLD, AND 37 SUBJECTS 40 TO 65 YEARS OLD (TEMPERATURE ON SKIN 35° TO 37°C)[84]

Segment	Age (yr)	n[a]	A Conduction Velocity (m/sec) Mean	95%	SD	n[a]	B Conduction Velocity (m/sec) Mean	95%	SD
N, peroneus superficialis									
Big toe—	15–25	19	46·1	39·0	4Ã1				
sup. ext. retinac.	40–65	17	42·2	36·0	6·3				
Sup. ext. retinac.	15–33	24	55·9	50·0	3·8	12	55·9	47·0	5·0
-capitul. fibul.	40–65	23	52·9	47·0	3·7				
Sup. ext. retinac.	15–30	15	56·3	50·0	3·7				
-poplit. fossa	40–65	11	53·0	48·0	2·9				
Capitul. fibul.	15–25					13	55·8	47·0	4·7
-poplit. fossa	40–65					11	53·5	46·0	5·2
N. suralis									
Dors. ped.-	15–30	16	51·2	42·0	4·5				
lat. malleol.	40–65	15	48·3	40·0	5·3				
Lat. malleol.	15–30	21	56·5	51·0	3·4	16	55·9	49·0	4·2
-sura	40–65	16	54·8	46·5	4·5	12	56·3	47·0	5·5
Lat. malleol.	15–30	19	57·3	52·0	3·5				
-poplit. fossa	40–65	12	53·3	47·5	4·1				
Sura-	15–30					18	57·6	52·0	3·0
poplit. fossa	40–65					10	54·3	47·0	4·8
N. tibialis posterior									
Bit toe-	15–30	23	46·1	39·0	3·5				
med. malleol.	40–65	10	43·4	37·0	3·8				
Med. malleol.	15–30	17	58·6[b]	52·5	3·8	22	56·4	51·0	4·0
-poplit. fossa	40–52	7	57·4[b]	51·5	4·5	6	54·0	47·0	4·4

A: calculated from the latency measured between onset of the stimulus and the initial peak of the sensory potential.
B: calculated from the difference of latencies, measured at two sites of recording.
[a]Number of nerves.
[b]Conduction velocity in fibers of mixed nerve.
Reprinted with permission from Behse F, Buchtal F. Normal sensory conduction in the nerves of leg in man. J Neurol Neurosurg Psychiatry. 1971; 34:408.

TABLE 6–23. MAXIMUM CONDUCTION VELOCITIES OF ULNAR NERVE FIBERS TO MUSCLES OF THE HYPOTHENAR EMINENCE AT VARIOUS AGES [85]

Age in Years	N[a]	Average Conduction Velocity	Standard Deviation
		m./sec.	
3.5–10	8	61.5	6.30
10–20	8	57.1	6.19
20–30	35	58.4	4.28
30–40	7	57.4	6.45
40–50	2	56.8	—
50–60	3	49.7	—
60–70	10	51.3	5.26
70–82[b]	10	51.5	7.26

[a]If more than one measurement was made on a single individual, the average only was used.
[b]Includes only one case above 80 years of age.
Reprinted with permission from Wagman I, Lesse H. Conduction velocity of ulnar nerve in human subjects of different ages & sizes. Fed Proc. 1950; 9:130.

TABLE 6–24. ASSESSMENT CATEGORIES WITH WHICH TO ELICIT RITUALS, BELIEFS, AND SYMBOLS OF CARE ACTIVITIES[80]

Sleep

Condition of room/environment: occupancy of room and bed/sleeping surface, kind of bed/sleeping surface and other furniture, condition of room (temperature, lights, doors and windows open or closed, other artifacts/symbols in room).

Kinds of covering, comforting materials: pillow/head support (height/number of supports used, type, positioning), covering (blanket type, sheet type, other).

Sleepwear: covering on head, body, legs, feet (type and variation by season or event).

Care of bed linen: kind of cleaning, frequency, how, by whom.

Bedtime ritual: time, tasks, others involved, food or liquid consumed, sensory stimulation, symbols/icons used.

Rules for sleeping: when, with whom, how, in what positions, where, beliefs related to rules.

Rules for awakening: by whom/what, how, mechanisms used.

Awakening rituals: time, tasks, others involved, food or liquid consumed, sensory stimulation, symbols/icons used.

Personal Hygiene

Tending one's body: rituals for mouth care (tools and substances used, time, who can assist); rituals for body and hair care (how, when, where, how often, substances used, taboos, gender rules, symbols, beliefs associated with aspects of ritual).

Associations with health/illness: care associated with body fluids/excretions, symbolism, body temperature, activities of tending one's body, substances used in rituals, seasonal/climate taboos, kinds of activities, time of day/year, gender rules, beliefs.

Eating

Kinds of foods: preferences, dislikes, specific to an event, ritual, specific to time of day/week/month/year, seasonal, rules or taboos for hot foods, cold foods, rules for amount, type, composition, beliefs, and symbolism associated with specific foods.

Schedule of foods: rules for when/when not to eat; amount related to time of day; healthy/ill status; associated with certain rituals, beliefs, symbols; before/after meal rituals, symbols/icons used/present.

Environment for eating: place, people, position, taboos/rules, symbols/icons used/present.

Implements/utensils: kind, number, rules for use of each, taboos, utensils as symbols.

Reprinted with permission from Rempusheski V. The role of ethnicity in elder care. Nurs Clin N Am. Sept 1989; 24(3):717–724.

CONCLUSION

Assessment is not simply a range of motion test. Assessment of the older person involves not only modification of the norms of classically used tools such as goniometry or nerve conduction velocities, but it also involves a thorough assessment, which requires evaluation of functional parameters as well. In addition, psychosocial and ethnic concerns may need to be addressed. This chapter has presented several valuable tools for each of these areas. It is the practitioner's responsibility to choose the one's best suited for their practice.

PEARLS

- Sample tools for assessing cognitive changes in mental status of the elderly are the Mini-Mental State Examination (MMSE) and the Mental Status Questionnaire (MSQ).

- The Zung, Popoff, Beck, and Geriatric Depression Scales are all useful tools for assessing depression in the elderly.

- The Holmes and Rahe Life Events Scale is one of the best known tools for assessing stress levels.

- Functional assessment is a method of measuring an individual's performance.

• Numerous functional assessment tools are available for evaluating older persons. Choose the tool best suited to the setting, clientele, mode of administration, and domain to be evaluated.

• Standard physical therapy measures, such as strength, range of motion, posture, and gait, change with age and may be better assessed with specific tools and norms designed for the elderly.

• Cardiopulmonary parameters, as well as nerve conduction velocity, change with age and require different normative values for assessment comparison.

• Assessing ethnicity of the elderly will help health professionals recognize bias and differences that may obstruct care.

REFERENCES

1. Manton KG. A longitudinal study of functional change and mortality in the United States. *Gerontology: Soc Sciences.* 1988; 43:S153–161.
2. Kasper JD. Using the long-term care surveys: longitudinal and cross-sectional analyses of disabled older people. *Proceedings of the 1987 Public Health Conference on Records and Statistics.* DHHS Pub. No. 88–1214. Hyattsville, Md: National Center for Health Statistics; 1988: 353–358.
3. Guralnik JM, Branch LG, Cummings SR, et. al. Physical performance measures in aging research. *J Gerontology: Med Sciences.* 1989; 44:M141–146.
4. Folstein M. Mini-mental state: a practice of method for grading the cognitive state of patients for the clinician. *Psychiatric Res.* 1975; 12:189–198.
5. Folstein M, Rabins P. Psychiatric evaluation of the elderly patients. *Primary Care.* September 1979; 6(3):609–619.
6. Kane R, Kane R. Measuring Mental Status. In: Kane R, Kane R: *Assessing the Elderly* Lexington, Mass: Lexington Books, 1981.
7. Kahn RL, Goldfarb AI, Pollack M, et al. Brief objective measures for the determination of mental status in the aged. *Am J Psychiatry.* 1960; 117:326.
8. Prestidge B, Lalle C. Prevalence and recognition of depression among primary care outpatients. *J Family Pract.* 1987; 25:67–72.
9. German P, Shapiro S, Skinner EA. Use of health and mental health services. *J Am Ger Soc.* 1985; 33:246–252.
10. Zung W, Richard D, Shrot M. Self-rating depression scale in an outpatient clinic. *Arch Ger Psy.* 1965; 13:508–515.
11. Freedman N, Bucci W, Elkowitz E. Depression in a family practice elderly population. *J Am Ger Soc.* 1982; 30:372–377.
12. Zung A. A self-rating depression scale. *Arch Gen Psy.* 1965; 12:63–70.
13. Popoff S. A simple method for diagnosis of depression by the family physician. *Clin Med.* 1969; 76:24–29.
14. Okimoto J, Barnes R, Yoith R, et al. Screening for depression in geriatric medical patients. *J Am Psy.* 1982; 139:799–802.
15. Gallagher D. The Beck depression inventory and older adults review of its development and utility. In: Brink T, ed. *Clinical Gerontology: A Guide to Assessment and Intervention.* New York: Haworth Press; 1986:149–163.
16. Nielson A, Williams T. Depression in ambulatory medical patients prevalence by self-report questionnaire and recognition by non-psychiatric physicians. *Arch Gen Psy.* 1980; 37:999–1004.
17. Kamerow D, Campbell T. Is screening for mental health problems worthwhile in family practice? *Postgrad Med.* 1972; 1:37–43.
18. Beck A, Beck R. Screening depressed patients in family practice: a rapid technique. *Postgrad Med.* 1972; 52:81–85.
19. Brink T, Yesavage J, Lum D, et al. Screening tests for geriatric depression. *Clin Gerontologist.* 1982; 1:37–42.
20. Yesavage J. The use of self-rating depression scales in the elderly. In: Poon E, ed. *Clinical Memory Assessment of Older Adults.* Washington, DC: American Psychological Association; 1986.

21. Holmes T, Rahe R. The social readjustment rating scale. *J Psychosomatic Res.* 1967; 11:213–218.
22. Intermediary Manual Part 3—Claims Process. Section 3904 Medical Review (MR) of Part 3 Intermediary Outpatient Physical Therapy (OPT) Bills [Edit], HCFA; 1988.
23. Tinetti M. Performance oriented assessment of mobility problems in elderly patients. *J Am Ger Soc.* 1986; 34(2):119–126.
24. Kane RL. Beyond caring: the challenge to geriatrics. *J Am Ger Soc.* 1988; 36(5):467–472.
25. Bohannon R, Andrews A, Smith M. Rehabilitation goals of patient with hemiplegia. *Int J Rehab Res.* 1988; 11(2):181–183.
26. Kane RL, Kane RA. *Assessing the Elderly.* Lexington, Mass: Lexington Books; 1981.
27. *Dorland's Medical Dictionary.* 26 ed. Philadelphia: Saunders; 1981.
28. Jette AM. State of the art of functional status assessment. In: Nothstein J, ed. *Measurement in Physical Therapy.* New York: Churchill Livingstone; 1988.
29. Mahoney FI, Barthel DW. Functional evaluation: the Barthel Index. *Md State Med J.* 1965; 14(2):61–65.
30. Katz S, Downs TD, Cash HR, et al. Progress in the development of the Index of ADL. *Gerontologist.* 1970; 10:20.
31. Katz S, Ford AB, Moskowitz RW, et al. Studies of illness in the aged. The Index of ADL: a standardized measure of biological and the psychosocial functions. *JAMA.* 1963; 185:914–919.
32. Schoening H, Anderson L, Bergstrom D, et al. Numerical scoring of self-care status of patients. *Arch Phys Med Rehab.* October 1965; 46:689.
33. Filenbaum G. Screening the elderly: a brief instrumental activities of daily living measure. *J Am Ger Soc.* 1985; 33:698–706.
34. Moskovitz E, McCann C. Classification of disability in the chronically ill and aging. *J Chron Dis.* 1957; 5:342.
35. Granger C, Greer DS. Functional status measure and medical rehabilitation outcomes. *Arch Phys Med Rehab.* 1976; 57:103.
36. Functional Independence Measure (FIM). *Uniform Data System for Med Rehab.* Buffalo, NY: Research Foundation of SUNY; 1990.
37. Jette AM. Functional Status Index: reliability of a chronic disease evaluation instrument. *Arch Phys Med Rehab.* September 1980; 61(9):395–401.
38. Jette A, Cleary PD, Rubenstein LV, et al. Functional Status Questionnaire reliability and validity when used in primary care. *J Gen Med.* May/June 1986; 1:143–149.
39. Branch LG, Meyers AR. Assessing physical function in the elderly. *Clin Geriatric Med.* 1987; 3(1):29–51.
40. Bishop C. Living arrangement choices of elderly singles. *Health Care Financing Review.* 1986; 7:65–73.
41. Wan TTH, Odell BG. Factors affecting the use of social and health services for the elderly. *Aging and Society.* 1981; 1:95–115.
42. Branch LG, Jette AM. A prospective study of long-term care institutionalization among the aged. *Am J Pub Health.* 1982; 72:1373–1379.
43. Branch LG, Jette AM, Evashwick C. Toward understanding elders' health service utilization. *J Comm Health.* 1981; 7:80–92.
44. Macken CL. A profile of functionally impaired elderly persons living in a community. *Health Care Financing Review.* 1986; 7:33–50.
45. Wiener JM, Hanley RJ, Clark R, et al. Measuring the activities of daily living: comparisons across national surveys. *J Gerton: Social Sciences.* 1990; 45(6):229–237.
46. Applegate W, Blass J, Williams F. Instruments for the functional assessment of older patients. *N Eng J Med.* April 26, 1990; 322(17):1207–1214.
47. Lachs M, Feinstein AR, Cooney LM, et al. A simple procedure for general screening for functional disability in elderly patients. *Annals of Int Med.* May 1990; 112(9):699–704.
48. Williams M. Why screen for functional disability in elderly persons? *Annals of Int Med.* May 1990; 112(9):639.
49. Tomanek R, Woo Y. Compensatory hypertrophy of the plantare muscle in relation to age. *J Gerontology.* 1970; 25(1):23–29.
50. Goldspink G, Howells K. Work induced hypertrophy in exercised normal muscles of different ages and the reversibility of hypertrophy after cessation of exercise. *Am J Physiol.* 1974; 239:179–193.
51. Moritani T, Devries HA. Potential for gross muscle hypertrophy in older men. *J Geron.* 1980; 35(5):673.

52. Rice C. Strength in an elderly population. *Arch Phys Med Rehab.* May 1989; 70(5):391–397.

53. Borges O. Isometric and isokinetic knee extension and flexion torque in men and women aged 20–70. *Scand J Rehab Med.* 1989; 21:45–53.

54. Vandervoort A, Hayes K. Plantarflexor muscle function in young and elderly women. *Eur J Appl Physiol.* 1989; 58:389–394.

55. Walker JSD, Walker JM, Sue D, et al. Active mobility of the extremities in older subjects. *Phys Ther.* June 1984; 64(6):914–923.

56. Frekany G, Leslie D. Effects of an exercise program on selected flexibility measurements of senior citizens. *Gerontologist.* 1975: 182–183.

57. James B, Parker A. Active and passive mobility of lower limb joints in elderly men and women. *Am J Phys Med Rehab.* August 1989; 68(4):162–167.

58. Lewis C. Musculoskeletal changes with age. In Lewis C, ed. *Aging: The Health Care Challenge.* Philadelphia: Davis; 1990: 135–160.

59. REEDCO Research. *REEDCO Posture Score Sheet.* Auburn, NY; 1978.

60. Murray MP. Gait as a total pattern of movement. *Am J Phys Med.* 1976; 46:290.

61. Murray MP, Kory RC, Clarkson BH. Walking patterns in healthy old men. *J Gerontol.* 1969; 24:169.

62. Andriacchi TP, Ogle JA, Galante JO. Walking speed as a basis of normal and abnormal gait measurements. *J Biomech.* 1977; 10:261.

63. Findley FR, Cody KA, Finizie RV. Locomotion patterns in elderly women. *Arch Phys Med Rehab.* 1967; 50:140.

64. Nelson A. Function ambulation profile. *Physical Ther.* 1974; 54:1061–1064.

65. Bohannon R, Larken PA, Cook AC, et al. Decrease in timed balance test scores with aging. *Physical Ther.* 1989; 64:1067.

66. Wolfson L, Whipple R, Amerman P. Gait assessment in the elderly. A gait abnormality rating scale and its relation to falls. *J Gerontol: Med Sciences.* 1990; 45(1):M14–M15.

67. Irwin S, Zadai C. Cardiopulmonary rehabilitation of the geriatric patient. In Lewis C, ed. *Aging: The Health Care Challenge.* 2nd ed. Philadelphia: Davis; 1990; 181–210.

68. Siebens H, Deconditioning. In: Kemp B, Brummel-Smith K, Ramsdell JD, eds. *Geriatric Rehabilitation.* Boston, Little, Brown & Co.; 1990: 177–191.

69. Serfass RC, Agre JC, Smith E. Exercise testing for the elderly, *Top Geriatric Rehab.* October 1985; 1(1):58–67.

70. Schaumburg H, Spencher P, Ochoa T. The aging human peripheral nervous system. In Katzman R, Terry R (eds).: *The Neurology of Aging.* Philadelphia: Davis: 1975; 442–444.

71. Buchtal F, Rosenflack A, Behse F. Sensory potentials of normal and diseased nerves. In: Dyck P, Thomas P, Lambert E. *Peripheral Neuropathy.* Philadelphia: Saunders; 1975: 433–446.

72. Dorfman L, Bosley T. Age-related changes in peripheral and central nerve conduction in man. *Neurology* 29:38–44, January 1979.

73. Rempusheski V. The Role of Ethnicity in Elder Care. *Nursing Clinics of North America* 24(3):717–724, September 1989.

74. Fitzgerald GK, Wynveen KJ, Rheult W, Rothschild B. Objective assessment with establishment of normal values for lumbar spine range of motion. *Phys Ther.* November 1983; 63(11):1778.

CHAPTER **7** SEVEN

Exploring Nutritional Needs

Nutrition is an area that is rarely considered when exercise is prescribed and functional levels are determined for activity in the elderly. Nutritional manifestations often overlap normal aging and disease and facilitate their progression. With the elderly, under- and overnutritional problems and concerns are of great importance in accurately determining the overall fitness and functional levels of activity in the elderly. In the Surgeon General's report from 1979, the goals for the 1980s aimed at improving the health and quality of life for all individuals over the age of 65.[1] This was hoped to be accomplished by encouraging healthy exercise and nutritional practices. It was anticipated that by providing a coordinated educational effort on federal, state, regional, and local levels that the average annual number of days of restricted activity resulting from acute and chronic health problems could be reduced by 20% (or to fewer than 30 days per year) by 1990.[2]

This chapter will address the changes related to aging that affect the nutritional well-being of the elderly by looking at common deficiencies and risk factors. Guidelines for good nutrition in the elderly and the impact of poor nutrition on the physical, emotional, and cognitive well-being of the elderly will also be addressed. In addition, components of nutritional programs for the elderly will be presented to provide the necessary guidelines for nutritional measures and the insights essential to assessing the nutritional status of the elderly to promote health, prevent or reduce risks of certain diseases, support other medical interventions, and improve the quality of life in old age.

There is no clear demarcation to indicate where on the spectrum of aging "healthy old age" begins and ends with respect of nutrition. There is clearly a state produced by normal aging, but there is great difficulty in identifying this conceptually "healthy" state in the absence of overt or occult disease. As each cohort ages, there is a progressive variability in biological efficiency. This variability is a result of a combination of the disparate influences of disease, environment, time, genetic profile, and nutrition on an individual's aging process.

AGE RELATED CHANGES IN THE GASTROINTESTINAL SYSTEM

Changes in the digestive system will have the most impact on nutritional status as the gastrointestinal tract is most directly involved in ingestion, absorption, transport, and excretion of food products.[3]

Several changes associated with aging affect the oral cavity. There is a decreased amount of saliva in the mouth coupled with the loss of natural teeth or ill-fitting dentures that inhibits the chewing of foods. It is estimated that approximately 50% of individuals are edentulous by the age of 65.[4] Poor dentition and decreased saliva can cause discomfort and poor mastication. As a result, the elderly tend to pick softer and moister foods. They eat fewer raw fruits and vegetables and less meat that requires chewing. These eating pattern changes appreciably diminish the gratification of eating. The inability to chew foods properly is often an embarrassment for the elder and decreases his or her desire to eat with others, thereby decreasing socialization.

There is a decrease in sensory input with aging.[5-7] Atrophy of gustatory papillae decrease taste, and a decrease in olfaction affects the sense of smell. Sensory losses in taste and smell may potentiate a poor appetite. Loss of dentition not only decreases chewing ability, thereby affecting appetite, but dentures also detract from the perceptual response and can negatively affect the desire to consume certain foods. In addition, depression, smoking, and medications can have an effect on sensory input, diminishing the pleasure of eating. Mulligan suggests that sensory changes may be the result of misuse, disuse, or pathology, and challenges the concept of sensory loss as a normal, age related change.[8]

The esophagus shows little change with age. Esophageal changes are generally related to pathology, such as a hiatal hernia. Swallowing and peristalsis remain relatively intact. Khan[9] suggests that the peristaltic amplitude and velocity of the upper third of the esophagus may decrease with advanced age.

The gastric mucosa shows age related atrophy.[10] As a result, fewer chief and parietal cells remain to provide sufficient pepsin, hydrochloric acid, and gastric mucus. These elements are essential to the absorption of vitamin B_{12} and iron, which are required to initiate protein digestion.[10] Horowitz[10] reported that there is a delay in gastric emptying of both solids and liquids with advancing age, though no clinical significance was found. The parietal cells of the stomach lose their ability to secrete hydrochloric acid and there is a general reduction in the secretion of digestive juices in old age. There is some evidence from testing with very large amounts of gastric and intestinal material that aging causes a relative insufficiency in the capacity to digest protein.[11] The clinical significance of this is the unavailability of protein for energy production and maintenance of healthy muscle tissue. The inability of the body to use ingested protein efficiently also impacts wound healing and tissue repair.

There is a reduction in the intestinal mobility and in the amount of digestive enzymes as a function of age, which are both associated with a reduction in carbohydrate absorption.[12] With a possible decrease in gastric emptying, reduced carbohydrate absorption, and a decrease in lipase excretion by the pancreas, absorption of dietary fat becomes very inefficient.[12] This decrease in the overall efficiency of the gastrointestinal tract can result in constipation and diverticular disease. The colon remains functionally intact,[13] though some changes appear to be age related. These changes include an increase in diverticula and decreases in motility, rectal wall elasticity, and sphincter tone.[14] The effect that aging might have on the absorption of food has been tested by using xylose as a marker substance. Though there is a gradual decrease in absorption of xylose after the age of 60, the most significantly impeded age group is over 80 years of age when the intestinal capacity to absorb xylose is influenced and diminished. Calcium absorption has been found to decrease with age.[12] Undernutrition or excesses in nutrient intake can contribute to these physiological gastrointestinal changes.[15] Psychologically, changes in the gastrointestinal tract can trigger overconcern and undue anxiety, especially about bowel function, to the extent that essential foods are excluded from the daily diet.

The kidneys show changes related to aging that directly affect the nutritional status of the elderly. Though not considered a part of the digestive system, the renal nephron is responsible for the provision of some essential nutrients to the blood.[15] With age, there is a decrease in renal blood flow affecting the return of nutrients. In addition, there is a decrease in glomerular filtration, sodium retention, urine concentration capacity (an increased water output decreasing hydration), and daily creatinine excretion. Combining these changes with the loss of nephrons with aging results in a decrease in efficiency and a possible kidney insufficiency. Diminished glucose resorption occurs, and often there is either excessively low or high sodium blood levels, reflections of the decrease in efficiency in kidney functioning.

Renal insufficiency is common in old age. Glomerular filtration rates, renal blood flow, and renal tubular function all decline in efficiency. Atrophy of renal mass is usual and especially pronounced in the cortex by a decline in the number of nephrons and by hypertrophy and sclerosis in the remaining nephrons. In addition, chronic degenerative diseases, including hypertension, diabetes mellitus, and kidney disease, also often give rise to kidney damage. In end stage renal disease, therapeutic diets are often prescribed to decrease the symptomatology and blood biochemistry disturbances. These include limitation of protein, sodium, and phosphorus.[16] The possibility that age related deterioration in kidney function is not inevitable but that it results in part from chronic protein overnutrition is receiving much attention.[17,18] The theory that protein restriction can decrease progression of chronic renal insufficiency is also being studied.

There is a decrease in liver enzyme activity with aging. This directly affects the metabolism of carbohydrates and the breakdown of drugs and alcohol in the system.

Other age related changes or chronic diseases influencing food habits are those affecting the musculoskeletal, neuromuscular, cardiovascular, and pulmonary systems. Problems creating pain, weakness, paralysis, breathing difficulties, or fatigue create loss of function and result in immobility. Shopping, opening food containers, and cooking can often become insurmountable obstacles.

Changes in body composition and weight and a decline in physical exercise and activity levels also influence nutritional needs. With aging, as with inactivity, there is an increase in adipose tissue, a decrease in lean body mass, a decrease in basal metabolism (only a problem from the prospective of obesity), a decrease in caloric requirements, and a decrease in total body water.[19]

AGE RELATED CHANGES THAT AFFECT NUTRITION

The biological, anatomical, and physiological changes that occur with aging were discussed in Chapter 3 and will only be discussed here as they relate to the nutritional status of the elderly. A progressive decline in the efficiency of many physiological organ functions and an inability to restore homeostasis once it is disrupted are both related to aging.[14] There are extraneous factors complicating the nutritional and homeostatic situation, such as age, frequency of disease and disabilities, multiple medications, hereditary, and genetic predispositions. The decline in physiological functioning shows considerable variation from one individual to the next, and it varies even among cells, tissues, and organs of the same individual.[3] For instance, in calculating body water content, there is a significant but normal change with age, and these changes can be compounded by dehydration or edema secondary to inflammatory processes from diseases or social factors. Table 7–1

TABLE 7–1. PHYSIOLOGICAL CHANGES AND NUTRITIONAL CONSIDERATIONS

Physiological Changes with Aging	Potential Functional Outcome	Probable Clinical Outcome
Musculoskeletal		
Decreased number and size of muscle fibers	Decrease in lean body mass	Decreased muscular strength, decreased mobility
Decreased bone density	Osteoporosis	Increased risk of fractures
Decreased joint mobility	Narrowing of joint space	Impaired mobility
Central Nervous System		
Cerebral atrophy, senile plaques, neurofibrillary tangles	Parkinson-like symptoms, supranuclear palsy	Confusion, diminished response and perception, memory loss, decreased ADLs, poor nutritional compliance
Decreased sensory function	Decreased reaction to pain, touch, heat, and cold	Decreased perception leading to accidental injury
Impaired proprioception	Diminished mechanisms controlling balance	Increased susceptibility to falls
Skin		
Thinning of epithelial and subcutaneous layer	Tissue and vascular fragility	Increased susceptibility to abrasions, bruises, and burns
Eye		
Sclerosis of lens	Cataract, decreased peripheral vision	Impaired peripheral vision, susceptibility to accidents
Degeneration of muscles of accommodation	Smaller pupils	Impaired visual acuity, decreased socialization
Degenerative changes in vitreous, retina, and choroid	Decreased color vision and decreased night vision	Susceptibility to accidents
Degeneration of intrinsic/extrinsic ocular muscles	Impaired upward gaze	Susceptibility to falling

(continued)

TABLE 7–1. PHYSIOLOGICAL CHANGES AND NUTRITIONAL CONSIDERATIONS (CONT.)

Physiological Changes with Aging	Potential Functional Outcome	Probable Clinical Outcome
Hearing		
Degeneration of organ of corti	Loss of high frequency tones	Decreased hearing, decreased socialization
Smell		
Atrophy of olfactory mechanism	Impaired sense of smell	Decreased appreciation of food
Oral Cavity		
Decreased salivary flow	Dry mouth	Poor oral hygiene, gingivitis, impaired food bolus formation
Resorption of gums and bony tissue surrounding teeth	Tooth loss, impaired force of bite	Preference for softer foods, malfunctioning dentures
Diminished taste bud sensory input	Increased salt and sugar consumption	Diet high in sugar and salt
Gastrointestinal		
Decrease in esophageal smooth muscle, dysfunction of lower esophageal sphincter	Decreased esophageal mobility	Difficulty swallowing, high-bulk foods, hiatal hernia
Decreased intestinal blood flow, decreased liver size	Impaired intestinal absorption and liver metabolism	Subclinical malnutrition
Decreased contractile function of smooth intestinal muscle	Decreased intestinal motility	Constipation
Decreased HCl secretion, decreased number of absorbing cells	Defective absorption of calcium and iron	Pernicious anemia, iron deficiency anemia, osteoporosis
Decreased gallbladder motility	Gallstones	Gastrointestinal upsets, fatty food intolerance
Renal		
Decrease in nephrons, atherosclerosis in combination with decreased cardiac output	Decreased ability to dilute and concentrate urine, diminished renal blood flow	Renal insufficiency, increased potential for dehydration
Endocrine		
Pancreatic beta cells, function and insulin end-organ responsiveness diminish	Progressive glucose intolerance with advancing age	Diabetes mellitus, susceptibility of hypoglycemia if on insulin or oral hypoglycemic drugs
Psychological		
Role changes	Retirement, loss of productivity, increased leisure time	Depression, decreased nutritional intake, decreased finances
Loss	Multiple physical cognitive, financial, and social loss	Depression isolation, decreased nutrient intake

Modified and used with permission from Foley CJ, Tideiksaar R.[61]

summarizes the common physiological changes accompanying aging, their potential functional outcome, and the probable clinical manifestations that may affect the nutritional status of an elderly individual.

BASAL METABOLIC RATE

The basal metabolic rate (BMR) declines rapidly from the time of birth to the age of 20. Further decrease in the BMR gradually occurs until approximately the age of 80. Cell mass and muscle mass slowly decline with age, and muscle mass is partially replaced by fat and connective tissue.[20,21] It is not known whether the slowing of the BMR is the result of a decline in cell mass or reflects an actual decrease in metabolic activity. Of interest is the fact that the decline in lean body mass is reflected in a 15% to 20% decrease in exchangeable potassium per kilogram from age 20 to 75.[22,23] This exchangeable body potassium is viewed as an indicator of lean body mass. The decline of BMR with advancing age parallels that of exchangeable potassium. Thus, energy requirements, as a reflection of BMR, appear proportional to lean body mass at all ages.[24]

In conjunction with the BMR decline, there is a gradual reduction in physical activity from the approximate age of 20 to 65.[20,21] Further advances in age do not appear to significantly influence energy expenditure unless there are additional variables, such as arthritis, a cerebral vascular accident, or cardiovascular or pulmonary diseases. An elderly person involved in moderately strenuous exercise requires significantly more energy output compared to younger individuals.[23] It has been hypothesized that this occurs because of the decrease in neuromuscular coordination and the resulting increase in muscular inefficiency. The consequence is "wasted energy." This potential for greater energy loss is balanced by a reduction in extraneous movements and less indulgence in activity on the part of the elder. Overall, the decrease in energy requirements superimposed on the decrease in demand on a reduced lean body mass results in decreasing caloric requirements with advancing age.

Other age related changes occur in body composition and function. On a cellular level, there is a decrease in nutrient uptake by cells, glucose and lipid metabolism decrease, and protein synthesis declines.[25] These changes have a direct effect on BMR as well as altering the energy requirements of activity in the elderly.

The optimal level of physical activity varies because of differences among the aged in their life-style, disability, and disease. Evidence is rapidly accumulating that marked declines in physical activity among the aged are undesirable from a health standpoint. Reasonable levels of physical activity improve physical conditioning, may improve some aspects of endocrine function, contribute positively to bone health, increase cerebral oxygenation and alertness, and prevent muscle atrophy.[26] Exercise can improve work capacity and cardiovascular function when it is undertaken with sufficient frequency, intensity, and duration. Body fat decreases, lean body mass increases, and endurance increases on aerobic programs with improvement in oxygen delivery and use.[14] Exercise also contributes to psychological and social health.

AGE RELATED CHANGES IN MUSCLE METABOLISM

Skeletal muscle mass declines with advancing age and is paralleled by a decrease in the total RNA concentration in muscle tissue,[27] which affects protein metabolism and production of essential amino acids for energy production. Additionally, it has been reported that there is a reduction in the protein–synthetic activity of muscle ribosomes with increasing age, a decrease in the proportion of polyribosomes, and a decline in the pH enzyme fraction, all of which contribute to alterations in tissue protein synthesis and energy production in muscle tissue with advancing age.[28]

Ultimately, studies of protein metabolism at the cellular and organ level have been evaluated in reference to the status of whole body protein metabolism. In this context, Waterlow and Stephen[29] observed that with increased age and body weight, the turnover of body protein decreased and affected both the liver and muscle cells. They concluded that there was a marked reduction in total body protein turnover in older subjects. Numerous studies have been undertaken to determine body protein in humans, and a few of these studies have dealt with the changes in body protein content with advancing years. Of special importance to the clinician is the catabolic and corresponding anabolic component of metabolism in the presence of infection. Anabolic responses occur not only during recovery but also in the early phase of illness when anabolism is associated with increased production of phagocytes and other leukocytes and the induction of several tissue enzymes and immunoglobulins. Overall liver protein synthesis is increased and skeletal muscle protein synthesis is decreased in response to an infectious episode.[6]

Cross-sectional, as well as longitudinal, studies reveal that there is a progressive decline in body potassium and a fall in intracellular fluid as aging progresses.[6] Because of possible changes in the intracellular concentration of potassium with age, the precise physiological significance of body potassium loss in later years is uncertain. Tissues with a high potassium content, such as skeletal muscle, may decrease relative to those with a lower potassium concentration, and the relative amount of connective tissue, which contains little potassium, may become greater. However, a loss of total body potassium is generally taken to indicate a decrease in total cellular protein mass, and this may be due, to a large extent, to a decrease in skeletal muscle protein mass with age.[22]

The motor function of the human body declines with age. It has already been noted that the number of functioning motor units decreases with age (see Chapter 3). The decline in number of muscle fibers is also associated with a decrease in speed of contraction and myofibrillar and myosin ATPase activity. The rate of calcium transport by the sarcoplasmic reticulum increases with age, which might relate to muscle dysfunction by making it difficult to obtain sufficient calcium in the myoplasm for the contractile requirements of the actomyosin system.[30] The age related decline in bone mass (osteoporosis) is highly correlated with the loss of skeletal muscle. Calcium is one of the most important elements in the body, with essential functions in muscle contraction, nerve conduction, and membrane transport. For body function, maintaining a serum calcium level greater that 6.0 mg/dL is far more important than maintaining skeletal mass. Although the body supply of calcium is almost exclusively from bone, calcium can be obtained from the diet. Calcium balance for homeostasis is, therefore, dependent on the skeletal mass and the dietary intake of calcium.

Creatinine excretion has been used as an index of muscle mass in children and adults and should have the same meaning in the elderly, even though creatine clearance is reduced with aging.[16] The total body protein synthesis per gram of creatinine excretion is considerably higher in the aged subject compared to that of young adults. Because muscle mass is reduced, the higher turnover per unit of creatinine excretion in the elderly may be interpreted to reflect a greater contribution by the active visceral tissues relative to whole body protein metabolism in the elderly. Research data suggest that not only is there a shift in the distribution of body protein synthesis with increasing age, but the rate of muscle protein breakdown and synthesis may decline at the same time. The net result of these concurrent changes is an increase in total body protein synthesis per unit of creatinine with a maintenance of the total body protein synthesis rate when expressed per unit of body cell mass (BCM).

This hypothesis of the changes in the quality and quantity of total body protein metabolism can be further supported by comparing urinary nitrogen and its related amino acid (3-methylhistidine) excretion in young adults and elderly subjects. This unusual amino acid (3-methylhistidine) is present in actin of all muscles and in myosin of "white" muscle fibers. It is quantitatively excreted in the urine, and, unlike the common amino acids of body proteins, it is not reused for purposes of protein synthesis. Preliminary comparative findings on the urinary output of this amino acid in young adults and elderly subjects suggest that the daily output of 3-methylhistidine is much lower in the elderly. This reflects the decreased muscle mass. In addition, when normalized for differences in creatinine excretion, the output of 3-methylhistidine is still quite different for the elderly. This observation suggests that, per unit of muscle mass, the rate of muscle protein breakdown appreciably declines with age.[6]

A relationship between the nutritional state and skeletal muscle function has long been suspected. During periods of either partial or total starvation, body protein is broken down to supply the required amino acids. As a labile pool of body protein is unavailable for this purpose, all the protein that is broken down serves either a functional or structural role, resulting in a loss of the BCM. Body cell mass represents the total mass of living, functioning cells, the component of the body composition that is metabolically active, and, therefore, the source for oxygen consumption and carbon dioxide production. Skeletal muscle accounts for 60% of BCM and is the largest source of endogenous amino acids. As a result, protein-calorie malnutrition is invariably accompanied by skeletal muscle wasting.[31] A relationship has been demonstrated between skeletal muscle function and nutritional state, and the validity of skeletal muscle function as a functional measure of nutritional state has been demonstrated.[31-34]

CHRONIC DISEASE AND NUTRITION IN THE ELDERLY

Aging processes and lifelong eating patterns are often associated with diseases and disorders that influence the life span, such as atherosclerosis, hypertension, osteoporosis, diabetes, cancer, renal disease, dental disease, and obesity. The prevalence of many chronic degenerative diseases increases with advancing age. These disease states may have synergistic negative effects on individuals whose physiological function is already compromised by the aging process. Many chronic conditions have dietary implications that alter the need for nutrients, the physical and metabolic form in which nutrients are delivered, and the activities of daily living (ADLs) related to food and eating. Modifications in the type or amount of energy, or the energy providing the nutrients, vitamins, and minerals may be called for in order to provide nutritional support or to control the progression of chronic degenerative diseases. Unfortunately, manifestations of malnutrition, such as cracks in the mouth or a bright red tongue, are overt signs of a problem that is far advanced. For example, physical signs of dehydration are usually not apparent until it is in its advanced stages. With a decreased nutrient intake, there is a gradual tissue depletion with evolving biochemical abnormalities before it surfaces in an overt deficiency. Table 7–2 summarizes the most frequently encountered conditions and the nutritional problems they give rise to.

NUTRITION AND DIABETES MELLITUS IN THE ELDERLY

Approximately 18% of the population between the ages of 65 and 74 years has diabetes mellitus.[35] In general, elderly individuals tend to have an impaired glucose tolerance when compared to younger individuals. Data suggest that only about 10% of the variance in total serum glucose response to an oral glucose load is attributable to age.[36] Body weight and the level of physical activity appear to have a more important role in the pathogenesis of hyperglycemia with aging. The major factors involved in hyperglycemia and the development of type II diabetes mellitus include a poor second-phase insulin secretion, failure to inhibit glucose production, a defect in the insulin receptor and postreceptor sites, obesity, and lack of physical activity. Regardless of the etiology of diabetes mellitus in the elderly, evidence reveals that control of glucose levels improves the quality of life and decreases morbidity and mortality rates in the elderly.

Impaired glucose tolerance of aging has been shown in cross-sectional studies to be related to the level of physical activity and fitness.[37] In a prospective trial of

TABLE 7–2. CHRONIC CONDITIONS AND RELATED NUTRITIONAL PROBLEMS

Chronic Condition	Related Nutritional Problems
Alzheimer's disease, other dementias	Cachexia and emaciation due to poor eating habits and self-care
Celiac sprue	Malabsorption, diarrhea, weight loss, malabsorption with secondary vitamin deficiencies
Cerebral vascular accident	Suppressed cough reflex, increased risk of choking, dysphagia
Chronic mesenteric ischemia	Abdominal pain after eating, weight loss, malabsorption
Constipation	Prolonged transit time especially with immobility, decreased colonic motility
Gastroenteritis	Gastrointestinal discomfort, vomiting, diarrhea, loss of appetite, weight loss, dehydration
Colitis	Decreased elasticity of rectal wall, abdominal discomfort, fecal impaction
Coronary artery disease	Dyspnea, drugs lead to suppressed appetite and constipation
Diabetes mellitus	Glucose intolerance, poor energy use
Diverticular disease	Gastrointestinal pain, bowel discomfort, possible bleeding, infection, lack of appetite, weight loss
Emphysema	Dyspnea leading to lack of appetite and difficulty eating
Gallbladder disease	Gallstones, cholecystitis, pancreatitis, food restriction, some foods repugnant, undernutrition
Gastritis/duodenitis	Malabsorption of vitamin B_{12} and iron, some food restrictions, other foods repugnant, undernutrition
Hiatal hernia	Gastroesophageal reflux, heartburn, dysphagia
Liver diseases	Foods repugnant, restricted protein, drug level changes
Obesity	Energy intakes usually low, need for essential nutrient intake
Osteoarthritis	Difficulty in food shopping and preparation
Osteoporosis	Dyspnea with vertebral collapse, distortion of thorax and abdominal compression, lack of appetite, difficulty eating, decreased intake
Peptic ulcer	Obstruction, bleeding, and perforation, dysphagia, dyspepsia, retrosternal discomfort, antacid overuse and undernutrition
Pernicious anemia	B_{12} deficiency, spinal cord degeneration
Renal disease	Limited ability to handle protein, sodium, potassium, and water

Modified and used with permission from Dwyer JT.[61]

the effects of exercise on glucose tolerance, Seals and associates[38] found that while glucose levels did not change, both insulin and C peptide levels decreased. In addition, high-density lipoprotein cholesterol levels increased, and triglyceride levels decreased. In elderly patients with type II diabetes mellitus, short-term exercise programs do not show a major advantage over dietary control of glucose intake.[39] However, long-term exercise programs did result in improvements of glucose tolerance.[40,41] In combination with dietary control, the possible benefits of exercise on glucose tolerance are evident. In addition, exercise may also improve cardiovascular function, lipid profiles, hypertension, osteopenia, and psychological components in diabetic elders.

There are a number of effects on vitamin and mineral status in diabetes mellitus.[42] Many of these changes are parallel to those seen with aging. Diabetes mellitus is associated with decreased zinc absorption and hyperzincuria.[43] Zinc deficiencies are associated with poor wound healing, poor immune function, immune dysfunction, and anorexia.[44] Supplementary zinc administration has been shown to improve immune function[45] and facilitate wound healing[46] in patients with zinc deficiencies.

Chromium plays a role in normal glucose homeostasis. Deficiency of chromium has been implicated in the glucose intolerance with aging.[47] Copper levels are elevated in type II diabetes mellitus.[48] The clinical significance of this is not clearly known, however, Klevay[48] demonstrated that experimentally induced copper deficiency resulted in elevation of cholesterol levels. Thiamine is essential for the transport of metabolized glucose into the Krebs' cycle. In type II diabetes mellitus, erythrocyte transketolase activity, an indirect measure of thiamine status, is elevated, which may be related to poor availability of intracellular glucose. Diabetes mellitus is also associated with pernicious anemia. Vitamin B_{12} deficiency is common in the diabetic and is associated with posterior column neuropathy and dementia.

OBESITY

Obesity is common in persons aged 65 years or older. A diet that is higher in calories than required for the body's energy needs leads to energy storage and fat deposition. Excess calories from fat, carbohydrate, and protein foods leads to obesity. Some drugs promote appetite (hyperphagic drugs) and lead to obesity because of increased food intake. Alcohol intake, in addition to a diet providing sufficient food energy to meet caloric needs, can also lead to obesity. Reduction in body weight in obese persons is commonly retarded or impeded by a disinclination for exercise. Exercise may also be restricted as a result of secondary effects of obesity, such as osteoarthritis leading to physical disabilities.

Obesity is associated with numerous medical disabilities. Causal relationships have been identified between obesity and the development of late-onset diabetes, essential hypertension, and hypertensive heart disease. Obesity increases the risk of cardiovascular disease. Data from the Framingham Heart Study demonstrated a continuous relationship between obesity and coronary morbidity and mortality (greater in men than in women). Obesity is associated with increased blood pressure and serum lipoprotein levels.[49] The effects of weight change on blood lipid profiles are considerable. The Framingham Study showed that weight reduction resulted in modest increases in high-density lipoprotein (HDL) cholesterol.[50] It appears that both blood lipids and blood pressure are sensitive to the degree of obesity.

Obesity is the most common nutritional problem of public health concern in the United States.[1] While gross obesity is uncommon in the very old (because persons who are morbidly obese are more likely to die at an earlier age), obesity is still a serious disability in the elderly.

Obesity is also associated with the development of abdominal hernias. Gallbladder disease and gout are more common in obese individuals, and most importantly, obesity is associated with increased symptoms of degenerative osteoarthritis. Other complications include varicose veins with stasis dermatitis and stasis ulcers and bacterial and yeast infections between fat folds.[49,50]

In general, obesity is a hindrance to independent living in the elderly. Despite the limitations of modern actuarial reports and experimental finding, the data do show that obesity shortens life span and that limitation in food or caloric intake can result in a longer life.[51]

OSTEOPOROSIS

Osteoporosis is a heterogeneous condition characterized by an absolute decrease in the amount of normal bone (i.e., loss of bone mass). It results from the failure of bone formation to keep pace with bone resorption. This is termed coupling. It is due neither to a lack of dietary calcium nor defective bone mineralization,[52] but rather to endosteal resorption, which is greater than the formation of new osteons or bone units.[53] Age related trabecular bone loss starts at age 35, and cortical bone loss from about age 40. The loss proceeds at about 0.5% per year, but, at female menopause, the accelerated rate is 2.0% to 8.0% due to (directly or indirectly) lowered estrogen production.[52]

Calcium supplementation does nothing to prevent postmenopausal bone loss in women undergoing menopause or who have undergone menopause within the past 5 years. In women who are postmenopausal by 6 or more years, calcium citrate malate can significantly reduce bone loss if given at a dosage of 800 mg/day.[54] Riis[55] suggests that calcium supplementation may have a minor effect on the loss of cortical bone but that it has no effect on the trabecular bone.

The importance of osteoporosis is in how it relates to the incidence of bone fractures in postmenopausal females. Women are postmenopausal for 40% of their lives. Symptomatic osteoporosis affects one in three of the older female population and results in more than 175,000 femur and 500,000 vertebral fractures per year in American women.[56] Fracture of the femur is a major contributor to mortality in the elderly. Activity (particularly weight-bearing activity), calcitonin, sodium flouride, calcium intake of 1500 mg/day, and vitamin D 400 to 600 IU/day may retard further bone loss.[56] Boron supplementation may reduce the urinary excretion of calcium and magnesium and elevate the concentration of 17 beta-estradiol,[57] thus, inhibiting the normal bone loss of aging. Calcium supplementation is thought to inhibit immunoreactive and parathyroid hormone (PTH) secretion as levels of PTH increase with age in response to diminished levels of extracellular fluid calcium. Estrogen replacement therapy may retard the normal bone loss of aging, but the protective effect may last no longer than 2 to 3 years after termination of treatment.[58]

CLINICAL EVALUATION OF NUTRITIONAL STATUS

There are several physical findings related to nutritional status and many of the normal changes of aging mimic clinical findings described as pathognomic of malnutritive states in the elderly.[59] Clinically overt malnutrition is rarely caused by a primary deficit in nutritional intake, rather it is more likely to be associated with gastrointestinal tract dysfunctions or with one of the chronic debilitating illnesses common to the elderly. In contrast, subclinical malnutrition,[59] by definition undetectable by physical findings on clinical evaluation, is probably frequent in certain at-risk elderly populations. These subgroups might include those who are institutionalized, those with mental disturbances or gross central nervous system disease, or those at or below the poverty level. In subclinical malnutritive states, an elderly individual may manifest depleted nutritional reserves as a failure to thrive. Diminished nutritional reserves may contribute to postoperative confusion, delayed recovery times of homeostatic function, slow wound healing, and increased susceptibility to infection.[60]

Anthropometric variables provide estimates of body composition that can be used as indicators of nutritional status. The most relevant of anthropometric measures are weight and skin fold thickness.[61] Weight is a measure of all the constituents of the body.[62] Weight, however, does not reflect any of the alterations or changes in the relative proportions of body constituents that accompany aging, specifically the increase in fat and the decline in lean muscle mass. Variables, such as food or fluid intake, constipation, or problems producing edema, are not accounted for by weight measures. Weight/height measures have been standardized to define "ideal" weights. Another measure using weight is a weight/stature measure. This measure provides a moderate correlation with the percent of body fat and a high degree of correlation with total body fat in the elderly.[63] A third weight measure is relative weight. Height decreases approximately 3 cm during an average life span as a result of postural changes, such as kyphosis, intervertebral disk shrinkage, or vertebral fractures. Because of the potential inaccuracies in the estimation of height, other related measures are employed. For example, recumbent length of arm span measures are used for comparison to actual height measures. Arm span is a reasonable equivalent to height during all stages of the life span except the aged. Relative weight is then determined using adjusted height tables that have been standardized to account for a possible height reduction adjusted for age.[64]

Other anthropometric measures include triceps/subscapular skin fold thickness and upper arm circumference. The accuracy of skin fold thickness measures in the elderly is questionable because of age related changes in the skin and altered skin compressibility. Upper arm circumference is a good measure of total body fat in edematous patients in cases where weight might be misleading. There are, however, progressive muscular changes associated with aging, specifically an increase in fibrous tissue, loss of muscle fibers, and an increase in intramuscular fat, that may confound this measure's accuracy. It is important to recognize that all of these anthropometric measures do not actually measure nutritional status, rather, they provide an indicator of nutritional status. When compared with standardized norms, these measures provide a percentile nutritional rank for the individual patient.

Functional assessment tools are also valuable in assessing the elderly individual's nutritional status. Increasingly, attention has been paid to the importance of maintaining essential ADLs among the aged. Simple questionnaires have been developed that appear to be closely associated with nutritional risk.[65] These provide another type of assessment tool that is important when assessing the patient's overall nutrition-related functional status. Functional assessment tools, such as those evaluating basic ADLs, and instrumental ADLs provide important insights into the well-being of the aged.[66]

The clinical or physical examination may reveal findings associated with nutritional deficiencies. Table 7–3 provides possible clinical manifestations of nutritional deficiencies that can occur in the aged. It is important to keep in mind that before ascribing any physical findings elicited on physical examination to nutritional problems, the clinician should consider whether the findings are consistent with normal aging or with an underlying disease state.

NUTRITIONAL REQUIREMENTS OF THE ELDERLY

Many nutritional studies have been done on institutionalized elders, but there are inherent difficulties in assessing the nutritional status of community elderly. As a group, there is very little information available relating to the nutritional quality of diets consumed by the elderly compared to any other age group. Major nationwide surveys, such as the USDA Food Consumption Surveys, the Department of Health and Human Services Ten State Nutrition Survey, and the Health and Nutrition Examination Survey (HANES), have been used to assess the nutritional status of the elderly. Findings vary depending on the age, sex, and economic status of the group surveyed and the methods used for study (i.e., clinical signs, biochemical measurements, or dietary intake surveys). These studies are hampered by the lack of anthropometric, biochemical, and clinical norms that are specific to the elderly.

In spite of this, some generalizations can be made. Diets of the elderly living independently in the community have been found to be more nutritionally adequate than those who are institutionalized or in nursing homes.[67] Dietary intake data reveal that a substantial portion of diets for the elderly are low in vitamins C and A, thiamine, calcium, iron, folate, and zinc compared to the recommended dietary allowances (RDA). The prevalence of nutritional problems among the aged arising from low dietary intakes appears to be quite high. In national population

TABLE 7–3. COMMON NUTRITIONAL DEFICIENCIES IN THE AGED

Nutritional Deficiency	Physical Signs
Vitamin A	**Eyes:** photophobia, decreases lacrimation, corneal ulceration, loss of light reflex, Bitot's spots (white spots) **Gums:** gingivitis **Skin:** dry, follicular hyperkeratosis (gooseflesh)
Vitamin C	**Gums:** gingival hypertrophy **Skin:** petechiae, purpura **Muscular:** intermuscular hematomas
Iron	**Eyes:** pale conjunctivae **Tongue:** atrophic, smooth, sore papillae **Skin:** pallor **Nails:** spoon-shaped koilonychia **Vulva:** vulvovaginitis
Folic acid	**Eyes:** pale conjunctivae **Mouth:** stomatitis **Tongue:** glossitis **Skin:** pallor
Riboflavin	**Eyes:** angular blepharitis **Nose:** nasolabial exfoliation **Lips:** cheilosis, inflammation of the mucous membranes **Gums:** gingivitis **Mouth:** angular stomatitis **Tongue:** atrophic lingual papillae
Magnesium	**CNS:** tremor, convulsions, behavioral disturbances
Niacin	**Gums:** gingivitis **Tongue:** raw, atrophic lingual papillae, fissures **Skin:** increased pigmentation, thick skin, atrophic in intertriginous areas, dermatitis **CNS:** dementia **GI:** diarrhea
Thiamine	**Muscular:** calf muscle tenderness and weakness **CNS:** hyporeflexia, foot and wrist drop, hyperesthesia, paresthesia
Protein	**Hair:** dry, brittle **Skin:** pitting edema **Muscular:** wasting, loss of subcutaneous fat **Liver:** hepatomegaly **GI:** diarrhea
Calcium	**Skeletal:** osteoporosis/osteomalacia, fracture
Lactose	**Body:** low weight **GI:** diarrhea
Fluoride	**Teeth:** caries **GI:** diarrhea
Vitamin B_{12}	**Eyes:** optic neuritis **CNS:** dementia **Muscular:** weakness **GI:** anorexia, diarrhea
Glucose	Tachycardia, sweating, fainting

Modified and used with permission from Dwyer JT.[172]

and community-based surveys, intakes were low among those 65 years of age, especially among the poor, for protein, calcium, thiamine, vitamin D, folic acid, vitamin B_6, and zinc.[68] Many diets were found to have very low caloric intakes. Twenty-one percent of the white population and 36% of the black population had daily intakes of less than 1000 calories. Conversely, 25% of the lower income black and white women aged 45 to 75 years of age were found to be obese. Protein was reported to be near or above the RDA with the exception of some low income groups. In fact, the elderly appear to maintain approximately the same ratio of protein, fat, and carbohydrate in their diets compared to younger cohorts, namely: 13% to 30% protein; 50% to 55% carbohydrate; and 30% to 35% fat. When biochemical methods were used, vitamins C, A, and B_6, thiamine, riboflavin, iron, zinc, and calcium were most likely to be below RDA standards.[68] Despite the reporting of the inadequate dietary intake of these nutrients, there was a relative lack of clinical symptoms indicating nutrient deficiencies. Clinical signs other than iron deficiency were infrequently found. This leads one to question the appropriateness of RDA standards for good nutrition in an elderly population.

The aged are highly vulnerable to malnutrition because there is little direct experimental evidence available from which to establish nutritional standards or necessary dietary intake, especially for those aged 85 years and over. Information on the nutritional needs of the elderly have been derived by extrapolation from investigations using young adults.[69] Table 7–4 provides the RDAs for individuals aged 51 years and older.

Lowenstein[70] reviewed the problems of lack of nutrient standards for the aged. It was found that the quality of the diet required by the aged is higher. Caloric needs decrease because of the elderly's reduced metabolic rates and lower levels of physical activity, while needs for protein, vitamins, and minerals stay more or less constant. Thus, nutrient density (i.e., nutrients per calorie) necessary to fulfill recommended dietary allowances is higher for the aged when compared to younger adults.[70] The fact that separate guidelines have not been established for advancing age (except for extrapolations for the 51+ age group) reflects the lack of

TABLE 7–4. RECOMMENDED DAILY DIETARY ALLOWANCES (REVISED 1989)

	Men Older than 51 Years	Women Older than 51 Years
Weight (kg)	70	55
Height (cm)	178	163
Protein (g)	56	44
Calcium (mg)	800	800
Phosphorus (mg)	800	800
Magnesium (mg)	350	300
Iron (mg)	10	10
Zinc (mg)	15	15
Iodine (μg)	150	150
Vitamin A (μg)	1000	800
Vitamin D (μg)	5	5
Vitamin E (mg)	10	8
Vitamin C (mg)	60	60
Thiamine (mg)	1.2	1.0
Riboflavin (mg)	1.4	1.2
Niacin (mg)	16	13
Vitamin B$_6$	2.2	2.0
Folacin (μg)	400	400
Vitamin B$_{12}$	3.0	3.0
Energy needs (kcal)		
Age 51–75	2400	1800
Age 76+	2050	1600

From Committee on Dietary Allowances of the Food and Nutrition Board of the National Academy of Sciences/Nutrition Research Council.

solid knowledge of the elderly's needs. When this is coupled with the fact that (1) the elderly population is much less uniform compared to other age groups with respect to biological, anatomical, and physiological aging; (2) they have an increased susceptibility to disease and chronic illness; and (3) there are a variety of other social and psychological influences that affect diet, which makes it unlikely that a specific standard can be devised that takes into account all of these factors.

The aged are vulnerable and at high risk for developing nutritional problems because of various social, psychological, and physical factors,[71] including social factors (such as age, living alone [especially if there has been a recent bereavement or significant negative life event], lack of an effective family or community support network, and low income). Psychological factors, such as depression, mental deterioration, and impaired self-concept, increase the risk of nutritional deficiencies. Physical factors, such as functional dependence, sensory impairment, and limited mobility (especially when associated with severe chronic degenerative diseases), also have a negative influence. Indices of nutritional risk using these factors are proving useful in identifying the aged with more nutritional deficits than their hospitalized or institutionalized peers.[72]

The elderly generally have a progressive decline in exercise levels and a proportional decrease in energy expenditure, which, when linked to the decrease in their BMR, suggest the need to reduce progressively caloric intake.

COMMON NUTRITIONAL DEFICIENCIES IN THE AGED

Nutrient requirements, according to the RDAs, remain relatively constant with advancing age. Studies have revealed, however, that calcium intake should more closely approximate 1200 mg/day (higher than current RDA), especially in women.[54] This will aid in preventing postmenopausal osteoporosis. In addition, since calcium maintains an inverse relationship to phosphorus, the ingestion of foods that have high levels of phosphorus, such as carbonated beverages and meats should be reduced. A reduction in dietary phosphorus could result in higher total body calcium and perhaps delay or reduce the rate of development of osteoporosis. Exercise has been shown to have a further beneficial effect.

The need for the 44 essential nutrients remains qualitatively similar over the life span. However, quantitative changes for some nutrient requirements are of importance to the elderly individual. When diet-related disorders are present, additional alterations in nutrients may also be necessary. When mean population intakes of a nutrient are below a standard, such as the RDA, nutritionists regard it as a "problem nutrient." Surveys of the aged reveal that mean intakes of calories and calcium are low and often problematic, and that, while mean intakes of protein are adequate, at least a third of those surveyed have intakes below the standard, especially in certain subgroups of the population.[68,73] Other vitamins and minerals present special problems for certain groups of the aged and will be discussed. Although vitamin and mineral deficiencies are presumed to be more common in the elderly, there is little experimental data on which to estimate exact daily requirements of these so-called micronutrients in the diet. Increased need, with age, for vitamins and minerals may result from less efficient absorption, altered metabolism and excretion, and increasing use of certain medications. It is important to remember that any nutrient may be insufficient or in excess and can constitute a problem for the elderly.

Calories/Energy Intake

The RDA for "energy intake" is just enough kilocalories to maintain an energy balance. As indicated in Table 7–4, the specific recommendations for calories from 51 to 75 years is 2400 kcal for men and 1800 kcal for women. The unstated range is from 2000 to 2800 and 1200 to 2000 kcal for men and women, respectively. For those aged 76 and older, the recommendation is 2050 kcal for men (range 1650 to 2450) and 1600 kcal for women (range 1200 to 2000).

Four major factors influence energy needs: (1) resting energy expenditure, (2) physical activity, (3) growth, and (4) thermogenesis (heat production secondary to food consumption, exercise, or cold stress). Resting energy expenditure and physical activity both decline with age, and therefore, energy needs are also lower. Linear growth does not occur in the aged organism, although during recovery, healing, and rehabilitation, lean body mass and fat may be laid down, which requires energy. Thermogenesis (heat production), a relatively minor contributor to energy needs at any age, is not known to differ between aged and younger persons. Resting metabolic rate differs with age chiefly because lean body mass, which is metabolically active tissue, decreases by about 3 kg per decade after age 50. Cellular metabolic rate also decreases with age. It is assumed that energy allowances should decrease by 6% from ages 51 to 75 years and by another 6% after age 76 to account for reductions in resting metabolism. Energy output in the form of physical activity declines with age. A decrease of 300 kcal for men and 200 kcal for women is recommended for ages 51 to 75 years, with an additional 500 kcal for men and 400 kcal for women substracted after age 76 years to account for reduced activity levels.

Surveys report that energy intakes among the aged are so low as to be inadequate for a significant proportion of the population.[73-75] One might conclude that, in view of such low intakes, a large proportion of the aged are extremely lean if not emaciated. However, median weights at age 76 are 5 kg higher in men and 7 kg higher in women as compared to younger cohorts.[76]

Certainly this argues against widespread starvation among the aged. One explanation for this discrepancy is that the energy intake standards are too high. Some evidence suggests that, in healthy individuals of desirable weight, energy intake recommendations and outputs should agree closely.[77] Many elderly are ill, and with increasing age and illness interindividual differences in energy requirements and body weight become more pronounced.[78] Limitations on physical activity caused by chronic diseases, such as arthritis, hip fractures, emphysema, osteoporosis, congestive heart failure, cerebral vascular accidents, peripheral vascular disease, and other degenerative conditions, limit physical activity, and consequently, reduce energy needs in at least one tenth of the population over 65 years of age.[67] Among the very old, especially those who are in nursing homes, energy needs are often only slightly above BMR. While the need for energy is lower in some aged, it is extremely high in others. When neuromuscular coordination declines, mechanical efficiency is reduced, and difficulties in balance control are increased, the energy cost of movement is greatly increased.

Protein/Energy Malnutrition

The RDA for protein is 0.8 g per kilogram of high quality protein per day. This amounts to 56 g for men and 44 g for women.[70,79] Protein requirements are more likely to be affected by stresses, such as disease, that may increase dietary protein requirements by two or more times. The reduced contribution of muscle to body protein metabolism in the aged may decrease the ability of the individual to adapt during periods of restricted dietary energy or protein intake, when protein synthesis in vital organs is maintained by mobilization of amino acids from the periphery.[27,80] The reduction in energy intake is likely to increase protein needs because the efficiency of protein use depends on energy balance. An allowance of 12% to 14% of total energy needs of the aged should come from protein sources.[27]

Clinical correlates of nutritional indicators for protein intake used in large surveys have not been well established. For example, a decrease in serum albumin does not occur early in protein deficiency states, however, declines are significant when a pure deficiency state exists. There is a gradual decline in serum albumin that normally accompanies advancing age,[81] but a drop in serum albumin does not usually occur in the initial stages of protein deficiency, rather, it shows significant declines only in the advanced stages of severe deficiency. This makes interpretation of lab results of serum albumin levels difficult with respect to the elderly. A serum albumin below the normal range for adults could be an indication of a normal age related change or of protein malnutrition.

Chronic protein-energy malnutrition is synonymous with cachexia. Cachexia usually results from low food intake secondary to anorexia. In the elderly, common causes of cachexia are cancer, chronic neurological disease with associated paralysis, end stage hepatic or renal disease, and cardiac cachexia resulting from high dosage digitalis therapy. While cachexia is mainly caused by reduced energy and protein intake, additional causes are the catabolic effects of disease and excessive losses of nutrients by malabsorption or through protein-losing enteropathy (any disease of the intestine).

Calcium/Vitamin D

Several factors negatively influence adequate calcium nutrition in the elderly. Intake of calcium among the aged is low and frequently does not meet the RDA.[75] Absorption of dietary calcium in the gut is poor,[82] and the ability to adapt to a low calcium diet decreases with age.[83] There are several possible explanations for this. Decreased sensitivity to parathyroid hormone decreases renal production of the vitamin calcitrol, which decreases serum levels of this vitamin and ultimately decreases calcium absorption from the gut.[84] Since passive absorption accounts for only half of the calcium absorbed by the gut and the active transport process of calcium absorption requires calcitrol, decreases in this vitamin decrease absorption with advancing age.[85] Thus, dietary calcium absorbed by the gut contributes less to the maintenance of serum calcium, and bone is resorbed to maintain serum calcium.

Other factors that increase the risk of poor calcium nutrition are large amounts of protein in the diet, which increases urinary calcium losses,[86] and high levels of phosphorus, which increase calcium fecal losses.[87] Protein has profound effects on urinary calcium levels and on calcium nutriture. Doubling of dietary protein has been found to increase urinary calcium by as much as 50%.[86] Since the kidney filters as much as 10 g of calcium per day, these differences may be of great consequence in calcium metabolism.[88] Protein increases the obligatory renal loss of calcium, and its sulfur containing amino acids are oxidized to sulfate during metabolism. The sulfates are then eliminated by a compensatory decrease in the tubular reabsorption of calcium. Even in the presence of large amounts of phosphorus in the diet, it has been found that the effect phosphorus has on decreasing urinary calcium is not enough to prevent protein's negative effect.[85]

Sodium also increases urinary calcium loss at the tubular level,[85] and very high levels of dietary fiber intake (e.g., > 30 g) may affect the absorption of calcium as well. Both dietary fiber and the phytic acid, which is often associated with the bran portion of cereals, decrease calcium absorption. Oxalic acid (found in rhubarb and spinach) also decreases calcium absorption.

Caffeine increases both the amount of calcium secreted in digestive juice and renal calcium losses. Alcohol also increases urinary calcium losses, and at very high levels, it may have an adverse effect on bone cell metabolism.

One significant hormonal event that influences calcium nutrition is menopause. Estrogens increase calcium absorption and decrease renal losses, so that on the same calcium intake, the estrogen-replete female uses dietary calcium better. Postmenopausal estrogen replacement therapy is helpful for preventing a negative calcium balance and osteoporosis. Growth hormones and hormonal events, such as pregnancy, also increase absorption and decrease renal losses.

Bone loss is significantly increased during the winter months secondary to the decrease in ultraviolet rays of the sun. One hypothesis says this is a result of a lack of vitamin D, which is necessary for calcium absorption. A vitamin D deficiency is defined biochemically as levels of calcitrol below 3.8 µg/mL. Among the institutionalized and housebound aged without vitamin D supplements, this biochemical indicator of vitamin D deficiency is relatively prevalent.[89] Osteomalacia, or undermineralized bone, sometimes contributes to the increased incidence of fractures among the aged.[90] Because several foods are fortified with vitamin D, however, intakes are higher and deficiencies somewhat rarer in the United States than in other countries.[91] It has been shown that an individual can get enough vitamin D from milk. The causes of osteomalacia include vitamin D disturbances due to inadequate exposure to sunlight, dietary deficiency, and altered absorption or metabolism of the vitamin due to disease.

Iron

The current RDA for iron is 10 mg/day for individuals 51 years and older. The need for iron declines with age among females. This is a postmenopausal event because iron is no longer lost through menstrual bleeding and childbearing. Counterbalancing decreased iron loss is some evidence that the efficiency of iron absorption may be decreased among the aged. This is due to the presence of atrophic gastritis, which makes the body less able to use the hydrochloric acid available to reduce the iron present in the oxidized (ferric) form to the absorbable form (ferrous).[92] Other factors that decrease iron absorption among the aged are the frequent use of antacids, calcium supplements, and tea, all of which form complexes with iron in the gut and decrease absorption. Some elderly individuals decrease their intakes of red meat and other animal flesh foods rich in highly bioavailable iron because of dental difficulties or limited incomes. Instead they rely on plant foods, which are generally lower in bioavailable iron. Some aged also decrease their intakes of ascorbic acid-rich foods and protein-rich foods, thereby decreasing intakes of ascorbic acid and amino acids, two enhancers of iron absorption.

Concerns about iron in the elderly usually focus on its role in blood production. Lack of iron is a causative factor of anemia, however, evidence that iron deficiency anemias are a normal part of aging is weak, though the incidence of anemia increases with age. Experimental animal models do not show that aging is accompanied by anemia, although hematopoietic reserve capacity, or the time it takes for hematocrit to recover after stress is increased.[93] Reductions in hematocrit that are not associated with dietary iron deficiency, chronic disease, or blood loss are usually a result of an abnormality in cellular proliferation.[94] Anemias due to other causes are common. Indeed, in contrast to popular belief, iron deficiency anemia is not the sole or major cause of anemia in the aged. In addition to lack of iron, nutritional anemias due to deficiency of ascorbic acid, vitamin B_6, vitamin B_{12}, folic acid, and protein–calorie malnutrition are also observed.[95] Blood losses of iron may be due to alcohol abuse, frequent use of aspirin, infection, neoplasms, and renal disease.

Vitamin B_{12}

Different surveys have found either no change or decreased levels of vitamin B_{12} in the elderly.[96,97] Achlorhydria, which decreases B_{12} absorption, occurs in 15% to 20% of persons over age 40.[98] In the elderly, a vitamin B_{12} deficiency is commonly due to lack of gastric intrinsic factor, which causes malabsorption of vitamin B_{12}. In pernicious anemia, a disease common in the elderly, the production of gastric intrinsic factor ceases, and there is a complete lack of gastric acid production (achlorhydria).[99] Pernicious anemia is an autoimmune disease in which megaloblastic and neurological signs are caused by vitamin B_{12} deficiency. Vitamin B_{12} from the diet cannot be absorbed in the absence of gastric intrinsic factor. The aging process increases the risk of autoimmune disease within the gut. B_{12} deficiency produces both megablastic anemia and neurological symptoms including mild dementia, sensory losses in the hands and feet, and a painful, red, smooth, and shiny tongue. In addition, a mildly jaundiced appearance is common in an individual with a vitamin B_{12} deficiency. Pernicious anemia represents one of the conditions associated with the syndrome of polyglandular failure (as described by Addison in 1955).[100] Thus, in elderly patients with B_{12} deficiency other associated diseases, such as hypothyroidism, diabetes mellitus, and Addison's disease (adrenal failure), are often found.

Folic Acid

Low folic acid levels have been found in depressed, institutionalized elderly and in elderly persons in general hospitals as well as among elderly living at home. Serum folate levels less than 3.0 mg/mL or red cell folate less than 140 mg/mL are indicative of folate deficiency that may be caused by inadequate dietary intake due to poor food choices that is often related to alcoholism; the use of drugs, such as anticonvulsants, that interfere with the absorption or metabolism of folate; the increased use of heat processed foods with reduced folate content; a restricted intake associated with poor dentition; gastrointestinal surgery that reduces folate absorption; or impaired folate metabolism. Intakes of 400 µg per day are usually sufficient to meet the needs of the older population. Garry and co-workers[96] found that among healthy elderly subjects low plasma folate and erythrocyte folate levels were common. The subjects, however, did not have significantly increased mean corpuscular volumes, which is a pathological consequence of folate deficiency (e.g., increased red blood cell production). Other studies of elderly people with low incomes or physical or mental deterioration have shown that folate deficiency is not uncommon in this group.[101] Further, Elsborg[102] has shown that in elderly subjects with nutritional folate deficiency, folate absorption is impaired. This malabsorption of folate appears to be related to the folate deficiency itself and can be reversed by treatment with folic acid. Besides its effect on red blood cells, it has been suggested that folate deficiency may produce mental dysfunction in the elderly.[103,104]

Vitamin C

Ascorbic acid is a potent nonenzymatic protector against free radical damage.[105] Spurred by the proclamations (and longevity) of Linus Pauling, megadoses of vitamin C have been touted as playing a protective role in upper respiratory tract infections[106] and neoplasms.[107] Schorah and associates[108] found that elderly individuals receiving vitamin C had small but statistically significant increases in body weight and plasma albumin and a reduction in purpura and petechial hemorrhages. No changes in mood or mobility were observed. The risks of megadoses of vitamin C include rebound scurvy when ascorbic acid is reduced to the RDA, reduced vitamin B_{12} absorption, oxalic acid renal calculi, false-negative fecal occult blood results—leading to delayed diagnosis of colonic cancer, and excessive absorption of dietary iron. It has been concluded that taking too much vitamin C is not worth these risks.[109]

An association between ascorbic acid and arteriosclerosis has been made. Early intimal changes seen in the arteries of patients with atherosclerosis are similar to those observed in patients with scurvy.[110] Coupled with the finding of low leukocyte ascorbic acid levels in patients with coronary atherosclerosis and acute myocardial infarction, these findings have led to the suggestion that vitamin C may be involved in the pathogenesis of atherosclerosis.[109] Numerous studies have documented lower ascorbic acid levels in plasma, leukocytes, and platelets in older subjects.[108,111,112] Not only do ascorbic acid levels fall with age, but the levels of free radicals associated with ascorbate also fall.[113] The decline in ascorbate radical levels with age may indicate a decline in the free radical defense mechanism.

Spindler[114] studied vitamin C status in elderly people with and without cognitive impairment. Leukocyte vitamin C levels are found to be unacceptably low in the impaired subjects but less so in the unimpaired subjects, though levels were still below those recommended. All of the subjects with low vitamin C levels were consuming at least 100% of the recommended dietary intake (RDI) of vitamin C.

Vitamin C levels were lower in men than in women, but in women the degree of cognitive impairment was related to their poor vitamin C status. The author suggested that the proposed RDA for vitamin C is below the intake levels required to support acceptable nutritional status in healthy elderly and that the RDA might be hazardous if applied indiscriminately as a standard for those who are cognitively impaired.[114]

Vitamin E

Early studies established that vitamin E levels decline with aging.[115] Vitamin E is necessary for the action of glutathione peroxidase, which prevents the formation of the hydroxyl radical by converting hydrogen peroxide to water. Besides its role as an antioxidant, vitamin E has been suggested to have some effect in the management of intermittent claudication.[116]

Vitamin E appears to play a central role in maintaining the structure and function of the human nervous system. According to Sokol,[117] vitamin E deficiency initiates and perpetuates a progressive neuromuscular degeneration with irreversible neurologic consequences if treatment is delayed.

Vitamin E may also be useful in the treatment of neurological disorders not associated with vitamin E deficiency. Its use is being investigated in Parkinson's disease, and it appears that vitamin E may help to prevent or retard the degeneration of nerves that occurs in this disease.[117]

Vitamin A

The main functions of vitamin A are its role in the eye's adaptation to the dark, maintaining epithelial integrity, and in hemoglobin synthesis. A significant decline in the light threshold in relation to aging has been demonstrated; however, this does not correlate with serum vitamin A levels and is not improved by vitamin A administration.[118] Follicular hyperkeratosis, a classic sign of vitamin A deficiency, is often seen in elderly subjects, but it does not appear to be related to a vitamin A deficiency.[119] There is no evidence that plasma vitamin A or the absorption of vitamin A is affected by aging. Vitamin A, however, is the second most commonly used nutritional supplement.[120]

In contrast to the rarity of symptoms from vitamin A deficiency in the elderly, vitamin A toxicity is more commonly seen. Symptoms include general malaise, headaches, liver dysfunction, leukopenia, and hypercalcemia.[121]

Zinc

Zinc deficiency in humans can lead to anorexia, impaired immune function, poor wound healing, decreased strength of muscle contraction, and possibly, altered taste acuity. The RDA for zinc in persons over 51 is set at 15 mg. On the basis of an analysis of the related literature, Sandstead and co-workers[122] estimated that the average daily intake of zinc in elderly persons in the United States ranged from 7 to 13 mg. On balance, it appears that serum zinc levels decrease with aging.[122–124] Similar decreases in hair zinc levels have also been demonstrated with aging.[122,125] Other studies have found that zinc concentration in bone[126] and kidney[127] also fall after the age of 50 years.

Zinc has been demonstrated to be necessary for adequate functioning of T cell lymphocytes.[128] Aging is associated with a progressive deterioration in T lymphocyte function.[129] The role of zinc in wound healing is now well established,[130] and zinc supplementation has been shown to accelerate the healing of leg ulcers in elderly subjects.[46,131]

The effect of zinc supplementation on enhancing appetite in elderly subjects has been clearly demonstrated,[132] and zinc deficiency may play a role in the anorexia of aging. Zinc deficiency decreases the responsiveness of neurotransmitters (including the opioid peptide dynorphin) that are potent stimulators of food intake.[132,133]

Impotence is extremely common in the elderly, and a strong correlation has been established between hyperzincuria, low serum zinc levels, and impotence in this population.[134] Zinc supplementation restored potency in a significant percentage of the elderly subjects studied.

It appears that zinc levels decline with age, possibly as the result of chronic, long-term marginal zinc intake. This situation can be further aggravated by the hyperzincuria associated with chronic diseases, such as diabetes mellitus, to which the elderly are particularly prone. Burnet[135] has hypothesized that zinc deficiency may also play a role in the pathogenesis of dementia based on zinc's essential role in enzyme production, such as DNA polymerases that are necessary for DNA replication, repair, and transcription. Research continues to substantiate lower levels of zinc in the central nervous system and brain in patients with Alzheimer's disease.[135]

Copper

Copper serves as a catalyst in the biochemistry of every organ system. In particular, copper plays a role in iron absorption and mobilization, which as was previously discussed, is particularly relevant to aging.[136] Copper is a catalyst for lysyloxidase, an enzyme important for the cross-linking of collagen and elastin,[137] and it plays a role in the conversion of dopamine to norepinephrine.[138] Klevay[48] found that copper deficiency increases serum cholesterol levels, possibly by increasing the rate of cholesterol release from the liver to the circulation. As high dietary zinc accentuates copper deficiency, Klevay[48] suggested that atherosclerosis is related to the ratio of zinc to copper. Despite the great theoretical interest in the role of copper in the aging process, there is little information concerning copper in the aged population. Yunice and associates[139] reported a small but significant increase in serum copper levels with aging. Bunker and co-workers[124] also found an increase in plasma copper with aging but no change in leukocyte copper levels. Copper absorption appears similar in aged and young subjects.[124,139]

Chromium

Chromium deficiency leads to hyperglycemia, hypercholesterolemia, and corneal opacities.[140] Tissue chromium levels decline with age and may do so more dramatically in Western societies that eat refined foods, which are somewhat deficient in chromium.[141] Preliminary studies have suggested that chromium-rich brewer's yeast improved glucose tolerance, insulin sensitivity, and cholesterol levels in elderly subjects.[142] Serum chromium levels have been reported to be lower in subjects with coronary artery disease.[143] At present, a role for chromium in diabetes mellitus or atherosclerosis has not been proved, although available studies have raised intriguing possibilities concerning chromium's role in some degenerative diseases of civilization.

Water Intake

Dehydration is the most common fluid and electrolyte disturbance in the elderly.[144] The threshold for recognition of thirst is higher in the elderly. In many instances, cognitive or physical disabilities also reduce the ability to recognize thirst, express thirst, or obtain access to water.[145] In addition, healthy elderly individuals seem to have reduced thirst in response to fluid deprivation.[144] Elderly individuals also produced less concentrated urine following fluid deprivation. Since elderly subjects had higher vasopressin levels in response to dehydration, the decreased ability to concentrate the urine is most likely occurring at the renal level.[144] Fluids, as well as solid foods, are essential to life. Approximately 1.5 qt of water or other fluid per day is a reasonable goal to strive for in the aged.

An increase in serum sodium concentration results from a loss of body water in excess of salt loss. Among elderly patients, hypernatremia (dehydration with elevated sodium levels in the serum) is most common in those who are bedridden and are not provided with sufficient water to satisfy their thirst or in those whose thirst sensation is diminished by an impaired central nervous system. A net deficit of water is associated with vomiting, diarrhea, diabetes insipidus, and hyperpyrexia (excessive sweating). In general, older patients appear to be predisposed to the development of hypernatremia. Surgery, febrile illnesses, infirmity, and diabetes mellitus account for most of these incidences.[146]

DRUG EFFECTS ON NUTRITION

The frequent use of pharmacological agents by the elderly increases their vulnerability to malnutrition. Drug–diet interactions occur at all ages but are more common in the elderly because of prescription and over-the-counter drug use on a regular basis. In addition, age related changes in gastrointestinal function, liver and renal function, and body composition alter drug and nutrient metabolism. Coexisting disease, undernutrition, and malnutrition may further complicate these interactions.[147,148]

Drugs may affect the nutritional status simply by their effect on appetite, but more commonly, absorption, metabolism, and excretion of dietary constituents are altered. Dietary factors, such as water consumption, amount of food consumed, timing of meals in relation to drug intake, and the constituents consumed, may affect absorption and oxidative drug metabolism.[147]

Commonly used drugs that increase the need for calcium include aluminum-containing antacids, which decrease phosphorus absorption, lower plasma phosphorus, and ultimately increase calcium excretion.[149] Thiazide diuretics, on the other hand, decrease calcium needs by decreasing urinary calcium losses and may have a positive effect on bone mass.[150]

ALCOHOL

Alcohol is both a drug and a food that provides substantial amounts of energy. It is widely abused by individuals of all ages. Among the aged, its abuse is especially easy since the risks of intoxication from a given dose of alcohol are elevated because lean body mass and total body water decrease with age. Consequently, the total volume of alcohol distribution is smaller and peak blood alcohol levels are higher in older persons.[151] Greater physiological sensitivity to the effects of alcohol and greater psychological vulnerability to alcohol abuse due to depression, loneliness, and a lack of meaningful roles combine to make alcohol abuse risks higher in the aged. Alcohol use should be avoided entirely among those with known dementia, chronic medication with psychoactive drugs, a previous history of alcohol abuse, or chronic and extreme depression.

Moderate alcohol use (e.g., one or two drinks per day) has been associated with some health benefits. Alcohol in moderation is an appetite stimulant and enhances the taste of food. It increases HDL cholesterol levels, thereby lowering atherosclerotic risks. Moderate alcohol intake is also associated with lowered congestive heart failure rates.[152] Since elderly energy intakes are already low, however, care must be taken to ensure that calories from alcohol do not displace other items in the diet that provide not only energy, but also protein, vitamins, and minerals.

THEORIES OF AGING RELATED TO NUTRITION

Though the mechanisms of aging are not clearly understood, there is evidence suggesting that nutrition influences the aging process. Since nutrients are obtained from the food we eat and used by the cells of the body, nutritional factors have been directly credited for their role in longevity. Malnutrition can contribute to chronic diseases. A combination of good nutrition and exercise leads to better health and energy levels and notably improves the person's capability of withstanding psychological and physical stresses.

Theories related to nutrition and longevity abound, for example, obesity has been correlated to shorter life span. Several studies have attempted to determine relationships between specific food components, chronic disease, and longevity. In 1935, a classic study by McCay demonstrated that laboratory rats lived significantly longer when their caloric intake was restricted at an early age.[153] Subsequent studies have confirmed that the leaner rats lived longer and that the onset of age related diseases was significantly later in the undernourished laboratory animals.[51]

There are many molecular theories of aging that relate specifically to nutrition. It has been proposed that the degenerative changes with age may be the result of free radical reactions with resulting damage to cell membranes and cell organelles.[154] Mechnikova hypothesized that the accumulation of toxins secreted by intestinal bacteria can in fact facilitate the aging process.[155] Some theories attribute aging to the gradual oxidation of lipid membranes throughout life and promote the consumption of foods with antioxidant properties. A number of in vivo and in vitro studies have explored the effects of both natural and synthetic sources of antioxidants, including vitamins A, C, E and selenium, in prolonging average maximal life span.[156] An increase in the average life span was observed; however, there is no evidence that any of these antioxidants delay the aging process or significantly extend the maximum life span.[157] Antioxidants have been demonstrated to decrease the effects of certain environmental and nutritional factors on the average life span.[158,159]

Energy produced from plant and animal nutrients is potential energy obtained by oxidation of carbohydrates, fats or lipids, and proteins.[160] This potential energy is converted by metabolic reactions to various forms of energy within the body systems. In essence, theories related to energy in nutrition and aging deal with the energy balance or homeostatic mechanisms. Electrical energy provides conduction of nerve impulses, mechanical energy for muscle contraction, chemical energy for anabolism and catabolism, and heat for the regulation of body temperature and the maintainance of homeostasis. Temperature regulation requires as much as 60% of the energy obtained from food, whereas anabolic processes require 30 to 40%.[161]

The body reaches a state of energy balance when the amount of energy expended is equal to the amount of energy consumed. If the energy intake exceeds the energy expended, a positive energy state exists, and energy is stored as glycogen or fat. When the expenditure of energy exceeds the amount of energy consumed, a negative energy state exists. This becomes an important consideration in the elderly as the ratio of intake to output is often unbalanced. The incidence of undernourishment in the elderly is quite high, as is the other end of the spectrum: obesity. In the elderly, physical activity and BMR decrease. Without a concommitant decrease in food intake, the chances of weight gains and diseases associated with inactivity increase substantially. Nutritional needs will vary according to body size and composition, rate of growth, and physical activity.[6]

At cell maturity, there is a cessation of growth. With aging, the catabolic rate (cell breakdown) slightly exceeds the anabolic rate (cell growth). The result of this is a gradual decrease in the total number of body cells.[162] Young[163] hypothesizes that at the cellular level, translational or posttranslational processes in protein metabolism may influence aging. The energy balance important to physical functioning is, therefore, affected by a progressive loss of cells, a decrease in mitotic capacity (protein metabolism), and an overall decrease in lean body mass. Enzymes and hormones also play a key role in metabolism. Genetics may influence enzyme activity, and hormonal activity changes the rate of metabolism in the elderly.

Although it appears that genetic factors play an important role in the nutrition of the elderly, environmental factors are also important. These include psychological, socioeconomic, cultural, and ecological factors. The nutritional adequacy of an elder could be affected by a number of factors, such as:

1. The ability of the elder to select appropriate nutrient sources (physical, cognitive, socioeconomic factors).
2. The ability of the elder to prepare meals (physical or cognitive problems).
3. The ability of the elder to ingest food (oral health, physical or cognitive changes).
4. The ability to digest ingested food.
5. The ability to absorb digested food.
6. The ability to metabolize absorbed nutrients.
7. The ability to use or store nutrients.
8. The ability to excrete metabolic waste products.

Another predominant theory in aging is that modulation of the age associated immune dysfunctions commonly occurring with advancing age can be altered by nutritional intervention. The immune theory of aging is covered extensively in Chapter 2.

Age related changes in life-style, socioeconomic status, and decreased basal metabolism make homeostasis a difficult state to achieve. Some studies have begun to examine the specific effect of environmental factors that influence nutritional requirements of the elderly.[63,164]

Preventively oriented nutritional strategies for the aged differ from those most effective for younger persons.[67] For instance, drug–diet interactions rarely cause malnutrition in younger adults, but they may in the elderly, and such causes of malnutrition are preventable. Several measures can keep the adverse interactions of nutrients and drugs to a minimum.[147] A review of the patient's medication schedule and over-the-counter drug use can eliminate harmful drug–drug and drug–diet effects. It is important to consider the abuse of antacids, drugs, or alcohol. Avoidance of drugs that are associated with unwanted nutritional effects, especially among the aged who are already malnourished due to disease processes is recommended.

Many nutritional measures involving health promotion will act at the level of primary prevention, as was previously discussed. Secondary preventions, such as the early detection of and the nutritional support and treatment for various chronic degenerative diseases; developing sensory deficits; cognitive and emotionally related eating and drinking problems; drug–diet interactions; and failures of the social support system for the aged, are vital components in intervention.[165] Special risk factors for nutritional problems include severe chronic illnesses, especially if housebound or confined to an institution; social isolation, depression, or other mental disability; severe dental and periodontal disease; and low socioeconomic status.[166,167]

Finally, nutritional support is an important part of tertiary prevention (rehabilitation). Since most of the aged suffer from one or more chronic degenerative diseases, this type of prevention is especially important.

NUTRITIONAL PROGRAMS FOR THE ELDERLY

Federal food assistance programs were the result of the Surgeon General's 1979 report. Excellent references are now available on community nutrition services for the aged.[168,169] They include food and nutrition services for the healthy aged, such as the elderly meal programs, meals for maintaining the dependent aged at home, and food and nutritional services for the aged in group care and health care facilities.

Under the auspices of the Older Americans Act, the federal government's Administration on Aging provides congregate and home-delivered meals to over 2.5 million Americans 65 years of age and older. Those who participate in the "Meals on Wheels" program for the homebound aged are often economically poor and have multiple diseases and have a relatively high prevalence of nutritional deficiencies that are correctable by the provision of adequate food and nutritional supplements.[170] The meals provide at least a third of the RDA, and in this sense, are helpful in sustaining the nutrition of the aged.

In addition, the opportunity for social interaction provided by congregate dining or regular visits to deliver meals to the homebound elderly is also important and may increase food intake as well as improve the quality of life. The elderly who attend congregate meals tend to be healthier than those receiving home-delivered services.[170] In addition to providing substantial amounts of daily nutrient intakes, the elderly who attend congregate meal sites can also be screened for referrals to other preventive services.

The federal food stamp programs, which provides coupons that increase food purchasing power, are available for the poor elderly. While only about 30% of the aged now participate in the program and the program benefits are only about $60 per month, the availability of this extra food money may be a great help in increasing diet quality. At present, many eligible elderly individuals fail to apply for or use this program.[171]

The aged who reside in group care or health care facilities are in especially fragile health and often have special nutritional needs or feeding requirements. Institutional conditions of participation in Medicare and Medicaid require the maintenance of certain standards with respect to food and nutritional services in order to obtain certification and licensure. Dietary and institutional consultants can assure that these standards are met, and they can plan and implement more extensive nutritional services in these institutions including appropriate menus that meet the RDA and therapeutic diet needs, dining rooms that are available and accessible for those who are to use them, feeding assistance where needed, and the attainment of food safety regulations.[169]

CONCLUSION

Although the majority of the elderly are not undernourished, they represent a particularly vulnerable segment of the population with a precarious nutritional balance that can easily be disturbed by illnesses, decreased mobility, or increased economic hardship. As such, it is essential that health professionals pay particular attention to the components of the nutritional status of the elderly. This includes patients in institutional settings where refusal of food or fluids may lead to unexpected nutritional deficiencies. Adequate nutrition is not a panacea. It is most useful as a preventive and therapeutic tool in combination with exercise, stress management, and education. It appears clear that the significance of nutritional adequacy will grow as it adds increasingly to the rehabilitation of community and institutionalized elders.

Much research is needed, and in particular, nutritional regimens for those elderly individuals in the community and institutions need to be implemented and evaluated for benefits, effectiveness, and harmful effects. Nutritional education should be at the top of the agenda for the population at large, for the elderly, and for health care professionals. Major recommendations from the National Research Council of the National Academy of Sciences on diet and health have suggested social, scientific, and clinical environments for implementation of dietary changes. What remains is to fill the gaps with research, look at nutrition from different perspectives, and translate these findings into improved health. Health promotion and disease prevention can delay, or possibly even eliminate, chronic disorders and the so-called "normal" aging process. Nutrition appears to have proved itself a crucial ally in the rehabilitation of the elderly.

PEARLS

- The age related changes in the gastrointestinal system, such as decreased saliva, poor dentition, decrements of taste and olfaction, gastromucosal atrophy, and reduced intestinal mobility will have the most impact on nutritional status because this system is directly involved in digestion.

- Basal metabolic rate declines rapidly from birth to age 20 and then gradually until age 80.

- Numerous chronic diseases that are more prevalent in the elderly, such as Alzheimer's disease, cerebral vascular accidents, and diabetes, demonstrate related nutritional problems.

- Obesity is common in the aged and can be due to decreased activity, medication, and a poorly balanced diet. This problem is associated with medical disabilities, such as diabetes, hypertension, and heart disease and can hinder an older person's independence.

- The clinical evaluation of nutritional states can be done by the use of anthropometric measures, functional assessment tools, physical signs of nutritional deficiencies, or a combination of these.

- The elderly require a higher quality, more nutrient dense (i.e., more nutrients per calorie) diet.

- The recommendation for calories from ages 51 to 75 years is 2400 kcal for men and 1800 kcal for women.

- Programs such as the Federal Food Assistance program, federal food stamps, and congregate and home delivered meals can assist the older person in attaining adequate nutrition.

REFERENCES

1. US Department of Health, Education and Welfare. *Public Health Service. Healthy People: The Surgeon General's Report on Health Promotion and Disease Prevention 1979.* Washington, DC: Government Printing Office; 1979.
2. Wartow NJ: The national initiative on health promotion for older persons: the role of the administration on aging. *Top Geriatr Rehabil.* 1990; 6(1):69–77.
3. Steen B. Body composition and aging. *Nutr Rev.* 1988; 46:45–51.
4. American Dietetic Association. Position of the American Dietetic Association: nutrition, aging and the continuum of health care. *J Am Diet Assoc.* 1987; 87:344–347.
5. Bidlack WR, Kirsch A, Meskin MS. Nutritional requirements of the elderly. *Food Technology.* 1988; 40:61–70.
6. Chernoff R. *Geriatric Nutrition: The Health Professionals Handbook.* Gaithersburg, Md: Aspen Publishers; 1991.
7. Murphy C. Chemical senses and nutrition in the elderly. In: Kare MR, Brand TG, eds. *Interaction of the Chemical Senses with Nutrition.* New York: Academic Press; 1986.
8. Mulligan R. Oral health: effect on nutrition and rehabilitation in older persons. *Top Geriatr Rehabil.* 1989; 5(1):27–35.
9. Khan TA, Shragge BW, Crispen JS, et al. Esophageal mobility in the elderly. *Am J Digestive Dis.* 1977; 22:1049–1054.
10. Horowitz M, Maddern GT, Chateron BE, et al. Changes in gastric emptying rates with age. *Clin Sci.* 1984; 67:213–218.
11. Werner I, Hambraeus L. Protein digestion insufficiency with aging. *Acta Soc Med Upsal.* 1970; 76:239.
12. Webster SGP, Wilkinson EM, Gowland E. A comparison of fat absorption in young and old subjects. *Age Aging.* 1977; 6:113–117.
13. Berman PM, Kirsner TB. The aging gut. II. Diseases of colon, pancreas, liver, and gall

bladder, functional bowel disease, and iatrogenic disease. *Geriatrics.* 1972; 27(4):117–124.

14. Shepard RJ. Nutrition and the physiology of aging. In: Young EA, ed. *Nutrition, Aging and Health.* New York: Alan R Liss; 1986.

15. Weg RB. Nutrition: a crucial "given" in rehabilitation. *Top Geriatr Rehabil.* 1989; 5(1):1–26.

16. Walser M. Renal system. In: Paige DM, ed. *Clinical Nutrition.* 2nd ed. St Louis: Mosby; 1988:227–241.

17. Rudman D. Kidney senescence: a model for aging. *Nutr Rev.* 1988; 46:209–214.

18. Mitch WE. Protein metabolism and the aging kidney. In: Mitch WE, Klahr S, eds. *Nutrition and the Kidney.* Boston: Little, Brown and Co.; 1988.

19. Chernoff R. Aging and nutrition. *Nutrition Today.* 1987; 22(2):4–11.

20. Tzanoff SP, Norris AH. Effect of muscle mass decrease on age related BMR changes. *J Appl Physiol.* 1977; 43:1001–1006.

21. Tzanoff SP, Norris AH. Longitudinal changes in basal metabolism in man. *J Appl Physiol.* 1978; 45:536–539.

22. Shizgal HM, Spanier AH, Humes J, Wood CD. Indirect measurement of total exchangeable potassium. *Am J Physiol.* 1977; 233(3):F253–259.

23. Forbes GB, Reina JC. Adult lean body mass declines with age: some longitudinal observations. *Metabolism.* 1980; 19:653–663.

24. McGandy RB, Barrows CH, Spanias A, et al. Nutrient intakes and energy expenditure in men of different ages. *J Gerontol.* 1966; 21:581–587.

25. Uauy R, Winterer JC, Bilmazes C, et al. The changing pattern of whole body protein metabolism in aging humans. *J Gerontol.* 1978; 33:663–671.

26. Shepard RJ. *Physical Activity and Aging.* Gaithersburg, Md: Aspen Publishers; 1987.

27. Young VR. Impact of aging on protein metabolism. In: Armbrecht HJ, Prendergast JM, Coe RM, eds. *Nutritional Intervention in the Aging Process.* New York: Springer Verlag; 1984:27–48.

28. Shizgal HM. Body composition. In: Fischer JE, ed. *Surgical Nutrition.* Boston, Little, Brown and Co.; 1983:3–17.

29. Waterlow JC, Stephen JML. The turnover of protein with aging. *Clin Sci.* 1967; 33:489–496.

30. Astrand PO, Rodahl K. *Textbook of Work Physiology.* San Francisco, London: McGraw-Hill Book Co., 1970.

31. Shizgal HM, Vasilevsky CA, Gardiner PF, et al. Nutritional assessment and skeletal muscle function. *Am J Clin Nutr.* 1986; 44:761–771.

32. Russell DM, Leiter LA, Whitwell J, et al. Skeletal-muscle function during hypocaloric diets and fasting: a comparison with standard nutritional assessment parameters. *Am J Clin Nutr.* 1983; 37:133–138.

33. Lopes J, Russell DM, Whitwell J, Jeejeebhoy KN. Skeletal muscle function in malnutrition. *Am J Clin Nutr.* 1982; 36:602–610.

34. Kelly SM, Roza A, Field S, et al. Inspiratory muscle strength and body composition in patients receiving total parenteral nutrition. *Am Rev Resp Dis.* 1984; 130:33–37.

35. Harris MI, Hadden WC, Knowler WC, et al. Prevalence of diabetes and impaired glucose tolerance and plasma glucose levels in US population aged 20–74 years. *Diabetes.* 1987; 4:523–534.

36. Zavaroni I, Dall'Aglio E, Bruschi F. Effect of age and environmental factors on glucose tolerance and insulin secretion in a worker population. *J Am Geriatr Soc.* 1986; 34:271–278.

37. Rosenthal MJ, Hartnell JM, Morley JE, et al. UCLA geriatric rounds: diabetes in the elderly. *J Am Geriatr Soc.* 1987; 35:435–447.

38. Seals DR, Hagberg JM, Hurley BF, et al. Effects of endurance training on glucose tolerance and plasma lipid levels in older men and women. *JAMA.* 1984; 252:645–649.

39. Krotkiewski M, Lonnroth P, Mandroukas K, et al. The effects of physical training on glucose metabolism in obesity in type II diabetes mellitus. *Diabetologia.* 1985; 28:881–890.

40. Saltin B, Lindgarde F, Houston M, et al. Physical training and glucose tolerance in middle-aged men with chemical diabetes. *Diabetes.* 1979; 28(suppl):30–32.

41. Bogardus C, Ravussin E, Robbins DC, et al. Effects of physical training and diet therapy on carbohydrate metabolism in patients with glucose intolerance and non insulin dependent diabetes mellitus. *Diabetes.* 1984;33:311–318.

42. Mooradin AD, Morley JE. Micronutrient status in diabetes mellitus. *Am J Clin Nutr.* 1987; 45:877–895.

43. Kinlaw WB, Levine AS, Morley JE, et al. Abnormal zinc metabolism in type II diabetes mellitus. *Am J Med.* 1983; 75:273–277.

44. Morley JE. Nutritional status of the elderly. *Am J Med.* 1986; 81:679–695.

45. Niewoehner CB, Allen JI, Boosalis M, et al. The role of zinc supplementation in type II diabetes mellitus. *Am J Med.* 1986; 81:63–68.

46. Hallbook T, Lanner E. Serum-zinc and healing of venous leg ulcers. *Lancet.* 1972; II:780–782.

47. Wallach S. Clinical and biochemical aspects of chromium deficiency. *J Am Coll Nutr.* 1985; 4:107–120.

48. Klevay LM. Hypercholesterolemia produced by an increase in the ratio of zinc to copper ingested. *Am J Clin Nutr.* 1978; 26:1060–1065.

49. Bosch JP, Saccaggi A, Lauer A, et al. Renal functional reserve in humans, effect of protein intake on glomerular filtration rate. *Am J Med.* 1984; 75:943–950.

50. Uchida S, Tsutsumi O, Hise MK, et al. Role of epidermal factor in compensatory renal hypertrophy in mice. *Kidney Int.* 1988; 33:387–392.

51. Ross M. Nutrition and longevity in experimental animals. In: Winick M, ed. *Nutrition and Aging.* New York: Wiley; 1976; 43–57.

52. Dowd T. The female climacteric. *Nat OB/GYN Group.* 1990; 6(1):32–54.

53. Giansiracusa DF, Kantrowitz FG. Metabolic bone disease. In: Keiber JB. *Manual of Orthopaedic Diagnosis and Intervention.* Baltimore, Md: Williams and Wilkins Co.; 1978.

54. Dawson-Hughes B, Dallal G, Krall E. A controlled trial of the effect of calcium supplement on bone density in postmenopausal women. *N Engl J Med.* 1990; 329(13):878–883.

55. Riis B, Thomsen K, Christiansen C. Does calcium supplementation prevent postmenopausal bone loss? *N Engl J Med.* 1987; 316(4):173–177.

56. Harrington T. Preventing osteoporosis in menopausal women. *J MSSK Med.* June, 1990.

57. Nielsen F, Hunt C, Mullen L, Hunt J. Effect of dietary boron on mineral, estrogen and testosterone metabolism in postmenopausal women. *J FASE B.* 1987; 1:394–397.

58. Pogrund H, Bloom R, Menczel J. Preventing osteoporosis: current practices and problems. *Geriatrics.* 1986; 41(5):55–71.

59. Exton-Smith AN. The problem of subclinical malnutrition in the elderly. In: Exton-Smith AN, Scott DL, eds. *Vitamins in the Elderly.* Briston, UK: Wright and Sons, Ltd.; 1968; 12–18.

60. Gambert SR, Guansing AR. Protein-calorie malnutrition in the elderly. *J Am Geriatr Soc.* 1980; 28:272–275.

61. Foley CJ, Tideiksaar R. Nutritional problems in the elderly. In: Gambert SR, ed. *Contemporary Geriatric Medicine.* New York: Plenum; 1980; I.

62. Dyer AR, Stamler J, Berkson DM, Lindberg HA. Relationship of relative weight and body mass index to 14-year mortality in the Chicago People Gas Co. study. *J Chronic Dis.* 1975; 28:109–123.

63. Natlow AB, Heslin J. *Geriatric Nutrition.* Boston: CBI Publishing Co.; 1980.

64. Master AM, Lasser RP, Beckman G. Tables of average weight and height of Americans aged 65–94 years. *JAMA.* 1960; 172:658–662.

65. Wolinsky FD, Coe RM, Chavez MN, et al. Further assessment of the reliability and validity of a nutritional risk index: analysis of a three wave panel to study elderly adults. *Health Services Res.* 1986; 20:977–990.

66. Fillenbaum GG. *The Well-being of the Elderly: Approaches to Multidimensional Assessment.* Geneva: World Health Organization; 1984. WHO Offset Publication No. 84.

67. Branch LG, Jette AM. Personal health practices and mortality among the elderly. *Am J Public Health.* 1984; 74:1126–1129.

68. O'Hanlon P, Kohrs MB. Dietary studies of older Americans. *Am J Clin Nutr.* 1988; 31:1257–1269.

69. National Research Council. *Committee Report on Dietary Allowances of the Food and Nutrition Board.* Washington, DC: National Academy of Sciences Publication; 1989.

70. Lowenstein FW. Nutritional requirements of the elderly. In: Young EA, ed. *Nutrition, Aging and Health.* New York: Alan R Liss; 1986; 61–89.

72. Wolinsky FD, Coe RM, Miller DK, et al. Measurement of global and functional dimensions of health status in the elderly. *J Gerontol.* 1984; 39:88–92.

73. Korhs MB, Czajka-Narins D. Assessing nutrition of the elderly. In: Young EA, ed. *Nutrition, Aging and Health.* New York: Alan R Liss; 1986:25–59.

74. Abraham S. Dietary intake findings, United States 1971–1974. In: *National Health Survey, Vital and Health Statistics*. US Department of Health, Education and Welfare, Public Health Service; 1977.

75. Carroll MD, Abraham S, Dresser CM. Dietary intake source data: United States 1976–1980. In: *The National Health Survey*. Washington, DC: Department of Health & Human Services; 1983. Series 11, NO. 231. DHHS Publication No. PHS-83–1681.

76. Abraham S. *Height and Weight of Adults*. Washington, DC: Department of Health Education and Welfare; DHEW Publication No. PHS-79–1659.

77. Calloway DH, Zanni E. Energy requirements and energy expenditure of elderly men. *Am J Clin Nutr*. 1980; 33:2088–2092.

78. Widdowson EM. How much food does man require? An evaluation of human energy needs. *Experientia*. 1983; 44(suppl):11–25.

79. Munro HN, Suter PM, Russell RM. Nutritional requirements of the elderly. *Ann Rev Nutr*. 1987; 7:23–49.

80. Cahill GF. Starvation in man. *N Engl J Med*. 1970; 282:668–675.

81. Greenblatt DJ. Reduced albumin concentration in the elderly: a report from the Boston collaborative drug surveillance program. *J Am Geriatr Soc*. 1979; 27:20–23.

82. Bullamore JR, Gallagher JC, Wilkinson R, Nordin BEC. Effect of age on calcium absorption. *Lancet*. 1990; II:535–537.

83. Ireland P, Fordtran JS. Effects of dietary calcium and age on jejunal calcium absorption in humans studied by intestinal perfusion. *J Clin Invest*. 1983; 52:2671–2681.

84. Armbrecht HJ. Changes in calcium and vitamin D metabolism with age. In: Armbrecht HJ, Prendergast JM, Coe RM, eds. *Nutritional Intervention in the Aging Process*. New York: Springer Verlag; 1984:69–86.

85. Heaney RP. Calcium intake, bone health, and aging. In: Young EA, ed. *Nutrition, Aging and Health*. New York: Alan R Liss; 1986:165–186.

86. Johnson NE, Alcantara EN, Linksweiler HN. Effect of level of protein intake on urinary and fecal calcium retention of young adults. *J Nutr*. 1990; 100:1425–1430.

87. Draper HH, Sie TL, Bergen JG. Osteoporosis in aging rats induced by high phosphorus diet. *J Nutr*. 1984; 102:1113–1142.

88. Heaney RP, Recker RR. Effects of nitrogen, phosphorus and caffeine on calcium balance in women. *J Lab Clin Med*. 1982; 99:46–55.

89. McKenna MJ, Freaney R, Meade A, Muldowney FP. Hypovitaminosis D and elevated serum alkaline phosphatase in elderly people. *Am J Clin Nutr*. 1985; 41:101–108.

90. Slovik DM, Adams JS, Weer RM, et al. Deficient production of 1,25 dihydroxyvitamin D in elderly osteoporotic patients. *N Engl J Med*. 1991; 305:372–374.

91. Baker MR, Peacock R, Nordin BEC: The decline in vitamin D status with age. *Age Aging*. 1980; 9:249–256.

92. Freiman R, Johnston FA. Iron absorption in the health of the aged. *Geriatrics*. 1983; 18:716–720.

93. Lipschitz DA, Mitchell CO, Thompson D. The anemia of senescence. *Am J Hematol*. 1986; 11:47–54.

94. Lipschitz DA, Udupa KB, Milton KY, Thompson D. The effect of age on hematopoiesis in man. *Blood*. 1984; 63:502–509.

95. Lipschitz DA, Mitchell CO. The correctability of the nutritional, immune and haematopoietic manifestations of protein-calorie malnutrition in the elderly. *J Am Coll Nutr*. 1982; 1:17–25.

96. Garry PJ, Goodwin JS, Hunt WC. Folate and vitamin B_{12} status in a healthy elderly population. *J Am Geriatr Soc*. 1984; 32:719–726.

97. Bailey LB, Wagner PA, Christakis GJ, et al. Vitamin B_{12} status of elderly persons from urban low-income households. *J Am Geriatr Soc*. 1990; 28:276–278.

98. Comfort MW. Gastric acidity before and after development of gastric cancer: its etiologic, diagnostic and prognostic significance. *Ann Intern Med*. 1991; 34:1331–1336.

99. Steinberg WM, Toskes PP. A practical approach to evaluating mal-digestion and malabsorption. *Geriatrics*. 1988; 33:73–85.

100. Trence DL, Morley JE, Handwerger BS. Polyglandular auto-immune syndromes. *Am J Med*. 1984; 77:107–116.

101. Read AE, Gough KR, Pardge JL, et al. Nutritional studies on the entrants to an old people's home, with particular reference to folic acid deficiency. *Br Med J*. 1985; 11:843–848.

102. Elsborg L. Reversible malabsorption of folic acid in the elderly with nutritional folate deficiency. *Acta Haematol*. 1986; 55:140–147.

103. Batata M, Spray GH, Bolton FG, et al. Blood and bone marrow changes in elderly patients, with special reference to folic acid, vitamin B_{12}, iron and ascorbic acid. *Br Med J.* 1987; 2:667–669.

104. Fox JH, Topel JL, Huckman MS. Dementia in the elderly—a search for treatable illnesses. *J Gerontol.* 1985; 30:557–564.

105. Leibovitz BE, Siegel BV. Aspects of free radical reactions in biological systems: aging. *J Gerontol.* 1990; 35:45–56.

106. Pauling LC. Vitamin C and the common cold. San Francisco: Freeman; 1970.

108. Schorah CJ, Tormey WP, Brooks GH, et al. The effect of vitamin C supplements on body weight, serum proteins, and general health of an elderly population. *Am J Clin Nutr.* 1981; 34:871–876.

109. Sauberlich HE. Ascorbic acid. In: Olson RE, ed. *Nutrition Reviews: Present Knowledge in Nutrition.* Washington, DC: Nutrition Foundation; 1984; 269–272.

110. Sulkin NM, Sulkin DF. Tissue changes induced by marginal vitamin C deficiency. *Ann NY Acad Sci.* 1975; 258:317–328.

111. Attwood EC, Robey E, Kramer JJ, et al. A survey of the haematological, nutritional, and biochemical state of the rural elderly with particular reference to vitamin C. *Age Aging.* 1988; 7:46–56.

112. Burr ML, Elwood PC, Hole DJ, et al. Plasma and leucocyte ascorbic acid levels in the elderly. *Am J Clin Nutr.* 1984; 27:144–151.

113. Susaki R, Kurokawa T, Tero-Kubota S. Ascorbate radical and ascorbic acid level in human serum and age. *J Gerontol.* 1983; 38:26–30.

114. Spindler AA. The role of Vitamin C in cognitive impairment in the elderly. *Nutr Rep Internatl.* 1989; 39:713–717.

115. Vatassery GT, Johnson GJ, Krezowski AM. Changes in vitamin E concentrations in human plasma and platelets with age. *J Am Coll Nutr.* 1983; 4:369–375.

116. Haeger K. Long-time treatment of intermittent claudication with vitamin E. *Am J Clin Nutr.* 1984; 27:1179–1181.

117. Sokol RJ. Vitamin E deficiencies in the elderly. *Free Radical Biol Med.* 1989; 6:189–193.

118. Birren JE, Bick MW, Fox C. Age changes in the light threshold of the dark-adapted eye. *J Gerontol.* 1988; 43:267–271.

119. Watkin DM. *Handbook of Nutrition, Health and Aging.* Park Ridge, NJ: Noyes Publications; 1983.

120. Read MH, Graney AS. Food supplement usage by the elderly. *J Am Diet Assoc.* 1982; 80:250–253.

122. Sandstead HH, Henriksen LK, Greger JL, et al. Zinc nutriture in the elderly in relation to taste acuity, immune response and wound healing. *Am J Clin Nutr.* 1982; 36:1046–1059.

123. Lindman RD, Clark ML, Colmore JP. Influence of age and sex on plasma and red-cell zinc concentrations. *J Gerontol.* 1991; 26:358–363.

124. Bunker VW, Hinks LJ, Lawson MS, et al. Assessment of zinc and copper status of healthy elderly people using metabolic balance studies and measurement of leucocyte concentrations. *Am J Clin Nutr.* 1984; 40:1096–1102.

125. Wagner PA, Krista ML, Bailey LB, et al. Zinc status of elderly black Americans from urban low-income households. *Am J Clin Nutr.* 1990; 33:1771–1777.

126. Alhava EM, Olkkonen H, Puittinen J, et al. Zinc content of human cancellous bone. *Acta Orthop Scand.* 1987; 48:1–4.

127. Schroeder HA, Nelson AP, Tipton IH, et al. Essential trace metals in man: zinc. Relation to environmental cadmium. *J Chronic Dis.* 1987; 20:179–210.

128. Blazsek I, Mathe G. Zinc and immunity. *Biomed Pharmacother.* 1984; 38:187–193.

129. Makinodan T, Yunis E, eds. *Immunology and Aging.* New York: Plenum Press; 1977; 1.

130. Wacker WEC. Role of zinc in wound healing: a critical review. In: Prasad AS, ed. *Trace Elements in Human Health and Disease.* New York: Academic Press; 1986: 107–114.

131. Haeger K, Lanner E, Magnusson PO. Oral zinc sulfate in the treatment of venous leg ulcer. In: Pories WJ, Strain WH, Hsu JM, Woosley RL, eds. *Clinical Applications of Zinc Metabolism.* Springfield, Ill: Charles C. Thomas; 1974:158–167.

132. Essatara M'B, Morley JE, Levine AS, et al. The role of the endogenous opiates in zinc deficiency anorexia. *Physiol Behav.* 1984; 32:475–478.

133. Morley JE, Levine AS. The pharmacology of eating behavior. *Ann Rev Pharmacol Toxicol.* 1985; 25:127–146.

134. Billington CJ, Levine AS, Morley JE. Zinc status in impotent patients. *Clin Res.* 1983; 31(abstr):714A.

135. Burnet FM. A possible role of zinc in the pathology of dementia. *Lancet.* 1991; 1:186–188.
136. Cartwright GE, Wintrobe MM. The question of copper deficiency in man. *Am J Clin Nutr.* 1984; 15:94–110.
137. Harris HD, O'Dell BL. Copper and amine oxidases in connective tissue metabolism. Protein-metal interaction. *Adv Exp Med Biol.* 1984; 48:267–284.
138. O'Dell BL. Biochemistry of physiology and copper in vertebrates. In: Prasad AS, ed. *Trace Elements in Human Health and Disease.* New York: Academic Press; 1986; I:391–413.
139. Yunice AA, Linedman RD, Czerwinski AW, et al. Influence of age and sex on serum copper and ceruloplasmin levels. *J Gerontol. 1984; 29:277–281.*
140. Schroeder HA. Serum cholesterol and glucose levels in rats fed refined and less refined sugars and chromium. *J Nutr.* 1989; 97:237–242.
141. Schroeder HA, Nason AP, Tipton IH. Chromium deficiency as a factor in atherosclerosis. *J Chronic Dis.* 1990; 23:123–142.
142. Offenbacher EG, Pi-Sunyer FX. Beneficial effects of chromium rich yeast on glucose tolerance and blood lipids in elderly subjects. *Diabetes.* 1980; 29:919–925.
143. Newman HAI, Leighton RF, Lanese RR, et al. Serum chromium and angiographically determined coronary artery disease. *Clin Chem.* 1978; 24:541–544.
144. Phillips PA, Rolls BJ, Ledingham JGG, et al. Reduced thirst after water deprivation in healthy elderly men. *N Engl J Med.* 1984; 311:753–759.
145. Miller PD, Krebs RA, Neal BJ, et al. Hypodipsia in geriatric patients. *Am J Med.* 1982; 73:354–356.
146. Lavizzo-Mourey R, Johnson J, Stolley P. Risk factors for dehydration among elderly nursing home residents. *J Am Geriatr Soc.* 1988; 36:213–218.
147. Roe DA. Therapeutic effects of drug-nutrient interactions in the elderly. *J Am Diet Assoc.* 1985; 85:174–178.
148. Smith CH, Bidlack WR. Dietary concerns associated with the use of medications. *J Am Diet Assoc.* 1984; 84:901–908.
149. Spencer H, Lender M. Adverse effects of aluminum-containing antacids on mineral metabolism. *Gastroenterology.* 1989; 76:603–606.
150. Wasnich R, Benfante R, Yanok-Heilbrun L, Vogel J. Thiazide effect on the mineral content of bone. *N Engl J Med.* 1983; 309:344–347.
151. Vestal RE, Norris AH, Tobin JD, et al. Antipyrin metabolism in man: influence of age, alcohol, caffeine and smoking. *Clin Pharm Ther.* 1975; 18:425–432.
152. Alderman E, Coltart D. Alcohol and the heart. *Br Med Bull.* 1982; 38:77–81.
153. McCay CM, Crowell MF, Maynard LA. The effect of retarded growth upon length of life span and ultimate body size. *J Nutr.* 1935; 10:63–79.
154. Harman D. Free radical of aging: dietary implications. *Am J Clin Nutr.* 1972; 25:839–843.
155. Mechnikova O. *Life of Elie Metchnikoff.* London: Constable and Company; 1921.
156. Young VR. Diet as modulator of aging and longevity. *Fed Proc.* 1979; 38:1994–2000.
157. Porta EA. Nutritional factors and aging. In: Robin RB, Mehlman MA, eds. *Advances in Modern Human Nutrition.* Park Forest South, Il: Pathotox; 1980;I:106–118.
158. Kohn RR. *Principles of Mammalian Aging.* Englewood Cliffs, NJ: Prentice Hall; 1978.
159. Shamberger RJ, Andreone TL, Willis CE. Antioxidants and cancer, I.V. initiating activity of malgnaldehyde as a carcinogen. *J Natl Cancer Inst.* 1963; 53:316–326.
160. Ordy JM. Nutrition as modulator of rate of aging, disease, and longevity. In: Ordy JM, Harman D, Alin-Slater RB, eds. *Nutrition in Gerontology.* New York: Raven Press; 1984; 26:1–17.
161. Hegsted DM. Energy needs and energy utilization. *Nutr Rev.* 1974; 32:33–45.
162. Kreutler PA. *Nutrition in Perspective.* Englewood Cliffs, NJ: Prentice Hall; 1980.
163. Young VR. Protein metabolism with aging. In: Munro HN, ed. *Mammalian Protein Metabolism.* New York: Academic Press; 1980; IV.
164. Weg RB. *Nutrition and the Later Years.* Los Angeles: University of Southern California Press; 1979.
165. Stultz BM. Preventive health care for the elderly. *Western J Med.* 1984; 141:832–845.
166. Kennie DC. Health maintenance in the elderly. *J Am Geriatr Soc.* 1984; 32:316–323.
167. Berkman LF. The assessment of social networks and social support in the elderly. *J Am Geriatr Soc.* 1983; 31:743–749.
168. Smiciklas-Wright H, Fosmire GJ. Government nutrition programs for the aged. In: Watson RR, ed. *CRC Handbook of Nutrition in the Aged.* Boca Raton, Fla: CRC Press; 1985; 323–334.

169. Fanelli MT, Kaufman M. Nutrition and older adults. In: Phillips HT, Gaylord SA, eds. *Aging and Public Health.* New York: Springer Publishing; 1985:76–100.

170. Lipschitz DA, Mitchell CO, Steele RW, Milton KY. Nutritional evaluation and supplementation of elderly subjects participating in a "Meals on Wheels" program. *J Parent Ent Nutr.* 1985; 9:343–347.

171. Villers Foundation. *On the Other Side of Easy Street: Myths and Facts About the Economics of Old Age.* Washington, DC: Villers Foundation; 1986.

CHAPTER **8** EIGHT

Pharmacology

Mrs Jones, a 98-year-old woman with Parkinson's disease who recently had an amputation above the knee, came to physical therapy late one day. Her therapist was busy in the gym with several other patients, but she handed Mrs Jones a black dumbbell weight, which Mrs Jones had frequently used to do her warm-up exercise. Instead of beginning her usual exercises, Mrs Jones raised the dumbbell to her ear and said, "Hello, Emily?" She continued to chat on what she thought was a phone. The therapist immediately went to the nurses' station and discovered that Mrs Jones was on a new medication, which had obviously profoundly confused her. Her medication was changed, and in a few days, she was her usual coherent self. This real-life example graphically depicts one of the many complications of administering drugs to older persons.

This chapter will explore the multiple aspects of medication management in the elderly. Drug disposition, response, and adverse reactions in the elderly patient will be discussed, as well as common drug regimens. Monitoring techniques and compliance issues will also be examined. Finally, frequently used medications, common pathologics, and drug reactions will be explored.

EPIDEMIOLOGICAL ISSUES

In the early 1980s people over 65 composed 11.4% of the population, and yet they consumed over 31% of all prescription medications.[1] The Department of Health and Human Services reported that in 1977 an average of 10.7 prescriptions were obtained per year by persons over the age 65 as compared to 4.3 per person for the population under the age of 65.[2]

Older persons tend to have more chronic problems and diseases that often involve a multisystem diagnosis. Both of these are causes for concern when managing medication for this age group. Chronicity of disease impels the prescribing physician to sample a wide array of medications for symptom relief. Physicians will, in most instances, consult a specialist for additional advice in management. Unfortunately, this additional management is usually accompanied by additional drugs. Since chronic problem management is not curative in nature, multiple and ongoing drug use may be prescribed to alleviate symptoms. This pharmacological behavior can easily cause complications unless someone coordinates all the medications.[3] The multiplicity of disease that is so commonly seen in the elderly also dictates polypharmacy management and, therefore, requires careful coordination.

CLINICAL IMPLICATIONS

It is important for physical therapists working with the elderly to understand the actions and interactions of drugs for several reasons. First, physical therapists design and monitor exercise programs that can adversely affect pharmacokinetics. Fat soluble drugs, for example, may be affected by a person's decrease in fat after participation in an exercise program, and, therefore, dosages will need to be adjusted accordingly. Second, physical therapists see patients on a regular basis and can easily note adverse reactions, such as dizziness, confusion, and slurred speech.

If educated in pharmacology, physical therapists can suggest modifications of drug regimens based on patient symptoms. A good example of this would be that of Mrs Jones. Noting her confused state, the therapist would be able to note her medications, find the offending drug (for example, benztropine, the drug for treatment of Parkinson's), and perhaps suggest that the physician prescribe another, nonconfusional drug for replacement or lower the present dosage of the drug.

Appropriate medication management is an interdisciplinary concern. Other health care team members, not just the physician, must take responsibility for the supervision and coordination of drug interventions.

PHARMACOKINETICS

Pharmacokinetics is the process by which the body handles drugs. Pharmacokinetics has four progressive stages: absorption, distribution, biotransformation, and excretion, and each stage can be affected by the aging process. Since the goal of drug administration is to reach a therapeutic level, the rate and efficiency of these stages of pharmacokinetics will be influential in achieving this goal.

Controversy exists as to whether aging or the effects of disease truly affect the absorption of drugs.[4,5] Absorption is the process by which a drug passes from the gastrointestinal tract to the bloodstream,[5] and because age related changes occur in the gastrointestinal tract, it has been hypothesized that they are one cause for a decrease in absorption that occurs in later life. These age related changes include decreases in the intestinal blood flow, the time needed for gastric emptying, and the mucosal cell absorbing area, which might delay or reduce absorption.[5] In addition, there is an alteration in gastric pH that may affect ionization and drug solubility.

Distribution, the next phase of pharmacokinetics, determines the concentration of a drug at its target site.[5] The nature of drugs will cause them to have an affinity for certain body components, such as water, fat, or protein, and this will affect their action at their target site.

Since a drug must go through the liver, be changed to enzymes, enter the circulation, bind to protein in the blood or cells, and eventually reach the target organs, it is easy to see that how well an organ is perfused affects the drug's distribution. The age related changes affecting this process are a decrease in lean body mass, total body water, and plasma albumin.[6] These changes will affect the concentration of the drug and the protein binding ability of the drug. In addition, the increase in body fat with increased age will affect the drug's accumulation in the fatty tissue and possibly prolong its action.[7] The results of these changes are that the elderly are more susceptible to toxicity and are more prone to have side effects of the drug.[8]

Biotransformation, the next phase of pharmacokinetics, is the process of metabolizing a drug to inactive or active metabolites.[8] This process determines the length of time that a drug stays in the body. Since the liver plays an integral role in biotransformation, age related changes in liver function will affect the efficiency of this process. The age changes related to biotransformation are a decrease in the size, blood flow, and hepatic enzyme activity of the liver,[9] and all of these changes will result in a decreased rate of hepatic metabolism. This decreased metabolism of the drug may cause a buildup of the drug and result in toxic effects.

The final phase of the pharmacokinetics process is excretion. Excretion is the elimination of a drug from the body. Most drugs are eliminated through the kidneys, although a small portion are excreted through the skin and feces, therefore, age changes in the kidney have a significant influence on the elimination of drugs. These age changes are a decrease in the renal blood flow, the glomerular filtration rate, and the tubular excretion.[10] The changes' effect is an overall reduction in excretion and the drugs' and drug metabolites' accumulation in the body. This accumulation, again, can lead to toxicity. In addition, common cardiac problems can increase the likelihood of drug toxicity because of the damaging effects of these diseases on renal functioning.

Pharmacokinetics will vary from person to person. The therapist should keep in mind the phases of this process and look for signs of drug toxicity and adverse reactions.

DRUG USE AND ADVERSE REACTIONS IN THE ELDERLY

The biggest drug users in this country are the population over the age of 65. In a study done by May, 88.6% of the older population were found to be using either prescribed or nonprescribed medication on a regular basis.[11] In the rehabilitation setting, the use of medications is probably even more prevalent. Most rehabilitation patients have multiple problems and consequently receive multiple medications. In addition, these patients may be taking self-prescribed over-the-counter medications to alleviate chronic symptoms associated with the diseases or inactivity due to the disease. The purpose of their behavior is to alleviate their symptoms and improve their functional status. Many times, however, adverse reactions or unwanted side effects occur. Therapists should be aware of the most commonly used drugs, therefore, and any adverse effects associated with them. These will be listed later in this chapter.

In a study done by the United States' government on prescription drugs used by Medicare patients, the top nine drugs were identified. They are listed in Table 8–1. The general medication use for noninstitutionalized older persons reveals different, common drugs (Table 8–2). It is obvious from such frequent and diverse drug taking behaviors that side effects are likely to occur, and drug taking behav-

TABLE 8–1. PRESCRIPTION DRUGS COMMONLY USED BY MEDICARE PATIENTS

Cardiovasculars	Tranquilizers	Diuretics	Benzodiazepines	Antibiotics	Analgesics	Anti-inflammatories	Diabetic Products	Antispasmodics
Antianginal	Minor	Thiazide	Temazepam	Erythromycin	Non-narcotic	NSAIDS	Insulin	Dicyclomine
Nitrates	Diazepam	Benzthiazide	*Restoril*	*E-Mycin*	Acetaminophen	Aspirin	preparations	hydrochlor-
Nitrodur	*Valium*	*Exna*	Triazolam	Amoxicillin	*Tylenol*	*Bufferin*	Oral	ide
Diltiazem hydrochloride	Lorazepam	Chlorothiazide	*Halcion*	*Amoxil*	Aspirin	*Anacin*	hypogly-	*Bentyl*
Cardizem	*Ativan*	*Diuril*	Flurazepam		*Bufferin*	Ibuprofen	cemics	
Antiarrhythmic	Major	Potassium sparing	*Dalmane*		*Anacin*	*Motrin*	Glipizide	
Quinidine	Phenothiazine	Triamterene			Narcotic	Naproxen	*Glucotrol*	
Duraquin	derivatives	*Dyrenium*			Codeine	*Naprosyn*		
Antihypertensive agents		Loop			Morphine	Adrenal corticosteroids		
Sympatholytics		Bumetanide				Dexamethasone		
Guanabenz		*Bumex*				*Decadron*		
Wytensin		Furosemide				Prednisone		
Clonidine		*Lasix*				*Deltasone*		
Catapres								
β-Blockers								
Propranolol								
Inderal								
Metroprolol								
Lopressor								
Atenolol								
Tenormin								
Acebutolol								
Sectral								
Vasodilators								
Minoxidil								
Loniten								
Nifedipine								
Procardia								
ACE inhibitors								
Captopril								
Capoten								
Enalapril								
Vasotec								
Antilipemic agents								
Cholestyramine								
Questran								
Cholestipol								
Colestic								
Cardiac glycosides								
Digoxin								
Digitoxin								

TABLE 8–2. DRUGS COMMONLY USED BY NONINSTITUTIONALIZED PERSONS

Vitamins	Nonnarcotic Analgesics	Cardiovasculars	Benzodiazepines	Diuretics	Cathartics	Antacids	Thyroidals	Anticoagulants
One-a-Day	Acetaminophen	Antianginal	Flurazepam	Thiazide	Castor Oil	Sodium bicarbonate	Thyroidal hormones	Coumadin
Geritol	*Tylenol*	Nitrates	*Dalmane*	Chlorothiazide	*Purge*	*Alka-Selzer*	Levothyroxine	*Panwarfarin*
and	Aspirin	*Nitrodur*	Temazepam	*Diuril*	Psyllium	and other over-the-	*Levothroid*	Heparin
other	*Bufferin*	Diltiazem	*Restoril*	Potassium sparing	*Fiberall*	counter	*Synthroid*	
over-the-	*Anacin*	hydrochloride	Triazolam	Amiloride		preparations	Liotrix	
counter	and other over-	*Cardizem*	*Halcion*	*Midamor*		Aluminum hydroxide	*Euthroid*	
prepara-	the-counter	Antiarrhythmic		Triamterene		*Basaljel*	Antithyroid agents	
tions	preparations	Quinidine		*Dyrenium*		*Alternagel*	Propylthiouracil	
		Duraquin		Loop		Aluminum and	*Propyl-Thyracil*	
		Lidocaine		Bumetanide		magnesium hydroxide	Methimazole	
		Xylocaine		*Bumex*		*Maalox*	*Tapazole*	
		Antihypertensive agents		Furosemide		*Mylanta*		
		diuretics		*Lasix*		and other over-the-		
		Triamterene				counter		
		Dyrenium				preparations		
		sympatholytics				Magaldrate		
		Guanabenz				*Riopan*		
		Wytensin						
		Clonidine						
		Catapres						
		vasodilators						
		Minoxidil						
		Loniten						
		Nifedipine						
		Procardia						
		β-blockers						
		Metroprolol						
		Lopressor						
		ACE inhibitors						
		Captopril						
		Capoten						
		Enalapril						
		Vasotec						
		Antilipemic agents						
		Cholestyramine						
		Questran						
		Cholestipol						
		Colestic						
		Cardiac glycosides						
		Digoxin						
		Digitoxin						

ior in relation to age related changes contributes to the occurrence of adverse reactions.

The adverse reactions or side effects of special concern to therapists are postural hypotension, fatigue and weakness, depression, confusion and dementia, movement disorders, incontinence, anticholinergic actions, dizziness, extrapyramidal signs, and fluid volume depletion.

Postural Hypotension

Postural hypotension is defined as a drop in systolic blood pressure upon assumption of an erect posture.[12] When blood pressure drops in this manner, the person often is more susceptible to falls and fractures, as well as to cardiac and cerebral infarcts, which the older person is already at risk for because of age related changes in the homeostatic mechanisms affecting this process.[13] Any additional impairment caused by a drug, for example, would put the person at further risk. Table 8–3 provides a list of drugs that can cause or contribute to postural hypotension.[5,13]

Fatigue and Weakness

Fatigue and weakness in older patients may have a pathological, pharmaceutical, or psychological cause.[13] The therapist can explore possible causes through consulting with both the physician and the patient to determine if any intervention would be successful. For psychological causes of fatigue and weakness consult Chapter 4. For cardiovascular disease, diabetes, and arthritis, the therapist should understand the limitations posed by these pathologies and respect and progress within those limits (see Chapter 5 for pathologies of aging). Drug administration may contribute to the psychological and pathological disease component.

Several drugs deserve to be mentioned when discussing fatigue and weakness. β-Blockers can cause fatigue because of their ability to slow down the heart and reduce blood flow. Diuretics decrease fluid volume and may cause dehydration, a decrease in cardiac output, or both, which can cause hyponatremia or hypokalemia. In addition, vasodilators, digitalis preparations, antihypertensives, and oral hypoglycemics may cause weakness and fatigue.[13]

Since fatigue and weakness are such important factors in a rehabilitation program, the therapist must work with the physician to alter the medication to fit the rehabilitation program or to alter the rehabilitation to fit the medication program.

Depression

Depression can be caused by any drug that has an adverse effect on brain function. If an individual is depressed, they lack the motivation and interest to participate in a rehabilitation program. In addition, they are unable to realistically assess their improvements. Therapists, again, must be involved with the doctor to manage these problems. Table 8–4 lists drugs that may cause depression.

Confusion and Dementia

Confusion and dementia are, unfortunately, caused by many drugs. Any drug that causes confusion with prolonged use can cause dementia.[14] The drugs that most frequently cause confusion are listed in Table 8–5. This list of drugs is frighteningly long. Therapists should become familiar with these drugs and consider drug toxicity when observing for confusional states in their patients.

Movement Disorders

Movement disorders caused by medication can be broken down into several types and causes. Drug-induced parkinsonism is characterized by bradykinesia, resting tremor and rigidity, is relatively common in the elderly, and is usually, but not

TABLE 8–3. DRUGS CAUSING POSTURAL HYPOTENSION AND PRIMARY INDICATION FOR DRUG USE

Tricyclic Antidepressants (depression)	Tranquilizers (psychotic behavior)	Antihypertensive Drugs (hypertension)	Diuretics (hypertension, CHF)	Nitrates (angina)	Narcotic Analgesics (pain)	Antiparkinsonians (Parkinson's)	Sedative–Hypnotics (insomnia, anxiety, behavioral disturbances)	Antiarrhythmic Drugs (cardiovascular disease)
Amitriptyline	Thiothixene	Sympatholitics	All	Nitroglycerin	All	Levodopa	Benzodiazepines	All
Elavil	_Navane_	Methyldopa		_Nitro-Dur,_			Florazepam	
Endep	Haloperidol	_Aldomet_		_Nitro-Bid_			_Dalmane_	
Desipramine	_Haldol_	Guanethidine		Erythrotyl			Temazepam	
Norpramin		_Esimil_		tetranitrate			_Restoril_	
Pertofrane		Peripheral α-blockers		_Cardilate_			Triazolam	
Doxepin		Phenoxybenzamine		Isosorbide			_Halcion_	
Adapin		_Dibenzyline_		dinitrite				
Sinequan		Phentolamine		_Dilatrate SR_				
Imipramine		_Regitine_						
Tofranil		Prazosin						
Nortriptyline		_Minipress_						
Aventyl		β-Adrenoreceptor						
Pamelor		blockers						
Protriptyline		Atenolol						
Vivactil		_Tenormin_						
Trimipramine		Pindolol						
Surmontil		_Visken_						
		Metroprolol						
		Lopressor						
		Timolol						
		Blocadren						
		ACE Inhibitors						
		Captopril						
		Capoten						
		Enlalapril						
		Vasotec						
		Vasodilators						
		Nifedipine						
		Procardia						
		Calcium channel						
		blockers						
		Nicardipine						
		Cardene						
		Isradipine						
		DynaCirc						
		Verapamil						
		Isoptin						
		Calan						

TABLE 8–4. DRUGS ASSOCIATED WITH DEPRESSIVE SIDE EFFECTS IN THE ELDERLY PATIENT

Antihypertensives	Anti-inflammatories	Antimycobacterial	Antiparkinson Drugs	Diuretics	H₂ Receptor Antagonist	Sedative–Hypnotics	Vasodilators
Sympatholytic	NSAIDs	Ethambutol	Levodopa	Acetazolamide	Cimetidine	Glutethimide	Hydralazine
Methyldopa	Naproxen	*Myambutol*	Levodopa-Carbidopa	*Diamox*	*Tagamet*	*Elrodorm*	*Apresoline*
Aldomet	*Naprosyn*		*Sinemet*	Methazolamide		Barbiturates	
Clonidine	Tolmetin		Amantadine	Neptazane		Phenobarbital	
Catapres	*Tolectin*		*Symmmetrel*	Hydrochlorothiazide		*Nembutal*	
Guanabenz	Indomethiacin		Bromocriptine	and deserpidine		Benzodiazepines	
Wytensin	*Indocin*		*Parlodel*	*Oreticyl*		Flurazepam	
Receptor Blockers	Meclofenamate					*Dalmane*	
α-Blockers	*Meclomen*					Temazepam	
Prazosin	Peroxicam					*Restoril*	
Minipress	*Feldene*					Triazolam	
β-Blockers	Steroidals					*Halcion*	
Nadolol	Prednisolone					Alcohol	
Corgard	*Meticortelone*					rum, etc.	
Propranolol							
Inderal							
Atenolol							
Tenormin							
Metaprolol							
Lopressor							
Pindolol							
Viskin							
ACE Inhibitors							
Guanethidine							
Esimil							
Reserpine							
Various derivatives							

TABLE 8–5. EXAMPLES OF DRUGS THAT CAUSE CONFUSIONAL STATES

Cardiac Glycosides	Antiparkinsonians	Antidepressants	Anticholinergics	Anti-inflammatories	Analgesics
Digitoxin *Cardigin* Digoxin *Digacin*	Benztropine *Cogentin* Levodopa Trihexylphenidyl *Artane* Amantadine *Symmetrel* Bromocriptine *Parlodel*	Tricyclics (See Table 8–3)	(See Table 8–7)	Indomethasin *Indosin* Salicylates *Bufferin* *Anacin* Phenylbutazone *Butazolidin* Oxyphenbutazone *Oxalid*	Hydromorphone *Dilaudid* Meperidine *Demerol* Methadone *Fenadone* Pentazocine *Talwin*

Sedative–Hypnotics	H$_2$ Receptor Antagonists	Diuretic	Hypoglycemic Agents	β-Blockers
Benzodiazepines Flurazepam *Dalmane* Temazepam *Restoril* Triazolam *Halcion* Barbiturates Phenobarbital *Nembutal* Secobarbital *Pramil*	Cimetidine *Tagamet*	Methyclothiazide *Aquatensen* Hydrochlorothiazide *Hydro-Diuril* Furosemide *Lasix*	Tolazamide *Tolinase* Tolbutamide *Orinase*	Propranolol *Inderal* Metroprolol *Lopressor* Atenolol *Tenormin* Acebutolol *Sectrol*

always, caused by antipsychotic medication. (See Table 8–6 for a list of drugs causing drug-induced parkinsonism.)[13]

Tardive dyskinesia is a neuroleptic-induced movement disorder that usually affects the lips, jaw, and tongue and can be induced or exacerbated by medications.[15] This disorder may occur as a late effect of antipsychotic drug treatments, the administration of anticholinergic medications, or from withdrawal from a medication.[16] Patients with preexisting brain damage are more likely to develop tardive dyskinesia.

Akathisia, or motor restlessness, is another neuroleptic movement disorder that may result from antipsychotic drug administration.

Finally, essential tremor, which is defined as quick oscillating movements around a joint when the limb is used for active movement, can be exacerbated by lithium carbonate, tricyclic antidepressants, and adrenergic drugs.[16]

Incontinence

Incontinence is another severe and embarrassing problem that can be caused and exacerbated by a variety of drugs. Drugs that depress cerebral function, such as benzodiazepines and barbiturates, can exaggerate a preexisting incontinence by depressing one's ability to inhibit bladder contractions. Stress incontinence, on the other hand, is exacerbated by thioridazine and chlorpromazine, both antipsychotic phenothiazines. Anticholinergic drugs relax the muscles of the bladder and may cause urinary retention and overflow incontinence. Therapists can encourage patients to schedule the administration of these drugs so that they coordinate with activities. Further, anticholinergic effects may be evidenced in cardiac abnormalities, dryness of the mouth, difficulty in swallowing, confusion, hallucinations, fa-

TABLE 8–6. DRUGS CAUSING DRUG-INDUCED PARKINSONISM

Antipsychotics	Sympatholytics
Phenothiazines	Centrally acting
Chlorpromazine	Methyldopa
Thorazine	*Aldomet*
Fluphenazine	Presynaptic adrenergic inhibitors
Permatil	Reserpine
Mesoridazine	*Crystoserpine*
Serentil	
Perphenazine	
Trilafon, Triavil	
Prochlorperazine	
Compazine	
Thioridazine	
Mellaril	
Trifluoperazine	
Stelazine	
Triflupromazine	
Vesprin	
Butyrophenone	
Haloperidol	
Haldol	
Dehydroindolone	
Molondone	
Moban	
Dibenzoxazepine	
Loxapine	
Loxitane	

TABLE 8–7. DRUGS WITH ANTICHOLINERGIC ACTION

Drug	Trade Name
Tricyclic antidepressants	
Amitriptyline	Elavil, Endep
Amoxapine	Asendin
Doxepin	Adapin, Sinequan
Imipramine	Tofranil
Maprotiline	Ludiomil
Nortryptyline	Pamelor, Aventyl
Protriptyline	Vivactil
Trimipramine	Surmontil
Antipsychotics	
Benztropine	Cogentin
Biperiden	Akineton
Chlorpromazine	Thorazine
Molindone	Moban
Thioidazine	Mellaril
Antihistamines	
Diphenhydramine	Benadryl
Antiparkinsonians	
Orphenadrine	Disipal
Trihexyphenidyl	Artane

tigue, difficulty in urination, and ataxia. Table 8–7 provides a list of drugs with potent anticholinergic action.[13,15]

Dizziness

Drugs may be the major cause of dizziness in people over age 60.[13] The number of drugs that can cause dizziness in older persons is almost as intimidating as those identified for confusion. The greatest contributors are given in Table 8–8. Since

TABLE 8–8. DRUGS THAT MAY CAUSE DIZZINESS

Cardiovascular Antillipemic Agents	Sedative–Hypnotics	Analgesics	Antihypertensives
Gemifibrozel *Lopid*	Barbiturates all	NSAIDs all	Vasodilators Diltiazem *Cardizem* Nifedipine *Procardia* Hydralazine *Apresoline*
Colestipol *Cholestid*	Benzodiazepines all		β-Blockers all
Clofibrate *Atromid-S*	Alcohol all		Sympatholytic Acting on CNS Clonidine *Catapres* Guanabenz *Wytensin* Methyldopa *Aldomet*
			Acting on postganglionic sympathetic neurons Guanethidine *Esimil* Phenoxybenzamine *Dibenzyline*
			α-Receptor blockers Phentolamine *Regitine* Prazosin *Minipress*
			β-Adrenoreceptor blockers Atenolol *Tenormin* Metaprolol *Lopressor* Timolol *Blocadren*
			ACE inhibitors Enlalapril *Vasotec* Captoril *Capoten* Lisinopril *Zestril, Prinvil*

TABLE 8–9. COMMONLY USED DIURETICS

Potassium Sparing Diuretics	Thiazides and Combinations
Spronolactone and hydrochlorothiazide	Polythiazide
Aldactazide	*Renese*
Spironolactone	Acetazolamide
Aldoctone	*Diamox*
Triamterene	Chlorthalidone
Dyazide	*Hygroton*
Dyrenium	Chlorothiazide
Amiloride	*Diuril*
Midamor	Methylclothiazide & crystenamine
Amiloride hydrochlorothiazide	*Diutensin*
Moduretic	Triamterene & hydrochlorothiazide
	Dyazide
	Hydrochlorthiazide
	Esidrix

therapists work so closely with patients on problems of coordination and balance, the adverse effects of these medications are important to understand. The therapist should remember that a patient will never improve on a balance program if a medication continues to make them dizzy.

Fluid Volume Depletion

Diuretics are the major cause of volume depletion in older persons. Volume depletion can cause decreased cardiac output and they may result in tiredness. Therapists should be aware of the diuretic use of their patients who are constantly tired. (See Table 8–9 for listing of diuretics.)

DRUG REGIMENS

Common drug regimens will be explored in the cardiovascular, neuromusculoskeletal, psychiatric, and gastrointestinal realms. A drug regimen is a method of administering a drug. Drug regimens must be altered for older persons. The following are brief descriptions of drug regimens.

Cardiovascular Regimens

Drug management for the cardiovascular system revolves around managing congestive heart failure (CHF), hypertension, angina pectoris, cardiac arrhythmias, and arteriosclerosis. Congestive heart failure is a condition in which the heart is unable to pump enough blood throughout the body based on the body's metabolic needs at that time. The symptoms of CHF are tiredness, shortness of breath, edema, and an inability to take a deep breath. Frequently, CHF is a problem in the elderly.

This problem is complicated by the fact that the most commonly used drugs to treat CHF are toxic. These drugs are digoxin and digitoxin (cardiac glycosides) or vasodilators. Under the influence of the glycosides, the weakened heart is able to pump more forcefully. The glycosides, however, are not curative and do not make any permanent changes in the heart muscle and, therefore, must be given for life.[17]

TABLE 8–10. COMMONLY USED VASODILATORS[27]

Drug	Trade Name
Hydralazine[a]	Apresoline
Minoxidil[a]	Loniten
Calcium channel blockers	Verapamil
	Nifedipine
	Diltiazem

[a]Primary vasodilators used.

Another problem with the glycosides, more so than with any other drug, is their narrow margin of safety. Even small changes, therefore, in the functioning of the body, such as an increase in an exercise program, may cause toxic effects in the older person. Another important point about this drug regimen is that it takes longer for the elimination of this drug from the system of the older person.[17] Early symptoms of toxicity from glycosides are blurred vision, slowed heart rate, and confusion. These can eventually lead to significant cardiac disturbances.[17] The clinician should be alert to these signs as a means of precluding more serious problems.

Vasodilators can also be used to treat CHF. They work by reducing the resistance of the vasculature. This causes the heart to work less; it pumps against less resistance and, therefore, pumps more efficiently. The vasodilators are less toxic than the glycosides, but they may also be less effective. Their toxic symptoms are very similar to the ones noted for glycosides. Table 8–10 provides a list of commonly used vasodilators.

Hypertension is another common problem in the older person. Unlike CHF, hypertension is virtually symptomless until it reaches the advanced stages. The main dangers are its possible sequelae: heart attack, stroke, and renal disease. Hypertension is difficult to define and may, therefore, be even more problematic to treat. The World Health Organization defines hypertension as diastolic blood pressure over 95 mm Hg.[18] The Framingham Study defined hypertension as diastolic over 95 mm Hg and systolic over 160 mm Hg.[19]

Before discussing the types of drugs used to treat hypertension, it should be noted that the physical therapist should realize that there is a question as to whether and when to treat patients who present with hypertension. Most physicians choose conservative methods as their first treatment course (i.e., weight control, smoking cessation, salt restriction, and exercise). If nondrug therapy is ineffective, the first reasonable step in drug therapy would be thiazide diuretics (e.g., chlorothiazide). Thiazide diuretics are slower acting (average duration of action 10 to 12 hours) and show no early peak effect. Therefore, the inconvenience (especially for the elderly patient) of an overwhelming urinary frequency produced by a faster acting diuretic is not a factor with this drug.[20]

Even though thiazide diuretics are tried first, they have adverse side effects that are particularly dangerous for older persons. Thiazides are likely to produce some degree of hyperglycemia, hypokalemia, and hyperuricemia. Because of the increased prevalence of late-onset diabetes, arrhythmias, and gout in older persons, the side effects of these drugs must be carefully monitored.[20]

Calcium channel blockers and β-adrenergic blockers are often the second stage of management for hypertension. Calcium channel blockers are more effective than the β-blockers in the older population because of their ability to lower arterial blood pressure without increasing total peripheral resistance (TPR). In the elderly patient TPR is typically increased and cardiac reserve is restricted. β-Blockers would be counterproductive because they lower blood pressure mainly by reducing cardiac output and somewhat increasing TPR in a patient whose TPR is already high. Both, however, have the liability that an overdose can slow or even stop the heart.

Figure 8–1 is based on the various stages for hypertension management of the elderly. Please note that the choice of drugs often depends on the other diagnoses the patient may have.

Angina pectoris requires two forms of drug management. Angina is a condition where the person suffers a sudden severe pain in the substernal area that is due to a temporary lack of oxygen to the heart. To manage this problem, the sufferer needs quick relief. Vasodilators, such as amyl nitrite and nitroglycerin, which are placed under the tongue, are absorbed quickly and travel rapidly to the heart. The other mode of drug management for angina is preventative. The drugs most beneficial for this are calcium channel blockers and β-blockers.[20] Table 8–11 provides a list of the commonly used antianginal agents with route, dose, and comments.

Management of arrhythmias is a controversial area in the treatment of the older person. Often the arrhythmia, or abnormal heart beat, is a manifestation of an underlying pathology and will resolve when the pathology is treated. Nevertheless, arrhythmias should not be overlooked in the older person because of the older person's inability to maintain a normal cardiac output between 40 and 170 beats per minute as can younger persons. In the aged, there is a reduction in this range to between 45 and 120 beats per minute. The drugs of choice depend on the rhythm alteration. Table 8–12 provides a list of some commonly used antiarrhythmic agents, with route, dose, and comments noted. In older persons, the rate of removal of procainamide, lidocaine, and quinidine are reduced. Disopyramide may cause voiding problems in older men.[16]

The final cardiovascular condition that is typically treated with drugs is atherosclerosis. Atherosclerosis is a buildup of plaque in the arteries, causing a thickening of the arterial walls and, therefore, diminishing the size of the lumen. Drug therapy for atherosclerosis is aimed at preventing the development of plaques by reducing the blood levels of certain lipids, especially cholesterol. The three most common drugs used for this problem are lovastatin, niacin, and cholestyramine.[14] At present lovastatin has little toxic effect. Niacin used in the high doses necessary for results may cause itching, flushing, and gastrointestinal distress. Cholestyramine is not absorbed into the body and acts by binding to cholesterol, thereby promoting its excretion in the feces. Cholestyramine may bind to fat soluble vitamins and cause a deficiency in an undernourished older person. Finally, it may be difficult to predict the effectiveness of this drug because of the amount of laxatives that older people tend to take.[13]

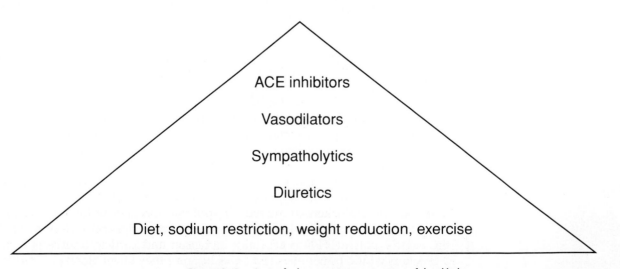

Figure 8–1. Stages for hypertension management of the elderly.

TABLE 8–11. ANTIANGINAL AGENTS

Drug	Trade Name	Method of Action	Side Effects	Drug Interactions
Nitroglycerin	Nitro-Bid	Relax smooth muscle in arterial and venous beds	Transient headache, nausea/vomiting, dizziness, flush on face/neck, rapid pulse	Alcohol, antihypertensives, dihydroergotamine, sympathomimetics, tricyclic antidepressants, vasodilators
	Nitro-Dur	Relax smooth muscle in arterial and venous beds	Skin rash, transient headache, tachycardia, nausea, hypotension, vomiting, rapid pulse, dizziness, flush	Antihypertensives, vasodilators, sympathomimetics
	Transderm nitro	Relax smooth muscle in arterial and venous beds	Transient headache, hypotension, nausea/vomiting, rapid pulse, dizziness, flush	Antihypertensives, vasodilators, sympathomimetics
Isosorbide dinitrate	Iso-Bid	Relax vascular smooth muscle in arterial and venous beds	Weakness, cutaneous vasodilation with flushing, hypotension	Antihypertensives, tricyclic antidepressants, vasodilators, sympathomimetics
Erythrityl tetranitrate	Cardilate	Direct dilation of coronary conductance vessels. Decreased myocardial oxygen demand (preload and afterload)	Headache, flushing, dizziness, weakness, signs of cerebral ischemia, associated hypotension (caused by overdosage)	Alcohol
Verapamil	Calan and Calan SR	Blocks active and inactive calcium channels	Hypotension, peripheral edema, dizziness, headache/fatigue, constipation/nausea	Disopyramide, carbamazepine, β-blocking agents, digoxin, calcium supplements
Diltiazem hydrochloride	Cardizem	Calcium channel block	Edema, decrease in blood pressure, occasional hypotension, headache, nausea, dizziness, rash, AV block	Digoxin, calcium supplements, β-blocking agents, disopyramide
Nifedipine	Procardia	Calcium channel block	Dizziness, lightheadedness, nausea, headache, weakness, transient hypotension	β-Blocking agents, cimetidine, digoxin, bentanyl, calcium supplements, long-acting nitrates
Nadolol	Corgard	Nonselective block of β-adrenergic receptors	Dizziness, fatigue, paresthesia, drowsiness, hypotension, conjunctive heart failure, peripheral vascular insufficiency	Epinephrine, lidocaine, indomethacin, oral hypoglycemics, catecholamine-depleting
Dipyridamole	Cardoxine	Selectively dilates coronary arteries resulting in increased oxygen supply to myocardium, also inhibits platelet aggregation	Dizziness, weak or syncope flushing, nausea/vomiting, skin rash, GI distress, headache	No known clinical significance
Pentaerythritol tetranitrate	Vasodiatol	Direct dilation of coronary conductive vessels	Flushing, headache, dizziness/weakness, postural hypotension	Norepinephrine, acetylcholine, histamine, alcohol

Neuromusculoskeletal Regimens

This section will discuss drug management of arthritis, neuralgias, stroke, and Parkinson's disease. Since arthritis is so common in the older population, the chances of an older patient taking some type of medication for the management of pain and inflammation are great. Physicians prescribing drugs for the management of arthritis must understand that this is not a comprehensive program. Both

TABLE 8–12. ANTIARRHYTHMIC DRUGS

Drug	Trade Name	Method of Action	Side Effects	Drug Interactions
Quinidine	Quinaglute	Depresses pacemaker rate, depresses conduction and excitability	Nausea/vomiting, abdominal pain, diarrhea, headache, tinnitus, disturbed vision, worsening arrythmia	Amiodarone, reserpine phenothiazine, digitalis glycosides, neuromuscular blocking agents, antacids, oral anticoagulants
Procainamide hydrochloride	Procan	Supresses automaticity, decreases conduction velocity, prolongs effective refractory period	Hypotension, worsening ventricular arrythmia, systemic lupus erythematosus symptoms, arthritis, arthralgia, fever, rash	Antiarrhythmic agents, anticholinergic agents, antihypertensive agents
Lidocaine	Xylocaine	Suppressor of abnormal cardiac activity, acting exclusively on sodium channels	Paresthesias, tremor, lightheadedness, convulsions, drowsiness	Oxytocic drugs
Propranolol	Inderal	Nonselective blockage of β-adrenergic receptors	Dizziness, fatigue, lightheadedness, nausea/vomiting, bronchospasm bradycardia, peripheral vascular insufficiency	Chlorpromazine, epinephrine, barbiturates, cimetidine, haloperidol, catecholamine-depleting, thioamines, rifampin
Verapamil	Calan	Coronary vasodilator, blocks both activated and inactivated calcium channels	Hypotension, peripheral edema, bradycardia, dizziness, headache/fatigue, constipation, nausea	Carbamazepine, β-adrenergic blocking agents, digoxin, calcium supplements, digitalis, disopyramide, antihypertensive agents, quinidine, methyldopa
Amiodarone hydrochloride	Cordarone, Miocard	Effective blocker of inactivated sodium channels, blocks α- and β-adrenoreceptors	Halo in peripheral vision fields, yellowing of cornea, photodermatitis, grayish/blue skin discoloration	Warfarin, theophylline, quinidine, procainamide, flecainide
Disopyramide phosphate	Norpace	See quinidine	Dry mouth, urinary retention, constipation, blurred vision, dry nose, eyes, bloating malaise, fatigue, muscle weakness	Alcohol, warfarin, phenytoin, digoxin
Quinidine polygalacturonate	Cardioquin	Slows conduction time, prolongs refractory period, depresses excitability of the heart muscle	Disturbed vision, headache, diarrhea, nausea/vomiting, abdominal pain, confusion, vertigo, fever, delirium, syncope, apprehension	Digoxin, potassium supplements, phenobarbital, phenytoin, anticholinergic drugs
Quinidine gluconate	Duraquin	Prolongation of refractory period, decrease in excitability of ectopic foci of the heart	Same as above	Potassium, coumarin, anticoagulants, thiazide diuretics, sodium bicarbonate, carbonic anhydrase inhibitors, other antiarrhythmic drugs
Isoproterenol	Isupren	Increases cardiac output, increases venous return to heart, lowers peripheral vascular resistance	Sweating, mild tremors, nervousness, tachycardia with palpitations	Diuretics, epinephrine, cyclopropane

environmental modifications and an appropriate physical therapy program that enhances independence must be addressed.

The most common drugs used in the management of osteoarthritis are analgesics and nonsteroidal anti-inflammatories. Even though osteoarthritis is a degenerative disease, the patient may have significant inflammation, often on the initial presentation, due to overuse and irritation of the joint. The use of anti-inflammatories at this point may help in the management of the disease. The most frequent nonsteroidal anti-inflammatory (NSAID) prescribed for osteoarthritis is aspirin. The dosage may vary, but it should be titrated to the individual. The patient should begin with one aspirin every 4 hours and increase the dosage to two aspirins every 4 hours until the relief of symptoms is achieved and before any adverse drug reactions (i.e., gastric irritability or tinnitus). If the older person does not tolerate aspirin, then another NSAID may be used. These drugs are more expensive and the many different types of NSAIDs abound. Table 8–13 provides a list of the most common NSAIDs on the market. The major problems with NSAIDs in the older population are the adverse reactions, which include frontal headaches, dizziness, light-headedness, confusion, and depression.[21] In addition to these reactions, NSAIDs may also cause renal dysfunction.

Combining analgesics with anti-inflammatory drugs, as well as using multiple analgesics, is relatively common in the older population.[22] The use of acetaminophen can be helpful for pain relief without an analgesic effect. It can also be combined with anti-inflammatories for episodes of severe pain.

Neuralgias can be defined as a sudden recurring pain that extends along the site of a nerve and affects the anatomical distribution of that nerve. The three most common types of neuralgia in older persons are postherpetic (shingles), glossopharyngeal, and trigeminal neuralgia. The pharmaceutical management of these problems revolves around pain management. For very mild cases, rest and analgesics, such as aspirin and acetaminophen, are suggested. Stronger drugs, such as carbamazepine and phenytoin, are effective for the trigeminal and glossopharyngeal neuralgias.[22] For the management of shingles in severe cases, morphine or codeine may be necessary. In addition, systemic adrenal steroids may be recommended for most elderly patients but are contraindicated for patients with neoplasms or any underlying disease and for patients on immunosuppressive therapy.[22]

Drugs that are used in the treatment of strokes are a quickly growing area of study. The current thought, however, is to protect the area of infarct. The concern is that even a slight fall in blood pressure may aggravate a cerebral ischemia and extend the infarct area. Nevertheless, studies continue to investigate the effects of the "intracerebral steal" and the "inverse steal" effects on the poststroke brain. In the first effect, the healthier cerebral arteries may dilate and take blood from the needy arteries and the infarct. In the "inverse steal," administration of vasoactive drugs may reduce the swelling of capillary walls, which occurs after stroke.[13]

Despite the controversy of the previously stated effects, certain drug regimens have been used for poststroke patients for the management of cerebral edema, cerebral emboli, and blood pressure. Corticosteroids can be used to reduce cerebral edema, and glycerol can be used to improve regional blood flow. Anticoagulants are indicated for the management of cerebral emboli. The management of the poststroke patient's blood pressure should be aimed at maintaining pressure in the acute phases. For older patients, the use of activity or stressing the postural response is preferable to drug management for maintaining blood pressure.[13]

The final neuromusculoskeletal drug to be discussed in this section is parkinsonism. Parkinsonism is a condition that reflects a deficiency of dopamine in the brain. Because dopamine does not cross the blood–brain barrier, L-dopa must be used. L-dopa is a dopamine precursor that crosses the blood–brain barrier and is converted to dopamine.[15] Unfortunately, large doses of dopamine are needed to achieve concentrations in the brain and these large doses lead to major side effects, such as involuntary movements, adverse mental changes, postural hypotension, and vomiting. Sinemet is the most widely used drug for the management of parkinsonism, and it is a combination of L-dopa and carbidopa. Carbidopa acts as an inhibitor to decarboxylase, which rapidly breaks down L-dopa thus allowing smaller doses of L-dopa to be effective. Long-term L-dopa therapy may lose its effect, and the results of this can be seen with the patient displaying end of dose "stiffness" or freezing, or swings in function.[15] The creative titration of this drug, as well as the use of dopaminergic derivatives and anticholinergic drugs, can be helpful. Table 8–14 lists the drugs commonly used to treat Parkinson's disease.[15]

TABLE 8–13. COMMONLY USED NSAIDS

Drug	Trade Name	Method of Action	Side Effects	Drug Interactions
Indole acetic acids				
Tolmetin	Tolectin	Inhibits cyclooxygenase resulting in biosynthesis of prostaglandin	GI symptoms, dizziness, drowsiness, depression, rash, pruritus, headache, nervousness, chest pain, hypertension, tinnitus, edema, nausea/vomiting, asthenia, heartburn	Warfarin
Sulindac	Clinoril	Inhibits cyclooxygenase resulting in biosynthesis of prostaglandin	GI symptoms, drowsiness, dizziness, headache, nausea/vomiting, pruritus, rash, diarrhea	Oral anticoagulants, salicylates, furosemide, lithium, probenecid, β-adrenergic blockers, methotrexate
Indomethacin	Indocin	Inhibits cyclooxygenase resulting in biosynthesis of prostaglandin	GI symptoms, drowsiness, dizziness, somnolence, depression, fatigue, nausea, tinnitus, headache, diarrhea, vomiting	Oral anticoagulants, salicylates, loop or thiazide diuretics, lithium, captopril, probenecid, diflunisal, β-adrenergic blockers
Fenamic acids				
Meclofenamic acid, sodium salt, mono-hydrate	Meclomen	Inhibits cyclooxygenase resulting in biosynthesis of prostaglandin	Dizziness, tinnitus, edema, headache, nausea/vomiting, diarrhea, rash	Warfarin, salicylates
Mefenamic acid	Ponstel	Inhibits cyclooxygenase resulting in biosynthesis of prostaglandin	Diarrhea, nausea/vomiting, abdominal pain, anorexia, pyrosis, drowsiness, dizziness, nervousness, headache, blurred vision, insomnia, rash	Anticoagulants
Propionic acids				
Ibuprofen	Motrin	Inhibits cyclooxygenase resulting in biosynthesis of prostaglandin	GI symptoms (cramps, constipation) pruritus, tinnitus, dizziness, anxiety, headache, nausea/vomiting, aseptic meningitis	Coumarin-type anticoagulants, aspirin
Fenoprofen	Nalfon	Inhibits cyclooxygenase resulting in biosynthesis of prostaglandin	GI symptoms, occult blood in stool, somnolence, dizziness, rash, tremor, pruritus, headache, nervousness, dyspnea, fatigue, insomnia, decreased hearing	Salicylates, phenobarbital, coumarin-type anticoagulants
Naproxen	Naprosyn	Inhibits cyclooxygenase resulting in biosynthesis of prostaglandin	Blurred vision, edema, anorexia, shortness of breath, indigestion, tinnitus, constipation, nausea, drowsiness, dizziness, headache	Oral anticoagulants, furosemide, lithium, β-adrenergic blockers
Naproxen sodium	Anaprox	Inhibits cyclooxygenase resulting in biosynthesis of prostaglandin	Shortness of breath, indigestion, tinnitus, edema, itching, dizziness, drowsiness, headache, nausea, vomiting	Oral anticoagulants, naproxen, methotrexate, furosemide, lithium, β-adrenergic blockers, salicylates, probenecid
Ketoprofen	Orudis	Inhibits cyclooxygenase resulting in biosynthesis of prostaglandin	GI symptoms, headache, dizziness, drowsiness, constipation, nausea, vomiting, tinnitus, visual disturbances, urinary tract infection	Antacids, aspirin, diuretics, digoxin, warfarin, probenecid, methotrexate, lithium
Pyrazoles				
Phenylbutazone	Butazolidin	Inhibits cyclooxygenase resulting in biosynthesis of prostaglandin	Aplastic anemia, edema, water retention, GI distress, nausea, dyspepsia, rash	Anti-inflammatory agents, phenytoin, oral antidiabetics, sulfonamides, sodium valproate, coumarin-type anticoagulants, digitoxin hexobarbital, cortisone

(continued)

TABLE 8–13. COMMONLY USED NSAIDS (CONT.)

Drug	Trade Name	Method of Action	Side Effects	Drug Interactions
Phenylacetic acids				
Diclofenac sodium	Voltaren	Inhibits cyclooxygenase resulting in biosynthesis of prostaglandin	Peptic ulceration, GI bleeding, abdominal cramps, headache, fluid retention, diarrhea, indigestion, constipation, dizziness, tinnitus, rash, pruritus	Aspirin, cyclosporine, methotrexate, digoxin, oral hypoglyemics
Oxicams				
Piroxicam	Feldene	Inhibits cyclooxygenase resulting in biosynthesis of prostaglandin	Stomatitis, anorexia, GI distress, nausea, constipation, flatulence, diarrhea, dizziness, somnolence, headache, malaise, tinnitus, anemia, leukopenia, eosinophilia, edema	Lithium, aspirin
Salicylates				
Diflunisal	Dolobid	Inhibits cyclooxygenase resulting in biosynthesis of prostaglandin	Abdominal cramps, diarrhea, rash, somnolence, insomnia, dizziness, nausea/vomiting, dyspepsia, fatigue, tinnitus	Aspirin, naproxen, hydrochlorothiazides, antacids, sulindac, indomethacin
Salsalate	Disalcid	Inhibits cyclooxygenase resulting in biosynthesis of prostaglandin	Tinnitus, abdominal pain, abnormal hepatic function, anaphylactic shock, angioedema, vertigo, rash, bronchohepatitis, hypotension, urticaria, nephritis	Aspirin, anticoagulant, drugs, penicillin, triiodothyronine, thiopental, thyroxine, naproxen, warfarin, corticosteroids, methotrexate, thyroid hormone, sulfinpyrazone
Aspirin	Bufferin	Inhibits cyclooxygenase resulting in biosynthesis of prostaglandin	Stomach pain, heartburn, nausea, vomiting, increased rate of GI distress	Acetazolamide, alcohol, ammonium chloride, tolbutamide, chlorpropamide, probenecid, methotrexate, NSAIDs, phenytoin, penicillin, spironolactone, heparin, corticosteroids

TABLE 8–14. ANTIPARKINSON DRUGS

Drug	Trade Name
Anticholinergics	
Diphenhydramine	Benadryl
Biperiden	Akineton
Procyclidine	Kemadrin
Ethopropazine	Parsidol
Trihexyphenidyl	Artane
Orphenadrine	Disipal
Levodopa	
Levodopa/carbidopa	Sinemet
Amantidine	Symmetrel
Bromocriptine	Parlodel
Deprenyl	Selegiline

Psychological Regimens

The incidence of psychological complications in the older person is a known problem, and the management of these problems has always been a challenge. The most important step in the pharmacological management is proper diagnosis. Unfortunately, it is often the case that the patient and the physician accept the psychological complication as a natural occurrence of aging. For the sake of simplicity the mental disorders to be discussed in this section are:

1. Adjustment disorders.
2. Affective disorders.
3. Organic brain disorders.
4. Anxiety disorders.
5. Schizophrenic disorders.
6. Personality disorders.
7. Substance abuse disorders.

Adjustment disorders are time-limited responses to psychosocial stressors, the most common of which is the death of a spouse. The treatment is a short-acting medication for the relief of anxiety, agitation, and sleep disturbances. Short-acting benzodiazepine-type sedative/hypnotic or antianxiety agents are appropriate versus the use of antidepressants or antipsychotic medications.[15] Table 8–15 lists the commonly used antianxiety agents.

An unresolved adjustment disorder may lead to an affective disorder. Affective disorders are composed of depressive and manic depressive disorders. The manifestations of these major depressive disorders are increased physical complaints, memory problems, guilt, hopelessness, agitation, appetite disturbances, decreased energy, helplessness, and suicidal thoughts. The first line of treatment for these problems are antidepressant medications. The next effective line of treatment, providing there are no contraindications, is electroconvulsive shock therapy, tricyclics, and monoamine oxidase inhibitors (MAO). Because of the side effects of severe orthostatic hypotension, MAOs may need to be avoided, as well as tricyclic antidepressants for cardiac condition defects.[15] Manic depressive illness is treated with lithium carbonate and carbamazepine. Drugs used in the treatment of affective disorders are listed in Table 8–16.

Organic brain disorders are treated symptomologically (see Chapter 3 for a full description). Cognitive agents that supposedly stop or reverse the dementia are of little or no value. The symptom most treated is agitation, and the treatment of choice is short-acting sedative/hypnotics and antianxiety agents.[15] (See Table 8–16.)

Schizophrenic disorders usually have their onset before 45 years of age and are characterized by delusions, hallucinations, social withdrawal, and an inappropriate and flattened affect. The primary treatment for schizophrenia is antipsychotic drugs, which are associated with blocking central dopamine receptors in the brain. Older persons with schizophrenic disorders are usually treated with lower doses of antipsychotic agents with relatively good outcomes.[15] Table 8–17 lists antipsychotic drugs used in the treatment of schizophrenia.

Anxiety disorders usually have their onset in the young to middle adult years. Interventions are usually psychological and behavioral. Psychotropic (i.e., antianxiety medications) can be used adjunctly in severe situations.[15]

Personality disorders are lifelong patterns of maladaptive ways of relating to the world. The treatment of choice is behavior modification and psychotherapy. Psychotropics may be used, but many times they are discouraged because of the potential for addiction.[15]

Substance abuse disorders are characterized by withdrawal symptoms and the inability to control the use of a substance. The primary treatment is psychotherapy and behavior modification. However psychotropics can be used in the initial stages and then tapered off.

TABLE 8–15. ANTIANXIETY AGENTS

Drug	Trade Name	Method of Action	Side Effects	Drug Interactions
Benzodiazepines				
Diazepam	Valium	Facilitates neurotransmitter action of γ-aminobutyric acid (GABA), which mediates both pre- and postsynaptic inhibition in all regions of the CNS	Ataxia, drowsiness	Alcohol and other CNS depressants
Chlordiazepoxide hydrochloride	Librium	Facilitates neurotransmitter actions of γ-aminobutyric acid (GABA), which mediates both pre- and postsynaptic inhibition in all regions of the CNS	Drowsiness, ataxia, confusion	Alcohol and other CNS depressants
Clorazepate, dipotassium salt	Tranxene	Facilitate neurotransmitter action of γ-aminobutyric acid (GABA), which mediates both pre- and postsynaptic inhibition in all regions of the CNS	Drowsiness, dizziness, nervousness, dry mouth, blurred vision, headache, confusion	Alcohol and other CNS depressants
Lorazepam	Activan	Facilitates neurotransmitter action of γ-aminobutyric acid (GABA), which mediates both pre- and postsynaptic inhibition in all regions of the CNS	Sedation, dizziness, weakness, unsteadiness, disorientation, depression	Alcohol and other CNS depressants
Oxazepam	Serax	Facilitates neurotransmitter action of γ-aminobutyric acid (GABA), which mediates both pre- and postsynaptic inhibition in all regions of the CNS	Drowsiness, dizziness, vertigo, headache	Alcohol and other CNS depressants
Alprozolam	Xanax	Facilitates neurotransmitter action of γ-aminobutyric acid (GABA), which mediates both pre- and postsynaptic inhibition in all regions of the CNS	Drowsiness, dizziness, dry mouth, hypotension	Alcohol and other CNS depressants
Prazepam	Centrax	Facilitates neurotransmitter action of γ-aminobutyric acid (GABA), which mediates both pre- and postsynaptic inhibition in all regions of the CNS	Fatigue, dizziness, drowsiness, weakness, lightheadedness, ataxia	Alcohol and other CNS depressants
Nonbenzodiazepines				
Buspironic	Buspar	Unknown	Dizziness, drowsiness, nervousness, nausea, headache, fatigue	Trazodone, haloperidol, CNS active drugs, MAO inhibitors, warfarin

Gastrointestinal Drugs

Understanding the types of gastrointestinal drugs is important to the rehabilitation professional because a large proportion of patients use them. According to Peura, 60% to 100% of chronically ill patients suffer some type of stress related stomach problem.[23]

The good news about gastrointestinal drugs is that they do not produce any significant side effects that may impair rehabilitation. The only potential side effect may occur with the administration of opiates for the treatment of diarrhea due to their addictive nature. The most common gastrointestinal problems are gastric ulcers, diarrhea, and constipation.

TABLE 8–16. DRUGS USED IN THE TREATMENT OF AFFECTIVE DISORDERS

Drug	Trade Name	Method of Action	Side Effects	Drug Interactions
Tricyclic Antidepressants				
Desipramine hydrochloride	Norpramine	Inhibits membrane pump mechanism responsible for the reuptake of norepinephrine and serotonin at presynaptic nerve postsynaptic terminals	Tachycardia, nausea, vomiting, dizziness, headache, constipation, weight gain	Alcohol, cimetidine, CNS depressants, MAO inhibitors, sympathomimetics, anticholinergics, guanethidine
Doxepine	Sinequan	Inhibits membrane pump mechanism responsible for the reuptake of norepinephrine and serotonin at presynaptic nerve terminals, potentiating activity at postsynaptic terminals	Tachycardia, dry mouth, blurred vision, nausea, vomiting, dizziness, weakness, headache, constipation, urinary retention, weight gain	CNS depressants, anticholinergics, MAO inhibitors, clonidine, cimetidine, sympathomimetics, dicumarol, guanethidine
Amitriptyline	Elavil	Inhibits membrane pump mechanism responsible for the reuptake of norepinephine and serotonin at presynaptic nerve terminals, potentiating activity at postsynaptic terminals	Tachycardia, dry mouth, blurred vision, nausea, weakness, headache, constipation, urinary retention, weight gain	CNS depressants, anticholinergics, MAO inhibitors, sympathomimetics, guanethidine
Imipramine	Trofanil	Blocks uptake of norepinephrine at nerve endings	Orthostatic hypotension, hypertension, tachycardia, confusional states, delusions, anxiety, numbness, tingling, incoordination, dry mouth, blurred vision, constipation, jaundice, nausea/vomiting	CNS depressants, guanethidine
Nortriptyline	Pamelor	Blocks uptake of norepinephrine at nerve endings	Orthostatic hypotension, hypertension, tachycardia, confusional states, delusions, anxiety, numbness, tingling, blurred vision, incoordination, dry mouth, constipation, nausea/vomiting	CNS depressants, thyroid medication, guanethidine and other antihypertensives
Trimipramine	Surmontil	Unknown	Hypotension, hypertension, confusional states, delusions, numbness, jaundice, tingling, blurred vision, rash, nausea/vomiting	Local decongestants, catecholamine, MAO inhibitors, anticholinergics, sympathomimetics, alcohol, cimetidine
Protriptyline	Vivactil	Unknown	Myocardial infarction, stroke, heart block, hypotension, confusional states, delusions, anxiety, incoordination, seizures, tremors, dizziness, drowsiness, jaundice, urinary retention, nausea/vomiting, anorexia	Guanethidine, thyroid medication, CNS depressants, neuroleptic, sympathomimetics, cimetidine
MAO inhibitors				
Isocarboxazid	Marplan	Potent inhibitor of amine oxidase	Orthostatic hypotension, dizziness, vertigo, disturbance in cardiac rate, headache, tremors and muscle twitches, mania, confusion, weakness, fatigue, blurred vision	Sympathomimetics, MAO inhibitors, caffeine, tryptophan, benzodiazepines, clomipramine hydrochloride, buspirone, CNS depressants

(continued)

TABLE 8–16. DRUGS USED IN THE TREATMENT OF AFFECTIVE DISORDERS (CONT.)

Drug	Trade Name	Method of Action	Side Effects	Drug Interactions
Maprotiline	Ludiomil	Blocks norepinephrine reuptake	Nervousness, drowsiness, dizziness, tremor, dry eyes and blurred vision, weakness, fatigue, headache, constipation	MAO inhibitors, general anesthetics, CNS depressants, sympathomimetics, thyroid sympathomimetics, guanethidine, phenothiazine, cimetidine
Tranylcypromine	Parnate	Nonhydrazine MAO inhibitors, increases concentration of norepinephrine and serotonin	Hypertensive crisis, headaches, restlessness, insomnia, weakness, drowsiness, dizziness, diarrhea, abdominal pain, tinnitus, muscle spasm, jerks	MAO inhibitors, benzodiazepines, CNS depressants, caffeine, antihistamine anaesthetic drugs, buspirone, meperidine, tyramine, antiparkinson drugs, dextromethorphan, antihypertensives
Phenelzine	Nardil	MAO inhibitors	Postural hypotension, dizziness, headache, drowsiness, fatigue, constipation, GI distress	MAO inhibitors, other antidepressants, fluoxetin, thiazide, diuretics, β-blockers, benzodiazepines, buspirone, antihypertensives
Amoxepine	Asendine	Blocks norepinephrine and serotonin reuptake	Drowsiness, blurred vision, anorexia, insomnia, nausea, dizziness, headache	Neuroleptic, MAO inhibitors, anticholinergic drugs, CNS depressants, cimetidine
Alprazolam	Xanax	Increases CNS GABA effects	Drowsiness, dizziness, hypotension, dry mouth	CNS depressants
Carbamazepine	Carbamazepine	Unknown	Dizziness, drowsiness, nausea, vomiting, unsteadiness, bone marrow depression, urticaria, congestive heart failure, edema, aggravation of hypertension, syncope, collapse, fever, pneumonia, aplastic anemia	Phenobarbital, primidone, warfarin, doxycycline, haloperidol, phenytoin, erythromycin, cimetidine, calcium-channel blockers, lithium propoxyphene, theophylline
Lithium carbonate	Carbolith	Alters sodium transport in nerve and muscle cells; it is not known how it controls mania	Blackout spells, tremor, muscle hyperirritability, ataxia, slurred speech, dizziness, vertigo, weight loss, cardiac arrhythmia, hypotension, anorexia, nausea/vomiting, blurred vision, fatigue, lethargy	Haloperidol, antipsychotic medications, neuromuscular blocking agents, indomethacin, piroxicam, NSAIDs, ACE inhibitors, enalapril, captopril

Gastric ulcers, or the hemorrhaging and ulceration of the stomach lining due to an above-normal amount of acids being produced, can be treated in a variety of ways. The main treatment is antacids. Other commonly used medications are H_2 receptor blockers, anticholinergics, and sucralfate. See Table 8–18 for dosages, side effects, and trade names.[20,23]

Antidiarrheal agents mainly take three forms: absorbants, bacterial cultures, and opiate derivatives. Absorbants, such as pectin and kaolin, have essentially no side effects and work by absorbing excess fluid. Bacterial cultures are used to replace specific active cultures that for some reason may be deficient. They do, however, have minor intestinal gas and flatulence as side effects. Finally, opiate derivatives are, perhaps, the most effective agents in the treatment of diarrhea.[22] They

TABLE 8–17. ANTIPSYCHOTIC DRUGS

Drug	Trade Name	Method of Action	Side Effects	Drug Interactions
Phenothiazine derivatives				
Chlorpromazine	Thorazine	Unknown, has actions at all levels of CNS, strong central adrenergic blocking activity	Tardive dyskinesia, drowsiness, jaundice, agranulocytosis, postural hypotension, tachycardia, fainting	CNS depressants (alcohol, barbiturates, etc.), oral anticoagulants
Trifluoperazine	Stelazine	Unknown, has actions at all levels of CNS, strong central adrenergic blocking activity	Tardive dyskinesia, jaundice, rash, pseudoparkinsonism, dystonias, motor restlessness, drowsiness, dizziness, dry mouth, fatigue, muscle weakness	CNS depressants, oral anticoagulants, propranolol, dilantin, guanethidine, other antihypertensives, thiazide, diuretics, amipaque
Fluphenazine	Prolixin	Unknown, has actions at all levels of CNS, strong central adrenergic blocking activity	Hypertension, nausea, salivation, polyuria, perspiration, dry mouth, headache, constipation, weight change	Epinephrine, alcohol, CNS depressants, anticholinergics
Mesordazine	Serentil	Acts indirectly on reticular formation; depression of hypothalamic centers	Drowsiness, hypotension, parkinsonism, dizziness, weakness, restlessness, dystonia, rigidity, dry mouth, blurred vision, nausea, slurring, fainting	CNS depressants
Promethazine	Phenergan	Unknown antitussive effect on the CNS; also has anticholinergic effects	Drowsiness, rash, nausea/vomiting, blurred vision, dry mouth, dizziness	Alcohol and other CNS depressants, anticholinergic agents, MAO inhibitors
Prochlorperazine	Compazine	Competitively blocks postsynaptic dopamine receptors in cerebral cortex, basal ganglia, hypothalamus, limbic system, medulla, and brain stem	Drowsiness, dizziness, blurred vision, hypourticaria, extrapyramidal reaction, tardive dyskinesia	Alcohol, metrizamide, CNS depressants, anticoagulants, anticholinergics, β-adrenergic blocking drugs, guanethidine
Thioridazine	Mellaril	Competitively blocks postsynaptic dopamine receptors in the cerebral cortex, basal ganglia, hypothalamus, limbic system, medulla, and brain stem	Drowsiness, dizziness, dry mouth, constipation, blurred vision, extrapyramidal reactions, tardive dyskinesia, dermatitis	CNS depressants, anticholinergics, guanethidine
Thioxanthene derivatives				
Thiothixene	Navane	Competitively blocks postsynaptic dopamine receptors in the cerebral cortex, hypothalamus, basal ganglia, limbic system, medulla, and brain stem	Tachycardia, extrapyramidal symptoms, drowsiness, tardive dyskinesia, urticaria, weakness, photosensitivity, diarrhea, pruritus	CNS depressants, anticholinergics
Butyrophenone derivatives				
Haloperidol	Haldol	Blocks postsynaptic dopamine receptors in the cerebral cortex basal ganglia, hypothalamus, limbic system, medulla, and brain stem	Hypotension, insomnia, tachycardia, restlessness, anxiety, lightheadedness, tardive dyskinesia, blurred vision, photosensitivity, nausea/vomiting, rash, pruritus	CNS depressants, guanethidine, anticonvulsants, lithium

TABLE 8–18. DRUG TREATMENTS FOR GASTRIC ULCERS

Drug	Trade Name	Method of Action	Dosages
Antacids			
Sodium bicarbonate	Alka-Selzer	Neutralization of gastric acid	1–2 tablets every 4 hr as needed
Aluminum hydroxide	Basaljel	Relief of hyperacidity	2 capsules as often as every 2 hr, up to twelve daily
	Amphogel	Relief of hyperacidity	2 tablets of 0.3 g or 1 tablet of 0.6 g strength five to six times daily
Aluminum hydroxide, magnesium	Maalox	Neutralization of acidity	1–2 tablets well chewed, or 1–2 tsp at meals and bedtime
	Mylanta	Neutralization of acidity	2–4 tablets well chewed, or 2–4 tsp after meals and at bedtime
Magaldrate	Riopan	Rapid and uniform buffering action	Chew or swallow 1–2 tablets or 1–2 tsp between meals and at bedtime
H receptor blockers			
Cimitedine	Tagamet	Inhibits histamine at the H receptors on gastric cells	300 mg four times/day
Ranitidine	Zantac	Inhibits histamine at the H receptors on gastric cells	100–150 mg two times daily
Famotidine	Pepcid	Inhibits histamine at the H receptors on gastric cells	40 mg once daily at bedtime
Anticholinergics Please see Table 8–7.			
Sucralfate	Carafate	Formation of ulcer adherent complex, which covers the ulcer site and protects it against further attack by acid, pepsin, and bile salts	1 g twice daily
Metoclopramide	Reglan	Stimulates motility in the upper GI tract	10–15 mg up to q.i.d. 30 min before a meal or bedtime

slow intestinal peristalsis, but offer such side effects as nausea, gastrointestinal disturbances, drowsiness, constipation, and fatigue.[23] Table 8–19 lists the common drugs, trade names, methods of action, and dosage for each.[22,23,24]

Laxatives, commonly used agents in the older population, are present in four different forms: bulk forming, stimulant, hyperostotic, and lubricant or stool softeners. Prior to using laxatives, the rehabilitation professional may want to encourage the patient to exercise. Decreased activity has been shown to lower gastric motility.[24] A major concern in laxative administration is the potential for abuse with long-term usage. Table 8–20 provides a list of a few of the common laxatives, their trade names, methods of action, and side effects.[24]

COMPLIANCE AND MOTIVATION IN DRUG REGIMENS

The issue of compliance must be addressed when discussing pharmaceutical management of disease. The use of medications in the management of physical illness

TABLE 18–9. ANTIDIARRHEAL AGENTS

Drugs	Trade Name	Method of Action	Dosages
Absorbants			
Kaolin, pectin	Kaelin	Absorption of excess fluid and causative agent	60–120 mL regular strength suspension after each loose bowel movement
Bacterial cultures			
Lactobacillus acidophilus	———	Administered to reestablish flora	2 capsules, 4 tablets, or 1 packet, 2–4 times daily
Lactobacillus bulgaris	———	Administered to reestablish flora	2 capsules, 4 tablets, or 1 packet, 2–4 times daily
Opiate derivatives			
Diphenoxylate	Lomotil	Binds to intestine opiate receptors, decreasing peristalsis	5 mg, 4 times daily
Loperamide	Imodium	Unknown	4 mg unit or 2 after each unformed stool

is only as useful as the patient's ability to adhere to the program. This final section will explore compliance behaviors of older patients.

Health professionals appear to believe that older persons are less compliant. In reality, older patients are no more noncompliant than younger patients.[25] However, a statistical relationship does exist between noncompliance and patients taking multiple drugs.[25] Other factors involved in noncompliance are unmanageable

TABLE 8–20. LAXATIVES

Drug	Trade Name	Method of Action	Side Effects
Bulk forming			
Psyllium	Metamucil	Polycarbophil absorbs water in the GI tract to form a gelatinous bulk that encourages a normal bowel movement	Powder may cause allergic reaction if inhaled
Perdiem	———	Vegetable mucilages soften stool and provide pain-free evacuation	Laxative dependance, excessive water and body salt loss
Stimulants			
Castor oil	Fleet-flavored castor oil	Works directly on small intestine to promote a bowel movement	Laxative dependance, excessive water and salt loss
Bisacodyl	Ducolax	Contact laxative directly on colonic mucosa to produce peristalsis through the large intestine	Abdominal cramps
Phenophthalein	Modane	Acts on large intestine to produce semifluid stool	Excess bowel activity, abdominal discomfort, cramps, weakness, dizziness, palpitations
Hyperosmotic			
Lactulose	Chronolac	Broken down in the colon to lactic acid, formic and acetic acids; causes an increase in stool water content	Intestinal cramps nausea/vomiting, flatulence
Sodium	Fleet	Versatile in action	Laxative dependance, sodium loss
Phosphate	Phospho-soda	As gentle laxative or purgative	
Lubricants & stool softeners			
Docusate	Pericolace, Disonate	Provides general peristaltic stimulation and helps keep stools soft	Nausea, abdominal cramping, rash, diarrhea
Mineral oil	Fleet mineral oil enema	Contact softens and lubricates hard stools	Abdominal pain

costs, physical weakness, and impaired vision or hearing.[26] These factors tend to be more prevalent in older persons and may be the reason health professionals see older persons in general as noncompliant. In recognizing noncompliance, the therapist should look at these factors as contributors to the problem instead of describing all older people as noncompliant.

The simplest initial step in enhancing patient compliance is giving clear, simple, and explicit instructions. Sometimes prescribing physicians omit this important information. Physical therapists can assist in assuring compliance by researching and reiterating the correct drug procedure in concise and easily understandable terms. Devices such as pill containers, charts, and booklets may enhance compliance. A therapist may suggest these alternatives to the physician of a noncompliant patient. The supplementation of the medication regimen with clear instructions and devices, though, may still not alleviate the noncompliance problem. The literature is still unclear as to what is the best answer in this case, and it appears that no program is completely effective.[25]

It appears that the best intervention for noncompliance is to understand why the patient does or does not comply. In this regard, an interesting group to study are the self-regulators. Often this group does better than the strict compliers. This information tells the therapist to respect the patient's input into designing and monitoring the rehabilitation program in both the medication and exercise aspects. In the medication aspect, the therapist can act as an advocate for the patient.

Finally, the practitioner–patient relationship is an extremely important factor in appropriate patient compliance.[25] When a practitioner questions a patient about compliance, the most honest and useful answers are obtained when the questions are nonthreatening. In addition, explanations on the importance of compliance are also enhanced when the practitioner uses a positive tone, explains clearly, and has a close relationship with the patient.[27]

PEARLS

- Even though the elderly compose less than 15% of the population, they consume 31% of all prescription medications.

- The four stages of pharmacokinetics (absorption, distribution, biotransformation, and excretion) are all diminished with age, which will affect the impact of a medication when taken by an older person.

- The most common adverse reactions or side effects of drug use seen in the elderly are postural hypotension, fatigue, weakness, depression, confusion, movement disorders, incontinence, anticholinergic actions, dizziness, extrapyramidal signs, and volume depletion.

- Cardiovascular regimens revolve around controlling congestive heart failure, hypertension, angina pectoris, cardiac arrhythmias, and arteriosclerosis.

- Common neuromusculoskeletal regimens are designed to manage arthritis, neuralgias, stroke, and Parkinson's disease.

- Psychological drug regimens can be used for adjustment, affective, organic brain, anxiety, schizophrenic, personality, and substance abuse disorders. The most important step in this area is proper diagnosis.

- Gastrointestinal drugs are commonly used by the elderly; they have minimal side effects that may impair rehabilitation.

- Compliance and motivation for using drugs appropriately by the aged can be enhanced by initially assessing the economic and physical decrements of the person and then providing clear and simple instructions.

REFERENCES

1. Baum C, Kennedy DL, Forbes MB, et al. Drug Use in the United States in 1981. *JAMA.* 1984; 251:1293–1297.
2. Simonson W. *Medications and the Elderly.* Rockville, Md: Aspen; 1984:7–41.
3. Yee B, Williams B, O'Hara N. Medication Management and Appropriate Substance Use for Elderly Persons. In Lewis, ed. *Aging: Health Care's Challenge,* 2nd ed. Philadelphia: F.A. Davis; 1990:298–330.
4. Krammer P. Influences of Aging in Drug Disposition and Response. *Top Geriatr Rehab.* 1987; 2(3):12–23.
5. White D, Lewis C. The older patient and the effects of drugs on rehabilitation. In: Malone T (ed.): *Physical and Occupational Therapy: Drug Implications of Practice.* Philadelphia: JB Lippincott; 1989:144–182.
6. Myers-Robfogel MW, Bosmann HB. Clinical pharmacology in the aged-aspects of pharmacokinetics and drug sensitivity. In: Williams TF (ed.): *Rehabilitation in the Aging.* New York: Raven Press; 1984:23–40.
7. Robertson D. Drug handling in old age. In: Brocklehurst JC (ed.): *Geriatric Pharmacology and Therapeutics.* Boston: Blackwell Scientific Publications; 1984:41–59.
8. Woo E. Drug treatment of the elderly. In: Walshe TM (ed.): *Manual of Clinical Problems in Geriatric Medicine.* Boston: Little, Brown; 1985:21–26.
9. Stevenson IH. Pharmacokinetics in advancing age. In: Barbagallo-Sangiorgi G, Exton-Smith AN (eds.): *Aging and Drug Therapy.* New York: Plenum Press; 1984:1–9.
10. Lamy PP: Comparative Pharmacokinetics Changes and Drug Therapy in an Older Population. *J Am Geriatr Soc.* 1982; 30:S11–S19.
11. May FE, Stewart RB, Hale W, et al.: Prescribed and nonprescribed drug use in an ambulatory elderly population. *South Med Journ* 1982; 75:522–528.
12. Davidson W. Treatment of orthostatic hypotension. In: Barbagallo-Sangiorgi G, Exton-Smith AN (eds.): *Aging and Drug Therapy.* New York: Plenum Press; 1984:345–355.
13. Chapron D, Besdine RW. Drugs as an obstacle to rehabilitation of the elderly: A primer for therapists. *Top Geriatr Rehab.* 1987; 2(3):63–81.
14. Eddy L. *Physical Therapy Pharmacology.* St. Louis: C.V. Mosby; 1991:71–99.
15. Eddy L. *Physical Therapy Pharmacology.* St. Louis: C.V. Mosby; 1991:99–115.
16. Chapron DJ. Clinical pharmacology in the elderly: Recognizing and preventing of adverse drug effects during rehabilitation. In Jackson O (ed.): *Physical Therapy of the Geriatric Patient,* 2nd ed. New York: Churchill Livingstone; 1989:145–173.
17. Lye M. Cardiovascular system—Digitalis glycosides. In Brockelhurst JC (ed.): *Geriatric Pharmacology and Therapeutics.* Boston: Blackwell Scientific Publications; 1984:71–86.
18. WHO Expert Committee. Arterial hypertension. Technical Report, Series 628. Geneva: World Health Organization; 1978.
19. Kannel W, Gordon T. *The Framingham Study: An Epidemiological Investigation of Cardiovascular Disease,* Washington, D.C.: U.S. Government Printing Office; 1970.
20. Ciccione C. *Pharmacology in Rehabilitation,* Vol. 4. Philadelphia: F.A. Davis; 1990:188–285.
21. Sack K: Update on NSAID's in the elderly. *Geriatrics.* 1989; 44(5):71–90.
22. Chapron DJ. Drug–drug interactions in the elderly: A potential consequence of polypharmacy. *Top Geriatr Rehab.* 1987; 2(3):54–62.
23. Peura D, Freston J. Introduction: Evolving perspectives on parenteral H_2 receptor antagonist therapy. *Am J Med.* 1987; 18:1–2(suppl 6a).
24. Ciccione C. *Pharmacology in Rehabilitation,* Vol. 4. Philadelphia: F.A. Davis; 1990:188–285.
25. Fuchinetti N. Adherence by patients to prescribed therapies: A social psycholic perspective. *Top Geriatr Rehab.* 1987; 2(3):33–45.
26. Haynes RB, Sackett DL, Taylor DW, et al. Manipulation of the therapeutic regime to improve compliance: Conceptions and misconceptions. *Clin Pharmacol Ther.* 1977; 22:125–130.
27. Becker MH. Patient adherence to prescribed therapies. *Med Care.* 1985; 23:539–555.

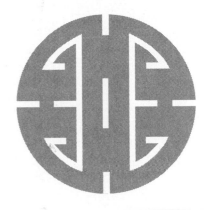

PART II

Patient Care Concepts

CHAPTER NINE

Principles and Practice in Geriatric Rehabilitation

Normal aging is not necessarily burdened with disability; even though almost all conditions that cause disability are more frequently seen in the older population. As a result, the aged are more likely to require assessment for rehabilitative services. The mutual exclusion of geriatrics and rehabilitation is unjustified, and functional assessment for needed rehabilitative services should be an essential part of routine evaluation by all health care disciplines working with the aged population. Geriatrics teaches that maximal functional capabilities be attained; therefore, it can be argued that rehabilitation is the foundation of geriatric care. The purpose of this chapter is to provide clinicians with a knowledge of rehabilitation principles and practices in working with the aged individual to help them apply interventions to provide high quality care.

The basis of geriatric rehabilitation is to assist the disabled aged in recovering lost physical, psychological, or social skills so that they may become more independent, live in personally satisfying environments, and maintain meaningful social interactions. This may be done in any number of settings, including acute and subacute care settings, rehabilitation centers, home and office settings, or in long-term care facilities, such as nursing homes.

Because of the complexity of the interventions needed in dealing with the aged, an interdisciplinary team approach is required for rehabilitation. The rehabilitation process also requires that the patients and their families be educated. Finally, rehabilitation is more than a medical intervention: It is a philosophical approach that recognizes that diagnoses and chronological age are poor predictors of functional abilities, that interventions directed at enhancing function are important, and that the "team" should always include patients and their families.

DISABILITY: A DEFINITION

The meaning of "disability" is key to an understanding of rehabilitation. When referring to alterations in people's function, three terms are often used interchangeably: impairment, disability, and handicap. A more distinct understanding of these concepts is useful in geriatric rehabilitation, and a "systems approach" is the most useful. In the systems approach a problem at the organ level (e.g., an infarct in the right hemisphere) must be viewed not only in terms of its effects on the brain, but also in terms of its effects on the person, the family, the society, and, ultimately, the nation. It goes beyond the pure "medical model," in which only the current medical problem is assessed to determine rehabilitative goals. From this perspective "impairment" refers to a loss of physical or physiological function at the organ level. This could include alterations in heart function, nerve conduction velocity, or muscle strength. Impairments usually do not affect the ability to function. However, if an impairment is so severe that it inhibits the ability to function normally, then it becomes a "disability." Rehabilitation interventions are most often oriented toward adaptation to or recovery from disabilities. Given the proper training or adaptive equipment, people with disabilities can pursue independent lives. Obstructions in the pursuit of independence can arise, however, when people with disabilities confront inaccessible buildings or situations that limit rehabilitation interventions, such as low toilet seats, buttons on an elevator that are too high, or signs that are not readable. In these cases a disability becomes a "handicap." Society's environment creates the handicap.

This chapter will be primarily concerned with the rehabilitative approaches employed to reduce disabilities.

DEMOGRAPHICS OF DISABILITY IN THE AGED

The aged are disproportionately affected by disabling conditions when compared to younger cohorts. According to Wedgewood,[1] the old-old age group (85 plus years of age) comprises the highest percentage of disabled persons; indeed, 40% of all disabled persons are over the age of 65. Three-fourths of all cerebrovascular accidents occur in persons over the age of 65[2]; the highest incidence of amputations have been reported in the aged[3]; and hip fractures occur the most frequently between the ages of 70 and 78, on the average.[4] The Federal Council on Aging has reported that, of all those persons studied over the age of 65, 86% have at least one chronic condition and 52% have limitations in their activities of daily living (ADLs).[5] It is the impact of these disabilities on the level of independence that needs to be considered, rather than the presence of an impairment or disability.

Disabilities in old age are associated with a higher mortality rate, a decreased life span, greater chronic health problems (e.g., cardiovascular, musculoskeletal, or neurological), and an increased expenditure for health care. Disabilities resulting in an inability to ambulate, feed oneself, or manage basic ADLs, like toileting or self-hygiene (e.g., bathing), are strong predictors of the loss of functional independence and an increased burden on care givers.[6] The greater the disability, the greater the risk of institutionalization. Rehabilitative measures can be cost effective when they enhance the patient's functional ability and help him or her to attain greater levels of independence. Higher functional capabilities and greater levels of independence have been associated with fewer hospitalizations and a lower mortality rate among the aged.[7,8]

Geriatric rehabilitation includes both institutional and noninstitutional services for the aged with chronic medical conditions that are marked by deviation from the normal state of health and manifested in physical impairment. Unless treated, these conditions can have the potential for causing substantial, and frequently cumulative, disability. The aged with disabilities need assistance with such daily functions as bathing, dressing, and walking. This increased need for help is often compounded when there is no spouse, nearby family, or friends able to assist the patient. With social isolation, which is common in the aged, continuing professional medical care is required to ward off the debilitating effects of inactivity and depression.

FUNCTIONAL ASSESSMENT OF THE AGED

The assessment of functional capabilities is the cornerstone of geriatric rehabilitation. The ability to walk, to transfer (e.g., from bed to chair or chair to toilet), and manage basic ADLs independently is often the determinant of whether hospitalized aged patients will be discharged home or to an extended-care facility. Functional assessment tools that are practical, reliable, and valid are necessary to assist all interdisciplinary team members in determining the need for rehabilitation or long-term care services. In the home care setting, precise assessment of the patient's functional level can detect early deterioration and allow for immediate intervention.

In response to the growing importance of chronic diseases and the need for long-term care, the Commission on Chronic Illness was established in 1949.[9] The Commission highlighted the importance of function and disability, and concluded that there was a need for a means of classifying functional ADLs.[10]

Since that time functional assessment tools have gone through many evolutional stages. Early in this evolution scales included such variables as locomotion and traveling, dressing, toileting, eating, and hand activities like managing coins or knitting.[11] Some assessment tools addressed bowel and bladder function,[12] while others had measures for muscle strength, overall functional capacity, communication, and behavior.

From these early efforts, a series of more sophisticated methodologic scales were developed under the direction and sponsorship of the National Institute on Aging, the Administration on Aging, and the National Center for Health Services Research. These studies were concerned with the reliability, validity, and usefulness of the various tools proposed. Among those who helped to clarify the theoretical framework for functional assessment, Lawton proposed a behavioral model in which function is viewed within a hierarchy of domains.[13] Each domain includes a set of functions that can be ordered along a continuum from simple to complex activities. For example, the simple task might be the act of picking up the telephone receiver while the more complex task would be picking up the telephone receiver and dialing a number. This model revealed the component ADLs covering more than one domain of self-maintainance functions within a broader set of functions. For instance, Lawton included mobility and ambulation (or locomotion) as basic self-maintainance functions that enabled an aged individual to adjust and adapt within their environment. For example, the ability to ambulate one block and ascend and descend four stairs would enable the aged person to walk to the bus stop and board a bus.

Lawton's conception of functional capacity defined three levels of ADLs: (1)

basic ADLs, including such self-care activities as bathing, dressing, toileting, continence, and feeding; (2) instrumental activities of daily living (IADLs), such as using the telephone, driving, shopping, housekeeping, cooking, laundry, managing money, and managing medications; (3) mobility, described as a more complicated combination of IADL activities, such as leaving one's residence and moving from one location to another by using public transportation. Mobility and IADL are more complex and are concerned with people's ability to cope with their environments. This classification of ADL, IADL, and mobility has become standard in most functional assessment tools.

As a clinical tool, functional assessment scales are invaluable. Initial assessment identifies areas of functional deficit and can assist the clinicians in developing treatment regimens that address specific needs. Subsequent assessments measure progress toward the rehabilitation's goals. On a broad scale, functional assessment can assist public policymakers in the provision of health care services by determining the level of need within a population. Demographically, it is apparent that Americans are living longer; the question is, are the additional years of life years of vigor and independence or years of frailty and dependence?

By design, functional assessment scales are meant to determine specific outcomes. Outcomes of interest to those working with the aged include mortality, hospitalization, institutionalization, special interventions, and declining physical function, to name a few. Numerous functional assessment tools are available to determine physical, emotional, cognitive, and social functioning in various care settings. Table 6–5 summarizes a number of ADL and IADL scales and indexes, including those summarized by Branch and Meyers.[14] Though this table of functional assessment tools is not exhaustive, it represents a relatively comprehensive reference list of existing scales. In reviewing this list, the reader will notice some tools include only basic ADL skills (more useful in the institutional setting), while others are comprehensive and include all three levels of functioning as defined by Lawton (more useful in discharge planning and the home care setting).

FUNCTIONAL ABILITIES OF THE CARE GIVER: A REHABILITATIVE CONSIDERATION

Aged patients, given a choice, would prefer to stay at home rather than recuperate and rehabilitate in an institutional setting. The aged have strong ties to their homes, and the help of spouses, relatives, and friends is a crucial component in making rehabilitation in the home possible. Home care by professionals can protect the health of informal care givers and maximize the patient's ability to perform ADLs by including a systematic assessment of the living environment as a key part of care planning. Provision of such assistance openly acknowledges that care givers (often aged themselves) have some decrease in physical ability that needs to be considered as it relates to caring for disabled relatives. It has been demonstrated that more than 90% of persons 75 to 84 years of age can manage, without help, to perform such tasks as grooming, bathing, dressing, and eating.[15] The more complicated skills of transferring and ambulation are more compromised, with more than 50% of persons aged 75 to 84 years of age presenting with limitations in their capabilities of performing these activities without assistance. These ADLs require greater assistive skills on the part of the care giver. Assessment of the home environment needs to incorporate the abilities (or disabilities) of the individual(s) providing care. Adaptive equipment, such as a sliding board for transfers or a rolling walker for ambulation, are available to assist the care giver in caring for a spouse, relative, or friend. Attention to the abilities of the care giver can facilitate the ease of care and decrease the burden placed on the care giver. The provision of home health care services may be necessitated when safety is an issue. Thorough evaluation of the functional capabilities of the aged individual and the care giver, in addition to assessment of the environmental obstacles that may be encountered, will increase the likelihood of a positive outcome.

PRINCIPLES OF GERIATRIC REHABILITATION

Three major principles are important in the rehabilitation of the aged. First, the variability of the aged must be considered. Variability of capabilities within an aged group is much more pronounced than within younger cohorts. What one 80 year old can do physically, cognitively, or motivationally, another may not be able to accomplish. Second, the concept of activity is key in rehabilitation of the aged. Many of the changes over time are attributable to disuse. And third, optimum health is directly related to optimum functional ability. In acute situations rehabilitation must be directed toward (1) stabilizing the primary problem(s); (2) preventing secondary complications, such as bed sores, pneumonias, and contractures; and (3) restoring lost functions. In chronic situations rehabilitation is directed primarily toward restoring lost functions. This can best be accomplished by promoting maximum health so that the aged are best able to adapt to their care environment and to their disabilities. Each of these principles—variability, inactivity, and optimum health—will be discussed in greater detail in the following sections.

Variability of the Aged

Unlike any other age group, the aged are more variable in their level of functional capabilities. In the clinic, we often see 65-year-old individuals who are severely physically disabled, and yet, sitting right alongside of that individual is a 65 year old who is still building houses and felling trees. Even in the old-old, variability in physical and cognitive functioning is remarkable. For example, at one end of the spectrum is John Kelly who, at the age of 87, is still running the Boston Marathon, while at the other end of the spectrum is a frail bedridden 87-year-old person in a nursing home who is not responsive to his or her environment. The differences that can be identified cognitively are just as remarkable. The spectrum moves from the demented institutionalized aged to those aged who are presidents and Supreme Court justices. Chronological age is a poor indicator of physical or cognitive function.

The impact of this variability is an important consideration when defining rehabilitation principles and the practices of the aged. A wide range of rehabilitative services has to be provided to address the varying needs of the aged population in different care settings. Awareness of this heterogeneity helps to combat the myths and stereotypes of aging and presents a foundation for developing creative rehabilitation programs for the aged. Older persons tend to be more different from themselves (as a collective group) than other segments of the population. Given this fact, interdisciplinary team members, policymakers, and planners in rehabilitation settings need to be prepared to design a wide range of services and treatment interventions. This becomes more difficult as the number of aged increase and the budget decreases, however, creating new and innovative rehabilitation programs could ultimately improve the functional capabilities and the resulting quality of life for many aged individuals.

Examples of Variability in Aging

Reaction time is one variable to be considered in the aged patient. In general, reaction time tends to slow with age,[16] but this is not necessarily a decline in the functioning of the nervous system. Such an assumption may result in inaccuracies such as decreasing the amount and intensity of exercise and rehabilitative measures that older persons require. Research indicates that those aged who are more physically active are capable of performing as well as, and in some cases better than, younger subjects on reaction time performance tasks.[17] Reaction time is a complex variable that may be affected by disease or social stigma. For example, an aged individual with arthritis may react slower because of stiff and painful joints. Their discomfort may lead to a sense of physical instability and inadequate physical adaptability, and it may result in a fear of falling. When evaluating functional capabilities, underlying pathologies or a sense of a social parameter (fear or discomfort) that may have an impact on a person's functioning may be discovered. Seeing variability in the older person in the area of reaction time may help to determine causes for functional declines in other areas.

There is a marked range of visual capabilities in the aged that also impacts on aged person's reaction time and ability to function safely in a given environment. Several changes normally occur within the aging eye:

1. The lens begins to thicken and becomes yellowed.
2. The muscles that control dilation of the pupil weaken.
3. The older eye needs three times the amount of light to function adequately.
4. The thickening of the lens and delayed pupil dilation means that the glare and reflections often encountered in the environment cannot be tolerated.[18]
5. The older person has difficulty with depth perception and color differentiation, which can interfere with ambulation, ADLs, and driving an automobile.

The combination of these visual changes presents many ramifications and creates many obstacles for the aged person. A decline in visual acuity may ultimately result in a decrease in function. Even when errors of the aged refraction are corrected, a loss of visual receptors in the aging retina or macula will result in a decrease of acuity. Fortunately, with modern technology, the majority of older people are able to maintain a high degree of visual function and independence. Research indicates that visual capabilities do not normally decline as part of aging. Instead, like so many other systems, the eyes are affected by nutritional deficits and environmental hazards, such as intense sunlight, poor lighting, and airborne contaminants, all of which are preventable causes of visual loss.[19,20]

Strength is another variable that directly affects an aged individual's ability to function at their maximum capability. Strength measures in a group of 70+ year olds compared to a group of 40 to 50 year olds (both male and female subjects) showed a greater range in strength values in the 70+ year group.[21] Part of the variability results from the difficulty in separating age dependent muscles changes from other factors that influence muscle strength, such as physical activity, disease, cardiovascular condition, and hormonal and neural influences. The younger group had fewer confounding factors. This variability in strength leads to different levels of functioning within an aged population and will be discussed further in the subsequent section of this chapter.

Mental ability is another area that varies greatly within an aged population and directly affects the rehabilitation potential of an aged individual. The presence of a pathology, such as Alzheimer's disease, can severely influence an aged individual's ability to safely function within their environment. In the absence of a pathology, however, an individual's cognitive abilities have been shown to undergo little or no change.[22]

What happens to intelligence and cognition with age? The answers are many, complex, and controversial. Some researchers say that cognition enters a process of irreversible decline in the adult years, because the brain becomes less and less efficient, just as do the heart, lungs, and other physical organs.[23] Other investigators say that intelligence and cognition is relatively stable throughout the adult years, with the brain providing more than enough capacity for any brain functioning necessary until serious disease begins late in life.[24] Yet, other researchers indicate that cognition declines in some respects (mental quickness, for example) and increases in others (knowledge about life, for example).[25]

The decline of intelligence and cognition over the age of 65 or 70 is variable and subject to several interpretations. In addition to notions of inevitable biological decrement, intellectual and cognitive decline can be attributed to social isolation, decreasing motivation to perform irrelevant tasks, disease, or a combination of these factors.

All in all, many researchers have begun to believe that the search for the curve of normal deterioration in mental abilities is a fruitless task.[26] In this view, there is too much variability in age trends to postulate a particular one as normal or basic. Some people decline in intellectual ability; others increase. Some abilities seem to be increasing with each new generation; others seem to be decreasing. An environmental event (the development of television, for example) can change age trends for some people and have little effect on others. Thus the search goes on, but it is a search now for the determinants of change or stability and much less for inevitable and irreversible decrements.

The principle of variability in geriatric rehabilitation is key to providing therapeutic interventions that address the range of mental capabilities in aged individuals. Though cognitive decline occurs in patients in the rehabilitative setting, it is possible that healthy aged individuals who maintain an active intellectual life will show little or no loss of intellectual abilities into their 80s and beyond.

Activity Versus Inactivity

The most common reason for losses in functional capabilities in the aged is inactivity or immobility. There are numerous reasons for the immobilization of the aged. "Acute immobilization" is often considered to be accidental immobilization. Acute catastrophic illnesses include severe blood loss, trauma, head injury, cerebral vascular accidents, burns, and hip fractures to name only a few. The patient's activity level is often severely curtailed until acute the illness becomes medically stable. "Chronic immobilization" may result from long-standing problems that are undertreated or are left untreated. Examples of chronic problems include cerebral vascular accidents (strokes), amputations, arthritis, Parkinson's disease, cardiac disease, pulmonary disease, and low back pain. Environmental barriers are a major cause of "accidental immobilization" in both the acute and chronic care settings. These include bed rails, the height of the bed, physical restraints, an inappropriate chair, no physical assistance available, fall precautions imposed by medical staff, no orders in the chart for mobilization, social isolation, and environmental obstacles (stairs or doorway thresholds are examples). Cognitive impairments, central nervous system (CNS) disorders (such as cerebral vascular accidents, Parkinson's disease, and multiple sclerosis), peripheral neuropathies resulting from diabetes, and pain with movement can also severely reduce mobility. Affective disorders, such as depression, anxiety, or fear of falling, may also lead to accidental immobilization. In addition, sensory changes, terminal illnesses (such as cancer or cirrhosis of the liver), acute episodes of illnesses like pneumonia or cellulitis, or an attitude of "I'm too sick to get up" can negatively affect mobility.

The process of deconditioning involves changes in multiple organ systems, including the neurological, cardiovascular, and musculoskeletal systems, to varying degrees. Deconditioning is probably best defined as the multiple changes in organ system physiology that are induced by inactivity and reversed by activity (i.e., exercise).[27] The degree of deconditioning depends on the degree of superimposed inactivity and the prior level of physical fitness. The term "hypokinetics" has been coined to describe the physiology of inactivity.[28] Deconditioning can occur at many levels of inactivity. For simplicity and clarity, two major categories of inactivity or hypokinetics will be examined: the acute hypokinetic effects of bed rest and the chronic inactivity induced by a sedentary life-style or by chronic disease.

Looking at the aging process with one eye on the adverse affects of bed rest or hypokinetics as a possible concommitant of deconditioning and disability can lead to discovering more about the potential use of exercise as one of the primary rehabilitation modalities. The phrase "use it or lose it" is a concept with tremendous ramifications for aging, especially in geriatric rehabilitation. Exercise has not been viewed as an important factor in health until recently. Until the 1950s the rate-of-living theory was promoted. According to this theory, the body would be worn out faster and life shortened by the expenditure of energy during exercise.[29] Conversely, studies in the past decade have shown that regular exercise does not shorten life span and may in fact increase it.[30] Exercise is becoming increasingly viewed as beneficial for both the primary and secondary prevention of disease.[31]

There are several challenges to understanding the interaction between inactivity and health in older persons. The first is that the process of aging itself causes some changes that parallel the consequences of hypokinetics or inactivity. Several studies have provided strong evidence that separates the aging process from a sedentary life-style.[32–35] It has been found that aged individuals can improve their flexibility, strength, and aerobic capacity to the same extent as younger individuals. The second challenge in studying inactivity is separating the effects of inactivity from those of disease.[36] It is obvious that some effects of aging can be directly related to inactivity. Many aged individuals who are deconditioned may also have superimposition of acute or chronic disease. Studies on younger subjects have helped to clarify some of the effects of inactivity alone (i.e., bed rest on physiological changes and functional performance).

Another challenge exists: the challenge of understanding the relationship between physiological decline and functional loss. Is the inability to climb stairs in an 85 year old primarily a result of cardiovascular deconditioning, muscle weakness, impaired balance secondary to sensory losses, or a sedentary life-style? Is there a new disease process beginning? Is this normal aging? An important concept in geriatric rehabilitation is that threshold values of physiological functioning may exist.[37] An aged person, who is below these thresholds, may suddenly lose an essential functional skill. An understanding of the consequences of inactivity is particularly important when addressing the rehabilitation needs of the aged individual.

Inactivity's effect on the nervous system has not been studied as intensely as other organ systems. Perhaps this is related to the complexity of the nervous system and the lack of assessment techniques. In younger individuals changes in the nervous system with inactivity are minimal. In the aged, however—especially those individuals with concurrent acute or chronic illnesses—the consequences of inactivity on the nervous system may be particularly extreme.[38]

Bed rest has been compared to the experience of sensory deprivation. Zubek and Wilgosh,[39] in a study of prolonged immobilization (i.e., immobilized during the day followed by bed rest at night), showed that occipital lobe frequencies on EEG were substantially decreased in awake subjects. Exercise prevented some of these changes.[40] In addition to physical changes, performance on several intellectual tests deteriorated, including verbal fluency, color discrimination, and reversible figures.

In another study on sensory deprivation, young subjects were put on bed rest and periodically stimulated by audiotapes of disjointed conversations.[41] Within a 3 hour test period, the subject's perception of time intervals became distorted, and several subjects described hallucinatory-like experiences. Social isolation was also very disconcerting to the subjects and made them feel uncomfortable. Frequent complaints included feelings of loneliness and the longing for some sign of recognition from the investigator. In young subjects, other emotions occur during prolonged bed rest, such as anxiety, irritability, and a depressed mood.[42] These dramatic feelings occurred in healthy young persons during a 3 hour bed rest period; reactions were more intense in subjects who were not allowed to exercise compared with those allowed to exercise three times a day.[43]

It has been found that bed rest also affects the EEG pattern of sleep. A longer period of time is spent in the deep stages of sleep, stages 3 and 4, in subjects on bed rest.[43] This was even more pronounced in individuals who were not allowed to perform light supine exercise. Rapid eye movement (REM) sleep periods also increased in subjects on bed rest. In addition, there was a noted increase in mental lethargy observed during waking hours. In conditioned subjects the onset of stage 3 sleep was sooner and the time spent in this deep slow wave sleep was longer than in subjects who were deconditioned.[44] These findings may have significant clinical implications in the aged person, especially one who is hypokinetic. Less time spent in deep sleep can lead to feelings of tiredness, depression, and lack of motivation. All of these sequelae could have a significant impact on an aged individual's level of functioning and rehabilitation potential.

Thermoregulation is also altered by bed rest.[45] Both oral and skin temperatures show a decline, which may have great clinical implications for the aged individual who already has decreased thermoregulatory responses.

Several neurological changes occur after bed rest that affect motor performance. Balance decrements are significant after 2 to 3 weeks of bed rest.[46] Muscle strengthening exercises during bed rest did not reverse this deterioration, but recovery of the balance losses was accomplished within 3 to 5 days following cessation of bed rest. Testing included assessment with the patient's eyes shut and open. Allowing visual cues greatly improved the relearning rate and overall performance scores.

Coordination was also found to decline with bed rest.[47] Pattern tracing skill tests were used to test coordination. Performance of these activities decreased in accuracy by 10% after 3 weeks of bed rest and resolved within 4 days of the resumption of activity.

Each of these changes has significant clinical implications for aged individuals on acute or chronic bed rest or severely restricted levels of activity. The neuropsychological consequences of a chronic level of inactivity, as in a sedentary life-style, are not easy to determine. Shepard[35] found that a moderate level of physical activity makes a person feel better, which leads to better intellectual and psychomotor development. The underlying mechanism may include increased arousal, improved self-esteem and body image, and a decreased level of anxiety, stress, and depression.

Chronic inactivity also negatively affects balance. Postural sway is known to increase with aging, and inactivity may contribute to the progression of this decline. Research indicates that balance is better in active, as compared to inactive, older women.[48] The results were similar for different types of exercise (i.e., golf, walking, range-of-motion exercise). In a study by Emes,[49] standing balanced on one foot was improved following a 12 week exercise program.

A sedentary life-style is also associated with prolonged reaction times.[33,48] A comparison between young versus older persons revealed an 8% decline in reaction and movement times when age was considered alone. A 22% decrement was present when nonactive young and old groups were compared. Spirduso[50] has proposed that "exercise prevents the cycle in which disuse increases brain metabolism leading to decreased blood flow and neuronal loss."

The summary of the effects of inactivity on the nervous system is of great significance in geriatric rehabilitation. Acute bed rest induces some cognitive changes including a distortion of time perception and decrements in some intellectual tests. Mood changes occur as well. Consequences on cognitive and emotional function of chronic inactivity may include a poorer sense of well-being. Balance is impaired after both acute and chronic inactivity. Prolonged reaction times are associated with chronic inactivity. Realizing the consequences of inactivity superimposed on the normal changes with aging should alert the rehabilitation team to the importance of maintaining activity and maximal functional capabilities in the aged person.

Changes in the cardiovascular system have been studied most in relation to inactivity versus activity. An aged individual in good physical condition responds to submaximal exercise levels without significant increases in heart rate or blood pressure. In contrast, a deconditioned person encountering a minimal to moderate activity level experiences a marked increase in these vital signs. Maximal work loads elicit similar increases in heart rate and blood pressure in both deconditioned and conditioned individuals, however, the recovery rate (i.e., the return to resting vital sign values) is slower in deconditioned individuals.

Within the first week of bed rest, there is a noted increase in resting heart rate.[35,51,52] In other words, the work of the heart is increased in spite of the fact that the body remains at rest. In very early studies on the effects of bed rest on cardiovascular function, it was found that by the end of the third week of bed rest the morning heart rate increased by as much as 21% and the evening heart rate by 33%. This is an average increase in resting heart rate of approximately 1 beat for every 2 bed rest days.[47] Other investigations showed approximately a 4 beat increase, documenting lesser increases in resting heart rate over a 1 week period.[52] In each of these studies, 6 weeks of submaximal exercise was necessary before the resting heart rate returned to its baseline value.

Total blood volume has been found to decrease after several weeks of bed rest.[53] These findings were based on studies of astronauts in the aerospace program, a presumably healthy group of individuals. It was determined that plasma volume decrements were greater than red cell mass decrements. Such a change could have significant import for older persons. There is a strong possibility that a decrease in total blood volume could be correlated with orthostatic hypotension in the aged, though this has not been studied in an elderly population to date.

Orthostatic hypotension occurs within the first week of inactivity in young subjects. This, and other cardiovascular signs of deconditioning, occur even with armchair rest.[54] Orthostasis resolves very slowly, even when the recovery period includes maximal exercise levels.

In addition to the deterioration of the cardiovascular system at rest, any level of activity above the resting level becomes more strenuous. At submaximal levels of exercise, heart rate increases of 10 to 20 beats are common in the deconditioned individual. In addition to an increase in the heart rate, the stroke volume tends to decrease, making the heart less efficient in delivering blood to the working muscles.[31,35] Delayed recovery rates also indicate an increased cardiac and metabolic stress. Before bed rest the return to the baseline heart rate in conditioned individuals occurs in less than 2 minutes and the systolic blood pressure returns to a resting level within 4 minutes. After 6 weeks of bed rest imposed on a healthy individual, it takes 3 to 6 minutes for the heart rate and 5 to 7 minutes for the systolic blood pressure to return to preexercise resting levels.[31]

Normal aging is accompanied by a 1% per year decline in oxygen uptake starting at the age of 30,[31,35] although it has been shown that oxygen uptake is improved with activity. There is less of a decrease in oxygen uptake in armchair rest versus bed rest. In one of the few studies involving older men, maximal oxygen uptake decreased 15% after 10 days of bed rest.[55] Oxygen uptake at submaximal levels of activity was approximately 10% less after bed rest despite an increase in heart rate. These oxygen uptake levels returned to their baseline within 1 month following the resumption of daily activities. Interestingly, recovery rates were similar for subjects who participated in an aerobic exercise program and those who just returned to their usual activities.

The cardiovascular system undergoes significant changes with bed rest. The alterations are noted even without activity by an increase in resting heart rate. Mere standing can be accompanied by orthostasis. Any level of activity stresses the heart and elicites a greater heart rate and a diminished stroke volume. These factors contribute to the overall decrease in maximal oxygen uptake resulting in decreased physical capabilities, decreased endurance, and lost function.

The cardiovascular consequences of chronic inactivity are similar to those seen in acute bed rest. Resting heart rates are higher. At submaximal activity levels, heart rate and blood pressure are greater than in physically fit individuals performing at the same intensity of exercise. Maximal oxygen uptake is lower than in individuals who exercise aerobically. The well-documented decline in maximal oxygen uptake with age is 50% less in physically active individuals as compared to inactive persons, and the latter's recovery rates are prolonged. The biggest difference in acute versus chronic inactivity's effects on the cardiovascular system are the cumulative effects of long-term inactivity. In other words, the longer an individual remains inactive, the more pronounced these cardiovascular changes are and the longer it takes to the body to return to a healthy, preconditioned baseline.

The skeletal muscle system of the body is the largest organ system by mass, and its physiological capabilities are closely related to levels of activity. Alterations in skeletal muscle with aging and with inactivity resemble those observed with denervation. The classic cross-innervation studies of Buller and associates[56] established the importance of the trophic influence on skeletal muscle function and demonstrated that the metabolic and physiological profile of a muscle fiber (i.e., the fiber type) was primarily determined by the type of neural innervation (phasic or tonic firing pattern and other trophic factors) it received. Adult skeletal muscle is composed of three distinct fiber types: type IIA (fast twitch, high oxidative fiber), type IIB (fast twitch, low oxidative fiber), and type I (slow twitch, high oxidative fiber). This heterogeneous fiber pattern is lost with aging and fibers become more homogeneous in respect to their physiological and metabolic profile.

It is well known that decreases in muscle mass occur with old age—with proximal muscles of the lower extremity being particularly affected. This decrease in muscle mass is due to a decrease in both fiber number and diameter. No change in the number of motor neural fibers has been found, but the size of the motor unit decreases due to the loss of muscle fibers. The reported decrease in fiber number primarily affects the red oxidative fiber, and the preponderance of evidence based on enzyme histochemistry and physiological properties suggest a greater loss in the fast type II fiber. This decrease occurs in both type IIA and IIB fibers such that the type IIB/IIA fiber ratio is unaltered with increasing age. As a result of this selective loss of type II fibers, the percentage of type I fibers increases from about 40% in 20- to 30-year-old persons to 55% in 60- to 65-year-old individuals.[31,35]

With aging and with inactivity, then, a loss of lean body mass is seen. The same changes are also observed in younger subjects on bed rest and in astronauts in a gravity-free environment.[42,43]

Exercise positively affects body composition. Bed rest imposes inactivity in a nonuniform way in muscle groups. Functionally, neck extensors and the antigravity muscles of the legs are the least exercised. Arm, back, and abdominal muscles may be used more frequently during positional changes and basic activities of care. During several weeks of bed rest in young men, grip strength, abdominal, and back muscle strength did not show any discernible change.[31] A decrease of 6% in shoulder and arm flexor muscles was observed. The tibialis anterior (the muscle that pulls the foot up) decreased in strength by 13%, and the gastrocsoleus complex (the muscle group that pulls the foot into a ballerina position and assists in flexion of the knee) lost 20% of its strength. Muller reported a loss of approximately 1.5% per day during a 2 week period of bed rest.[57]

Most of the studies on bed rest's effects on skeletal muscle have been done on younger subjects, therefore, the amount of strength lost by aged persons during bed rest has not been extensively studied. Inactivity superimposed on the normal aging process previously mentioned, however, is likely to have significant disabling consequences. The decrement in strength associated with aging is likely to be due partially to inactivity. Exercise programs have been found to improve strength in all age groups.[35]

The skeletal system functions to support, protect, and shape the body. Additionally, bone has the metabolic functions of blood cell production, the storage of calcium, and a role in acid-base balance.

Cortical thickening starts to decline at approximately age 35 and becomes 20% less in men and 30% less in women in the eighth and ninth decades. While exercise improves bone mineralization, bed rest or a lack of weight bearing activities produces bone loss. Astronauts lost 4 g of calcium during 84 day space flight simulation.[42,43]

The most commonly known age related change involving bone is the calcium related loss of mass and density. This loss ultimately causes the pathological condition osteoporosis. Bone density is lost from within by a process termed reabsorption. As the body ages, an imbalance occurs between osteoblast activity (bone buildup) and osteoclast activity (breaks down bone). Osteoclast activity proves to be the stronger. As one ages, a decline in circulating levels of activated vitamin D_3 occurs,[58] and this causes less calcium to be absorbed from the gut and more calcium to be absorbed from the bones to meet body needs. In postmenopausal women, decreased estrogen levels influence parathormone and calcitonin to increase bone reabsorption, which decreases bone mass. Certain factors, such as immobility, decreased estrogens, steroid therapy, and hyperthyroidism are known to accelerate bone erosion to pathological levels. Easily occurring fractures are the most common result.[59,60]

Bone mass and strength decline with age. Osteoporosis is a major bone mineral disorder in the older adult. This bone loss has been characterized by a decreased bone mineral composition, an enlarged medullary cavity, a normal mineral composition, and biochemical normalities in plasma and urine. The rate of bone loss is about 1% per year for women starting at age 30 to 35 and for men at age 50 to 55. In elderly subjects, regions of devitalized tissue with osteocyte lacunae and haversian canals containing amorphous mineral deposits have been described indicating a change in the bone mass/mineral ratio. These have been identified as micropetrotic regions and are noted to increase in frequency in the skeleton with age. Thus, it is clear that the mineral content of bone qualitatively changes with age.

Qualitatively, osteoporotic bone exhibits a reduction in bone mass with a resulting decrease in bone strength. There is some evidence, however, that alterations occur in the composition and structure of bone in the aged. Evans[61] observed that the tensile strength of bone in man is related to the number and size of osteons. It has been found that bone from older humans have smaller osteons and fragments and more cement lines than younger bone. This would account for some of the reduced bone strength of the older bone specimens. The remaining difference in strength results from the geometric structure of the bone in its distribution per unit area as a response to environmental stress placed on the bone. According to Wolff's law, bone is layed down in the direction of the stresses it must withstand. In the absence of stress (i.e., bed rest or varying levels of inactivity), the composition of bone becomes diffuse rather than uniform and loses its tensile strength.

Throughout life, red blood cells continue to be replaced after a life span of about 120 days. Some morphological changes do occur with aging, however. Red cells become slightly smaller and more fragile. Blood volume, however, is maintained until approximately 80 years of age. In the absence of pathology, few changes are seen in the white blood cells or in the platelet count. What is lost with aging is the functional reserve to quickly accelerate the production of red blood cells when needed,[61] and this inability is further accentuated by inactivity.

In the pulmonary system, age changes and those associated with inactivity can be organized according to mechanical properties, changes in flow, changes in volume, alterations in gas exchange, and impairments of lung defense. Decreases in chest wall compliance and lung elastic recoil tendency are two mechanical properties that are altered with age. Increased calcification of the ribs, a decline in intercostal muscle strength, and changes in the spinal curvature (resulting from osteoporotic collapse of the thoracic vertebrae) all result in a lower compliance and an increase in the work of breathing.

At normal lung volume, airway resistance is not increased, however, normal aging results in a reduction of maximum voluntary ventilation, maximum expiratory flow, and forced expiratory volume in 1 second (alone and in relation to forced vital capacity). Though tidal volume remains fairly constant throughout life, vital capacity decreases while residual volume increases. Bed rest has a relatively small effect on pulmonary function in healthy subjects,[52] however, chronic inactivity may cause some reversible decrement in vital capacity, and exercise training leads to a more efficient respiratory function.[34]

Ventilation, diffusion, and pulmonary circulation are the three major components of the respiratory system that lose efficiency with age. There is an increased thickening of the supporting membranes between the alveoli and the capillaries, a decline in total lung capacity, an increase in residual volume, a reduced vital capacity, and a decrease in the resiliency of the lungs. It is difficult to completely separate pulmonary changes resulting with age from those associated with the pathology of emphysema or chronic bronchitis. Throughout a lifetime, exposure to occupational and environmental inhalants, as well as cigarette smoke, may result in chronic pulmonary changes and lung pathologies. These disease states closely parallel those of the aging process and also increase in incidence with advancing age.[62] Normal pulmonary aging includes a loss of elastic tissue leading to expiratory collapse of the larger airways, difficulty with expiration, and dilatation of the terminal air passages.[63]

Aging and inactivity also affect the diffusion efficiency of the peripheral vascular system. Starting with the pulmonary system, impairment of gas exchange is illustrated by reduced diffusing capacity of carbon monoxide, a lower resting arterial oxygen tension, and an increased alveolar–arterial oxygen gradient. Aveolar surface area and pulmonary capillary blood volume diminish with age. As a result, the oxygen dissociation curve shifts to the left, which makes oxygen less available at the tissue level.

The ability to provide oxygen to working tissues diminishes with inactivity. Normal aging affects the cardiopulmonary system in a variety of ways, however, in the absence of pathology, the heart and lungs can generally meet the body's needs. The most evident change in the cardiovascular and cardiopulmonary functioning with bed rest is that the reserve capacities are diminished. In other words, with any challenge, the body's demand for oxygen and perfusion may exceed the available supply.

Of clinical importance in an older person is an impairment of pulmonary defenses resulting from normal aging changes and a decreased level of mobility. Cilia are reduced in number, and those that remain become less strong. The "mucus escalator" and alveolar macrophages (the germ killers) become less effective in removing inhaled particulate matter. In the absence of physiological challenges, the system does maintain fairly adequate defenses; however, an older individual who is chronically exposed to particle-laden air in addition to inactivity, which in essence diminishes the efficiency of the lungs, will be at risk for pulmonary dysfunction.[59,64]

As previously mentioned, the postexercise recovery period following effort is prolonged. Among other factors, this reflects a greater relative work rate, an increased proportion of anaerobic metabolism, a slower heat elimination, and a lower level of physical fitness.

Extremes of immobilization can lead to a decrease in joint range of motion secondary to connective tissue changes. There are many types of connective tissue in the body (loose, adipose, fibrous, etc.), but it is loose connective tissue that functions to bind organs together while holding tissue fluids and permitting cellular–

molecular diffusion. "Loose connective tissue" is located beneath most layers of epithelium and fills the spaces between muscles (fascia). The most common type of cell in loose connective tissue are fibroblasts. Fibroblasts work to produce protein fibers called collagen and elastin.[65]

In youth, collagen fibers are strong and flexible and are arranged in bundles that criss-cross to form structure in the body. As a person ages, there is an increased criss-crossing or cross-linkage of the fibers resulting in denser extracelluar matrices. The collagen structure becomes stiffer as it becomes denser. This increased density also impairs the movement of molecular nutrients and wastes at the cellular level.[66]

Structurally, elastin fibers also develop increased cross-linkage with age. Water and elasticity are lost. The elastin fibers become more rigid, may tend to fray, and in some cases, are replaced by collagen completely.[59]

The clinical significance of this increased cross-linking is seen in resultant collagenous contractures. Bonds between adjacent collagen strands can produce shortening and distortion of the collagen fibers. This shortening may result in contractures with a progressive restriction in tissue mobility.[67] Collagen fiber contractures are tough and inelastic, and their bonds cannot be broken by mechanical stretching forces.

Fibrinous adhesions have great clinical implications in working with the elderly. Fibrinogen, a soluble plasma protein is a normal molecular exudate within the capillary. When this substance passes through the capillary wall into the surrounding tissues, it is converted to strands of insoluble fibrin.[68] Fibrin strands can adhere to tissue structures and restrict movement of these structures. Normally, fibrin is removed as debris, but with age, the exudation of fibrinogen into the surrounding tissues is increased,[69] and with reduced activity levels, complete breakdown of fibrin may not occur. This leads to the accumulation of fibrin, which restricts movement and may result in adhesions.

Fibrinogin also accumulates at the site of tissue damage following an injury (traumatic or surgically induced). If activity is limited, these strands can consolidate and create an adhesion.[70] Some decrements in flexibility can be reversed by exercise,[35] but the most effective means of maintaining mobility is early intervention using bed exercises. What is not lost does not need to be regained, therefore, the prevention of contractures is of extreme importance in geriatric rehabilitation, and the only way to accomplish this is to maintain activity (even if an aged person is on bed rest).

Other connective tissue are also affected by aging and inactivity, including hyaline cartilage, elastic cartilage, and articular cartilage. Hyaline cartilage is found in the nose and the rings of the respiratory passages as well as in the joints. Elastic cartilage is found in parts of the larynx and the outer ear. Articular cartilage is found between the intervertebral discs, between the bones of the pelvic girdle, and at most articular joint surfaces.[71] With aging, cartilage tends to dehydrate, become stiffer, and thins in weight bearing areas.

Cartilage is formed when its cells are subjected to compressive forces (weight bearing) in an environment of low oxygen concentration. Cartilage is a unique connective tissue in that it has no direct blood supply. Blood flow in adjacent bones and synovial fluid provide nutrients to the cartilage. A strong osmotic force attracts water with dissolved gases, inorganic salts, and organic materials into the cartilage, thereby providing the materials necessary for normal metabolism. The concentration of glycoproteins in the matrix of the cartilage determines the amount of fluid drawn into the cartilage. Normal aging is accompanied by a reduction in the amount of glycoproteins produced,[72] resulting in a decrease in osmotic attraction forces and impairment in the ability of the cartilage to attract and retain fluids.

Nutrients enter the matrix of the cartilage only when compressive forces are absent.[35] In a loaded or compressed state, fluid and nutrient substances are squeezed out. To provide regular movement of substances in and out of the cartilage, it is necessary that alternating application and release of compressive forces occur. Metabolites remain in the cartilage in the absence of compression, and the presence of metabolites reduces the oxygen content, resulting in a reduction of the secretion of glycoproteins.[35] The destruction of the joint becomes a vicious cycle in the absence of activity.

In synovial joints, the articular surfaces are covered by hyaline cartilage. Lubrication at the interface of the hyaline cartilage is provided by the secretion of hyaluronic acid. Hyaluronic acid molecules form a viscous layer covering the hyaline cartilage. Compression facilitates the production of hyaluronic acid, which ensures the continual lubrication of the joint during movement.[73] The secretion of hyaluronic acid decreases with age, and in the absence of weight bearing activity, the efficiency of the lubrication system of the joint is reduced.[74] Degenerative changes of the cartilage are not reversible and rehabilitation efforts need to be directed toward regular (but not excessive) compression and release of compression in the aging joint. Normal weight bearing exercises are recommended to maintain cartilagenous health.

The cartilage that covers body joints thins and deteriorates with aging. This occurs especially in the weight bearing areas. Because cartilage has no blood supply or nerves, erosion within the joint is often advanced before symptoms of pain, crepitation, and limitation of movement are perceived. Decreased hydration, reduced elasticity, and increased fibrous growth around bony prominances all contribute to increased stiffness and decreased functioning. Advanced stages of cartilage–joint deterioration are commonly known as osteoarthritis.[59,65,75]

Since some types of connective tissue exist almost everywhere in the body, the effects of aging superimposed on inactivity are widespread. Increased rigidity of collagenous and elastin fibers results in a greater amount of energy being needed to produce a given stretch. Skin becomes less elastic and more wrinkled. Lungs lose some recoil tendency, arteries become more rigid, and the heart becomes less distensible. Joints become stiffer while decreased hydration in the intravertebral discs results in vertebral compaction and height shrinkage. Cellular repair, nutrition, and waste removal are impaired.[59] All of these consequences of inactivity and aging have been shown to be preventable with exercise.[35]

The changes in bowel and bladder function with aging have been discussed in Chapter 3, and lack of activity or deconditioning per se do not appear to directly impair these functions. Of note in considering inactivity on an acute basis, however, is the increased incidence of constipation.[76] The effect of chronic inactivity is less clear. It is difficult to sort out effects solely related to inactivity from dietary and functional problems.

The effects of bed rest on metabolic function include an increased excretion of calcium within the first 2 days of bed rest[42,43] (perhaps indicative of skeletal changes) peaking in the fourth week of immobilization.[51] Calcium losses stabilize by the fifth week of activity resumption. Negative nitrogen balance can start by the fifth day of bed rest. This is indicative of protein degradation, primarily in the skeletal muscle. Following a return to activity, normal levels are reached by the sixth week of exercise. Accelerated loss of calcium and nitrogen induced by bed rest has important implications with regard to the high incidence of osteoporosis and the loss of lean muscle tissue with aging.

It seems obvious from these body systems that the evaluation and treatment of hypokinetics is crucial in the total care of the elderly. Passive range of motion (PROM) or active–assistive range of motion (A-AROM) is appropriate even in the most immobilized patients to prevent the consequences of immobilization. Aging and inactivity are both associated with a loss of lean body mass and a gain in body fat.[33,35] Some degree of changes associated with aging are directly related to inactivity. Active aged individuals show lesser degrees of these changes, and exercise programs in sedentary aged persons have been shown to positively modify those changes associated with aging. Exercise has been shown to reverse the physiological changes of inactivity, including a return of cardiovascular and cardiopulmonary response to pre-bed rest base lines, and a return of muscle strength and flexibility.[31] A mnemonic representation of the effects of bed rest is helpful for remembering the overall effects of inactivity on functional capabilities:

B— Bladder and bowel incontinence and retention; bedsores.
E— Emotional trauma; potential electrolyte imbalances.
D— Deconditioning of muscles and nerves; depression; demineralization of bones.
R— ROM loss and contractures; restlessness; renal dysfunction.
E— Energy depletion.
S— Sensory deprivation; sleep disorders.
T— Trouble.

Optimal Health

The last principle in geriatric rehabilitation is the principle of "optimal health." The great English statesman, Benjamin Disraeli, said, "The health of people is really the foundation upon which all their happiness and their powers as a state depend." The World Health Organization defines health as a state of complete physical, mental, and social well-being, not merely the absence of disease or infirmity.[77] The existence of complete physical health refers to the absence of a pathology, impairment, or disability. Physical health is quite achievable. Mental and social well-being are closely related and are possibly less obtainable in this day and age. Mental health as defined by the World Health Organization would include cognitive and intellectual intactness as well as emotional well-being. The social components of health would include living situation, social roles (i.e., mother, daughter, vocation), and economic status.

As seen in Chapter 3, there are some cummulative biologicaly, physiological, and anatomical effects that may eventually lead to clinical symptoms. It has also been noted in this chapter that some of these changes are associated with inactivity and are not a result of progressive aging effects. In light of this, a preventive approach to physical health needs to be in the foreground when addressing the needs of the aged.

Preventing impairment and disability is a key principle in geriatric rehabilitation. It is reasonable to assume that the health status of individuals in their 70s and during subsequent decades of life is in a suboptimal range. Thus, the scope of health status for the aged should be focused toward preventing the complications that could result from suboptimal health. When considering suboptimal health then, the goal of geriatric rehabilitation should be to strive for relative optimal health (i.e., the maximal functional and physical capabilities of the aged individual considering their current health status).

In reviewing the importance of promoting relative optimal health in terms of the musculoskeletal, sensory, or cardiopulmonary systems, an example of an aged woman with a hip fracture may help.

The patient may be in suboptimal health and suffering from osteoporosis; however, she is not treated until she fractures her hip. The resulting complications could include pneumonia, decubitus from bed rest, all of the changes previously noted in relation to inactivity, and the possibility of death. Intervention at the suboptimal level was needed here rather than waiting for an illness or disability to occur. This intervention could include weight bearing exercises to enhance the strength of the bone, strengthening exercises of the lower extremities to provide adequate stability and endurance, balance exercises to facilitate effective balance reactions and safety, education in nutrition, and the modification of her living environment to ensure added safety in hopes of avoiding the kind of fall that results in a hip fracture.

Another excellent example of preventive intervention to maintain optimal health would be in the case of the diabetic aged individual. It is known that sensory loss in the lower extremities resulting from diabetes mellitus often predisposes diabetic individuals to ulcerations of the foot. An ill-fitting shoe or a wrinkle in a sock may go unnoticed and lead to friction, skin breakdown, and a foot ulcer. If undetected, even the smallest ulcer may lead to the amputation of a lower extremity. Screening the foot during an evaluation can prevent this devastating loss. Intervention could include education of the aged individual in foot inspection (or education of a family member or friend if the diabetic aged individual's eyesight is compromised), shoes properly fitted, and techniques for dealing with sensory loss (i.e., as temperature sensation diminishes, the individual needs to test bath water temperature with a thermometer, or have their spouse test the water before they put their insensitive feet into a steamy bath). With proper skin care and professional (podiatric) care of the nails and calluses, there is less likelihood that injury will occur. The cost of a therapeutic diabetic shoe (the P.W. Minor Thermold shoe, for example) is $130 to $160 per pair and provides protection and ample room for the forefoot. Compare this to the cost of ulcer care, which averages $6000, and the cost of hospitalization and rehabilitation for amputation, which averages $30,000.[78]

The principle of obtaining relative optimal health in geriatric rehabilitation is not only cost effective but would lead to an overall improvement in the quality of life. Encouraging healthy behaviors, such as decreasing obesity, stress, and smoking, and increasing activity, could be the elements necessary for maintaining health and striving for optimal health as defined by the World Health Organization.

Health care professionals involved in geriatric rehabilitation need to be good *evaluators* and *screeners*. Good investigative skills could detect a minor problem with the potential of developing into a major problem. Thorough assessment of physical, cognitive, and social needs could help to modify rehabilitation programs accordingly and would improve the health and functional ability of the aged client.

REHABILITATION MEASURES

Rehabilitation should be directed at preventing premature disability. A deconditioned aged individual is less capable of performing activities than a conditioned aged individual. For example, the speed of walking is positively correlated to the level of physical fitness in an aged person.[79] When cardiovascular capabilities are diminished (i.e., maximum aerobic capacity), walking speeds are adjusted by the aged person to levels of comfort. Himann[79] found that exercise programs geared for improving cardiovascular fitness improved the speed of walking. The more conditioned the individual, the faster the walking pace.

If disease and physical disability are superimposed on hypokinetic sequalae, the functional consequences can be disastrous, because pain often prevents mobility. For instance, the pain experienced by an aged individual with an acute exacerbation of an osteoarthritic knee accompanied by inflammation of the knee capsule may reflexively inhibit quadriceps contraction. While the quadriceps strength may have been poor in the first place due to inactivity, the absence of pain still permitted this individual to rise from a chair or ascend shallow steps. Now, with the presence of acute pain, these activities cause severe discomfort and threaten the capability of maintaining an independent life-style. In this situation, rehabilitation efforts should focus medically on

- Reducing the inflammation through drugs or ice (physician or nurse).
- Maintaining the joint's mobility during the acute phases by the joint mobilization techniques of oscillation and low grade passive range in addition to modalities, such as interferential current, to assist in reducing the edema, and decreasing the discomfort (physical therapy).
- Joint protection techniques and prescription of adaptive equipment, such as a walker, to protect the joint (occupational and physical therapy).

- Provision for proper nutrition in light of medications/nutrient (pharmacist/dietician) effects and evidence that vitamin C is a crucial component in health of the synovium.[74]
- Social and psychological support (social worker, psychologist, religious personnel) to provide emotional and motivational support.

These interventions to prevent the debilitating effects of bed rest highlight the need for an interdisciplinary approach when addressing geriatric rehabilitation.

Rehabilitation of the aged individual should emphasize functional activity to maintain functional mobility and capability, improvement of balance through exercise and functional activity programs (i.e., weight shifting exercises, ambulation with direction and elevation changes, and reaching activities, to name a few), good nutrition and good general care (including hygiene, hydration, bowel and bladder considerations, and rest), as well as social and emotional support.

It is important to optimize overall health status by implementing independence. The more an individual does for his- or herself, the more he or she is capable of doing independently. The more that is done for an aged individual, the less capable he or she is of functioning on an optimal independent level and the more likely the progression of a disability.

The advancing stages of disabilities increase the individual's vulnerability to illness, emotional stress, and injury. An aged person's subjective appraisal of his or her health status influences how he or she reacts to his or her symptoms, how vulnerable he or she considers his- or herself and when he or she decides an activity can no longer be accomplished. Often an aged person's self-appraisal of her or his health is a good predictor to a rehabilitation clinician's evaluation of health and functional status, but such assessments may also differ in many ways. In older persons, perceptions of one's health may be determined in large part by one's level of psychological well-being and by whether or not one continues in rewarding roles and activities.[80]

Because an aged individual's perception of their health status is an important motivator in compliance with a rehabilitation program, it is important to discuss this further. One interesting study showed that even when age, sex, and health status (as evaluated by physicians) were controlled for, perceived health and mortality from heart disease were strongly related.[81] Those who rated their health as poor were two to three times as likely to die as those who rated their health as excellent. A Canadian longitudinal study of persons over 65 produced similar results.[82] Over 3 years, the mortality of those who described their health as poor at the beginning of the study was about three times that of those who initially described their health as good.

Yet, despite this apparent awareness among older persons of their actual state of health, the aged are known to fail to report serious symptoms and wait longer than younger persons to seek help. Rehabilitation professionals need to listen carefully to their aged clients with this in mind. It appears that, contrary to the popular view that older individuals are somewhat hypochondriacal, the aged generally deserve serious attention when they bring complaints to their care givers.

The aged's perceived level of health will greatly impact the outcomes of functional goals in the geriatric rehabilitation setting whether it be acute, rehabilitative, home, or chronic care. Rosillo and Fagel[83] found that improvement in rehabilitation tasks correlated well with the patient's own appraisal of her or his potential for recovery but not with others' appraisals. Stoedefalke[84] reported that positive reinforcement (frequent positive feedback) for older persons in rehabilitation greatly improved their performance and feelings of success. This indicates that aged persons can improve in their physical functioning when modifications in therapeutic interventions provide feedback more often. Some research indicates that older persons with chronic illnesses have low initial aspirations with regard to their ability to perform various tasks.[85] As situations in which they succeeded or failed occurred, their aspirations changed to more closely reflect their abilities.

Older persons may have different beliefs about their abilities compared to younger persons.[86] When subjects were given an unsolvable problem, younger subjects ascribed their failure to not trying hard enough, while older subjects ascribed their failure to inability. On subsequent tests, younger individuals tried harder and older subjects gave up. This holds extreme importance in the rehabilitation potential of an aged person. If the cause of failure is seen as an immutable characteristic by the person, then little effort in the future can be expected.

Aged individuals may have a higher anxiety level in rehabilitation situations because they fear failure or are afraid of "looking bad" to their family or therapist.[87] Eisdorfer[87] found that if anxiety is high enough, then the behavior is redirected toward reducing the anxiety rather than accomplishing the task. Weinberg[88] found that subjects set their own goals for task achievement, even if they are directed to adopt the therapist's goals. In another study, Mento, Steel, and Karren[89] found that the best performance at difficult tasks, as many rehabilitation tasks are, occurs when the aged person sets a very specific goal, such as walking 10 feet with a walker. If the person simply tries to "do better," then performance is not improved as much. These are important motivational components to keep in mind when working with an aged client. Perhaps the clinician's therapeutic approach may have the greatest impact on the successful functional outcomes in a geriatric rehabilitation setting.

Exercise programs have potential for improving physical fitness, agility, and speed of response.[35] They also serve to improve muscle strength, flexibility, bone health, cardiovascular and respiratory response, and tolerance to activity.[90] Evidence suggests that reaction time is better in elders who engage in physical exercise than in those who are sedentary.[91] Stelmach and Worringham[91] showed a positive correlation between an individual's ability to maintain their balance when stressed and their level of fitness. Initial test scores on reaction time were significantly improved following a 6 week stretching and calisthenics program in individuals 65 years of age and older. This has great clinical significance when considering the increasing incidence of falls with age (an area to be discussed in more detail in a subsequent section of this chapter).

In addition, exercise has been shown to provide social and psychological benefits affecting the quality of life and the sense of well-being in the elderly.[92] Intuitively, it would appear plausible that an aged individual who is in better physical condition will experience less functional decline and maintain a higher level of independence and a resulting improvement in their perceived quality of life. The risks of encouraging physical activity are small and can be minimized through careful evaluation. While all the exercise and activity programs that constitute therapeutic exercise cannot be described in detail in this chapter, Table 9–1 summarizes therapies for various conditions seen most frequently in geriatric rehabilitation settings.

Specialized exercise techniques, such as proprioceptive neuromuscular facilitation (PNF), Bobath, and sensory integration techniques are very useful in regaining and maintaining functional mobility and strength and improving sensory awareness in elderly individuals.[93] Though these therapeutic exercises vary in application techniques, the concept of integrating sensory and motor function is consistent in each.

These exercise techniques are methods of placing specific demands on the sensory motor system in order to obtain a desired response. Facilitation by definition implies the promotion or hastening of any natural process—the reverse of inhibition. Specifically, it is the effect produced in nerve cells by the introduction of an impulse. Thus, these techniques, though highly complex and requiring specialized training to employ, may simply be defined as methods of promoting or hastening the response of the neuromuscular mechanism through stimulation of the proprioceptors.[94]

The normal neuromuscular mechanism is capable of a wide range of motor activities within the limits of the anatomical structure, the developmental level,

TABLE 9–1. REHABILITATION THERAPIES FOR COMMON CONDITIONS

Cerebral Vascular Accident (Stroke)

Physical Therapy	Occupational Therapy	Speech Therapy
Pregait activities (if individual is not ambulatory)	Training in activities of daily living (grooming, dressing, cooking, etc.)	Language production work
Gait training (if individual is ambulatory)	Transfer training (toilet, bathtub, car, etc.)	Reading, writing, and math retraining
Provision of assistive ambulatory devices (quad cane, hemi-walker)	Activities and exercise to enhance function of upper extremities	Functional skills practice (checkbook balancing, making change)
Ambulation on different types of surfaces (stairs, ramps)	Training to compensate for visual–perceptual problems	Therapy for swallowing disorders
Provision of appropriate shoe gear and orthotics	Provision of adaptive devices (reachers, special eating utensils)	Oral muscular strengthening
Education and provision of appropriate bracing		
Range of motion, strengthening, coordination exercises		
Proprioceptive neuromuscular facilitation		
Bobath techniques to modify tone		
Sensory integration		
Joint mobilization techniques (when appropriate)		
Functional electrical stimulation (when appropriate)		
Positioning and posturing (chair, feeding needs)		
Family and patient education for home management		

Parkinson's Disease

Physical Therapy	Occupational Therapy	Speech Therapy
Gait training	Fine/gross motor coordination of upper extremities	Improving respiratory control
Provision for appropriate shoe gear and orthotics	Provision of adaptive equipment	Improving coordination between speech and respiration
Training in position changes	Basic self-care activity training	Improving control of rate of speech
General conditioning, strengthening, coordination, and range-of-motion exercises	Transfer training	Use of voice amplifiers and/or alternate communication devices
Breathing exercises		
Training in functional instrumental activities of daily living		
Proprioceptive neuromuscular facilitation		
Sensory integration		

Arthritis

Physical Therapy	Occupational Therapy
Joint protection techniques	Range-of-motion and strengthening exercises for upper extremities
Joint mobilization for pain control and mobility	Splinting to protect involved joints, decrease inflammation, and prevent deformity
Conditioning, strengthening, and range-of-motion exercises	Joint protection techniques
Gait training	Provision of adaptive devices to promote independence and avoid undue stress on involved joints
Provision of proper shoe gear and orthotics	
Modalities to decrease pain and edema, and break up adhesions	
Provision of assistive ambulatory devices (when appropriate)	

TABLE 9–1. REHABILITATION THERAPIES FOR COMMON CONDITIONS (CONT.)

Amputees

Physical Therapy	Occupational Therapy
Fitting and provision of temporary and permanent prosthetic devices	Teaching donning and doffing of prostheses
Teaching donning and doffing of prostheses	Training in stump care
Progressive ambulation	Transfer training
Provision of assistive ambulatory devices	Training in activities of daily living
Training in stump care	
Wound care (when appropriate)	
Provision of shoe gear and protective orthotic for uninvolved extremity	
Instruction of range-of-motion, strengthening, and endurance activities for both involved and uninvolved extremities	
Balance activities	
Transfer training	
Buerger-Allen exercises	

Cardiac Disease

Physical Therapy	Occupational Therapy
Patient education	Labor-saving techniques
Conditioning and endurance exercises (walking, biking, etc.)	Improving overall endurance for participation in activities of daily living
Breathing and relaxation exercises	Monitoring patient's participation in activities of daily living
Strengthening and flexibility exercises	
Monitoring of patient's vital signs during exercise	

Pulmonary Disease

Physical Therapy	Occupational Therapy
Patient education	Training in labor-saving techniques
Breathing control exercises	Monitoring of participation in activities of daily living
Chest physical therapy	Improving endurance of upper extremities
Conditioning exercises	
Joint mobilization of rib cage	

Low Back Pain

Physical Therapy	Occupational Therapy
Joint mobilization/stabilization	Training in labor-saving techniques
Modalities to decrease pain and improve tissue mobility	
Strengthening and flexibility exercises	
Instruction in proper body mechanics for lifting, sitting, and sleeping	
Provision of proper shoe gear an shock absorbing orthotics	
Correction of leg length discrepancy (when appropriate)	

(continued)

TABLE 9–1. REHABILITATION THERAPIES FOR COMMON CONDITIONS (CONT.)

Alzheimer's Disease

Physical Therapy	Occupational Therapy
Sensory integration techniques	Sensory integration techniques
Gait training (when appropriate)	Activities of daily living (grooming, feeding, etc.)
Balance activities	Reality orientation activities/validation techniques
Provision of proper shoe gear and orthotics	
General conditioning exercises	
Reality orientation activities/validation techniques	

Hip Fractures

Physical Therapy	Occupational Therapy
Range-of-motion, strengthening, and conditioning exercises	Activities of daily living
Positioning	
Progressive weight bearing and gait training	
Provision of assistive ambulation devices	
Provision of proper shoe gear, lift on the involved side and orthotics for shock absorption	
Balance activities	
Transfer training	

and inherent and previously learned neuromuscular responses. The normal neuromuscular mechanism becomes integrated and efficient without awareness of individual muscle action, reflex activity, and a multitude of other neurophysiological reactions. Variations occur in relation to coordination, strength, rate of movement, and endurance, but these variations do not prevent adequate response to the ordinary demands of life.

The deficient neuromuscular mechanism is inadequate to meet the demands of life in proportion to the degree of the deficiency. Responses may be limited in aged persons by the faulty neuromuscular response previously discussed as a sequala of the aging process, inactivity, trauma, or disease of the nervous or musculoskeletal systems.

Deficiencies present themselves in terms of limitation of movement as evidenced by weakness, incoordination, adaptive muscle or connective tissue shortening, or immobility of joints, muscle spasm, or spasticity. It is the deficient neuromuscular mechanism that becomes the concern of the rehabilitation team in a geriatric setting. These techniques are very useful in successfully retraining the neuromuscular system in the aged person. Specific demands placed on the patient by a physical or occupational therapist have a facilitating effect on the individual's neuromuscular mechanism. The facilitating effects of these therapeutic exercises are the means used in physical and occupational therapy to reverse limitations of the aged person.[94]

A general measure to ensure the highest functional capacity should encourage early resumption of daily activities following trauma or acute illness. Safety measures to prevent falls and avoid accidents should include reinforcing the use of properly fitted shoes with good soles, low broad heels, and heel cups or orthotics to stabilize the foot during ambulation, the importance of wearing prescription eyeglasses needs to be stressed, and the staff and family should be educated in reducing potential hazards within the patient's living environment (i.e., decreasing the amount of furniture, securing all loose carpetings, obtaining a commode, installing handrails around the toilet and tub areas and railings in the hallways as needed). These are just a few examples of safety proofing the environment in which the elder lives so that the individual may function at their maximum level. Adapting the environment to improve safety is essential in geriatric rehabilitation and will be discussed more thoroughly in a subsequent section of this chapter.

Pain management is a very important factor in geriatric rehabilitation, but it is one of the most difficult pathophysiological phenomena to define. Pain is the human perception or recognition of a noxious stimulus. In geriatric rehabilitation, two basic types of pain—acute and chronic—are dealt with. Chronic pain can be broken down even further into two subcategories—acute–chronic and chronic–chronic.

Treatment of acute pain may include medications to reduce inflammation, ice, heat, or compression (also to reduce edema when warranted), rest, and gentle mobility exercises (low-grade oscillation techniques of joint mobilization are very helpful in pain relief and maintenance of joint mobility). Rarely are modalities, such as ultrasound or electrical currents (high galvanic current reduces edema, interferential current neutralizes the tissue and assists in fluid removal), used in the acute pain situation in the aged individual, although they are widely used in acute sports related injuries in younger populations. The reasons for this are not documented, though this author's clinical experience teaches that the more conservative approaches of rest, ice, compression or elevation, and gentle exercise in combination with nonnarcotic analgesics seem to be quite effective in treating acute pain in the older person.

Chronic pain is more frequently observed in the aged and is more difficult to control. Chronic pain may not always correspond with objective findings. It is well recognized that emotional and socioeconomic factors play a role in chronic pain. Tension and anxiety often lead to muscle tension and decreased activity, and this can be a vicious cycle. Situational depression may exacerbate this type of pain. In management of acute-chronic pain, such as an acute osteoarthritic condition, treatment is similar to acute pain management with the exception of the inclusion of various modalities. For instance, ultrasound may be used to break up a tissue adhesion, and interferential or high galvanic electrical stimulation may be used to break up adhesions, reduce swelling, and enhance the circulation to the painful area. Joint mobilization techniques are often employed to improve and maintain mobility. Nonnarcotic analgesics can be prescribed, but the aged are more susceptible to the cumulative effects, as well as the side effects, of the long term use of these drugs.

Foot pain and discomfort from boney changes, such as those induced by a lifelong use of ill-fitting shoes, arthritic changes, or age related shifting of the fat pads under the heel and the metatarsal heads, can severely curtail the ambulatory abilities of the aged. Proper shoe gear and shock absorbing orthotics that place the foot in a neutral position have been clinically observed to facilitate ambulation and prevent disability.

Though few studies have documented this effect of reducing plantar foot pressures or altering the weight bearing pattern of the foot during gait in aged individuals, this author[95] has completed one study (currently unpublished) that clearly demonstrates a decrease in discomfort as a result of reduced pressure and alteration in the weight bearing pattern and an increase in walking distance and functional capabilities. This has important ramifications in the area of geriatric rehabilitation.

Assistive devices, such as a cane, a quad cane (a more stable four legged cane), or a walker can also be prescribed to improve stability during ambulation and reduce the stresses on painful joints.

Wheelchair prescription may be necessary for longer distances (usually recommended for use outside the home) or when ambulation is no longer possible (i.e., in the case of a bilateral amputation or severe diabetic neuropathy). Wheelchairs should be prescribed to meet the specific needs of the aged individual. For instance, removable arms may be needed to enhance the ease of transfers, or elevating leg rests may be prescribed for lower extremity elevation when severe cardiac disease results in lower extremity edema.

Likewise, if upper extremity capabilities are limited by advanced rheumatoid arthritis or quadriplegia, an electric wheelchair will greatly improve that individual's capabilities of locomotion. Other considerations may be a one arm, manual drive chair for a hemiplegic or a "weighted" chair to shift the center of gravity and improve the stability of the chair in transfers for the bilateral amputee. All of these considerations necessitate a team approach for obtaining the equipment that best suits the individual's needs.

Proper positioning and seating for the aged individual who must sit for extended periods is required to decrease discomfort and keep pressures off of boney prominences, provide adequate postural support, facilitate feeding, and prevent progression of joint contractures and deformities. Many "geri-chairs" are on the market that address specific positioning needs. Armchairs that assist in rising from a seated position include higher chairs that decrease the work of the lower extremities for standing or electric "ejection" chairs that actually extend to bring the individual to a near standing position. Functional assessment of the aged person is vital in the prescription of these specialized devices.

SPECIAL GERIATRIC REHABILITATION CONSIDERATIONS

While the present design of active rehabilitation programs, which involves learning and problem solving on the part of the aged individual, may not be realistic in severe dementias, such as that encountered in Alzheimer's disease because of impaired cognition, inability to learn new tasks, and difficulty in cooperating or participating in a regimented physical exercise program, functional capabilities can be maintained. Until the end stages of Alzheimer's physical functioning remain relatively intact. It is the integration of movement, the motor planning (for instance, putting the sock on before the shoe), and the judgment required for safe functioning that becomes distorted.

The body communicates through its nervous system, which relays information and initiates motor activity. A breakdown in the system can lead to less efficient communication and a slowing of the body's responses. Thus, it is important to consider the degenerative effects on the body of an aging nervous system. Neuromuscular changes with aging include deficits in coordination, strength, and speed of motion.

Changes in the sensory system with age provide less information to the CNS, which results from a decrease in sensory perception. With the loss of sensory input in combination with dementia of any degree, the aged individual is less able to assess their environment accurately, and this leads to incorrect choices. Diminished hearing can also lead to incorrect choices due to inaccurately received and perceived communications. As a result of normal aging, older patients all experience changes in their ability to hear. For example, aged individuals experience a decreased ability to separate one sound or voice from background noises. Specific effects of aging on the auditory system include a decrease in auditory acuity and poorer speech discrimination skills based on their pure tonal losses.[96] In other words, as the ear ages, there is a greater distortion of auditory signals. In the aged person with dementia, these changes can add to confusion. Sensory losses and cognitive impairments, in addition to the physical changes associated with aging, need to be given special consideration in geriatric rehabilitation (specific interventions will be discussed in the subsequent section on adapting the environment).

With aging there is a loss of neurons, because neurons are postmitotic cells and do not duplicate themselves.[97] This cell loss results in the narrowing of the convolutions and widening of the sulci in the aging brain. In fact, brain mass itself decreases by 10% to 20% by 90 years of age.[98] The areas of the brain that show the greatest loss of neurons with normal aging are the frontal lobe (which is the area of cognition), the superior area of the temporal lobe (the main auditory area), the occipital area (the visual area), and the prefrontal gyrus (the major sensorimotor area of the brain).[99] A loss of neurons can be equated with a decrease in function if the losses are significant in any one area of the brain, and the rehabilitation of an elderly individual is directly affected by these changes. In the special case of Alzheimer's patients, the transcortical pathways are affected by the disease process and result in an inability to integrate activity. For instance, normally aging individuals know instinctively to alternate feet when walking. This may not be an automatic response for an individual with Alzheimer's disease, especially in the later stages of the disease.

Compensation for cognitive, hearing, and visual decrements needs to be incorporated into rehabilitation programs. (These changes will be readdressed in the subsequent section on adapting the environment.)

Diminished tactile sense often accompanies aging. Although vision and hearing are the predominant means of communication, touch is an important physical sensoricommunicator and should be considered when designing a rehabilitation program for aged patients. Information from receptors in muscles, joints, and the inner ear aid in movement and positioning. Decreased kinesthetic sensitivity owing to a general slowing and loss of receptor sensitivity with aging results in postural instability and difficulty in reacting to bodily changes in space.

Muscle strength determined by neurological function is defined by the rate of motor unit firing, the number and frequency of motor unit recruitment, and the cross-sectional diameter of the muscle.[28] The effects of the aging process on the neuromuscular system are seen clinically in the deterioration of strength, speed, motor coordination, and gait. Muscular atrophy may be attributed to a decrease in the number of muscle fibers as previously described.[100] Other changes include a decrease in the clear differentiation of fiber type functioning.[101,102] It has been suggested that muscle weakness in aging is a result of the replacement of skeletal muscle by fibrous tissue rather than free fat,[103] however, there is great variability in loss of strength. Despite the obvious relationship between neuromuscular changes and loss of strength, disuse appears to play a very important role.[28] Changes in lifestyle as one ages apparently contribute to the disuse of the muscles. As a result, aging changes of the muscle system closely parallel those discussed in the section on activity versus inactivity.[104]

Activity not only decreases but slows with aging and with disuse, and the aged exhibit slower reaction times. Nerve conduction velocity decreases at approximately 0.4% per year starting at 20 years of age,[98] but reaction time is a very complex response pattern to measure. The pathways involved include CNS processing, afferent nerve pathways, and the effector organ (muscles). Sensory stimuli and cognitive functioning are intimately involved in reaction time, and these factors must be considered when developing a rehabilitation program for the aged.

There are significant differences between the young and the old on tests measuring coordination and fine motor skills.[105] An increase in "sway" as a normal balance correction that diminishes the ability to maintain balance is observed in the aged population. As a result, gait changes are observed. To compensate for the loss of balance, a wider base of support (a greater distance between feet) is employed. Declines in sensory input due to inactivity also lead to sensorimotor deficits that alter gait in other ways.

Neurological assessment must include psychological factors and physiological pathologies. The changes seen in the aging nervous system compound disabilities resulting from physiological or cognitive decline.

Musculoskeletal changes that occur with aging influence flexibility, strength, posture, and gait. Functional changes in life-style and activity add to these age related changes.

Collagen, the supportive protein in skin, tendon, bone, cartilage, and connective tissue, changes with aging.[90] The collagen fibers become irregular in shape as a result of increased cross-linking, and this decreases the elasticity of the collagen fibers, thereby decreasing the mobility of all the body tissues.

Inactivity, too, has been shown to decrease muscle and tendon flexibility. Full immobilization in bed results in a loss in strength of approximately 3% per day.[98] Increased time spent sitting significantly affects the body's flexor muscles, as adhesions are more likely to develop if the flexors of the body are maintained in a shortened position for extended periods of time. This has been observed in studies of astronauts, which demonstrates the relationship between what is known to result from aging, and the effects of "disuse."[106]

A decrease in lean muscle mass and changes in muscular function result from a variety of factors, including a decrease in the efficiency of the cardiovascular system to deliver nutrients and oxygen to the working muscles and changes in the chemical composition of the muscle. Glycoproteins, which produce an osmotic force important in maintaining the fluid content of muscle tissues, are reduced in aging.[107] The inability of the muscle tissues to retain fluid causes the hypotrophic changes observed in aging muscles, and there is a decrease in the permeability of the muscle cell membrane, which makes the cell less efficient. At rest, high concentrations of potassium, magnesium, and phosphate ions are found in the sarcoplasm, while sodium, chloride, and bicarbonate ions are prevented from entering the cell. In the senescent muscle, there is a shift in this resting balance with a decrease in potassium. Lack of potassium in the aging muscle reduces the maximum force of contractions generated by the muscle.[102] Clinically, tiredness and lethargy result from a depletion of potassium stores.

A decrease in total bone mass, or osteoporosis, is a characteristic change with age. Four times more women than men and 30% of women over the age of 65 years are osteoporotic.[99] The older the person and the poorer the nutritional history, the greater the risk for this condition. Hormonal changes (as seen with menopause in women) and circulatory changes (as seen with decreased activity) also play a role. Though often asymptomatic, osteoporosis can be a major cause of pain, fractures, and postural changes in the musculoskeletal system.[28]

Balance, flexibility, and strength provide the posture necessary to ensure efficient ambulation. In aging, poor posture results from a decline in flexibility and strength and from bony changes in the vertebral spine, which results in less safe gait patterns. Gait is the functional application of motion. Changes in the gait cycle seen in the aged include (1) mild rigidity (greater proximally than distally), producing less body movement; (2) fewer automatic movements with a decreased amplitude and speed, such as arm swing; (3) less accuracy of foot placement and speed of cadence (step rate per minute); (4) shorter steps due to changes in kinesthetic sense and slower rate of motor unit firing; (5) wider stride width (broad based gait) in the attempt to enhance safety; (6) decrease in swing-to-stance ratio, which improves safety by allowing more time in the double support phase (i.e., both feet in contact with the ground at the same time); (7) decrease in vertical displacement which is the up and down movement created by pushing off from the toes for forward propulsion and the alternate heel strike, usually secondary to stiffness (a distinct push-off and heel strike are not observed in the aged); (8) decrease in toe-to-floor clearance; (9) decrease in excursion of the leg during swing phase; (10) decrease in the heel-to-floor angle (usually due to the lack of flexibility of the plantar flexor muscles and weakness of dorsiflexors); (11) slower cadence (another safety mechanism); and (12) decrease in velocity of limb motions during gait.[28]

Exercise is a physical stimulus that produces a metabolic increase above the resting level of vital signs. In a healthy, young individual, the cardiovascular system responds quickly to increase the metabolic rate by increasing heart rate, stroke volume (the amount of blood delivered to the system with each heart beat), and peripheral blood flow to deliver oxygen to the working muscles. In the aged, response time of the cardiovascular system is delayed when restoring homeostasis when the level of physical activity has been increased.[35] The aged have a lower resting cardiac output and basal metabolic rate primarily due to age related loss of lean body mass[90] and inactivity.[34] Heart rate and stroke volume decrease 0.7% per year after 30 years of age, decreasing from approximately 5 L/min at 30 years to 3.5 L/min at 75 years. As exercise levels increase, this is manifested as a reduced oxygen uptake.[104] In respiration, there is a 50% decrease in the maximum volume of ventilation and a 40% decrease in the vital capacity by the age of 85.[98] These limitations in oxygen transport capability translate directly into a reduced physical work capacity.

Understanding and managing a patient's sensation of fatigue is essential in any exercise program. Fatigue, a word understood by everyone, lacks precise definition. Darling[108] likened the concept of fatigue to the concept of pain. Both must be considered from physiological and psychological points of view. Physiological types of fatigue include "muscle" fatigue from prolonged use of a muscle group, "circulatory" fatigue associated with elevated blood lactate levels during prolonged activity, and "metabolic" fatigue in which exercise depletes glycogen (energy) stores. General fatigue is related to more subtle factors like interest, reward, and motivation.

Given these definitions, it is easy to understand why a deconditioned person can experience fatigue. From a treatment perspective it is essential to determine what sensation the aged individual is describing as fatigue. Elevated vital signs and progressively weak muscle contractions suggest that rest is needed. A vaguer complaint of fatigue in the absence of these changes would not necessarily be a basis for reducing exercise. In fact, poor aerobic fitness may be related to an otherwise healthy aged person's complaint of fatigue.[109]

In providing activity and exercise programs for the aged, normal aging changes in the musculoskeletal, neuromuscular, cardiovascular, and pulmonary systems will affect functional capacity. In addition, confusion, decreased sensory awareness, postural changes, cardiovascular limitations resulting from deconditioning, motivation, and preceived levels of fatigue all affect the potential for rehabilitation and the need to be assessed prior to implementing activity or exercise programs. More specific exercise recommendations are included in a subsequent section on fall prevention.

NUTRITIONAL CONSIDERATIONS

Nutrition in the aged has been extensively discussed in Chapter 7. Nutrition is reviewed here only as it impacts on functional capabilities.

A car needs gas in order to run; a human being needs adequate energy sources in order to function at an optimal level. Nutritional levels need close monitoring in relation to energy needs and functional activity levels. Increased feeding difficulties may be secondary to decreased appetite, poor oral status, visual or sensorimotor agnosia, cognitive declines (decreasing attentiveness), and physical limitations. Environmental cues and adaptive eating equipment can often be employed to facilitate feeding. Postural considerations need to be addressed as well. A poor sitting posture can further decrease the ease of feeding by preventing upper extremity movement or making chewing and swallowing difficult as a result of head position. For example, an elderly woman with severe osteoporosis and resulting kyphosis is at a postural disadvantage for feeding. Seated in an upright chair, her entire upper trunk will be forced forward and her face directed downward. Gravity only serves to allow the food to drop out of her mouth, especially if dentures are loose, she is edentuous, or oral motor skills are compromised.

Specialized feeding programs may be necessitated if there is neuromuscular involvement. For instance, an aged person sustaining a cerebral vascular accident may have difficulty swallowing or closing the mouth due to weakness in the muscles needed for these activities. In these cases, specialized muscle facilitation techniques can be employed to promote swallowing and facilitate mouth closure. The feeding needs of a neurologically involved individual can be comprehensively addressed by what is commonly called termed a "dysphasia team," which is made up of nursing, dietary, speech, physical, and occupational therapy. In the geriatric rehabilitation setting, this team is a vital component for obtaining maximal functional capabilities. They function to promote adequate nutrition through neuromuscular facilitation techniques, proper posturing and supportive seating, and adaptive eating utensils. Ultimately, the goal of the team is to permit independent feeding by the aged person.

FALLS IN THE AGED

Falls are not part of the normal aging process, but are due to an interaction of underlying physical dysfunctions, medications, and environmental hazards.[110] Poor health status, impaired mobility from inactivity or chronic illness, postural instability, and a history of previous falls are observable risk factors. The ultimate goals of rehabilitation are to combat the inactivity and loss of mobility that predisposes a person to falls.

Some of the ad hoc measures used to prevent falls, such as physical restraints and medications to reduce activity, are now suspected of increasing the patient's risk of falling.[110]

Medical conditions are often a cause of falling. A pathological fracture secondary to severe osteoporosis may result in a fall (rather than the fracture resulting from the fall), or an arrhythmia may induce dizziness. Certain drugs, such as the digoxin that is used for treating an arrhythmia, may also induce dizziness or fatigue.

The fear of falling is often a cause for inactivity and is commonly seen in an individual who has sustained a previous fall. The guarding patterns that aged individuals use as a result of this fear (i.e., grabbing furniture that may not be stable or supportive) may in fact lead to further danger. Intervention by a psychiatrist or psychologist is often necessary to diminish this fear.

Functionally, the limitations of a reduced range of motion, decreased muscle strength and joint mobility, coordination problems, or gait deviations can predispose an aged individual to falling. Specific strengthening and gait training programs help to prevent falls by improving overall strength and coordination, balance responses and reaction time, and awareness of safe ambulation practices (for example, freeing one hand to use on a handrail when carrying packages up the stairs). Some individuals will have inadequate strength and balance to ambulate without an assistive device, or assistive ambulatory devices may provide a safer mode for locomotion. Walking aids, such as canes and walkers, are beneficial for prevention of falls in some cases,[111] whereas, in other cases, they actually contribute to the cause of the fall.[112] Assess the appropriateness of the assistive device, and ensure that the aged individual is using it properly. With proper instruction, the aged person can usually function safely within his or her environment without falling.

Gait evaluation is one of the most important components in fall prevention. The "get up and go" test is a method often used to test strength, balance, coordination, and safety during gait. The aged individual is asked to get up out of a chair without using his or her hands, walk approximately 20 feet down the hall, turn around, come back to the chair, and then stand still. While standing still the eyes are closed, then a gentle push on the sternum can be given to test the patient's righting reflexes. Finally, the individual is directed to sit down without using the hands. Each component of the test is analyzed. For instance, the inability to arise from the chair without the assistance of the hands is indicative of hip extensor, quadriceps weakness, or both. If step symmetry is absent (i.e., the individual is taking irregular steps), the cause can often be pinpointed just by observation. A leg length discrepancy may be present or the hip abductors may be weak. These alterations in anatomical structure or muscle status can easily be determined by close evaluation of the gait pattern. Lower extremity pain may also result in non-rhythmical steps as the individual attempts to avoid the painful extremity. A tendency to veer, lose balance, or hold on to surrounding objects may be indicative of dizziness, muscle weakness, or poor vision. A loss of balance while turning or a stiff, disjointed turn may alert the clinician to the possibility of neurological disorders, such as Parkinson's disease or drug-induced muscle rigidity (often seen in aged individuals on haloperidol).

With good basic patient and family education and modification of the environment to reduce hazards, it is possible to prevent falls through methods that do not undermine mobility or autonomy. It is important to identify and treat reversible medical conditions, as well as physical impairments in gait and balance. Many falls can be prevented through proper exercise to maintain strength, sensory integration techniques to promote all functional activities by improving balance and coordination, good shoes and orthotics to provide a proper base of support and gait training activities, and modifications to safety proof the living environment.

Rehabilitation specialists have an important role in recommending interventions to prevent falls. When disease states and medication responses are stable, an individualized program of safety education, environmental adaptations, lower extremity strengthening exercises, balance exercises, and gait training should be implemented.

Safety education is an important first step in the prevention of falls. Many older individuals are not aware that they are at risk for falling. Often, simple instructions about environmental adaptations and encouraging a person to allow plenty of time for functional activities is all that is needed to facilitate their safety. Many aged people feel the need to rush to answer a phone or doorbell. They should be discouraged from rushing, because it could result in a fall. Care givers and visitors should also be a part of the safety education process. They are often able to remind the person who is at risk for falling of the need for added precaution.

Aged persons who complain of dizziness during changes of position should be evaluated for postural hypotension. These individuals should be taught to change positions slowly and to wait before moving to another position in order to allow the blood pressure to accommodate to the change.

Any aged individual who has fallen is at risk for falling again. In fact, a cluster of falls has been seen in some older individuals during the months preceding death.[113] Inability to rise or lack of assistance after a fall can produce devastating consequences. In one study, half of the aged persons who lay on the floor for longer than 6 hours after a fall died within 6 months.[114] Having a phone in every room may be a necessity for aged persons who live alone. A "buddy system" in which aged persons call each other regularly during the day is a means of "checking up" and can result in an early detection of a fall. Individuals at risk can also be provided with a device, such as the "life-line," that summons emergency personnel by pushing a button.

Eighty-five percent of all falls occur at home,[115] most commonly on stairs,[116,117] on the way to and from the bathroom,[118] and in the bedroom.[119] Environmental evaluation and adaptation is needed for those aged individuals who have fallen or are at risk for falling.

Safety evaluation should address such questions as, "Are the carpets tacked down?" "Is the pathway from the bed to the bathroom obstacle free?" and "Is there night time lighting?" Additional environmental suggestions include adaptive equipment for the shower or bathtub (i.e., using a tub seat and a hand held shower head can improve safety and independence while bathing. Adaptations may also be necessary in order to avoid falls in route to the bathroom. Individuals with urinary urgency, evening fatigue, or disorientation in the middle of the night should be encouraged to use a bedside commode.

The purpose of strengthening exercises to prevent falls is to provide adequate force production of the lower extremities and trunk muscles for support of posture and control of balance. Some aged individuals will tolerate a progressive resistive exercise program. Others will derive greater benefit from a more functional approach to strengthening exercises. For example, practicing sit-to-stand movements and the reverse is a functional means of strengthening extensors and flexors of the lower extremity. Going up and down stairs one stair at a time requires less strength, range of motion, and balance than walking step over step. A functional way to progress this activity, then, is to begin with one stair at a time and progress to step over step. Marching in place while standing can also be a lower extremity flexor strengthening activity. It can be progressed by asking the individual to hold the leg in flexion for a count of three. During this activity, isometric strengthening also occurs in the extensors, abductors, and adductors of the stance leg. Aged individuals should hold on to the back of a chair or the rim of the kitchen counter during this exercise for safety.

No matter which approach is selected for strengthening, the following precautions are recommended:

1. Many aged individuals have osteoporosis. Resistance and unilateral weight bearing may be excessive for them. It is possible to fracture an osteoporotic bone during strengthening exercises.
2. Many aged individuals have osteoarthritis. Isometric exercise may be less painful for them. Prolonging the amount of time that the contraction is held is an effective way to increase strength without adding external resistance.[120]
3. It is especially important for aged individuals to avoid holding their breath (Valsalva's maneuver) during exercise. Counting outloud helps to avoid this problem.
4. The aged individual should be taught to monitor their heart rate during exercise.

Therapeutic exercises designed to improve balance are an important part of fall prevention. Balance exercises address three areas of posture control: response to perturbation, weight-shifting, and anticipatory adjustments to limb movements.[121] Individuals must be able to respond to an external perturbation, such as a push to the shoulder or sternum, with a postural adjustment that brings the center of gravity back over the base of support. The usual response to a lateral perturbation will be extension of the weight bearing leg along with elongation of the trunk on the weight bearing side. Flexion and abduction of the nonweight-bearing leg will also be seen.[122] A small backward force should stimulate the reaction of the dorsiflexors at the ankles and flexion at the hips, whereas a small forward push should be followed by plantarflexion at the ankles and extension at the hips.[123]

Weight shifting of the entire body during standing involve muscular activity similar to that used in response to a perturbation; however, during weight shifting, the muscle activation occurs voluntarily. Balance must also be controlled when a limb movement occurs, such as reaching with the upper extremity or swinging with the lower extremity. In this case, the postural adjustment actually occurs in anticipation of the limb movement in order to prevent the center of gravity from moving outside of the base of support. For example, a forward movement of the arm should be preceded by ankle plantar flexion and hip extension. In this way, a small backward movement of the center of gravity counteracts the forward displacement caused by the moving arm. Practicing each of these activities, that is, the response to perturbation, voluntary weight shifting, and postural adjustments in anticipation of limb movement when standing, will help prepare the aged individual to use postural adjustment effectively during functional standing activities, such as cooking, transfers, and ambulation. These activities are directed toward improvement of the motor component of balance.

Altering the sensory conditions during balance activities encourages the aged person to attend to the support surface or visual information selectively. Balancing in bare feet with the eyes open or closed helps maximize the amount of somatosensory information that is available from the soles of the feet. On the other hand, balancing while standing on a piece of foam[124] disrupts information from the sole of the foot and from stretch receptors in the ankle muscles and forces the individual to practice using visual input to stabilize posture. Maintaining balance while turning the head from side to side or nodding the head is also important. Many aged people report falling during head movements[125] or while looking up to hang curtains or change a light bulb. Aged individuals should be instructed to use caution during upward head movements.

When an individual is unable to control standing balance and is about to fall, the normal response is protective extension of the arms or legs. Protective reactions, such as arm extension and the stepping response, should also be practiced. Upper extremity protective extension can be practiced both forward and sideways against the wall in the standing position.[126] Lower extremity protective reactions should be practiced when standing in forward, sideways, and backward directions. Brisk and accurately directed limb extension is the goal.

Balance exercises can be incorporated into functional activities for the aged. Moving from sit-to-stand and from stand-to-sit are examples of controlled voluntary weight shifting. Shifting the trunk forward and back and from side to side while sitting are also examples of voluntary weight shifting. Voluntary weight shifting while standing with the individual's back to a wall is a safe way to facilitate the control of balance. Dancing has also been recommended as a functional activity to improve balance for prevention of falls.[127] Postural adjustments in anticipation of arm movements can be practiced during functional activities by standing and reaching for objects on the kitchen or closet shelves. Reaching should be practiced in a variety of directions.

Ambulation requires weight shifting. Manual guidance during ambulation helps to organize the time and direction of weight shifting.[126] Functional ambulation requires interaction with a variety of different support surfaces, therefore, it should be practiced on smooth as well as uneven surfaces and on levels as well as inclines, curbs, and stairs. Varying the amount of available light and background noise also stimulates realistic environmental conditions. If step lengths are irregular, footprints on the floor make good targets for foot placement.

Manual guidance is also useful for improving ambulation speed. A variety of ambulation speeds is necessary for function. Challenging activities, like crossing a busy street, can be made less threatening if the aged individual practices with the therapist or care giver.

Risk factors for falling among the aged suggest that falling should not be considered a normal concommitant of aging; rather, it should alert the health care professional to the possibility of underlying disease or accelerated sensory or neuromuscular degeneration secondary to disuse. Secondary or multiple diagnoses, the use of multiple medications, especially diuretics and barbituates, decreased vision and lower extremity somatosensation, and decreased lower extremity strength all appear to contribute to balance and gait deficits, which in turn can result in falls. Prevention of falls depends on addressing the specific problem area for each individual at risk. A team approach is the most effective way of preventing falls in the aged.

ADAPTING THE ENVIRONMENT

The process of adapting to the environment, or of adapting the environment to the aged person, is especially important in geriatric rehabilitation. With decreased physiological reserves the aged person may not be able to continue an activity that is extremely demanding. For instance, an older person with a stroke and underlying cardiac insufficiency may need to learn wheelchair mobility skills. Therefore, the environment will need significant modification. Doors may need to be widened, ramps installed, and counters lowered. Opportunities for obtaining new housing or adapting the present home may be restricted by financial concerns and personal preferences.

The interaction between the aged person and his or her environment becomes potentially precarious as one ages. These interactions are affected by the aged person's underlying physical status, their living surroundings, and the social systems. Of course, all persons interact with their environment. As one ages, however, the physiological reserves, underlying medical problems, affective states, and a host of other factors complicate the relationship between the aged individual and the environment.

The purpose of rehabilitation providers is to manipulate the environment to make it safer. Assistive walking devices or modifications of the home may be recommended, but even these interventions are subject to differences when dealing with aging persons. The aged person with a disability may view such aids as unattractive or demeaning. The individual has a choice in when selecting eyeglasses, which may enhance their appearance, but walkers or chrome-plated grab bars seem to project an image of illness and disability, which the aged person may try to avoid. The older person may also have difficulty finding someone who can install home modifications. Some retired senior volunteer programs (RSVPs) have carpenters available for this purpose, but many communities lack such support services.

Tasks are carried out within a physical and social context that has the potential for facilitating or hindering the use of functional capabilities. Push-button controls placed at the front of a range assist aged individuals with low vision, whereas dials situated at the back of the range handicap them. Similarly, care givers can enhance functional independence by providing aged individuals with adaptive equipment, such as plate guards, bath brushes with elongated handles, and sock aids, or they can promote dependence by feeding, bathing, and dressing the individual.

Evaluation of the environment is more difficult than task analysis because the environment of concern is the one in which the individual actually lives and has to function, rather than a hospital or nursing home. Evaluation of a physical space aims at ascertaining architectural barriers, safety and functional features, and the extent to which available equipment can be operated by the aged individual. Evaluation of the social context probes the availability of care givers, their skills in rendering care and their need for training, their attitudes toward functional independence, and their experience of care giver burden.

Those with disabilities or physiological or anatomical changes resulting from inactivity and aging may experience memory loss, disorientation, decreased ability to perform normal physical activity, a deteriorating ability to remember details, difficulty in verbal expression, and impairment in judgment. Each of these factors is important when modifying the physical and social environment to meet the rehabilitation needs of the aged. Recent US government hearings and reports suggest that social and organizational characteristics of institutions and the home setting could postpone the time when aged people become bedridden and require skilled nursing care.[128,129]

It is reasonable for the direct care giver to seek advice about practical strategies that could reduce confusion or injury on the part of the disabled aged to prolong care at home. Environmental designs for aged patients have been studied, and several factors are consistently identified as environmental hazards, including poor illumination; inadequate color differentiation; cluttered furnishings; confusing layout, such as a table in a dimly lit hallway; bland, nondistinct textiles; architectural features, such as split level rooms; and climate control.[130] Certain environmental features are a threat to safety, can produce anxiety, and amplify cognitive deficits.[131] Cohen[132] found that behavioral approaches, (i.e., using environmental cues like color coding or labeling objects) had advantages over drugs in the treatment of cognitive impairments. Additional studies emphasized that encouragement of independence, self-sufficiency, and social interaction is critical to prolonging cognitive functions.[133]

The aged individual's environment may have some negative effects on their communication. Older people living alone are often isolated in home or community settings; that is, in an environment in which few opportunities for successful, meaningful communication are available.[134] This can result in impairment in their communication skills. An aged person needs an environment that stimulates and reinforces communication. Geriatric rehabilitation should encourage participation in a variety of activities that can serve as a basis for conversation and interaction. Providing socially stimulating environments within a hospital, rehabilitation, or long-term care setting can be provided by organized recreational and social therapies. This becomes more difficult in the home setting, though often resources, such as church, community groups, or senior centers, can facilitate social interaction. Meaningful conversation is a crucial component in enhancing and reinforcing cognitive functioning and a sense of well-being for the aged individual.[133,134]

Visual limitations, such as farsightedness, decreased ability to adapt to changes in lighting conditions requiring increased illumination to see, and an increased sensitivity to glare, are not uncommon in the elderly patient.

Several changes normally occur within the aging eye that affect safety within their environment, and they need to be considered when adapting that environment. The lens of the eye begins to thicken and yellow, and the muscles that control dilation of the pupil weaken. The thickening of the lens and delayed pupil dilation means that the glare and reflections often encountered in the environment cannot be tolerated.[135] In fact, the older eye needs approximately three times the amount of light to function adequately. The older person also has difficulty with depth perception and color differentiation that can interfere with ambulation (poor judgment in distance), ADLs, and driving an automobile. Color vision deficiencies in the aged have been described by Andreasen.[135] He found that the aged individual has difficulty distinguishing between shades of blue-green, blue, and violet and is unable to distinguish between two shades of a similar color. The aged person maintains his or her ability to differentiate between brighter colors, such as orange and red.[18] Several authors suggest the need for large pattern designs or solid bright colors in upholstery and textiles to enhance visability, interest, and appeal (reducing the likelihood of bumping into or falling over furniture). Small patterns can produce blurring of vision and eye fatigue.[135]

Independence can be facilitated by bright and sharply contrasting colors. Considering the poorer differentiation of similar colors, if an aged individual is in a poorly lit living room with a blue carpet, light blue walls, and lavender and blue flowered furniture and draperies, they are in trouble. Contrasting colors or better lighting, which is economically more feasible, could positively facilitate safety in that room. Color coding of walls and corridors in hospitals and nursing homes using bright colors can aid aged persons to find their own rooms, bathrooms, sitting rooms, and so on. Contrasting colors are extremely important, because they can eliminate the difficulty of independently managing a stairwell or a poorly lit hall where shadows can be hazards. Often this contrast can be accomplished through the use of fluorescent colors of tape (orange, lime green, or red).

Different colors have differing effects on an individual's emotional state.[135] The colors red, yellow, and orange have been associated with excitement, stimulation, and aggression.[135] Red increases muscular tension and blood pressure. It could be used as a visual stimulant with the elderly to alert them of environmental changes or hazards, such as stairs or level changes. Although elderly persons often need to be stimulated, the elderly individual with a dementia requires soothing, and warm colors, such as light oranges and blues, in their living quarters will enhance relaxation and comfort.

Higher, reasonably firm, supportive, and comfortable chairs with high backs allow rising from a sitting position with minimal assistance. Wide armrests, either wooden or metal, allow identification by touch when eyesight is poor or trunk rotation is limited. An aged individual should always be instructed to feel the chair seat with the back of the legs before attempting to sit down.

Human beings have a great propensity for adapting to less than ideal conditions. The aged, particularly those with a severe disability, have much more difficulty than average, though. Sensory stimulation should be incorporated into every aspect of rehabilitation. Repetitive visual cues using graphics, color, and lighting encourage independence, thereby increasing pride and self-esteem.

Hellbrandt[136] proposed a focus on the maintenance of good health and residual mental function, the latter through socialization, physical, and recreational activities. The relationship between physical condition and behavior is particularly important in patients with dementia. Changes in environmental design can accommodate the normal physiological changes of aging and prevent the effects of disuse. If the older person cannot manage the environment safely, his or her independence, socialization, and ADLs are hindered.

CONCLUSION

Rehabilitation of the aged patient is one of the most challenging tasks for health care professionals. It is often difficult to separate the physiological aspect of aging and disability from cognitive changes when designing a rehabilitation treatment program. With increased knowledge, the natural history of normal aging may eventually be altered. Until then, the rehabilitation of aged individuals needs to focus on obtaining the maximal functional capacity within the care environment by simplifying that environment and providing activity to ensure that disabilities do not result from disuse. To maintain the highest level of functional ability for the longest amount of time, a decline in all sensory integration and physical functioning capabilities must be considered when providing rehabilitative care. One of the most salient aspects of geriatric rehabilitation is the simultaneous management of multiple conditions. For the rehabilitation specialist, these multiple diagnoses translate into multiple, and often multidimensional, impairments that complicate ADLs and maximal functional capabilities.

Rehabilitation is a process that is not determined by a specific diagnosis or the care setting in which services are provided but by multidiagnostic circumstances and the aged individual's level of motivation. The primary goal of rehabilitation is to promote independent living, as defined by the aged themselves. When working with aged people, rehabilitation specialists need to be aware of the number of factors that make caring for them more complex, more challenging, and more fulfilling.

PEARLS

- The purpose of geriatric rehabilitation is to assist the disabled aged in recovering lost physical, psychological, or social skills so that they may become more independent.

- Forty percent of all disabled persons are over age 65; the old-old (over 85) compose the highest percentage of disabled persons.

- Lawton[137,138] defines three levels of ADL as: (1) basic ADL, such as self-care activities; (2) instrumental ADL, such as cooking and cleaning; (3) mobility, a more complicated form of ADL, such as using public transportation.

- Three major principles influence geriatric rehabilitation. These are variability, hypokinetics, and optimal health. The influence of these can be seen in the systems of the body and should be differentiated from normal versus pathological aging.

- Rehabilitation of the aged should emphasize maintenance of functional mobility, improvement of balance, good nutrition, and general care, as well as social and emotional support.

- Special geriatric rehabilitation considerations must be implemented for patients with cognitive, sensory, and generalized physical decline.

- Managing falls in the aged requires recognizing that falls are not a normal part of aging and may be due to medication, fear of falling, inactivity, chronic illness, postural instability, or a combination of these.

- The goals for adapting an environment for the older person are to ensure safety, increase mobility, and enhance comfort and communication.

REFERENCES

1. Wedgewood J. The place of rehabilitation in geriatric medicine: an overview. *Int Rehabil Med.* 1985; 7;107.
2. Warshaw GA, Moore JT, Friedman SW, et al. Functional disability in the hospitalized elderly. *JAMA.* 1982; 248(7):847–850.
3. Clark G, Blue B, and Bearer J. Rehabilitation of the elderly amputee. *J Am Geriatr Soc.* 1983; 31:439.
4. Kumar VN, Redford JB. Rehabilitation of hip fractures in the elderly. *Am Fam Physician.* 1984; 29:173.
5. Federal Council on the Aging. *The Need for Long-Term Care. A Chartbook of the Federal Council on Aging.* Washington, DC: US Government Printing Office; 1981. US Department of Health and Human Services publication No. (OHDS) 81–20704, 29.
6. Enright RB, Friss L. Employed care-givers of brain-damaged adults: an assessment of the dual role. Unpublished thesis, University of Arizona. 1987.
7. Lehman JF, Guy AW, Stonebridge JB, et al. Stroke: does rehabilitation affect outcome? *Arch Phys Med Rehabil.* 1975; 56;375.
8. Rubenstein LZ, Josephson KR, Gurland B. Effectiveness of a geriatric evaluation unit: a randomized trial. *N Engl J Med.* 1984; 311:1664.
9. Commission on Chronic Illness. *Chronic Illness in the United States: Prevention of Chronic Illness.* Cambridge, Mass: Harvard University Press; 1957: 1; 285–311.
10. Trussel RD, Elinson J. *Chronic Illness in the United States: Chronic Illness in a Rural Area.* Cambridge, Mass: Harvard University Press; 1959:3.
11. Dinken H. Physical treatment of the hemiplegic patient in general practice. In: Krusen FH, ed. *Physical Medicine and Rehabilitation for the Clinician.* Philadelphia: Saunders; 1951; 205.
12. Heather AJ. *Manual of Care for the Disabled Patient.* New York: Macmillan; 1960; 12–15.
13. Rusk H. *Rehabilitation Medicine.* St Louis; Mosby Co.; 1958; 40–44.
14. Branch LG, Meyers AR. Assessing physical function in the elderly. *Clin Ger Med.* 1987; 3(1):29–51.
15. Branch L, Jette A. The Framingham Disability Study: social disability among the aging. *Am J Public Health.* 1981;71:1202.
16. Woollacott MJ. Changes in posture and voluntary control in the elderly: research findings and rehabilitation. *Top Geriatr Rehabil.* 1990; 5(2):1–11.
17. Woollacott MJ. Response preparation and posture control: neuromuscular changes in the older adult. *Ann NY Acad Sci.* 1988; 51 5:42–53.
18. Andreasen MK. Making a safe environment by design. *J Gerontol Nurs.* 1985; 11(6):18–22.
19. Boyer GG. Vision problems. In: Carnevali P, Patrick B, eds. *Nursing Management for the Elderly.* Philadelphia; Lippincott; 1989; 482–484.
20. Kasper RL. Eye problems of the aged. In: Reichel W, ed. *Clinical Aspects of Aging.* Baltimore, Md: Williams and Wilkins Co.; 1988; 393–395.
21. Fitts RH. Aging and skeletal muscle. In: Smith EL, Serfass RC, eds. *Exercise and Aging: The Scientific Basis.* Hillside, NJ: Enslow Publishers; 1980.

22. Schaie KW. Historical time and cohort effects. In: McCluskey KA, Reese HW, eds. *Life-span Developmental Psychology: Historical and Generational Effects.* New York; Academic Press; 1984.
23. Wechsler D. "Hold" and "Don't hold" tests. In: Chown SM, ed. *Human Aging.* New York; Penguin Press; 1972.
24. Siegler IC. Psychological aspects of the Duke longitudinal studies. In: Schaie KW, ed. *Longitudinal Studies of Adult Psychological Development.* New York; Guilford Press; 1983.
25. Botwinick J. *Aging and Behavior.* 2nd ed, New York; Springer Publishing Co., 1987.
26. Baltes PB, Schaie KW. On the plasticity of intelligence in adulthood and old age. *Am Psychol.* 1986. 31; 720–725.
27. Lewis CB. *Aging: The Health Care Challenge.* Philadelphia: Davis; 1985.
28. Siebens AW, Schmedt JF, Eckberg DL, et al. Homodynamic consequences of cardiovascular deconditioning—functional effects. *Circulation.* 1990; 82(4):694.
29. Holloszy JO. Exercise, health, and aging: a need for more information. *Med Sci Sports Exerc.* 1983; 15:1.
30. Schneider El, Reed JD. Modulations of aging processes. In: Finch Ce, Schneider EL, eds. *Handbook of the Biology of Aging.* New York; Academic Press; 1985.
31. Astrand PO. Exercise physiology and its role in disease prevention and in rehabilitation. *Arch Phys Med Rehabil.* 1987; 68:305.
32. Bruce RA. Exercise, functional aerobic capacity, and aging—another viewpoint. *Med Sci Sports Exerc.* 1984;16:8–15.
33. Buskirk ER. Health maintenance and longevity; exercise. In: Finch CE, Schneider EL, eds. *Handbook of the Biology of Aging.* New York; Academic Press, 1985.
34. Shepard RJ. *Physical Activity and Aging.* Chicago; Year Book; 1978.
35. Shepard RJ. *Physical Activity and Aging.* 2nd ed. Rockland, Md: Aspen Publishers, Inc.; 1987.
36. Bortz WB. Disuse and aging. *JAMA.* 1982; 248:1203.
37. Young A. Exercise physiology in geriatric practice. *Acta Med Scand.* 1986; 711 (suppl):227.
38. Miller MB. Iatrogenic and nursigenic effects of prolonged immobilization of the ill aged. *J Am Geriatr Soc.* 1975; 33:360.
39. Zubek JP, Wilgosh L. Prolonged immobilization of the body: changes in performance and in the electroencephalogram. *Science.*1963; 140:306.
40. Zubek JP. Counteracting effects of physical exercise performed during prolonged perceptual deprivation. *Science.* 1963; 142:504.
41. Downs F. Bed rest and sensory disturbances. *Am J Nurs.* 1974; 74:434–438.
42. Ryback RS, Lewis OF, Sewab RS, Blum K. Psychobiologic effects of prolonged weightlessness (bed rest) in young healthy volunteers. *Aerospace Med.* 1971; 42:408.
43. Ryback RS, Lewis OF, Lessard CS. Psychobiologic effects of prolonged bed rest (weightless) in young, healthy volunteers (study II). *Aerospace Med.* 1971; 42;529.
44. Griffin SJ, Trinder J. Physical fitness, exercise, and human sleep. *Psychophysiology.* 1978; 19:447–451.
45. Greenleaf JE, Reese RD. Exercise themoregulation after 14 days of bed rest. *J Appl Physiol.* 1980; 48:72–77.
46. Haines RF. Effect of bed rest and exercise on body balance. *J Appl Physiol.* 1974; 36:323.
47. Taylor HL, Henschel JB, Keys A. Effects of bed rest on cardiovascular function and work performance. *J Am Physiol.* 1949; 2:223.
48. Rikli R, Busch S. Motor performance of women as a function of age and physical activity level. *J Gerontol.* 1986; 41:645.
49. Emes CG. The effects of a regular program of light exercise on seniors. *J Sports Med.* 1979;19:185.
50. Spiraduso WW. Physical fitness, aging, and psychomotor speed: a review. *J Gerontol.* 1980; 35; 850.
51. Dietrick JE, Whedon GD, Shorr E. Effects of immobilization upon various metabolic and physiologic functions of normal men. *Am J Med.* 1948; 4:3–9.
52. Saltin B, Astrand PO, Grover RF, et al. Response to exercise after bed rest and after training. *Circulation.* 1968; 38(suppl 7):1.
53. Miller PB, Johnson RL, Lamb LE. Effects of four weeks of absolute bed rest on circulatory functions in man. *Aerospace Med.* 1964; 35:1194.
54. Lamb LE, Stevens PM, Johnson RL. Hypokinesia secondary to chair rest from 4 to 10 days. *Aerospace Med.* 1965; 36, 755.

55. DeBusk RF, Convertino VA, Hung J, Goldwater D. Exercise conditioning in middle-aged men after 10 days of bed rest. *Circulation*. 1983; 68:245.

56. Buller AJ, Eccles JC, Eccles RM. Interaction between motor neurons and muscles in respect of the characteristic speeds of their responses. *J Physiol*. 1960; 150:417–419.

57. Muller EA. Influence of training and of inactivity on muscle strength. *Arch Phys Med Rehabil*. 1970; 51:449.

58. Fugiswawa Y, Kida K, Matsuda H. Role of change in vitamin D metabolism with age in calcium and phosphorus metabolism in normal subjects. *J Clin Endocrinol Metab*. 1984;59:719–726.

59. Kenney RA. *Physiology of Aging: A Synopsis*. Chicago; Year Book Medical Publishers, Inc.; 1982.

60. Ham RJ, Marcy ML. Normal aging: a review of systems/the maintenance of health. In: Wright J, ed. *Primary Care Geriatrics*. Boston; PSG, Inc.; 1983.

61. Evans CE, Galasko CS, Ward, C. Effect of donor age on the growth in vitro of cells obtained from human trabecular bone. *J Orthop Res*. 1990; 8(2):234–237.

62. Zadai CC. Cardiopulmonary issues in the geriatric population: implications for rehabilitation. *Top Geriatr Rehabil*. 1986; 2(1):1–9.

63. Cummings G, Semple SG. *Disorders of the Respiratory System*. Oxford, England; Blackwell; 1973.

64. Wynne JW. Pulmonary disease in the elderly. In: Rossman I, ed. *Clinical Geriatrics*. 2nd ed. Philadelphia; Lippincott; 1979.

65. Goldman R. Decline in organ function with age. In: Rossman I, ed. *Clinical Geriatrics*. 2nd ed. Philadelphia; Lippincott; 1979.

66. Ham RJ, Marcy ML, Holtzman JM. The aging process: biological and social aspects. In: Wright J, ed. *Primary Care Geriatrics*. Boston; PSG, Inc.; 1983.

67. Hamlin CR, Luschin JH, Kohn RR. Aging of collagen: comparative rates in four mammalian species. *Exp Gerontol*. 1980; 15:393–398.

68. Astrand PO, Rodahl K. *Textbook of Work Physiology*. San Francisco, London; McGraw-Hill Book Co.; 1970.

69. Meyer K, Hoffman P, Linker A. Mucopolysacchrides of costal cartilage. *Science*. 1958; 128:896.

70. Pickles LW. Effects of aging on connective tissues. *Geriatrics*. 1983; 38(1):71–78.

71. Hole JW. *Human Anatomy and Physiology*. Iowa; WC Brown Co.; 1978.

72. Kaplan D, Mayer K. Distribution of alkaline phosphatase. *Nature*. 1959; 183:1262–1263.

73. Calliet R. Mechanisms of joints. In: Licht S, ed. *Arthiritis and Physical Medicine*. Baltimore; Waverly Press; 1969.

74. Palmoski MJ, Colyer RA, Brandt KD. Joint motion in the absence of normal loading does not maintain normal articular cartilage. *Arthritis Rheum*. 1985; 23:325.

75. Gardner DL. Aging of articular cartilage In: Brockehurst JC, ed. *Textbook of Geriatric Medicine and Gerontology*. New York: Longman Group Ltd., 1978.

76. Larson EB, Bruce RA. Health benefits of exercise in an aging society. *Arch Intern Med*. 1987; 147:353.

77. World Health Organization. *Constitution of the World Health Organization*. Geneva; World Health Organization; 1964.

78. American Diabetes Association. *Direct and Indirect Costs of Diabetes in the United States in 1987*. Alexandria, Va: American Diabetes Association Report; 1988.

79. Himann JE, et al. Age-related changes in speed of walking. *Med Sci Sports Exerc*. 1988; 20:161.

80. Siegler IC, Costa PT, Jr. Health behavior relationships. In: Birren JE, Schaie KW, eds. *Handbook of the Psychology of Aging*. 2nd ed. New York; Van Nostrand Reinhold; 1985.

81. Kaplan E. Psychological factors and ischemic heart disease mortality: a focal role for perceived health. Paper presented at the annual meeting of the American Psychological Association, Washington, DC; 1982.

82. Mossey JM, Shapiro E. Self-rated health: a predictor of mortality among the elderly. *Am J Public Health*. 1982; 72:800–808.

83. Rosillo RA, Fagel ML. Correlation of psychologic variables and progress in physical therapy: I. degree of disability and denial of illness. *Arch Phys Med Rehabil*. 1970; 51:227.

84. Stoedefalke KG. Motivating and sustaining the older adult in an exercise program. *Top Geriatr Rehabil*. 1985; 1;78.

85. Nader IM, et al. Level of aspiration and performance of chronic psychiatric patients on a simple motor task. *Percept Mot Skills*. 1985; 60:767.

86. Prohaska T, Pontiam IA, Teitleman J. Age differences in attributions to causality: implications for intellection assessment. *Exp Aging Res.* 1984; 10:111.

87. Eisdorder L. Arousal and performance: experiments in verbal learning and a tentative theory. In: Talland GA, ed. *Human Aging and Behavior.* New York: Academic Press; 1968.

88. Weinberg R, Bruya L, Jackson A. The effects of goal proximity and goal specificity on endurance performance. *J Soc Psychol.* 1985; 7:296.

89. Mento A, Steele RP, Karren RJ. A metaanalytic study of the effects of goal setting on task performance: 1966–1984. *Organ Behav Hum Decis Process.* 1987; 39:52.

90. Smith E, Serfass R. *Exercise and Aging: The Scientific Basis.* Hillside, NJ; Hillside, NJ; Enslow Publishers; 1981.

91. Stelmach CE, Worringham CJ. Sensorimotor deficits related to postural stability: implications for falling in the elderly. In: Radebaugh TS, et al., eds. *Clinics of Geriatric Medicine.* Philadelphia: Saunders; 1985:1(3).

92. McPherson BD, ed. *Sport and Aging: The 1984 Olympic Scientific Congress Proceedings.* Champaign, Ill: Human Kinetics Publishers, Inc.; 1986:5.

93. Seltzer B, Rheaume Y, Volicer L, et al. The short-term effects of in-hospital respite on the patient with Alzheimer's disease. *Gerontologist.* 1988; 28(1):121–124.

94. Knott M, Voss DE. *Proprioceptive Nuromuscular Facilitation: Patterns of Techniques.* 2nd ed. New York; Harper and Row Publishers; 1968.

95. Bottomley JM. *Am J Phys Ther.* (in press).

96. Marshall L. Auditory processing in aging listeners. *J Speech Hear Disord.* 1981; 46:226–238.

97. Gutman E. *Age Changes in the Neuromuscular System.* Great Britain; Bristol, Ltd.; 1972.

98. Payton OD, Poland JL. Aging process: implications for clinical practice. *Phys Ther.* 1983; 63(1):41–48.

99. Brody H. Kliemer lecture, Gerontological Society Meeting. *Gerontology News.* Washington, DC: Gerontological Society of America. November, 1979.

100. McCarter R. Effects of age on contraction of mammalian skeletal muscle. In: Kalkor G, DiBattista J, eds. *Aging in Muscle.* New York; Raven; 1978; 1–22.

101. Moritani T. Training adaptations in the muscles of older men. In: Smith EL, Serfass RC. *Exercise and Aging: The Scientific Basis.* Hillside, NJ; Enslow Publishers; 1981; 149–166.

102. Gutman E, Hanzlikova V. Fast and slow motor units in aging. *Gerontology.* 1976; 22:280–300.

103. MacLennan WJ, Hall MRP, Timothy JI. Postural hypotension in old age: is it a disorder of the nervous system or of blood vessels? *Age Aging.* 1980; 9:25–32.

104. Ragen PB, Mitchell J. The effects of aging on the cardiovascular response to dynamic and static exercise. In: Weisfelt ML, ed. *The Aging Heart.* New York: Raven; 1980; 269–296.

105. Murray MP. Normal postural stability and steadiness: quantitative assessment. *J Bone Joint Surg (Am).* June, 1975; 57(A):510.

107. Carlson KE, Alston W, Feldman DJ. Electromyographic study of aging skeletal muscle. *Am J Phys Med.* 1964; 43:141–152.

108. Darling RC. Fatigue. In: Downey JA, Darling RC, eds. *Physiological Basis of Rehabilitation Medicine.* Philadelphia: Saunders; 1971.

109. Kohl HW, Moorefield DL, Blair SN. Is cardiorespiratory fitness associated with general chronic fatigue in apparently healthy men and women? *Med Sci Sports Exerc.* 1987; 19(S6).

110. Christiansen J, Juhl E, eds. The prevention of falls in later life. *Danish Med Bull.* 1987; 34(Suppl) (4):1–24.

111. Kalchthaler T, Bascon RA, Quintos V. Falls in the institutionalized elderly. *J Am Geriatr Soc.* 1978; 26:424.

112. Tinetti ME. Factors associated with serious injury during falls by ambulatory nursing home residents. *J Am Geriatr Soc.* 1987; 35:644.

113. Gryfe CI, Amies A, Ashley MJ. A longitudinal study of falls in an elderly population: I. incidence and morbidity. *Age Aging.* 1977; 6:201.

114. Wild D, Nayak US, Isaacs B. How dangerous are falls in old people at home? *Br Med J.* 1981; 282:266.

115. Tideiksaar R. Fall prevention in the home. *Top Geriatr Rehabil.* 1987; 3(1):57–64.

116. Droller H. Falls among elderly people living at home. *Geriatrics.* 1955;10:239–244.

117. Archea JC. Environmental factors associated with stair accidents by the elderly. *Clin Geriatr Med.* 1985; 1:555.

118. Ashley MJ, Gryfe CT, Aimes A. A longitudinal study of falls in an elderly population. II. Some circumstances of falling. *Age Aging.* 1977; 6:211.

119. Louis M. Falls and their causes. *J Gerontol Nurs.* 1983; 9:142.

120. Lawrence MS. Strengthening the quadriceps: progressively prolonged isometric tension method. *Phys Ther Rev.* 1956; 36:658.

121. Horak FB. Clinical measurement of posture control in adults. *Phys Ther.* 1987; 67:1881.

122. Bobath B. *Adult Hemiplegia: Evaluation and Treatment.* 2nd ed. London: Heineman Medical Books; 1978.

123. Woollacott MJ, Shumway-Cook A, Nashner L. Aging and posture control. *Int J Aging Hum Devel.* 1986; 23:97.

124. Shumway-Cook A, Horak FB. Assessing the influence of sensory interaction on balance. *Phys Ther.* 1986; 66:1548.

125. Stout RW. Falls and disorders of postural balance. *Age Aging.* 1978; 7:134.

126. Carr JH, Shepard RB. *A Motor Relearning Program for Stroke.* 2nd ed. Rockville, Md; Aspen Publishers; 1987.

127. Gabell A. Falls in the elderly: will dance reduce their incidence? *Human Movement Studies.* 1986; 12:119.

128. Government Document. *Alzheimer's disease: Report of the Secretaries Task Force on Alzheimer's Disease.* Washington, DC; US Government Printing Office; 1984. Rockville, Md; US Department of Health and Human Services, Public Health Service, Alcohol, Drug Abuse, and Mental Health Administration. DHHS pub. no. (ADM) 84–1323.

129. Government Document. *Alzheimer's Disease.* Washington, DC: US Government Printing Office; 1984. Joint hearing before the Subcommittee on Health and Long-Term Care of the Select Committee on Aging and the Subcommittee on Energy and Commerce. House of Representatives, 98th Congress, first session.

130. Liebowitz B, Lawton MP, Waldman A. Evaluation: designing for confused elderly people. *AIA Journal.* 1979; 2:59–61.

131. Weldon S, Yesavage JA. Behavioral improvement with relaxation training in senile dementia. *Clinical Gerontologist.* 1982; 1(1):45–49.

132. Cohen GD. The mental health professional and Alzheimer's patient. Hosp Community Psychiatry. 1984; 35(2):115–116, 122.

133. Reifler BV, Wu S. Managing families of the demented elderly. *J Fam Pract.* 1982; 14(6):1051–1056.

134. Lubinski R. Speech, language, and audiology programs in home health care agencies and nursing homes. In: Beasley DS, Davis GA, eds. *Aging: Communication Processes and Disorders.* New York; Grune and Stratton; 1981.

135. Sharpe DT. *The Psychology of Color and Design.* Chicago: Nelson-Hall Co.; 1974.

136. Hellebrandt FA. The senile dement in our midst: a look at the other side of the coin. *Gerontologist.* 1978; 18:67–70.

137. Lawton MP. Assessing the competence of older people. In: Kent D, Kastenbaum R, Sherwood S, eds. *Research Planning and Action for the Elderly.* New York; Behavioral Publications; 1972.

138. Lawton MP, Brody EM. Assessment of older people: self-maintaining and instrumental activities of daily living. *Gerontologist.* 1969;9:179–186.

Patient Evaluation

Preparation	Pain Assessment
Setting	Physical Assessment—How To
Tools	Environmental Assessment
Timing	Psychosocial Assessment
Expectations	Conclusion
Interview	Appendices
Physical Assessment	

Of all the elements of patient care, evaluation is the most crucial. A comprehensive evaluation provides the practitioner with all the necessary information for designing an appropriate program. Since older patients often present with complex problems because of multiple pathologies and the effects of aging, a thorough evaluation may be more difficult. Nevertheless, it is even more important to determine the exact nature of the problem. This chapter divides evaluation into six main components: preparation, expectations, the interview, physical assessment, environmental assessment, and psychosocial assessment. Assessment will be covered briefly here in terms of the initial evaluation. For a more detailed account, please refer to Chapter 6.

PREPARATION

Setting

What background is essential for a good evaluation of older patients? A quiet noncompeting environment is important because there is a high probability that the patient will have some hearing loss,[1] and background noise will make it difficult for the patient to hear questions. In addition, many older persons suffer from vision loss. Therefore, examination areas should be well lit and nonglare. Therapists should provide enough room for movement, and doorways and room space should be large enough to be wheelchair accessible. The room should have a comfortable, sturdy, 18-inch (or higher) chair available.[1] Optimally, the bed or treatment table should be automatically adjustable for height. The floor should have a low pile carpet or a low gloss nonslippery floor. Finally, the colors in the room should be those that make the older person most at ease, such as reds, oranges, gold, and beige. These colors should also be contrasted to avoid visual misinterpretation.[2] This scenario is for a clinical setting; however, many evaluations are done in the home. In the home setting try to imitate this background as closely as possible.

Tools

Any general evaluation form can be sufficient for the initial evaluation visit; however, specific forms for functional, physical (orthopedic, neurological, and cardiopulmonary), environmental, and psychosocial assessment are helpful and often cue the clinician to ask appropriate questions. It should be noted that many of the functional evaluation forms listed in Chapter 6 can be given to the patient prior to the evaluation. Forms for different diagnoses can be used by the clinician to look for specific problems. (See Appendix A for orthopedic, neurological, and cardiopulmonary forms.)

Timing

When is the best time to do an evaluation? There are times during the day when people perform better. It would be impossible to schedule evaluations to fit each patient's peak performance; however, a thorough clinician should ask the patient when he or she performs the best and note it. Only one time is contraindicated for an initial evaluation, and that is immediately following a large meal.[3] This is due to the decrease in blood flow to the brain for 1 hour after a large meal, which is most apparent in older patients.[3] Therefore, it is not good to overtax the system by doing an evaluation immediately after a large meal.

EXPECTATIONS

A clinician unfamiliar with treating geriatric patients can expect different levels of performance from an older person in an initial evaluation as compared to a younger person. Clinical experience shows that the older patient cannot tolerate a similar history taking session as younger patients. Initial evaluation may need some modification, especially in the physical performance area. Robin McKenzie, for example, requests that his patients both extend and flex the trunk approximately ten times.[4] This type of repetition is too rigorous for most older persons. Physically, most older persons can tolerate one or two repetitions of a movement, and can tolerate rolling into different positions one to two times. For these reasons, a clinician may need to anticipate two sessions to complete a thorough evaluation.

INTERVIEW

Though a great deal of information can be collected from the interview process, much of it is not useful. Limiting responses and directing questions is the key to a successful interview.

A good way to start an interview is to ask the patient, "Why are you here to see me?" A good follow-up to this question is, "What do you expect from physical therapy?" These two questions give the interviewer the main problem (usually in functional terms) and the patient's goals (again, in functional terms).

The next important piece of information is the relevant history. One way to get this information is to ask, "How did this happen?" Follow-up questions along this line are, "Have you had anything similar to this before?" or, "What do you think contributed to this?" To obtain additional medical history information that could impact the rehabilitation progress ask, "What other medical problems do you have that I need to know about?" or, "What other medical problems do you have that may affect your progress?"

Other important information that can easily be gathered in the initial interview is the patient's social support system. for example, a question like, "Do you live alone?" followed by, "Who is the main person that helps you when you are ill or having difficulties with any of your daily activities?" will give the clinician important insight into the patient's social support. Age, weight, and medication usage can all be asked in the initial interview.

The initial interview session can also be used to gather information on subjective areas. Pain assessments are the major subjective tests used by the geriatric physical therapist. When assessing pain in the elderly person the clinician should be aware of two different presentations of symptoms in the older patient from the younger. First, older people tend to underreport pain, and second, they are less sensitive to pain.[5,6] There are several pain ratings available for assessing pain in the elderly; some are better than others.

PHYSICAL ASSESSMENT

Physical assessment is probably the most important aspect of the physical therapist's time with a patient. Physical assessment will provide the therapist with both subjective and objective data from which to develop and monitor a treatment program. Appendix A contains sample forms for the orthopedic, neurological, and cardiopulmonary assessment. Chapter 6 provides specific information on aging changes that will affect some of the outcome measures in the tools listed in Appendix A.

The application of physical assessment tools in the geriatric patient is similar to younger patients except for the variables listed in the beginning of the chapter as well as the following:

1. The therapist should relate physical findings to function. For example, what is the patient unable to do with shoulder flexion limited to 90°?
2. An entire assessment may need to be broken up and conducted in several sessions. The older person may not have the endurance to complete an entire physical assessment.
3. Psychosocial components must be considered along with physical parameters (see subsequent section).
4. Pain can be a major component and should be assessed thoroughly in an older person (see next section).

Pain Assessment

Pain evaluation tools can be divided into four categories. The first includes general pain evaluation tools. (For example, asking a patient to rate his or her pain as severe, moderate, or mild.) Pain diagrams are the second type of pain evaluation tools. An example of a pain diagram is the visual analog scale, which is simply a 100 mm line with a label at top and bottom.[7] Figure 10–1 is an example of a visual analog scale. To use this scale, the older person simply marks the place that corresponds to their pain. The clinician then measures the distance from no pain to the mark. For example, on an initial evaluation a patient may have 67 mm of pain on the visual analog scale and 2 weeks later they mark their pain as 23 mm. How-

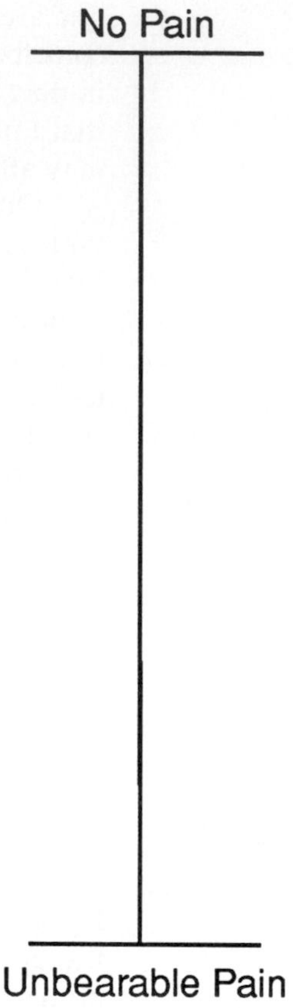

No Pain

Figure 10–1. *Visual analog scale.* Unbearable Pain

ever, pain diagrams pose potential problems for older patients. The tests require abstract thinking, and older persons do not tend to perform as well on tests of this nature.[6]

The third group of pain assessment tools are pain language tools. A good example of a pain language tool is the McGill-Melzak Pain Questionnaire.[8] This one-page questionnaire uses different pain descriptors to rank the person's pain. This particular test has been used with older populations; however, specific reliability and validity for this test and the older population has not been demonstrated.

The final type of pain tool is a pain diary, which is a running record of the person's pain. There are pros and cons for this tool. A pain diary can be useful, because it helps the patient focus and become aware of how pain affects their life.[9] A major drawback of it is that the patient often becomes too focused on his or her pain as a result.[10]

The interview process can provide a wealth of information for the clinician. According to Rothstein and associates the information synthesizing process begins in the interview process, even before the clinician lays hands on the patient.[11]

Physical Assessment—How To

Once the interview session is over, the physical process begins. If a treatment session could be extended to 4 hours, it would be possible to evaluate every aspect of the person during the physical assessment session. In reality, though, treatment sessions often last less than an hour, and it becomes crucial that the clinician choose to assess the areas that may affect the problem. The other reason for focusing on the major problem area is that the older person may have limited stamina.[12]

TABLE 10–1. PROBLEMS MORE COMMON OR SEVERE IN THE ELDERLY

1. Falls	18. Spinal stenosis
2. Syncope	19. Diabetic hyperosmolar nonketotic coma
3. Hip fracture	20. Inappropriate antidiuretic hormone secretion
4. Urinary incontinence	21. Accidental hypothermia
5. Fecal incontinence	22. Chronic lymphatic leukemia
6. Fecal impaction	23. Basal cell carcinoma
7. Pressure sores	24. Angioimmunoblastic lymphadenopathy with dysproteinemia
8. Hearing and vision impairment	
9. Stroke	25. Solid tumors
10. Dementia syndrome	26. Tuberculosis
11. Parkinsonism	27. Herpes zoster
12. Normal pressure hydrocephalus	28. Arteriosclerosis
13. Polymyalgia rheumatica/giant cell arteritis	29. Amyloidosis
14. Osteoporosis	30. Colonic angiodysplasia
15. Osteoarthritis	31. Isolated systolic hypertension
16. Paget's disease	32. Postural hypotension
17. Carpal tunnel syndrome	

Reprinted with permission from Besdine RW. Clinical approach to the elderly. In: Rowe JW, Besdine RW. Geriatric Medicine. ed 2. Boston: Little Brown & Co.; 1988: Table 3–5:30.

Appendix A contains many different types of evaluation forms. The first group of forms are orthopedic forms that can be used for the different body parts. For example, if a patient complains of neck pain, the therapist should evaluate the pain using a neck evaluation form. The forms included in Appendix A were specifically developed in a geriatric clinic.[13] The neurological forms look at various functional problems related to mobility. Appendix A contains forms to evaluate problems with bed mobility, sitting, standing, gait, and balance. In addition, stroke and Parkinson's evaluation forms are included.

The final area for evaluation is the cardiopulmonary system. A specific cardiopulmonary evaluation form is provided in Appendix A. Even though the physical assessment forms are divided into specific areas, it is often necessary to assess the patient's cardiopulmonary status, even if treating the patient for neck pain. Therefore, the wise clinician will use different pieces of various forms depending on individual patient needs.

Table 10–1 lists the more common problems among older people that a clinician should be aware of during an initial evaluation.[14]

ENVIRONMENTAL ASSESSMENT

Because there are so many changes that are common among the older population, environmental assessments may be necessary for the institution or the home. Appendix B contains an environmental assessment form for the home and the institution. These forms can be used by the clinician, family, or patient.

Assessing the environment should not be taken lightly. Lawton's "environmental docility hypothesis" states that the proportion of the behavior attributable to the environment increases as the person's competence decreases.[15] In addition, the older person has diminished senses and, therefore, reacts less to the environment. This results in a cascade of internalization and a decrease in reality and function.[16] Some evidence shows that enriched environments can favorably affect older persons.[17,18]

The assessment of color and lighting is an extremely important aspect of the environmental evaluation. The use of appropriate color can minimize the adverse effects of sensory deprivation, enhance mood, and improve function.[19] Color usage follows several simple rules:

1. Increase lighting as much as possible (up to three times as much as for younger persons).[20]
2. Use matte surfaces. Avoid glare on any surface.
3. Use contrasting colors as much as possible (that is, light and dark, different hues, cold and warm colors).
4. Use cues; however, make sure they are of adequate size and are clear and visible.
5. Use daylight fluorescent light. This light offers a broader distribution of light.[21]

PSYCHOSOCIAL ASSESSMENT

Specific psychosocial assessment forms are described in Chapters 4 and 6, therefore, this section will discuss when a psychosocial assessment is appropriate. The areas most important to the outcome of rehabilitation are depression and dementia. Depression is important because it will affect the participant's assessment and expectation of the rehabilitation program. The depressed client will have lower expectations and tend to underassess progress. In addition, depression can cause lethargy, which may discourage the client from participating in an exercise program.[22] Therefore, if the astute clinician senses depression from the global signs (i.e., pessimism, low self-esteem, loss of interest, and preoccupation with body aches), administering a depression test may be beneficial. The Geriatric Depression Scale is a good tool for assessing the older population. (See Chapters 4 and 6 for further discussion.) Once the clinician has determined that depression is a major problem, he or she should be aware that complaints of lethargy may only be a manifestation of depression. In addition, the clinician can also be on guard for subjective ratings of improvement or lack thereof.

Dementia, or brain syndrome, may also require special considerations in the rehabilitation program. If the clinician notices that the client has difficulty remembering during the initial questioning, then dementia may be the cause. Any of the brain syndrome screening tools may be administered at this time. (See Chapters 4 and 6.) If a patient does have a dementia, then the clinician must modify and simplify the treatment program so that the patient will derive the most benefit. Making the program more familiar, shorter, simpler, and more dependent on automatic responses will assist the patient with dementia. In addition, providing instruction to the care giver is crucial.

The final aspect of applying a psychological assessment is implementation. Many patients will resent being asked psychosocial questions in a physical therapy setting. A good approach is to say, "I am going to ask you a few questions that will measure mental processes. The questions may seem silly, but if we begin an exercise program that is too stressful for you, one of the first areas to show a change is your mental processing. Therefore, I need to get an initial assessment." Finally, as stated above, psychological assessments can be used to measure exercise tolerance.

CONCLUSION

Patient evaluation provides be some of the most valuable time a therapist spends with a patient. The initial evaluation provides the clinician with information that will enable him or her to design the most appropriate rehabilitation program. Once a thorough evaluation has been done, the rehabilitation program can begin. The next step is to conduct periodic reevaluations.

PEARLS

- The essential setting for evaluating an older person is a noncompeting environment that is well lit, has non-glare surfaces, is wheelchair accessible, and is color contrasted with low pile carpet or nonslip floors.

- The initial interview should focus on functional decrements and include questions on history, social support, and subjective findings.

- When physically assessing the aged, consider breaking up the initial evaluation into several visits.

- When assessing pain in the elderly, use additional pain tools, such as pain diagram, pain diaries, pain language tools, and general pain evaluations.

- The environment should be assessed for safety and optimal functioning because as the older person becomes frailer, they become more dependent on the environment.

- Psychosocial aspects of an older person may be awkward for the physical therapist to assess; however, using the straightforward approach will be easiest.

REFERENCES

1. Cooper BA. Model of implementing color contrast in the environment of the elderly. *Am J Occup Ther.* 1985; 39:253–258.
2. Cristarella M. Visual functions of the elderly. *Am J Occup Ther.* 1977; 31:432–440.
3. Lipsitz L, Fullerton R. Post prandial blood pressure reduction in healthy elderly. *J Am Ger Soc.* 1986; 34(4):267–270.
4. McKenzie R. *The Lumbar Spine: Mechanical Diagnosis and Therapy.* Waikanee, New Zealand: Spinal Public; 1981.
5. Harkins S, Kiventis J, Price D. Pain and the elderly. In: Benedette C, et al., eds. *Advances in Pain Management in the Elderly.* New York: Raven; 1984.
6. Ferrel B. Pain management in the elderly. *J Am Ger Soc.* 1991; 36–64–73.
7. Lewis C. *Documentation: Physical Therapists Course in Successful Reimbursement.* Bethesda, Md: Professional Health Educators; 1987.
8. Melzak R. *The Puzzle of Pain.* New York: Basic Books; 1973.
9. Mannheimer J. *Clinical Transculaneous Nerve Stimulation.* Philadelphia: Davis; 1984.
10. Woodruff L. Pain and Aging. Paper presented at APTA June Conference; 1990.
11. Echternach J, Rothstein J. Hypothesis-oriented algorithms. *Phys Ther.* 1989; 69–559–564.
12. Haines RF. Effect of bed rest and exercise on body balance. *J Appl Physiol.* 1974; 36:323.
13. Lewis C. Forms from physical therapy services of Washington, DC, Inc., 1990.
14. Besdine RW. Clinical approach to the elderly. In: Rowe JW, Besdine RW. *Geriatric Medicine.* 2nd ed. Boston: Little Brown & Co.; 1988.
15. Lawton MP. Assessment, integration and environments for older people. *Gerontologist.* 1970; 10:38–46.
16. Kraus A, Spasoff R, Beattie E. Elderly applicants to long-term care institutions: their characteristics, health problems and state of mind. *J Am Ger Soc.* 1976; 24(3):117–125.
17. Birren F. Human response to color and light. *Hospitals.* 1979, 53(14):93–96.
18. Whelihan W. Geriatric centers environment fosters interaction. *Hosp Prog.* 1980; 61:50–55.
19. Hiatt L. Care and design for color and use of color in environments for older persons. *Nursing Homes.* 1981; 30:18–22.
20. Corso J. Sensory processes and age effects in normal adults. *J Gerontol.* 1971; 26:90–105.
21. Sylvania GTE. Engineering Bulletin 0–341. Fluorescent Lamps. Montreal, Canada.
22. Zarit S. Aging and mental disorders. In: *A Psychological Approach to Assessment and Treatment.* New York: The Free Press; 1980.

Appendix A Orthopedic, Neurological, and Cardiopulmonary Evaluation Forms

Orthopedic Evaluation Forms
  Hip Pain Evaluation
  Hip Fractures
  Knee Evaluation
  Foot Assessment
  Shoulder Evaluation
  Neck Evaluation
  Back Evaluation
Neurological Evaluation Forms
  Hemiplegic Evaluation
  Coordination Evaluation

Mobility Assessments
  Transfer Evaluation
  Balance and Falls Assessment
Cardiopulmonary Evaluation Forms
Cardiopulmonary Evaluation
  Step Test
  Medical History Form
  Physical Activity Questionnaire
  Exercise Data Sheet

ORTHOPEDIC EVALUATION FORMS

Hip Pain Evaluation

Name _____ Age: _____ Sex: _____

Diagnosis _____

History _____

Precautions _____

Function _____

Pain
    Character _____

    When _____

    Where _____

    What increases _____

    What decreases _____

    Position of comfort _____

Low back check
    History _____

    ROM _____

    Pain _____

    Movement _____

Range of motion and strength

	ROM		STRENGTH	
	L	R	L	R
Hip Flexion				
Extension				
Adduction				
Abduction				
IR				
ER				
Knee Flexion				
Knee Extension				
Unilateral Stance				

Tenderness or Spasm _____

    Hip _____

    Thigh _____

    Knee _____

Posture _____

Gait _____

Sensation _____

Other _____

Figure 10A–1. (© *Carole B Lewis, Geriatric Orthopedics Handout.*)

Physical Therapy Evaluation and Treatment Report for Patients with Hip Fracture in Extended Care Settings

Name _____ Date _____ Record # _____

Age _____ Sex _____ Referring Physician _____

Description of fracture _____

Onset _____ Fixation used _____

Surgery date _____ Additional diagnoses _____

_____

Medications potentially impacting rehab performance _____

Other significant medications _____

Current weight bearing orders _____

Preinjury living arrangements _____

Preinjury functional/ADL status _____

Social support available _____

Bowel and bladder control _____

HOSPITAL DISCHARGE PHYSICAL THERAPY STATUS

Exercise program _____

Assistive devices used _____

Distance ambulating _____

Equipment brought to facility _____

SKIN EVALUATION

At risk bony prominences (heel of affected leg, sacrum, trochanters) _____

_____

General skin condition; other bony prominences _____

_____

Suture line _____

PHYSICAL AND FUNCTIONAL EVALUATION

Ability to go sitting to supine _____

Ability to relieve pressure from affected heel _____

Ability to roll to either side _____

Range of Motion

Affected Limb:

Hip _____

Knee _____ Ankle _____

Other Extremities and Trunk _____

_____

Leg length comparison _____

Ability to go supine to sitting _____

Manual Muscle Testing

	(R) arm	(L) arm		Unaffected Leg	Affected Leg
Shoulder flexors	_____	_____	Hip flexors	_____	Not tested
Serratus Antenor	_____	_____	Hip extensors	_____	Not tested
Biceps	_____	_____	Hip abductors	_____	Not tested
Triceps	_____	_____	Knee extensors	_____	_____
Wrist extensors	_____	_____	Knee flexors	_____	_____
			Ankle dorsiflexors	_____	_____
			Ankle plantarflexors	_____	_____

Continued

Continued from previous page

Tool for Physical Therapy Evaluation

Transfer ability: to horizontal surface _____
_____ to toilet _____
_____
Ability to come to standing _____
Gait Analysis (Address device, distance, ability to maintain weight bearing orders, posture, gait deviations, endurance, balance, etc.)

Discomfort in the affected limb _____
Other pain/discomfort _____
Wheelchair safety _____
Wheelchair mobility _____
Ability to stair climb _____

SENSORY AND EMOTIONAL EVALUATION
Vision _____ Hearing _____
Emotional state _____
Motivation _____
Ability to follow instructions _____

OTHER SIGNIFICANT FINDINGS

ASSESSMENT/REHABILITATION POTENTIAL
Short-range Goals:

Long-range Goals:

Treatment Plan:

_____
Physician's Comments: Therapist's Signature

Physician's Certification/Recertification

I certify _____ re-certify _____ that I have examined the patient and physical therapy is necessary and that service will be furthered while the patient is under my care, and that the plan is established and will be reviewed every 30 days or more often if the patient's condition requires. I estimate that these services will be needed for about _____ (specify no. of days, weeks, or months)

Physician's name	Physician's Signature	Date	Telephone

Figure 10A–2. *(Reprinted with permission from Hielema F, Mitchell R, Dyster R. A tool for the physical therapy evaluation of patients with hip fractures in the extended care setting. Top Ger Rehab. 1989; 4(2):56–57.)*

Knee Evaluation

Date _____

Name _____ Age and Sex _____

Diagnosis _____

History _____

Pain _____

Functional activities _____

   Sitting to Standing _____

   Ambulation (device & assistance needed) _____

   Approximate distance ambulates before resting _____

   Elevations (stairs, curbs, & ramps) _____

Range of motion—muscle strength

	(R) - ROM - (L)	(R) - MS - (L)
Hip Flexion		
Abduction		
External Rotation		
Internal Rotation		
Straight Leg Raise		
Knee Flexion		
Extension/Extension lag		
Ankle Plantarflexion		
Dorsiflexion		

Crepitations _____

Patellar Tracking _____

Leg length (ASIS —Med. Malleolus) (R) _____ (L) _____

Gait and posture

   Summary gait analysis _____

   Standing Time _____ Bilateral _____ Left _____ Right _____ 8 Steps _____

   Genu valgus or varus _____

   Sensation _____

Girth

	Left	Right
0 cm		
5 cm		
10 cm		
15 cm		
15 cm		

Swelling _____

Skin _____

Medication _____

Mentation _____

Goals _____

Treatment plan _____

Additional comments _____

Figure 10A–3. *(© Carole B Lewis, Geriatric Orthopedics Handout.)*

Assessment of the Foot

Name _____ Age _____ Assistive Device _____

Past Medical History _____

Current Medications _____

Complaints of Pain   Type _____   Location _____

At rest _____ Incessant _____ On movement _____

Light Touch Sensation: L4 _____   L5 _____   S1 _____

Vibratory Sensation _____

Inspection   Swelling? Volumetric measurements skin (ulcers? bunion? color, temp, nails, dryness, calluses?)

_____ R.A. Nodules? _____

Circulatory Status   Pulses: Posterior Tibialis _____   Dorsal Pedalis _____

Posture of Foot   Hallux Valgus/Varus _____   Foot Pronation _____

Forefoot Splaying _____ Lesser Toe Deformities _____

Calcaneal Valgus _____ Other _____

		Active	Passive	Resistive	(Pain) (Strength)
Ankle ROM	Dorsiflexion	_____			
	Plantarflexion	_____			
Subtalar Motion	Supination	_____			
	Pronation	_____			
Midtarsal Motion	Inversion/Eversion	_____			
	ABduction/ADDuction	_____			

Abductor Halluxes   Strength: _____

ROM: _____

Hallux Extension/Flexion   Strength: _____

ROM: _____

Digit Extension/Flexion   Strength: _____

ROM: _____

Digit Addubction   Strength: _____

Strength/ROM Deficits in   Hip _____

Figure 10A–4.   *(© Carole B Lewis, Geriatric Orthopedics Handout.)*

Shoulder Evaluation

Name: _____   Date: _____

Age: _____   Diagnosis:_____

_____

History:

1. Where is your pain?

_____

2. Was there an injury?

_____

3. How long have you had your problem?

_____

4. Have any other joints been affected?

_____

5. Has your pain spread?

_____

6. When does your pain occur?

_____

Observation: (check symmetry, atrophy or subluxation)

1. A-C Joint: _____   2. Superior border
of scapula: _____

3. Inferior angle of   4. Other areas: _____
Scapula: _____   _____

Palpation:

1. A-C joint (place arm in abduction past 90°, then horizontally adduct in forward flexion)
Pain _____   No Pain _____

2. Rotator Cuff Insertion (Place arm in internal rotation, extension and adduction)
Pain _____   No Pain _____

3. Crepitus
Yes _____   No _____

(FR = Full Range; LR = Limited Range; P = Pain; NP = No Pain)

——————Continued——————

━━━━ *Continued from previous page* ━━━━

4. Temperature (state whether hot, warm, cool; compare to other side) _____

	Active Movements	Passive Movements	Resisted Movements
Forward Flexion			
Abduction			
External Rotation			
Internal Rotation			
Extension			

Special Tests

Drop Arm Test: (Abduct arm to 90°, patient should be able to lower arm slowly down; if test is positive, patient unable to control arm)

Positive: _____   Negative: _____

Arthrogram Results: _____

_____

X-Ray Findings: _____

_____

Figure 10A–5.   *(© Carole B Lewis, Geriatric Orthopedics Handout.)*

Neck Evaluation

Date: _____ Age: _____ Sex: _____

Name: _____

Diagnosis:_____

Precautions:_____

History: _____

Function:_____

Range of Motion	Strength		Passive		Normal	Active		Comments
	Left	Right	Left	Right		Left	Right	
Flexion					0–30			
Extension					0–35			
Lat Flexion					0–40			
Rotation					0–130			

Shoulder ROM _____

Description of pain:

_____ Localized   _____ Sharp   _____ VAS

_____ Diffuse   _____ Prolonged; Intense

_____ Other   _____ Burning   Posture:

Forward Head _____

Scoliosis _____

Kyphosis _____

Shoulder Radiation_____

Related Pain _____

  When pain occurs _____

  Frequency and duration _____

  Position of comfort _____

Abnormal Sensation _____

Spasms (indicate position tested, area and degree) _____

Medication _____

Vocation or Avocation _____

Sleep position _____

Goals _____

Treatment _____

Additional Comments _____

Figure 10A–6. *(© Carole B Lewis, Geriatric Orthopedics Handout.)*

Low Back Evaluation

Patient: _____   Date: _____

Diagnosis: _____

HX: _____

I. Pain Description

  A. Where: _____

  B. How long: _____

  C. At rest: _____

        Sitting: _____

        Standing: _____

        Lying: _____

        Other: _____

  D. With activity: _____

        Walking: _____

        Lifting: _____

        Bending: _____

        Other: _____

  E. Character: _____

        Sharp: _____

        Dull: _____

        Radiating: _____

  F. Spinal Tenderness: _____

        Locale: _____

  G. Muscle Spasm: _____

        Locale: _____

II. Muscle Strength & ROM

	ROM		STRENGTH	
	L	R	L	R
Lumbar Flexion				
Lumbar Extension				
Hip Flexors				
Hip Extensors				
Int. Rotators				
Ext. Rotators				
Knee Flexors				
Knee Extensors				
Ankle Dorsiflexors				
Ankle Plantar Flexors				
Ankle Invertors				
Ankle Extensors				
Toe Flexors				
Toe Extensors				

Continued

Continued from previous page

Postural Examination

HEAD
Forward _____
Level   _____
Other   _____

HIPS
High   _____
Low   _____
Other   _____

ABNORMALITIES
SPINAL
Kyphosis _____
Lordosis _____
Scoliosis _____

SHOULDERS
High _____
Low _____
Other _____

LEG LENGTH
Supine _____
Upright _____

LOWER EXTREMITIES
Normal _____
Genu Valgum _____
Genu Varum _____
Genu Recurvatum _____
Tibial Torsion _____

Functional Evaluation

How is the patient's pain affecting his activities of daily living?

What makes you feel better?

_____ PT

Figure 10A–7. *(© Carole B Lewis, Geriatric Orthopedics Handout.)*

NEUROLOGICAL EVALUATION FORMS

Hemiplegic Evaluation

General Observations

1. Sitting (symmetry)_____ Leg position _____ Arm _____

2. Up from sit

3. Standing (with cane) _____ (without) _____

   Wiggle bottom _____ Leg (Wt) _____ Shoulder _____

4. Gait   Control _____   2 Gaits? _____

                 Turns _____   Backward _____

                 Side Step _____   Push-faster
   Spontaneous _____

                 Push pull _____   Spontaneous _____

                 Wiggle bottom _____

5. Standing

                 Bend strong side _____

                 Shoulder with elbow extension _____

                 Tone   hand wrist _____

                 Shoulder abduction _____

6. Undress

                 Arm _____

                 Leg _____

7. Sitting—left arm _____

          left leg _____

          tickle foot _____

          arm clasp _____

          cross leg _____

          uncross _____

          cross leg & clasp _____

Figure 10A–8. *(© Carole B Lewis, Geriatric Neurology Handout.)*

Coordination Evaluation

By each item, briefly describe deficits, abnormal posturing, etc. Put "N" beside each item that is normal. Put "—" in those categories not tested.

ITEM	DESCRIPTION

I. LOW LEVEL COORDINATION

A. Shoulder and UE

1. Weight shifting in prone on elbows (forward and backward, side to side)_____

2. Weight shifting sitting propped on hands (side to side)_____

B. Pelvis and LE

1. Weight shifting in bridging (forward and backward, side to side)_____

2. Pelvic tilt (anterior and posterior) in supine_____

3. Hip abduction and adduction in supine_____

4. Alternate knee to chest in supine_____

5. Weight shifting in kneeling (forward and back, side to side, diagonals)_____

6. Weight shifting in 1/2 kneeling (forward and back, side to side, diagonals)_____

7. Weight shifting in standing (forward and back, side to side, diagonals)_____

C. Combined UE and LE

1. Weight shifting in quadruped (forward and back, side to side, diagonals)_____

2. Jumping jack motion in supine_____

II. MIDDLE LEVEL COORDINATION

A. Shoulder and UE

1. Reaching in prone on elbows (forward and sideways)_____

2. Chopping and lifting patterns in kneeling_____

3. Alternate UE lifts in quadruped_____

—Continued—

Continued from previous page

ITEM	DESCRIPTION

B. Pelvis and LE

1. Unilateral bridging with other LE extended _____

2. Alternate LE lifts in quadruped _____

3. Kneel-walking (forward and back, sideways) _____

4. Heel slides opposite knee to ankle along tibial crest _____

5. Making circles with extended LE _____

6. Walking (forward, backward, sideways) _____

C. Combined UE and LE

1. Creeping _____

2. Alternate UE and LE lifts in quadruped (opposite sides, same sides) _____

III. HIGH LEVEL COORDINATION

A. UE

1. Bouncing ball (same hand, alternate hands) _____

2. Catching and throwing a ball _____

3. Finger to nose _____

4. Alternate forearm pronation/supination (same direction, opposite direction) _____

B. LE (upright)

1. One limb balance (right and left) _____

2. Two-foot hop _____

3. Jogging in place _____

4. One-foot hop (right and left) _____

5. Crossover walking (right and left) _____

6. Balance beam walking (forward, backward, sideways) _____

7. Foot tapping (right and left) _____

8. Tracing shapes with feet (right and left) _____

C. Combined UE and LE

1. Jumping rope _____

2. Jumping jacks _____

3. Crab walking _____

Figure 10A–9. *(Reprinted with permission from Cruz, V. Evaluation of Coordination—a clinical model. Clin management. 1986; 6(3):6–10. Reprinted with permission of the American Physical Therapy Association.)*

Mobility Assessment

Name _____ Date _____
Functional Problem _____
Goals _____
History _____
_____

Physical Evaluation _____
      Skin _____
         Cardiopulmonary BP _____ HR _____
         Pathology _____
        Musculoskeletal
           ROM _____
           STR _____
           FEET _____
        Neurological
           Reflexes _____ Proprioception _____
           Vibration _____ Sway _____
           Tremor _____ Tone _____
Psychological
        Motivation _____ Depression _____
        Dementia _____ Falling Fear _____
Drugs _____
        Prescribed _____ OTC _____
Environment _____
Mobility Grade
        Bed _____ Sitting _____
        Transfer _____ Wheelchair _____
        Standing _____
        Gait _____
Support System _____
MISC _____

Figure 10A–10. (© Carole B Lewis, Geriatric Neurology Handout.)

Transfer Evaluation

Cardiopulmonary Status
　　　HR _____
　　　BP _____
　　　Sit to Stand _____
Neuromusculoskeletal
　　　Tone _____
　　　Strength _____
　　　Flexibility _____
　　　Phsychosocial _____
　　　Personal _____
　　　Support System _____
Transfer Position

	Initial	Mid	Ending
Head			
Neck			
Trunk			
Hips			
Pelvis			
Knees			
Feet			

Figure 10A–11.   *(© Carole B Lewis, Geriatric Neurology Handout.)*

Balance and Falls Assessment

1. Current medical problems _____
   _____

2. Medications _____
   _____

3. History of Falls _____
   _____

       Frequency _____
       Time of day _____
       Position _____
       Activity _____
       Circumstances _____

4. Balance with eyes open _____
   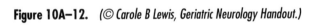
   Balance with eyes closed _____

5. Push balance recovery _____
   _____

6. Balance actuator _____
   _____

7. VAS _____
   _____

8. Lying to sit _____
   _____

9. Sit to stand _____
   _____

10. Flexibility _____
    _____

Figure 10A–12.   *(© Carole B Lewis, Geriatric Neurology Handout.)*

CARDIOPULMONARY EVALUATION FORMS

Cardiopulmonary Evaluation

Name _____

Date _____

RHR _____

RBP _____

RR _____

Current Activity Level _____

Posture

      C-Spine _____

      T-Spine _____

      Shoulders _____

Meds _____

Mental Status _____

History _____

_____

Pain _____

_____

Stress Level _____

Chair Step Test

		HR	BP
6"	2 min.		
	5 min.		
12"	2 min.		
	5 min.		
18"	2 min.		
	5 min.		
18" &	2 min.		
arms	5 min.		

Comments _____

Figure 10A–13.   *(© Carole B Lewis.)*

Step Test Data Sheet

Name _____

Age/DOB_____   Date _____

Weight _____   Examiner _____

Target Heart Rate Range (circle appropriate level)

Age	Target HR
61–70	114–132
71–80	108–125
81–90	102–118

Workload			HR	BP	Comments (symptoms)
Rest					
Step Test					
Step height	Steps/min	Met level			
0"	13	2			
8"	10	3			
8"	15	4			
8"	20	5			
8"	26	6			
Recovery					
3 minutes					
6 minutes					

Figure 10A–14.

Medical History Form

Have you ever had any indications of, or been treated for, any of the following? (underline applicable item)

	YES	NO
1. High blood pressure? (If "yes", list drugs prescribed and dates taken)	___	___
2. Disorders of the heart or blood vessels, such as rheumatic fever, heart murmur or irregular pulse?	___	___
3. Disorders of the lungs, such as asthma, tuberculosis, bronchitis or emphysema?	___	___
4. Cancer, tumor, cyst, or any disorder of the thyroid, skin or lymph glands?	___	___
5. Diabetes or anemia, or other blood disorder?	___	___
6. Sugar, albumin, blood or pus in the urine, or venereal disease?	___	___
7. Any disorder of the kidney, bladder, prostate, breast or reproductive organs?	___	___
8. Ulcer, intestinal bleeding, hepatitis, colitis or other disorder of the stomach, intestine, spleen, pancreas, liver or gall bladder?	___	___
9. Fainting, convulsions, migraine headache, paralysis, epilepsy or any mental or nervous disorder?	___	___
10. Arthritis, gout, amputation, sciatica, back pain or other disorder of the muscles, bones, or joints?	___	___
11. Disorder of the eyes, ears, nose, throat or sinuses?	___	___
12. Varicose veins, hemorrhoids, hernia or rectal disorder?	___	___
13. Alcoholism or drug habit?	___	___

HAVE YOU:

	YES	NO
14. Had, or been advised to have, an x-ray, cardiogram, blood or other diagnostic test in the past 5 years?	___	___
15. Been a patient in a hospital, clinic, or other medical facility in the past 5 years?	___	___
16. Ever had a surgical operation performed or advised?	___	___
17. Had any oral or respiratory infections in the past week?	___	___

Give details of "yes" answers on reverse, including number of attacks and dates.

Figure 10A–15.

Physical Activity Questionnaire

1. How often do you take walks?
   a. 4 or more times per week
   b. about 3 times per week
   c. very infrequently or never (Do not answer question 2 if your answer is c)
2. Of the walks you take at least three times per week, how far do you walk?
   a. less than 1/2 mile
   b. 1/2 mile or more, but less than 1 mile
   c. 1 mile or more, but less than 2 miles
   d. 2 miles or more
3. How many hours a day are you on your feet working in your apartment?
   a. 0–1 hour
   b. 1–2 hours
   c. 2–3 hours
   d. more than 3 hours
4. Do you do your own grocery shopping and carry your groceries? (May use wheeled cart to bring them home)
   a. frequently
   b. sometimes
   c. very infrequently or never
5. Do you do your own laundry?
   a. frequently
   b. sometimes
   c. very infrequently or never
6. Do you do any volunteer work or physical activity outside the building?
   a. frequently
   b. sometimes
   c. very infrequently or never
7. Do you go out of your apartment to socialize?
   a. frequently
   b. sometimes
   c. very infrequently or never
8. Do you invite friends and relatives over to socialize?
   a. frequently
   b. sometimes
   c. very infrequently or never

Continued

Continued from previous page

Indicate how often you do each activity on the list below using the following scores:

0 = never or almost never
1 = once a month or every other month
2 = 2 or 3 times a month
3 = 1 to 5 times a week
4 = about every day
5 = more than once a day

_____ Play cards, bingo, other games
_____ Watch television
_____ Sing
_____ Socialize
_____ Play billiards
_____ Ride stationary bike
_____ Read
_____ Take care of plants
_____ Shop
_____ Do needle work, art, crafts
_____ Eat
_____ Do crossword puzzles
_____ Travel
_____ Go to church

_____ Cook
_____ Sleep
_____ Iron, do laundry
_____ Listen to radio or music
_____ Work in apartment
_____ Sit
_____ Walk
_____ Watch sports
_____ Write letters
_____ Exercise
_____ Babysit
_____ Participate in organizations, committees
_____ Dance

Figure 10A–16.

Exercise Data Sheet

MD_____ Date_____

Admission Date _____ Age _____ Sex_____

Diagnosis _____ Marital Status _____ # of Children_____

Apt. or House_____ # of Stairs _____ Family Assess._____

Significant PMH: _____

Risk Factors _____

Complications: _____

Present Hx _____

Telemetry _____ CPK _____ MB _____ E.F. _____

Medications _____

Psych. Status _____

Date	Pre-Exercise BP & HR	Distance	Post Exercise BP & HR	Initials	Comments

Assessment:

Discharge:

Figure 10A–17.

Appendix B Environmental Evaluation Forms

Institutional Environmental
Evaluation

General Sensory Evaluation

Home Assessment Checklist for
Fall Hazards

General Environmental
Evaluation

Institutional Environmental Evaluation

Instructions: evaluate the resident's environment, checking either yes, no, or D/A (does not apply). Then check if the area needs work (NW). At the end, list all areas for correction.

Resident's Room	YES	NO	D/A	N/W
Colors				
1. Are the colors contrasted?				
2. Are reds predominant and blues and greens pale?				
Objects				
1. Are rugs and/or carpets secured safely?				
2. Are chairs or tables secure enough to support weight if needed?				
3. Is there any clutter or unsafe objects (i.e. low furniture)?				
4. Is ADT equipment (i.e. telephone, etc) easily accessible?				
5. Are grab bars or rails secure and accessible?				
Lighting				
1. Is lighting bright enough and from multiple sources?				
2. Are lights glare free and properly situated?				
3. Are glare situations minimized (i.e. mirrors)?				
Dangerous areas				
1. Are objects easily seen and reached without excessive reaching, stooping?				
2. Are doorways wide enough and trip-proof?				
3. Are bathtubs or showers furnished with skid proof surfaces?				
4. Is a night light used?				
Miscellaneous				
1. Is the room adequately sound-proofed?				
Exterior				
1. Are steps and edges clearly marked?				
2. Are color-contrasted handrails present in hallways and stairs?				
3. Are rooms, signs, etc. marked with sufficiently large and well spaced letters and written on a color contrasted background?				
4. Are social areas far from outside noise areas?				
5. Is background noise in general low-level?				
6. Are walkways and steps in good repair and free of cracks or bulges?				
7. Is adequate diffuse lighting available in all public areas?				
8. If music is playing, is it in the lower tones?				
9. Are foods presented on color contrasting plates and mats?				

Areas for improvement:

_____

_____

_____

_____

Figure 10B–1.

General Sensory Evaluation

Name _____

Place _____

Date _____

Vision

Color Contrasting _____

Food _____   Table _____   Plates _____

Pills _____

Rugs, Floors, Chairs _____

Stairs _____   Doorways _____

Glare

Windows _____

Floors _____

Furniture _____

Night Lighting _____

Reading Material _____

Lighting _____

Aids _____

Hearing

The Person

Aids _____   Motivation _____

Vision _____   Stress _____

Skills _____   Social Activities _____

_____

Figure 10B–2.

Home Assessment Checklist for Fall Hazards

Exterior
- Are step surfaces nonslip?
- Are step edges visually marked to avoid tripping?
- Are steps in good repair?
- Are stairway handrails present? Are handrails securely fastened to fittings?
- Are walkways covered with a nonslip surface and free of objects that could be tripped over?
- Is there sufficient outdoor lighting to provide safe ambulation at night?

Interior
- Are lights bright enough to compensate for limited vision? Are light switches accessible to the patient before entering rooms?
- Are lights glare free?
- Are stairways adequately lighted?
- Are handrails present on both sides of staircases?
- Are handrails securely fastened to walls?
- Are step edges outlined with colored adhesive tape and slip resistant?
- Are throw rugs secured with nonslip backing?
- Are carpet edges taped or tacked down?
- Are rooms uncluttered to permit unobstructed mobility?
- Are chairs throughout home strong enough to provide support during transfers? Are armrests present on chairs to provide assistance while transferring?
- Are tables (dining room, kitchen, etc) secure enough to provide support if leaned on?
- Do low-lying objects (coffee tables, step stools, etc) present a tripping hazard?
- Are telephones accessible?

Kitchen
- Are storage areas easily reached without having to stand on tiptoe or a chair?
- Are linoleum floors slippery?
- Is there a nonslip mat in the sink area to soak up spilled water?
- Are chairs wheelfree, armrest equipped, and of the proper height to allow for safe transfers?
- If the pilot light goes out on the gas stove, is the gas odor strong enough to alert the patient?
- Are step stools strong enough to provide support? Are stool treads in good repair and slip resistant?

Bathroom
- Are doors wide enough to provide unobstructed entering with or without a device?
- Do door thresholds present tripping hazards?
- Are floors slippery, especially when wet?
- Are skid-proof strips or mats in place in the tub or shower?
- Are tub and toilet grab bars available? Are grab bars securely fastened to the walls?
- Are toilets low in height? Is an elevated toilet seat available to assist in toilet transfers?
- Is there sufficient, accessible, and glare-free light available?

Bedroom
- Is there adequate and accessible lighting available? Are night-lights and/or bedside lamps available for nighttime bathroom trips?
- Is the pathway from the bed to the bathroom clear to provide unobstructed mobility (especially at night)?
- Are beds of appropriate height to allow for safe on and off transfers?
- Are floors covered with a nonslip surface and free of objects that could be tripped over?
- Can patient reach objects from closet shelves without standing on tiptoe or a chair?

Figure 10B–3. *(Reprinted with permission from Tideiksaar R. Fall prevention in the home.* Top Ger Rehab. *1987;3(1):59. Permission from Aspen Publishers, Inc.)*

General Environmental Evaluation

	Yes	No	D/A
Lighting:			
Does each room have multiple sources of light?			
Is the lighting diffuse?			
Is the lighting sufficiently bright?			
Are there blinds, drapes, sheer curtains across windows through which bright light shines?			
Are mirrors placed so that they do not reflect blinding amounts of light?			
Are older people seated so that bright sources of light are to the side of them?			
Colors:			
Do wall colors contrast with the colors of floors and rugs?			
Are the predominant colors red, orange, pink, and yellow?			
Are the blues and greens intense rather than pale?			
Are colors used to mark the edges of steps, curbs?			
Do small rugs contrast sharply in color with their floors?			
Is the paper used in making announcements, pamphlets, etc., a beige, off-white, yellow, or other warm color?			
Lettering:			
Are rooms, offices, signs, elevators, mailboxes, menus, notices, schedules, and so on, marked with sufficiently large and well spaced lettering?			
Are letters and numbers in sharp contrast to their background?			
Is the print easy to read for the older person?			
Are the markings on appliances easily discerned, such as OFF/ON, or HOT/COLD?			
Are personal letters to older people written in large, legible script or in large type?			
Hearing Environment:			
Is background noise reduced as much as possible?			
Are frequent interruptions by phones, people, or noises minimized?			
Are rooms adequately sound-proofed to facilitate conversation?			
Are conversational areas separated from areas containing noise-generating equipment?			
Communication:			
Are your voice tones moderate?			
Do you avoid shouting?			
Is your speech moderate in pace?			
Do you enunciate your words?			
Do you directly face older people and catch their attention?			
Do you inform the hard-of-hearing person of changes in conversation?			
Are you seated within three to five feet of the older person?			
Are children instructed about ways of interacting with older people?			
Are phone amplifiers available?			

Continued

Continued from previous page

Are receivers available in public halls, churches, etc.?

Is adequate lighting available for the older person to see lips and facial expressions?

Touch:

Does the environment contain a rich variety of textures that are easily accessible for the older person to feel?

Does the environment contain a rich variety of objects that are interesting to touch?

Do you and others shake hands warmly with older persons being welcomed into your setting?

Do you know what forms of touch are appreciated by older persons with whom you interact?

Dangerous Areas:

Are the edges of individual steps marked with a bright, contrasting color?

Are protrusions on walls or floors carefully marked?

Are curbs and driveways clearly marked?

Are kitchen appliances, showers, baths, and so on, clearly marked as to on/off or hot/cold positions?

Figure 10B–4. *(Reprinted with permission and adapted from* The Sixth Sense. The National Council on Aging. Washington, DC; 1985.)

Orthopedic Treatment Considerations

The principles of geriatric rehabilitation, posed in *Archives of Physical Medicine and Rehabilitation*, stated that approximately 30% of all geriatric patients consult their physicians because of musculoskeletal problems.[1] Therefore, it appears that orthopedics are a primary concern to physical therapists working with the elderly. This chapter will briefly explore the changes with age in the musculoskeletal system. Then, a joint by joint approach will be taken that will examine evaluation and treatment.

STRENGTH

Numerous studies cite the loss of strength with age.[2-4] The greatest loss appears to be in the type 2 muscle fibers, which are the fast-twitch fibers. Studies relate the loss of strength to several variables. (For further information on strength changes with age see Chapter 3). The clinical implications of some of these changes are

1. If the loss of strength is due to a decrease in the neuromuscular junction contact, it is suggested that the patient do frequent exercise repetitions, which will help keep the remaining neuromuscular junction intact.
2. If the decrease in strength is due to a lack of cardiovascular nutrients, then an increase in the cardiovascular flow to the muscle by aerobic conditioning will positively affect the muscle tissue.
3. If the decrease in strength is due to swelling (i.e., reflex inhibition due to joint distention), then the swelling and subsequent strength loss can be alleviated by using modalities and anti-inflammatory medication prior to joint strength training.[5]

Other major reasons for strength's decline with age are pathological in nature and appear to be more prevalent in the elderly. The clinician is cautioned to look for systemic problems that may cause weakness.[6] An example of this is polymyalgia rheumatica, a systemic disease of multiple joints, which causes pain and weakness, as well as other neurological and systemic rheumatological problems. If a person has an overlying pathology in addition to normal changes with age, the overlying pathology must be treated first.

FLEXIBILITY

Another major area of functional change with age is flexibility. As a person ages, the muscles tend to become less flexible. This is due to a decrease and change in the elastin and collagen of the muscle tissue (see also Chapter 10). The clinical implication for the loss of flexibility are

1. Heat the muscle prior to stretching.[7]
2. Stretch the muscle for at least 30 seconds.[8]
3. Maintain the muscle length in a functional activity.[9]
4. Cool down the muscle in its lengthened position.[7]
5. Set goals to recognize that older persons take longer to achieve benefits of a stretching program.[10]

Therapists should apply these principles of stretching to older patients to achieve the best results. Stretching contractures in older persons also requires special consideration. Figure 11–1 illustrates a protocol for stretching contractures.

Protocol For Stretching Contractures

1. Place the limb in the most lengthened position to be stretched.

2. Place hot pack on muscles to be stretched while in position #1 for 10 minutes.

3. Add weight (0.5% of patient's body weight) to distal part of limb in position #1 with heat still on for 5 minutes.

4. Remove heat and return part to neutral position for 1 minute.

5. Repeat steps 1–4 two more times.

Figure 11–1. (Lentell G. Hetherington T, Eagan J, Morgan M: The Use of Thermal Agents to Influence the Effectiveness of Low-Load Prolonged Stretch. JOSPT. 1992; 16(5). Light K, Nuzik S, Personius W, Barstrom A: Low-load prolonged stretch vs. high-load brief stretch in treating knee contracture. Phys Ther. 1984; 64:330–333.)

POSTURE

The third area of orthopedic functional change is posture. As people age, posture changes. As noted in Figure 11–2, normal posture, absected with a plumb line running from the ankle up to the ear, should fall through:

1. The middle of the earlobe.
2. The middle of the acromion process.
3. The middle of the greater trochanter.
4. Posterior to the patella but anterior to the center of the knee joint.
5. Slightly anterior to the lateral malleolus.

The most common posture changes with age are forward head, rounded shoulders, decreased lumbar lordosis, and increased flexion in the hips and knees (see also Fig. 10–3).[11]

To evaluate these postural deficits, the therapist can use a plumb line, as shown in Figure 11–2. Treatment for posture in the elderly is to work on the various body parts that have deviated from the norm. This will be discussed in the following sections on each body joint. Note that work on posture requires frequent repetition.[12]

After reviewing strength, posture, and flexibility changes with age, it is im-

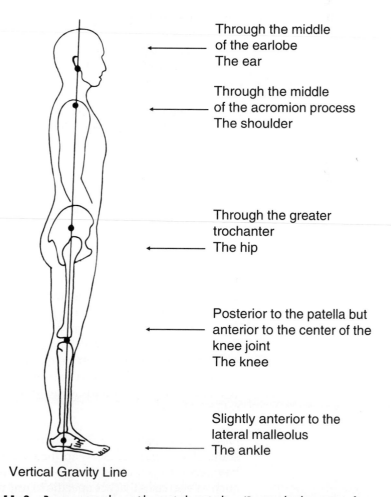

Through the middle
of the earlobe
The ear

Through the middle
of the acromion process
The shoulder

Through the greater
trochanter
The hip

Posterior to the patella but
anterior to the center of the
knee joint
The knee

Slightly anterior to the
lateral malleolus
The ankle

Vertical Gravity Line

Figure 11–2.   Proper posture shown with a vertical gravity line. *(Reprinted with permission from Lewis C, Bottomley J. Musculoskeletal changes with age. In: Lewis C, ed. Aging: the Health Care Challenge. Philadelphia: F.A. Davis; 1990.)*

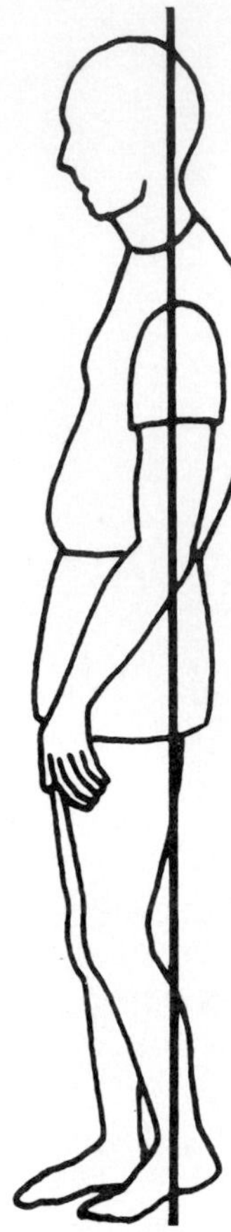

Changes in posture
(more forward head
and kyphosis)

Demineralization of
the bone (especially
dangerous in the
spine—may lead
to fractures)

Decreased flexibility
(especially in hips and
knees)

Loss of strength;
greater difficulty
in doing functional
activities

Changes in gait
patterns; less motion
and strength, causing
less toe off and floor
clearance

Figure 11–3.   Posture changes with age. *(Reprinted with permission from Lewis CB. What's so different about rehabilitating the older person? Clin Manage. May–June 1984; 4(3):12.)*

portant to note that there are several musculoskeletal orthopedic pathologies that are extremely prevalent in the elderly.

OSTEOARTHRITIS

The most prevalent orthopedic pathology is osteoarthritis. It occurs in 50% of the people aged 65, and 70% of the people over the age of 75.[12] It is defined as a noninflammatory progressive disorder of moveable articulations, especially the weight bearing joints, and is characterized by deterioration of articular cartilage and formation of new bone at joint margins and subcondoral areas.[13] Osteoarthritis most commonly occurs in the carpometacarpal joint, the knees, and the hips. The patient will complain of pain during weight bearing in the joints, and the pain tends to be relieved by rest.

Classic treatment consists of nonsteroidal anti-inflammatory drugs (NSAIDs). However, nonsteroidal anti-inflammatories for older persons have received a somewhat negative review in the current medical literature.[14] Liang and Fortin[14] have encouraged physicians to use more local and specific approach modalities, such as exercises that are specific to improve a person's functioning in the osteoarthritic joints. The works of Radin,[15] Fisher and associates,[16] and Kreindler and Lewis[17] suggest that strengthening around an osteoarthritic joint can alleviate some of the pain, as well as increase the strength and improve the functional mobility of arthritic patients. The clinical implication of these studies is that therapists should work with these patients on stretching and strengthening exercises, frequently throughout the day. Specific techniques for the various joints of the body will be given in subsequent sections.

RHEUMATOID ARTHRITIS

Rheumatoid arthritis is the second major orthopedic pathology that is seen in the elderly.[18] Rheumatoid arthritis (RA) classically affects young women; however, the second largest population to be affected are people over the age of 65.[19] The major differences between late onset RA and early onset are that the exacerbations tend to be more severe and the remissions tend to be much better. Therefore, the therapist must be cautious during the exacerbation phases and limit therapy to active assistive and active exercises. During the remission phases, the therapist can be much more aggressive when designing a strengthening and stretching program for an older patient than one for a younger person.

THE AGING SPINE

Pain in the neck and back is not uncommon in the older population. Although there is a higher prevalence of this problem in the population aged 35 to 55,[20] older persons do have a relatively high incidence of back and neck dysfunction.[21] Some of the major changes that are considered to be part of the normal aging process for the neck and back are

1. Muscles are less flexible, resilient and strong.[20,21] Nevertheless, Rider and Daly did find that they do respond to flexibility training.[21] In their study, a group of older women whose average age was 72 were put on a spinal mobility program and their mobility improved significantly.[21]
2. The bone tends to become slightly thinner due to osteoporosis, and as a result the older person will tend to lose some height. Approximately 20% is lost by the thinning of the disc, but the majority of the height loss is caused by the collapse of the cartilaginous end plates secondary to decrease in bone density and ballooning in the disc area.[22]
3. Joints are more prone to osteophytes. Twomey[22] states that the layer fat pads in older joints act as cushions against osteophytes, and that these vascular systems are more highly innervated, which may cause more pain and sensitivity. If joint congruity is not maintained by the tone of the multifidus, there is a chance that torn portions of the cartilage would be displaced—particularly with sudden rotatory movement. Manipulative techniques, therefore, would be particularly successful in freeing the torn pieces of cartilage; however, if the techniques are too strong, they may gap the joints and conceivably exacerbate the damage due to shearing of articular cartilage in the joint capsules.[23]
4. Aging changes in the cervical spine mean that older patients suffer from osteophyte formations and decreased range of motion with age. This was proven in an excellent study done by Hayashi and associates.[21] In addition, older patients experience a higher incidence of vertebral anterolisthesis and retrolisthesis, and a slight decrease in the diameter of the spinal cord, which was not enough, however, to cause any neurological symptomology.[22]

The implication of these changes is that the therapist needs to work on strengthening and the appropriate manual techniques to alleviate the patient's symptoms. Strengthening and flexibility would be the most helpful techniques for these problems.

SPINAL PATHOLOGY OF THE ELDERLY

There are many pathologies that can affect the spine of an older person. The first spinal pathology to be discussed is lumbar stenosis, which is a multilevel impingement on structures in the lumbar spine ligaments, usually by osteophytes.[23] Pain may be in the back, hip, or legs,[24] and it worsens when the person walks or extends their lumbar spine. It is usually partially or completely relieved with flexion. Lumbar stenosis rarely affects anyone under the age of 60.[24]

Treatment for lumbar stenosis consists of:

1. Rest for 1 to 2 hours in the afternoon with the knees higher than the hips.
2. Flexion type exercises (i.e., William's).
3. Heat and massage to decrease muscle spasm.
4. Teaching and enforcing posterior pelvic tilting in all positions.

Vertebral compression fractures usually affect the spinal areas of the lower thoracic and upper lumbar spine. Fractures can occur during any kind of routine activity, such as bending, lifting, or rising from a chair. The patient often complains of immediate, severe local back pain. The pain may subside in several months, but in some cases, it may continue for years. Other vertebral compression fractures, however, may cause no pain at all. Finally, the fracture may also be gradual, asymptomatic, and only able to be diagnosed by radiographs.[25]

Multiple vertebral compression fractures will cause shortening of the spine, which will lead to alveolar hyperventilation and retention of bronchial secretions. Eventually, the person may develop repeated episodes of pneumonia, abdominal symptoms, bloating, and constipation.[26]

Treatment for acute compression fractures is bed rest, but the patient must get out of bed every hour for 10 minutes to work on stabilization of the back.[25] Pain relief modalities may be helpful, such as heat, ice, TENS, or electrical stimulation, to relieve some of the symptoms.[27] Once the person can tolerate exercise, extension exercises should be used extensively.[26] Any type of extension exercises to the thoracolumbar spine is helpful.[27]

One of the pathologies affecting the neck of an older person is cervical spondylosis, which is defined as degenerative changes in the cervical spine. Symptoms of this are pain in the cervical spine with possible radiculitis into the shoulder, arms, or fingers.[28] The treatment for this include anti-inflammatories, keeping the neck in neutral or slightly flexed position, traction, heat, range of motion, and progressive resistive exercises that the patient can tolerate.[29]

A second pathology of the neck is vertebral artery syndrome (VAS). An encroachment on the vertebral foramina results in VAS, and this can be caused by a multitude of things. The most likely cause is the combination of a narrowing of the disc, osteophyte formation from osteoarthritis, and a forward head position.[30] The symptoms of VAS are dizziness, tinnitus, and blurred vision that occur in conjunction with neck motion and extension. The treatment for VAS is wearing a cervical collar, axial extension exercises, and cervical isometric exercises.[30]

A third pathology causing problems in the neck is RA. Patients who have RA with subsequent neck pain will tend to experience the pain in the middle area and the posterior aspect of the cervical spine. Therapists should check the x-rays for atlanto-occipital subluxation to be sure that no additional problems appear. If there is any question of subluxation, then the therapist should not use any manual techniques that could further exacerbate it (i.e., mobilization, traction, or occipital release).[30] Proper treatment includes supporting the neck with a cervical collar, heat, ultrasound, gentle massage, and range of motion and progressive resistive exercises.[30]

The fourth pathology of the neck is ossification of the posterior longitudinal ligament (OPLL). In OPLL, the ligament tends to ossify, usually over several segments of the cervical spine. This causes limitation in neck flexion and radiculopathy.[31] The treatment for OPLL consists of heat, cervical traction, and rest from sedentary static activities such as knitting, reading, computer, or desk work. In addition, stretching and range of motion or progressive resistive exercises are helpful.

In all of these pathologies, the therapist must first check the person's environment. Frequently, adding pillows between the knees while the person sleeps in the side lying position can provide relief. In addition, putting a lumbar pillow in a wheelchair or changing the level of the footrests can provide relief for the entire spine. Since older patients spend so much time sitting, and wheelchair patients are so often bound to their chairs, the therapist must check their environments to make sure they are not exacerbating any spinal symptoms. Often a simple modification can provide tremendous relief.

THE SHOULDER

As noted in the Chapter 3, range of motion in the shoulder does decline with age. Despite the fact that studies have documented age changes,[32,33] clinically there is evidence to show that if a person uses the shoulder more frequently, the range of motion decrease will be less. The aging shoulder is more prone to certain pathologies, such as the ones discussed here: osteoarthritis, bursitis, and rotator cuff tears.

The first pathology, osteoarthritis, is very rare and may be over diagnosed. Only 2% of shoulder problems in the elderly are truly osteoarthritis.[34] The symptoms of true osteoarthritis are a constant ache, crepitus, difficulty sleeping, and weakness. When the therapist moves the shoulder, there is a hard-end felt with joint movement. In addition, there will be a grinding and a dryness with shoulder movement.[35]

Osteoarthritis

Treatment of osteoarthritis, when the patient has severe joint pain, is rest, gentle pain-free range of motion exercises and anti-inflammatories.[35] Once the patient can move through range with less pain, however, heat or ice, functional adaptation, joint mobility, gentle weight bearing isometrics, and range of motion exercises can be helpful. In addition, the modalities, such as ultrasound and ice, can be very helpful in alleviating pain.

Bursitis

The second shoulder problem, which is more commonly seen than osteoarthritis in the elderly population, is bursitis. The symptoms of bursitis are

1. A palpable tenderness in the area of the inflamed bursa.
2. Pain with movement of the muscle affected by the temporary bursa.
3. Symptom relief with rest.[36]

The patient will usually have a late history of overuse of the shoulder prior to the initial onset of symptoms.[37]

Treatment for bursitis is heat or ice, ultrasound, and energy conservation. Painful movements should be avoided, and the patient should begin pain-free isometrics when he or she can tolerate them. No exercise should be done that exacerbates the pain, but having the patient exercise below and above a painful arc will be useful.

Rotator Cuff

The third shoulder pathology, and the one most commonly seen in the elderly, is rotator cuff problems. The rotator cuff is composed of the infraspinous, the supraspinatus, subscapularis, and teres minor. X-ray of the subacromial space of less than 5 mm is diagnostic of a rotator cuff tear.[37]

With the rotator cuff, the patient will complain of pain when sleeping on the shoulder. He or she will be positive on the impingement sign when the arm is brought to full passive flexion, and pain will be present for the last 10 to 20 degrees. Crepitus and catching sensations due to fibrosis and scarring may also be present. If the problem progresses, the patient may even have atrophy of the rotator cuff muscles and definite weakness in the shoulder abductors and flexors.[38]

Treatment for impingement, tears, and tendonitis of the rotator cuff is symptomological management. If the person has pain throughout an arc, the therapist should avoid range of motion exercises that use the arc and irritates the pain. The patient can be instructed to passively move the shoulder through that range and to do some end-range stretching and strengthening exercises. Heat, ultrasound, and electric stimulation may help decrease the inflammation. Passive active assistive stretching exercises can also be helpful, as will isometrics that do not encourage tightness in the shoulder musculature. The person must exercise the arm at least twice a day to see significant improvement.

Adhesive Capsulitis

Rotator cuff dysfunctions can become more irritating problems if the person develops a frozen shoulder. Although frozen shoulders are not always preceded by rotator cuff problems, it is a common occurrence in the aged. With frozen shoulders or adhesive capsulitis a person may or may not experience pain. A capsular pattern, where external rotation is most limited and abduction, flexion and internal rotation of the shoulder are also limited, is a symptom of adhesive capsulitis. The person may display a protracted scapula and atrophy of the deltoid, rotator cuff, biceps, and triceps. Tenderness of the anterior joint may also be present.[37]

Treatment for a frozen shoulder is heat or ice, depending on how painful the joint is and how well the person tolerates ice. Extremely painful joints may need the numbing effect of ice. Ultrasound can also be used to relieve some inflammation. Joint mobilization must be done in all limited directions, followed by active assistive or passive range of motion and contract–relaxed stretching. Posture work and scapular retraction exercises are also helpful.

Humeral Fracture

Humeral fractures are the final pathology to be discussed here. Classically, they will either be displaced or nondisplaced. Slightly more nondisplaced fractures occur, and they usually require pinning or wires. A fractured humerus usually requires that the patient use a sling for 1 week. After that time, the patient can remove the sling to work on general pendulum exercises, shoulder shrugs and circles, protraction and retraction, and any active motion exercises for the hand or wrist. At this point, the person should be doing no passive range of motion. For the first week, the patient should also learn ways of writing, eating, and performing daily ADLs without stressing the shoulder.[36]

By the third week the patient can begin gentle isometrics, either against the wall or using a Theraband. Active range of motion in the pain-free ranges can begin at this point as well, and the person should begin doing scapular humeral rhythm motion in front of the mirror, that is elevating the arms without raising the shoulder. This type of activity can also be used for all the previously noted shoulder pathologies. One of the most prevalent problems is that patients with shoulder pathologies have poor scapular humeral rhythm. Normally, they do not achieve full range of motion, because they are never taught how to properly move the shoulder. Simply working with patients in front of a mirror and encouraging them not to lift the shoulders as the arm is lifted is adequate for attaining the desired results.

By the sixth or eighth week, if the patient is healed, joint mobilization can begin. Passive range of motion can also begin, but scapular humeral rhythm should be stressed.

THE LOWER JOINTS OF THE UPPER EXTREMITY

The joints of the upper extremity (the elbows, wrists, and hands) show minimal changes in the range of motion with age. However, as seen in Chapter 6, grip strength does decline.[38,39,40] The practitioner should be careful when looking at grip strength measures in the elderly, because studies have shown that the older patient's grip and pinch strength may be influenced by extraneous variables. These variables range from mental status to gait. Therefore, grip strength may not be a true indicator of strength in the older population.[41,42]

Elbow

Almost one quarter of all elbow traumas and one third of elbow fractures are fractures of the radial head,[25] which usually are stabilized with an internal fixation device. For the first 3 weeks, the patient is immobilized in a hinged splint with the forearm held neutral. The patient can do range of motion exercises with the hand and shoulder, and to control swelling, cold packs can be applied for 10 minutes every hour. At day 21, active range of motion exercises can be started and passive range and progressive resistive exercises (PRE) can be increased gently as the patient tolerates. This regimen is followed slowly until 12 to 15 weeks.[43]

It is important to note that since this is such a painful fracture, practice and skill acquisition on a visual level may be beneficial. According to Marring,[44] the experimental group who visualized a forearm activity did much better than the control group who did not.[44]

Wrist

The most common pathology of the wrist is Colles' fracture, which is a fracture of the distal radius as a result of a fall on the hand. It can be treated by closed reduction, or it can be reduced by screws.[45] The therapist will usually see the patient once while the extremity is in a cast for instruction in edema control and for range of motion exercises for the uncasted upper extremity joints. After 4 weeks, the cast is usually removed, and at that time the therapist can use modalities as needed, such as heat, ice, and electrical stimulation to control swelling and increase circulation. Gentle joint mobilizations to the carpal joints, active range of motion, and gentle passive and resistive exercises can be started at this time. By 6 weeks, when the person is completely healed, the therapist can begin work on more vigorous passive resistive, contract–relax stretching exercises, or both. The therapist should be sure to reinforce the exercises with daily, functional activities at home.

Hand

The most common pathologies in the aging hand are (1) rheumatoid arthritis (RA) (2) Osteoarthritis and (3) Dupuytren's. In rheumatoid arthritis, the synovial fluid in the joints of the hand get particularly painful, and the person may develop ulnar drifting and significant deformities of the hand. The patient can undergo surgery or arthroplasty for severe deformities. Nevertheless, the therapist can work on light exercises and splinting to help alleviate pain symptoms, as well as range of motion deficits.[46] Osteoarthritis of the hand is more common than RA. It most commonly involves the interphalangeal joints and the carpometacarpal joint of the thumb. Since the thumb is so important for functioning, this particular problem can be devastating. The patient will present with pain, swelling, and weakness, possibly due to overuse of the hand. The treatment will involve joint protection, splinting to stabilize the thumb, and exercise. Heat, ice, and ultrasound can also give relief from pain and inflammation.[46,47]

The final pathology of the hand is Dupuytren's contracture, which is relatively uncommon in people under 50. It is caused by excessive collagen formation around tendons, nerves, and blood vessels in the palm of the hand, and it can cause minimal or permanent flexion of the fingers, usually of the proximal interphalangeal joints. It is usually not painful, and, therefore, people often delay treatment. However, treating the problem early can be extremely effective. Heat and ultrasound to the fascia of the hand followed by unidirectional transverse friction massage, stretching, and splinting in a stretched position can be extremely helpful. Patients are encouraged to continue the friction massage, range of motion and heating at home to enhance the benefits of the therapeutic regimen.[46]

THE HIP

The hip shows a decrease in range of motion similar to the other joints of the body, as demonstrated in the work of James and Parker[48] (see Chapter 6). In addition, Kramer and co-workers[49] found that older women have 61% less force in their hip abductors than younger women.[49]

The normal changes with age of decreased range of motion and strength will have a significant impact on an older person's gait, stability, and balance and may lead to a downward spiral for some of the pathologies that are commonly seen by therapists. The three major pathologies to be discussed in this section are hip fractures, osteoarthritis, and total hip replacements.

Hip Osteoarthritis

Patients with hip osteoarthritis may constantly complain of pain around or over the hip area. Even if a patient has radiographic evidence of hip osteoarthritis, the patient may have an inflamed bursa or tensor fascia lata tendinitis that relates pain to the hip.[16] It is imperative that the therapist assess this to treat it appropriately. If the patient's hip abductors are weak, they may be carrying the body's weight differently and irritating the bursas or the tendons around the hip area.[50] A thorough examination of these areas will help achieve an appropriate targeted treatment plan.

In arthritis of the hip, the patient will complain of an aching sensation, especially with weight bearing by the hip; there will be corresponding radiographic evidence. The treatment for hip osteoarthritis includes alleviating stress, such as through the use of a cane, to decrease weight bearing until a person increases his or her strength. This can be followed by strengthening exercises to the areas around the hip, especially for the abductors and extensors, to increase the shock absorbing system of the hip joint.[46]

Proper range of motion, stretching to the joint capsule, and ergonometric modifications may also be helpful, as can biomechanical alterations. According to Neumann and associates[50] a patient can decrease the hip force by carrying loads on one same side or with both hands. If a patient is carrying a purse on the uninvolved side, it may actually increase the pain felt by the patient.[50] Strengthening and range of motion exercises have also been shown to be very beneficial for patients with osteoarthritis.[18,19]

Hip Fracture

Hip fracture is the most common acute orthopedic condition of the elderly. Tinetti et al[51] found that active elderly persons fell less frequently than inactive, but when they did fall, it was more serious. Kampa[52] said, "Every 10 minutes someone dies from a hip fracture, and one out of every 20 women over 65 will suffer hip fracture."[52] In the United States, there are 267,000 fractures per year, and 97% of these involve persons 65 years or older, and two-thirds are women. It cost the United States $33.8 billion dollars in 1989.[53]

Cummings' and Nevitt's [53] study raised some interesting points about the relationship of osteoporosis to falls. They found that osteoporosis alone does not explain the exponential increase in the incidence of falls among the elderly.[53] They proposed that four conditions cause elderly people to fall and fracture their hips:

1. The faller is oriented so that impact occurs near the hip.
2. The faller's protective responses fail.
3. Local soft tissue absorbs less shock than necessary to prevent the fall.
4. The residual energy of the fall exceeds the strength of the femur.

Frequently, a fracture in older people occurs in the neck and intertrochanteric area of the femur where there is slightly less blood supply and the bone is of the cancellous rather than the cortical type. Subtrochanteric fractures occur with very high velocity falls and thus are rarely seen in the elderly population. The orthopedic surgeon has a multitude of choices in the types of fixation used, ranging from screws, to pins, to rods and plates. Table 11–1 lists some of these devices and the method of weight bearing progression that can be used by therapists.[54] It is imperative that the therapist gets the older patient to bear weight on the limb as soon as possible so as to enhance normal walking patterns, proprioception, and the integrity of the bone.[55]

Hip fractures are usually treated on a protocol basis. A total hip fracture protocol that is commonly used in departments around the United States is provided in Appendix A. In addition, Baker and co-workers[56] showed that treadmill gait

TABLE 11–1. MOST FREQUENTLY USED HIP FIXATION DEVICES

Name	Characteristics	Weight Bearing Precautions	Comments
Rods Enders	Three rods stabilize hip fracture. Rods are inserted into femoral condyle to knee joint	PWB—PO day 2 FWB—as patient tolerates pain, progress rapidly	Can cause toe-out posture. Rehabilitation of hip and knee joints is critical
Nails Jewett Smith-Peterson	Long stainless steel rods are used to stabilize intertrochanteric fracture	TDWB—PO days 2–5 FWB—when totally healed	Strict weight bearing secondary to fixation possibly piercing femoral head
Pins Knowles	Sharp stainless steel rod used to reduce non-comminuted intracapsular fracture	TDWB—PO days 2–5 FWB—by week 6 or 7	Strict weight bearing secondary to fixation possibly piercing femoral head
Screws and plates Richard's Compression	Most commonly chosen device for intertrochanteric fixation	PWB—PO day 2 FWB—by week 6 or 7	The screwing mechanism enhances healing

PWB, partial weight bearing; TDWB, touch down weight bearing; FWB, full weight bering; PO, postoperative.
Reproduced with permission from Zimmer Product Encyclopedia. Warsaw, Ind: Zimmer USA; December, 1981.[54]

retraining following a fracture of the neck of the femur showed significant increases in gait strength in those trained in this manner.[56]

Total Hip Replacement

The third hip pathology of the elderly is total hip replacements. Total hip replacements may be used for hip fractures, as well as for patients who have very severe rheumatoid arthritis, osteoarthritis, or carcinomas. Patients receiving total hip replacements tend to do well. They are usually put on a specific protocol procedure. For an example of this protocol, please see Appendix A. Depending on the approach used by the surgeon, various simultaneous motions need to be avoided by the patient so as not to cause dislocation. Unfortunately, there is no definitive time frame for dislocation, and some orthopedic surgeons may put patients on precaution protocols for anywhere from 3 months to the rest of their lives.

Some of the best predictors of outcomes for both hip fractures and total hip replacements are the number of visits that the patient makes to physical therapy.[57,58,59] It is imperative that patients who have had hip replacements or hip fractures receive adequate instruction in both exercise, activities of daily living, and proper precautions and methods of improving their weight bearing status. See Appendix A for a total hip protocol.

THE KNEE

The knee, similar to the hip, has been shown to lose strength with age.[60] According to Borges,[60] older patients showed a significant decrease in torque values likely to be generated at the knee. The knee, however, shows only a very slight decrease in range of motion with age.[48]

Osteoarthritis

Osteoarthritis of the knee is defined as a wearing away of the articular cartilage of the knee.[61] The articular cartilage softens, fissures occur, osteophytes form, and the synovium becomes fibrous. The capsule also thickens.[61] Barrett and associates[62] found that older patients tend to have a slight decrease of proprioception in the knee; however, there was a significant decrease in patients who had osteoarthritis of the knee in this study. They also found that when a patient received a joint replacement, they have an improvement in proprioception in the knee, but it is still not at the same level as normal.[62]

The important points to consider in osteoarthritis of the knee are the pain and other difficulties encountered by the patient. Frequently, the pain will occur with weight bearing, and the patient will have difficulty with gait activities and simple weight bearing. Therapists, again, need to work on decreasing forces on the knee joint until the patient is strong enough for daily activities.

According to the work of Radin,[15] the major shock absorbing mechanism of the joint is not the cartilage but is in fact the muscle, which absorbs 80% of the shock. Therefore, a very comprehensive exercise program to improve the strength around the joint will be helpful. According to the work of Fisher and associates[16] and Kriendler and Lewis,[17] strengthening around the joint can improve range of motion and strength. Therefore, a nonweight bearing strengthening program should be initiated early.

An article by Steinlan and co-workers[63] showed that infrared therapy helps to decrease pain in patients with osteoarthritis of the knee. In this study, patients used home infrared units for 20 minutes every 8 hours with significant pain relief.[63]

According to Liang and Fortin,[14] when therapists evaluate osteoarthritis problems of the knee, they must consider other causes for the pain, such as patellar–femoral problems, bursitis, as well as tendonitis and inflammation of the ligament around the knee. If it is a patellar–femoral problem, the patient needs to work on

Sit or lie on a flat surface with your legs straight out. With a rolled towel between your knees, push knees together. Then, still keeping your knees together, tighten the muscles in the front of your thigh by forcing your knee straight. Hold for 10 seconds. Do _____ times. Count out loud and breathe while holding.

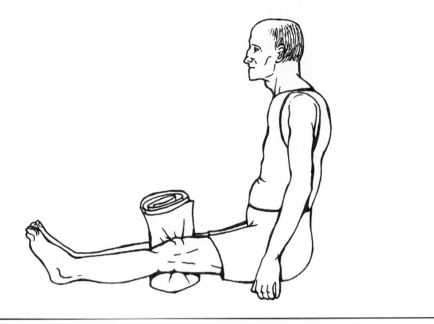

Figure 11–4.

patella–femoral tracking exercises to stimulate the vastus medialis.[64] The simplest exercise to facilitate this is a combination hip abduction with quadricep setting (Fig. 11–4).

Prior to starting any strengthening program, however, the therapist must consider decreasing the swelling of the knee joint. This treatment is based on reflex inhibition due to joint extension that may cause difficulty initiating a proper contraction.[5] This can be achieved with ice or electrical modalities.

In addition, the person may complain of stiffness after sitting for long periods of time. This may be caused by an inflammatory response in the knee joint, causing cross-linking of the collagen or synovial thickening. Simply having the person roll the foot back and forth on a soda bottle or something similar can help to increase extensibility of this tissue.

Total Knee Replacements

The next pathology to be discussed here is total knee replacements. Total knee replacements have been extremely successful in the United States.[65] In Appendix A are protocols for total knee replacements. These protocols are particularly specific and work with patients on active range of motion and various passive exercises, as well as strengthening exercises to improve the range of motion.

For the older patients, it is extremely important to encourage frequent but small bouts of exercise and to emphasize range of motion. Therapists need to be aware that total knee replacements are very painful operations and are more prone to infection than total hip replacements.[65] Therefore, the therapist needs to not only work on range of motion and strength but to check for infection and pain management techniques. Frequently, the use of ice and various weight bearing protocols have been shown to be effective.[64]

THE FOOT AND ANKLE

The foot requires a special introduction from Arthur Helfand:

> Have you ever imagined the difficulties you might encounter if your feet were in such condition that you could not walk or stand without chronic pain? The foot has received less attention than any other part of the human anatomy, possibly because injuries, disorders of the foot are seldom causes of mortality.[66]

White and Mulley found that 30% of community-dwelling elderly complain of pain in their feet.[67]

When evaluating feet, therapists must first check the skin for dryness and calluses. If they note that they are dry, rough, or callused, the therapist should encourage the person to use creams, unless there are open lesions. The therapist should also check the skin for the integrity of vibratory, temperature, and protective sensation; hair growth, and color to determine diminished circulation or of changes consistent with metabolic disorders such as diabetes.

The feet's skin should be checked for corns and calluses. These are layers of compacted skin that have built up over irritated areas. Calluses are usually found on the soles of the feet or heels. Corns are cone-shaped areas that occur on the toes and appear to be caused by friction and pressure from the skin rubbing against bony areas, such as when the patient wears ill-fitting shoes.[69] The person should be encouraged to wear shoes that fit properly.

The boney alignment of the foot also should be checked. The therapist should check for lesser toe deformities such as clawlike or overlapping toes. These lesser toe deformities are usually the result of weakness and the soft tissue surrounding metatarsal heads, which can lead to tendonitis or capsulitis. Treatment is aimed at relieving pressure. Interventions, such as metatarsal bars, intrinsic exercises to strengthen the foot, such as toe spreads and stretches, as well as anti-inflammatory medication can be very helpful.[69] Hallux valgus, another bone deformity, is an inward deviation of the first metatarsal, coupled with an outward deviation and rotational deformity of the great toe.[66] A person can develop osseous enlargements and joint pain. Treatments include: ultrasound, whirlpool, iontophoresis, joint mobilization and exercise to the great toe. Orthotics are extremely important for assisting these patients.

Circulation and sensation should be checked in the foot. Patients complaining of cramping and fatigue should receive special attention. For these patients, it is important that they inspect their feet, keep them warm and dry, do not wear circular garters, and are careful about any type of medication used on their feet, so as to not cause skin damage. Buerger-Allen exercises may be helpful in improving circulation in the aging foot. Figure 11–5 provides a sample of Buerger-Allen exercises for improving circulation.

There are strength and joint mobility changes in the foot, as noted in Chapter 6. Vandervoort and Hayes[70] showed a slowing and a decrease in torque generation applied to foot and ankle flexors in young versus old persons of 71%.[70] This means that older people will be significantly weaker in their plantarflexion strength, which may be a very important factor in balance. (See also Chapter 3.) In addition, ankle and foot range of motion decrease with age, decreasing the adaptability of the foot to changing walking surfaces.[48]

The treatment for foot problems is a thorough evaluation, and then treatment of the appropriate problem with modalities and exercises as needed. The importance of properly fitting shoes cannot be stressed enough. Frequently, older persons have been purchasing inappropriately sized shoes for many years, and it will be difficult to convince them they need appropriately sized shoes. To instruct an older person in the proper shoe fit, the following criteria should be used: When a person stands, a finger should fit from the end of the toe to the end of the shoe. When the therapist squeezes the person's shoe (while they are standing) at the metatarsal head, a slight give should be felt prior to feeling the metatarsal heads. In

First cycle of protocol: Buerger-Allen regimen

1. Lie supine with feet elevated and circumduct ankle until pain begins in the calf or until foot is cold and white if pain does not occur.
2. Sit with ankles crossed; press ankles together for a count of six, then relax. Repeat this until feet are warm and red.
3. Lie supine for 2 minutes.

This cycle is repeated twice.
Second cycle of protocol: Contrast bath

1. 2 minutes at 100°.
2. 1 minute at 55°.

This is repeated three times ending with the warm bath.
Buerger-Allen cycle is repeated twice, and patient should then walk until pain noted. Finish regimen with two cycles of Buerger-Allen exercises.
Patient should also perform the Buerger-Allen exercises twice daily at home. Improvement has been seen after approximately 2 weeks of treatment.

Figure 11–5.   Buerger-Allen Exercise Program.

approximately 99% of cases, patients have poor fitting shoes. In addition, the shoes should have a strong, supportive sole made of rubber or crepe, so that they do not slip. The sole should have a wide base, and high heels should be strongly discouraged.

CONCLUSION

Even though this chapter has divided orthopedic treatment into various joints, any thorough evaluation and treatment program must look at the person as a whole. This chapter is meant to provide information on specific changes with age in the musculoskeletal system, as well as pathologies that may occur orthopedically in the older person. General treatment suggestions have been provided (see Chapter 10).

PEARLS

- Thirty percent of all geriatric patients consult their physicians because of musculoskeletal problems.
- Therapists should assess the cause of strength declines (i.e., neuromuscular, cardiovascular, or joint swelling) and treat the strength defect with this in mind.
- Treatment suggestions for flexibility decrements in the aged are to heat the muscle, stretch it for at least 30 seconds, reinforce the stretch by doing functional activities, and to cool it down in the lengthened position.
- Normal changes of the spine include less flexible muscles, thinner bones with more osteophytes, and disc space narrowing.
- Lumbar stenosis can be treated with flexion exercises and environmental modifications, whereas vertebral compression fractures are treated with extension.

- Pathologies of old age seen in the shoulder are rotator cuff tears, adhesive capsulitis, fractures, and osteoarthritis.

- Aging causes a decrease in motion of almost all the body joints. Nevertheless, until pathological problems, such as fractures or arthritis ensue, the older person can be independent. Arthritis and fractures of any joint in the body, as well as many other pathologies, respond well to specific rehabilitation and exercise programs.

REFERENCES

1. Steinberg FU. Principles of geriatric rehabilitation. *Arch Phys Med Rehabil.* 1989; 70(1):67–68.
2. Eva P, Lyyra AL, Viitasalo, JT, et al. Determinants of isometric muscle strength in men of different ages. *Eur J Appl Physiol.* 1992; 64:84–91.
3. Frontera W, Hughes VA, Lutz KS, et al. A cross-sectional study of muscle strength and mass in 45- to 78-year-old men and women. *J Appl Physiol.* 1992; 72(2):644–650.
4. Hakkinen K, Hakkinen A. Muscle cross-sectional area, force production and relaxation characteristics in women at different ages. *Eur J Appl Physiol.* 1991; 62:410–414.
5. de Andrade J, Grant C, Dixon A, et al. Joint distension and reflex muscle inhibition in the knee. *J Bone Joint Surg.* 47-A(2):312–322.
6. Healy L. Late-onset rheumatoid arthritis vs. polymyalgia rheumatica in blacks may be an artifact. *J Am Ger Soc.* 1990; 38:824–826.
7. Sapega AA, Fuldenfeld TC, Moyer RA, et al. Biophysical factors in range of motion exercises. *Phys Sports Med.* December 1981; 9(12):57–65.
8. Gustavsen R. *Training Therapy: Prophylaxis and Rehabilitation.* New York: Georg Thieme Verlag; 1985.
9. Lesser M. The effects of rhythmic exercise on the range of motion in older adults. *Am Corr Ther J.* July/August 1978; 32(4):118–122.
10. Frekang G, Leslie D. Effects of an exercise program on selected flexibility measurements of senior citizens. *Gerontologist.* April 1978; 182–183.
11. Lewis C, Bottomley JM. Musculoskeletal changes with age: clinical implications. In: Lewis CB, ed. *Aging: Health Care's Challenge.* 2nd ed. Philadelphia: Davis; 1990: 135–160.
12. Verbrugge L, Lepkowski JM, Konkol LL, et al. Levels of disability among United States adults with disability. *J Gerontology.* 1991; 46(3):S71–S83.
13. The American Rheumatism Association Section of the American Arthritis Foundation. *Primer of Rheumatic Disease.* New York: The Arthritis Foundation; 1973.
14. Liang MH, Fortin P. Management of osteoarthritis of the hip and knee. *N Eng J Med.* July 11, 1991; 325(2):125–126.
15. Radin E. Mechanical aspects of osteoarthritis. *Bull Rheumatic Dis.* 1975–1976; 26(7):862–865.
16. Fisher N, Pendergast DR, Calkins EC, et al. Maximal isometric torque of the knee extension as a function of muscle length in subjects of advancing age. *Arch Phys Med Rehabil.* September 1990; 71:729–734.
17. Kreindler H, Lewis C. The effects of three exercise protocols on osteoarthritis of the knees. *Top Ger Rehab.* April 1989; 4(3):389–409.
18. Nesher G, Moor, TL, Zuckner J, et al. Rheumatoid arthritis in the elderly. *J Am Ger Soc.* March 1991; 39(3):284–294.
19. Rider R, Daly J. Effects of flex training of enhancing spinal mobility in older women. *J Sports Med and Phys Fit.* June 1991; 3(2):213–217.
20. Gandy S, Payne R. Back pain in the elderly: updated diagnosis and management. *Geriatrics.* December 1986; 41(12):59–72.
21. Hayashi, Okada K, Hamada M, et al. Etiological factors of mylopathy: a radiographic evaluation of the aging changes in the cervical spine. *Clin Ortho.* January 1987; 214:200–209.
22. Twomey LT, Tayor JR. *Physical Therapy of the Low Back.* New York: Churchill Livingstone; 1987.
23. Fast A. Low back disorders conservative management. *Arch Phys Med Rehabil.* October 1988; 69:880–891.
24. Frost H. Clinical management of the symptomatic osteoporotic patient. *Ortho Clin N Am.* July 1981; 12(3):671–681.

25. Turner P. Osteoporotic back pain—its prevention and treatment. *Physiotherapy*. September 1991; 77(9):642–646.
26. Sinaki M, Mikkelsen B. Postmenopausal spinal osteoporosis: flexion vs. extension exercises. *Arch Phys Med Rehabil*. October 1984; 65:593–596.
27. Sinaki M, McPhee MC, Hodgson SF, et al. Relationship between bone mineral density of spin and strength of back extensors in healthy postmenopausal women. *Mayo Clin Proc*. 1986; 61:116–122.
28. Payne R. Neck pain in the elderly: a management review, part I. *Geriatrics*. January 1987; 42(1):59–65.
29. Payne R. Neck pain in the elderly: a management review, part II. *Geriatrics*. February 1987; 42(2):71–73.
30. Lewis CB, McNerney T. Neck pain and the elderly. *Phys Ther Practice*. 1992; 1(1):43–53.
31. Harsh G, Sypert GW, Weinstein PR, et al. Cervical spine stenosis secondary to ossification of the posterior longitudinal ligament. *J Neurosurg*. 1987; 67:349–357.
32. Bassey E, Morgan K, Dalloso HM, et al. Flexibility of the shoulder joint measured at range of abduction in a large representative sample of men and women over 65 years of age. *Eur J Appl Physiol*. 1989; 58:353–360.
33. Faulkner C, Jensen RH, Nosse L. The aging rotator cuff: internal/external rotation torques for youth vs. senior citizens. *Phys Ther*. June 1991; 71(6):(suppl S75).
34. Sundstrom W. Painful shoulders: diagnosis and management. *Geriatrics*. March 1983; 38(3):77–96.
35. Warren R, O'Brien S. Shoulder pain in the geriatric patient, part II: treatment options. *Ortho Rev*. February 1989; 18(2):248–263.
36. Warren R, O'Brien S. Shoulder pain in the geriatric patient, part I: evaluation and pathophysiology. *Ortho Rev*. January 1989; 18(1):129–135.
37. Simon E, Hill J. Rotator cuff injuries. *J Orthop Sport Ther*. April 1989; 10(10):394–399.
38. Harrell L, Massey E. Hand weakness in the elderly. *J Am Ger Soc*. April 1983; 31:223–227.
39. Imrhan S. Trends in finger pinch strength in children, adults and elderly. *Human Factors*. 1989; 31(6):689–701.
40. Kallman D, Plato CC, Tobin JD, et al. The role of muscle loss in the aging related decline of grip strength cross-sectional and longitudinal perspectives. *J Gerontol*. 1990; 45(3):M82–M88.
41. Denham M, Modkinson MH, Furesh KN, et al. Loss of grip in the elderly. *Gerontol Clin*. 1973; 15:286–271.
42. Balogun J, Akinloye AH, Adeneola SA, et al. Grip strength as a function of height, body weight and quetelet index. *Physiotherapy Theory and Practice*. 1991; 7:111–119.
43. Sobel JS. Elbow injuries—a rehabilitation perspective. In: Lewis CB, Knortz K, eds. *Geriatric Orthopedics: Surgical and Rehabilitative Management*. St. Louis: Mosby Year Book; 1992.
44. Maring J. Effects of mental practice on rate of skill acquisition. *Phys Ther*. March 1990; 70(3):165–172.
45. Villar R, Marsh D, Rushton N, et al. Three Years After Colles' Fracture. *J Bone Joint Surg*. August 1987; 69-B(4):635–638.
46. Douvall S. Hand injuries—a rehabilitation perspective. In Lewis CB, Knortz K, eds. *Geriatric Orthopedics: Surgical and Rehabilitative Management*. St. Louis: Mosby Year Book; 1992.
47. Maddali Bongi S, Giuidi G, Cencett A, et al. Treatment of carpo-metacarpal joint osteoarthritis by means of a personalized splint. *Pain Clinic*. 1991; 4(2):119–123.
48. James B, Parker A. Active and passive mobility of lower limb joints in elderly men and women. *Am J Phys Med Rehabil*. August 1989; 68(4):165.
49. Kramer J, Vaz MD, Vandervoort AA, et al. Reliability of isometric hip abductor torques during examiner and belt-resisted tests. *J Gerontol*. 1991; 46(2):M47–M51.
50. Neumann D, Cook TM, Sholty RL, et al. An electromyographic analysis of hip abductor muscle activity when subjects are carrying loads in one or both hands. *Phys Ther*. March 1992; 72(3):207–217.
51. Tinetti ME, Williams TF, Mayewski R. Fall risk index for elderly patients based on number of chronic disabilities. *Am J Med*. 1986; 80(3):429–434.
52. Kampa K. Mortality of hip fracture patients within one year of fracture . . . an overview. *Geritopics*. April 1989; 14(1):10–11.
53. Cummings S, Nevitt M. A hypothesis: the causes of hip fractures. *J Gerontol Med Sciences*. 1989; 44(4):M107–M111.
54. *Zimmer Product Encyclopedia*. Warsaw, Ind: Zimmer USA; December 1981.

55. Zuckerman JD, Zetterber C, Kummer FJ, Frankel VH. Weight bearing following hip fractures in geriatric patients. *Top Ger Rehab*. December 1990; 6(2):34–50.
56. Baker P, Evans OM, Lee C, et al. Treadmill gait retraining following fractured neck-of-femur. *Arch Phys Med Rehabil*. August 1991; 72:649–652.
57. Barnes B, Dumovan K. Physical therapy discharge outcomes after hip fracture. *Phys Ther*. July 1987; 2(4):45–51.
58. Barnes B, Dunovan K. Functional outcomes after hip fracture. *Phys Ther*. November 1987; 67(11):1675–179.
59. Bonar S, Tinetti ME, Speechley M, et al. Factors associated with short versus long-term skilled nursing facility placement among community living hip fracture patients. *J Am Ger Soc*. October 1990; 38(10):1139–1144.
60. Borges O. Isometric and isokinetic knee extension and flexion torque in men and women aged 20–70. *Scand J Rehab Med*. 1989; 21:45–53.
61. Altman R, et al. Development of criteria for the classification and reporting of osteoarthritis of the knee. *Arthritis and Rheumatism*. August 1986; 29(8):1039–1049.
62. Barrett D, et al. Joint proprioception in normal osteoarthritis and replaced knees. *J Bone Joint Surg*. January 1991; 73-B(1):53–56.
63. Steinlan J, Gil I, Habot B, et al. Improvement of pain and disability in elderly patients with degenerative osteoarthritis of the knee treated with narrow-band light therapy. *J Am Ger Soc*. January 1992; 40(1):23–26.
64. Knortz K. Knee injuries—A rehabilitation perspective. In: Lewis CB, Knortz K, eds. *Geriatric Orthopedics: Surgical and Rehabilitation Management*. St. Louis: Mosby Year Book; 1992.
65. Berry G. Assessment and treatment of knee injuries with particular attention to the hamstring muscles and joint swelling. *Physiotherapy*. 1989; 75:690–693.
66. Helfand A. Podiatry in a total geriatric health program: common foot problems of the aged. *J Am Ger Soc*. June 1967; 15(6):593–599.
67. White EG, Mulley GP. Foot care for very elderly people: a community survey. *Age and Aging*. 1989; 18(4):275–279.
68. Evans S, Nixon BP, Lee I, et al. The prevalence and nature of podiatric problems in elderly diabetic patients. *J Am Ger Soc*. March 1991; 39(3):241–245.
69. Helfand A. The aging foot. *Focus on Ger Care and Rehab*. April 1989; 2(10).
70. Vandervoort A. Hayes K. Plantarflexor muscle function in young and elderly women. *Eur J of Appl Physiol*. 1989; 58:389–394.

Appendix A   Orthopedic Replacement Protocol

Total Knee Replacement Exercises

Total Hip Arthroplasty Protocol

Physical Therapy Protocol for Total Hip Arthroplasty

Hip Arthroplasty: General Instructions

TOTAL KNEE REPLACEMENT
HOME INSTRUCTIONS AND EXERCISE PROGRAM

GENERAL INSTRUCTIONS

1. It is very common to note swelling of the lower leg when first home. Do not be concerned as long as the swelling is down in the morning.

2. Do contact your physician if you have any evidence of infection in any part of your body (i.e., redness, edema, or increased heat in a joint).

3. Sit or stand with the operative leg out in front of the other leg.

4. Never pivot or twist on your operative leg when turning; take small steps to turn.

5. Wear your knee splint at night unless your surgeon discontinues its use.

6. You may sit for 30 minutes with your knee bent, but then you must stretch your knee muscles by walking approximately 5 minutes or by practicing your exercises.

7. Avoid low chairs! A straight back chair (kitchen type) is best for getting up and down comfortably.

8. As tolerated, walk in short sessions to gradually improve your physical endurance. Continue to use your walker or crutches until your surgeon specifies otherwise.

9. Stairs: when ascending stairs, the nonoperative leg goes up first, followed by the operative leg and your crutches. When descending stairs, the crutches and operative leg go first, then the nonoperative leg.

EXERCISE PROGRAM

- Exercises are to be performed two to three times per day building up to 20 repetitions of each exercise.
- Do not place any resistance on your ankle or foot when doing your exercises (i.e., remove heavy shoes, use no ankle weights).

1. **SUPINE:** Lying on your back on a firm, flat surface; exercise both legs!

   a. Tighten the muscles on the top of the thighs pushing the back of the knees down into the bed. Hold 5 seconds. Relax; repeat.

   b. Tighten buttock muscles. Hold 5 seconds. Relax.

   c. Slowly make circles with your ankles moving your feet in clockwise and counterclockwise directions. Only your foot should move, not the entire leg.

   d. Tighten your knee and bend your ankle so that your toes point toward your face. Lift your leg straight up in the air. Tighten the knee again before slowly lowering your leg to the bed, making the back of your knee hit the bed first.

   e. With one leg straight, bring the opposite knee to your chest allowing your knee to bend as much as possible. Hold your thigh up with your hands or a towel as you kick your foot in the air to straighten your knee. Lower your leg to the bed with the knee straight.

   f. Place a large towel roll (12 inches in diameter) under your thigh. Straighten your knee by lifting your foot up toward the ceiling and by tightening your knee cap. Do not lift your thigh or upper leg off the roll. Hold 5 seconds. Relax.

2. **LONG SITTING:** Sit in the bed with your back straight. Stretch your legs out in front of you. Push the back of your knees down into the bed and bend your ankle by pulling your toes toward your face. Keeping knees tight, reach forward toward your toes in order to feel stretching in the back of your knees. Hold 5 seconds. Relax.

Continued

Continued from previous page

3. **SITTING:** Sit on a firm surface with a small towel under your knee. Straighten the operative leg, using the foot of the nonoperative leg for support if necessary. Let your operative leg drop by gravity slowly, then force it to bend using the other foot to exert pressure on top of the ankle within limits of pain tolerance.

4. **PRONE:**
   a. Roll over your operative knee to get on your stomach. Lie on your stomach, feet hanging over the edge of the bed, and thigh rolls in place. Assume this position for 15 minutes twice each day. You may wear your shoes to give an added stretch to the muscles behind the knee.
   b. After resting, bend your operative knee as much as is possible. Hold 5 seconds. Relax.
      *Discontinue this exercise if it is too painful.

5. **BIKING:** Gradually increase your bike riding endurance to two 15 minute sessions per day. Initially adjust the seat to the height determined in the hospital.* Once riding the bike comfortably at that seat height, lower the seat 1/4 inch each week.

   *Seat height at discharge: _____. Measure from the tip of the seat to the top of the pedal at its lowest point.

   Note—NO RESISTANCE IN BIKING!!!

   If you have any questions or problems with your exercises, please contact your therapist.

   _____ RPT

Figure 11A–1. *(Reprinted with permission from Vanderbilt University Hospital, Physical Therapy Department.)*

Total Hip Arthroplasty Protocol

Purpose

To guide patients through the pre- and postoperative phases of rehabilitation following total hip arthroplasty to assist the patient in becoming functionally independent following surgery.

Indications

Patients who have been admitted for or who have acutely undergone total hip arthroplasty.

Contraindications

Any surgical or postoperative complications as stated by the attending orthopedic surgeon.

Physical Therapy Goals

1. Increase range of motion of the operative hip with progression towards full anatomical range of motion and limited only by the prosthetic design and the patient's potential.

2. Muscle strengthening primarily of the hip abductor muscle groups. These exercises are not to be instituted until approximately 2–6 weeks after surgery and without the use of ankle weights.

3. Gait training. Assistive devices are used to enable the patient to achieve the proper weight bearing status on the operative extremity and to assist with balance. These devices are ultimately discontinued at the discretion of the attending orthopaedic surgeon.

Physical Therapy Program Shall Consist of

1. Preoperative instruction via "Total Hip Information" class.

2. Preoperative evaluation and teaching.

3. Postoperative rehabilitation.

4. Home instructions prior to discharge.

5. Home/outpatient physical therapy follow-up.

6. Progression in outpatient therapy per and with the attending orthopedic surgeon in the orthopedic clinic on follow-up clinic visits.

Preoperative Physical Therapy Evaluation

History

Mentation

Range of motion of both lower extremities

Muscle function and strength

Pain

Sensation

Skin, including edema, erythema, increased heat or cold

Posture

Leg length measurements. Taken with the patient supine, measure from ASIS to the medial malleolus

Gait analysis

Functional abilities of the patient

Equipment used by the patient

Other medical problems

Continued

Continued from previous page

Statement of physical therapy goals. Long- and short-term goals are set and reviewed with the patient

Prognosis, duration, and frequency of physical therapy.

Physical Therapy Preoperative Teaching

1. Explanation of the role of physical therapy in total hip arthroplasty rehabilitation.

2. Statement of physical therapy goals for total hip arthroplasty.
3. Step-by-step explanation, instruction, and demonstration of postoperative physical therapy treatments.
4. Answering of general questions regarding the actual surgical procedure and rehabilitation following total hip arthroplasty.

Generaly Precautions in Hip Arthroplasty

1. No combination movements of the operative lower extremity. Patients are allowed to flex, extend, rotate, and so forth their operative hip to tolerance (i.e., no limitations on range of motion), but are not to combine any of these motions. All ranges of motion exercises are done in single planes of movement.

2. No straight leg raises.

3. No use of ankle weights with any of the prescribed exercises.

4. No sleeping on the operative hip for 6 weeks.

5. Low, soft, contour-type furniture (i.e., sofas, chairs) is to be avoided.

6. Patients may resume driving at 10 weeks from the date of surgery.

7. Patient may return to work at the discretion of the surgeon.

8. Sexual activity may be resumed when comfortable. Specific literature on this subject is available from the nursing staff upon request.

9. Ambulation guidelines.

   a. **Cemented Protheses:** WBAT ambulation. Patients will be required to ambulate using a walker/crutches for a total of 6 weeks following their surgery. At that time, they are begun on ambulation programs using a cane with emphasis on strengthening their hip abductor muscle groups. At the time they are able to ambulate without a Trendelenburg limp, the cane may be discontinued, and they are encouraged to ambulate without any assistive device.

   b. **Uncemented Prosthesis:** TDWB ambulation. Patients are to ambulate using walker/crutches with TDWB status for a total of 6 weeks. At 6 weeks postop, the patient is begun on a progressive weight bearing program using the walker/crutches. Patients begin by bearing 1/3 of their body weight on the operative extermity; in 2 weeks, they progress to 2/3 body weight on the operative extremity (continuing to use their assistive device); in 2 weeks, they are allowed full weight bearing on the operative extremity for a total of 2 more weeks. At the end of these 2 weeks, 12 weeks from the date of surgery, walker/crutches are discontinued and cane ambulation is begun. Patients are to continue ambulating using a cane until they are able to ambulate without a Trendelenburg limp. At this time, the cane may be discontinued, and patients are encouraged to ambulate without any assistive device.

Figure 11A-2. (Reprinted with permission from Vanderbilt University Hospital, Physical Therapy Depratsment.)

Physical Therapy Treatment Protocol for Total Hip Arthroplasty

Preoperative: 1 Month Prior to Hospitalization

1. Attend total joint class on hip arthroplasty. Material covered in the class includes discussions on anatomy of normal and abnormal hip joint components and types of hip prosthesis, admission procedures for VUH, inpatient preoperative care, intraoperative sequence of events, identification of postoperative complications and preventative measures, inpatient/home rehabilitation via physical therapy, and occupational therapy and postdischarge needs. Class personnel includes nursing, PT, OT, and SW.

Preoperative: Day of Admission

1. Preoperative evaluation of range of motion, strength, limb length discrepancy, pain, gait, etc.
2. Review basic precautions and instruct in immediate postoperative exercises.
3. Fit walker/crutches and instruct in appropriate gait pattern. Three-point gait if one extremity is involved, four-point gait if both lower extremities are involved: WBAT if cemented prosthesis is to be used, TDWB if noncemented prosthesis is used.

Postop Day 1

1. Begin lower extremity isometrics and ankle pumping exercises.
2. Initiate bilateral upper extremity and contralateral limb strengthening exercises.
3. Begin bed-to-chair transfers with assistance to a chair of appropriate height. Patients are not required to "slouch" sit and may sit in an upright position if comfortable.

Postop Day 2

1. Review lower extremity isometrics and ankle pumping exercises.
2. Begin active-assisted lower extremity range of motion exercises to the operative extremity in bed. Operative limb motions should be to the patients tolerance and the limb should be kept in a single plane of motion.
3. Begin assisted walker/crutch ambulation with weight bearing status dependent on prosthesis design and implantation.

Postop Days 3–5

1. Continue supine exercises.
2. Instruct patient in sitting exercises.
3. Instruct in bathroom transfers. Patients are to use an over-the-commode chair that the nursing staff will secure for their use while hospitalized.
4. Continue gait training on level surfaces.

Postop Days 6–Discharge

1. Review and reinforce supine and sitting exercises.
2. Reinforce postoperative precautions.
3. Further gait refinement to achieve maximum, safe, energy-efficient gait pattern with appropriate weight bearing status.
4. Instruct in stair climbing.
5. Begin and complete discharge plans and arrangements for follow-up home/outpatient physical therapy (follow-up physical therapy services arranged for 6 weeks with three sessions per week).
6. Review home instructions and exercise program with patient and family members.

Continued

Continued from previous page

After Discharge

First clinic follow-up visit. Approximately 2 to 3 weeks from hospital discharge; seen in orthopedic clinic with surgeon.

1. Review home instructions and exercise program.
2. Instruct in hip abduction exercises—standing only, and instruct in supine IT band stretches.
3. Continue walker/crutch ambulation with appropriate weight bearing status.

Second clinic follow-up visit. Approximately 6 weeks postop.

1. Review complete exercise program.
2. Instruct in hip abduction exercises, side-lying and instruct in supine IT band stretches.
3. Instruct in increased activity schedule.
4. If cemented prosthesis, can begin ambulation. Continue to use the cane until patient is able to ambulate without a Trendelenburg limp.
5. If noncemented prosthesis, begin on progressive weight bearing program using walker/crutches.

Third clinic follow-up visit. Approximately 12 weeks postop.

1. Review complete exercise and activity program.
2. Noncemented prothesis, begin can ambulation. Continue to use cane until patient able to ambulate without a Trendelenburg limp.

All other clinic follow-up visits.

1. Continue to review and reinforce exercises and activity regimens.

Figure 11A–3. *(Reprinted with permission from Vanderbilt University Hospital, Physical Therapy Department.)*

Hip Arthroplasty
General Instructions

1. The exercise program should be carried out two to three times per day building up to 20 repetitions of each exercise.

2. You may sit for up to 30 minutes at one time, as often as desired, as long as you walk or lie flat on your back or stomach for a few minutes between sitting periods.

3. It is very common to note swelling of the lower leg when first home; do not be concerned as long as the swelling is down in the morning.

4. Do not sleep on your operative side until approved by your surgeon.

5. Sexual activity may be resumed when comfortable.

6. Try to keep your operative leg positioned in bed so that the toes and kneecap point upwards toward the ceiling when you are backlying.

7. When advised by your surgeon, you may take a shower (tub baths are not advised). You may wish to put a chair in your shower to sit on while bathing (mesh lawn chairs work well).

8. Low, soft contour-type chairs should be avoided.

9. Dining out: Do not sit in booths or low chairs.

10. Walk in short sessions as tolerated to gradually improve your physical endurance. You may walk out of doors when stamina and strength are adequate.

11. You may return to work at the discretion of your surgeon.

12. Walking

    a. Keep erect posture at all times with buttocks tucked under shoulders.

    b. Look straight ahead.

    c. Walk in a heel-to-toe sequence, with toes pointed straight ahead.

    d. Tighten your buttocks and the knee of the supporting leg until the heel of the moving leg hits the ground.

   e. Never lean on your crutches. Distribute your weight on the hand grips.

13. Stairs

    UP: Step up with your _____ leg first. Lean slightly forward and push down on your crutches. Raise your other leg. After both feet are firmly on the stair above, raise your crutches.

    DOWN: Come to the edge; lower your crutches to the stair below as you bend your knees. Lower your_____ leg, then lower your other leg.

Additional Comments:

Figure 11A–4. *(Reprinted with permission from Vanderbilt University Hospital, Physical Therapy Department)*

Neurological Treatment Considerations

Parkinson's Disease	Evaluation
Evaluation	Treatment Interventions
Treatment Considerations	Conclusion
Stroke	

This chapter will build upon the discussion of specific biological changes that occur with age or pathology, as developed in Chapters 3 and 5. This section will discuss a model for looking at neurological dysfunction, followed by sections on mobility, balance and coordination, weakness, and tremor. The two major pathologies that will be discussed are cerebral vascular accidents (CVA) and Parkinson's disease, which will be discussed in terms of prevalence, efficacy of treatment interventions, evaluation, and treatment strategies.

The model for neurological dysfunction used is that of Schenkman and Butler.[1] Figure 12–1 illustrates the progression of the stages that result in ultimate disability.

This model is best explained using an example; therefore, a patient with a CVA in which the neuroanatomic pathology is a parietal lobe lesion will be discussed. The impairment's direct effects might include a motor loss from the parietal lesion resulting in hypotonicity of the shoulder. An indirect pathological effect could be a rotator cuff tear, and the resulting impairment would be a subluxed shoulder. The impairment's composite effects would be a decreased use of the upper extremity and pain on movement, as well as movement dysfunction in the upper and lower extremities. The resultant functional disability is this individual's inability to dress or walk independently, sleep without discomfort, or any of these.

The therapist can then use this model to examine where physical therapy can benefit the patient. In this example, the therapist may have little effect on the insult or neuroanatomic pathology. The therapist, however, could positively affect the other areas. Using this information, the therapist can choose the most effective intervention for the problem. This problem solving model should be kept in mind when reviewing the subsequent dysfunctions.

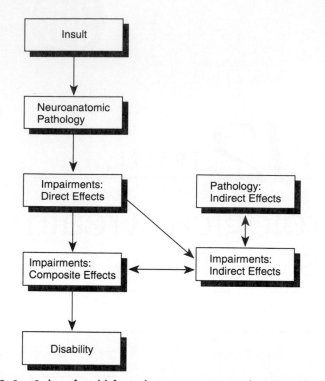

Figure 12–1. Outline of model for evaluating, interpreting, and treating individuals with neurologic dysfunction. *(Reprinted with permission from Schenkman M, Butler RB. A model for multisystem evaluation, interpretation and treatment of individuals with neurologic dysfunction. Physical Therapy. July 1989; 69(7):538–547.)*

PARKINSON'S DISEASE

Parkinson's disease is the primary neurological disease of the elderly.[2] It affects 1% of people over 50 years of age, and 50,000 new cases are diagnosed annually.[2] The description of Parkinson's disease and its causes are discussed in further detail in Chapter 5. The most common symptoms in Parkinson's disease are

1. Slowness in ambulation and dressing.
2. Difficulty in getting out of a chair and in turning in bed.
3. Shuffling.
4. Stooping when walking or falling to one side when sitting.
5. Difficulty with speech.
6. Tremor and handwriting changes.
7. Difficulty initiating movements.[3]

Medical management of Parkinson's disease revolves mainly around the use of drugs such as L-dopa. More information is available on the use of L-dopa in Chapter 8. It is important to note that the side effects associated with L-dopa's use are less in the elderly and, therefore, it can be prescribed at the onset.[4] The literature is filled with controversy as to dosage and side effects of anti-Parkinson medications (again see Chapter 8 for the side effects). The most noteworthy and deleterious side effects in the elderly are mental side effects, such as disorientation and confusion.[5]

The medical management of Parkinson's disease depends on the stage of disability. The Hoehn and Yahr stages are as follows:

- Stage I: Is characterized by minimal or no functional impairment and unilateral involvement only.
- Stage II: Is characterized by bilateral involvement without any type of balance impairment.
- Stage III: Is characterized by mild to moderate disability and here the pa-

tient may lose righting reflexes as evidenced by unsteadiness on turns.

- Stage IV: Is characterized by moderate to severe disability. The patient can still walk and stand unassisted but is not stable.
- Stage V: Is severe disability and here the patient is confined to bed or a wheelchair.[6]

The medical literature has shown that medication alone is not adequate treatment for this disease and that physical therapy is an important adjunct to medical treatment.[4-8]

Physical therapy has been shown to be efficacious for these patients.[8] In a study by Banks, Parkinson's patients with all degrees of impairment and duration of the disease improved in walking and other mobility skills after physical therapy.[8]

Evaluation

Schenkman and Butler have developed a model for the evaluation of patients with Parkinson's disease (Fig. 12–2).[9]

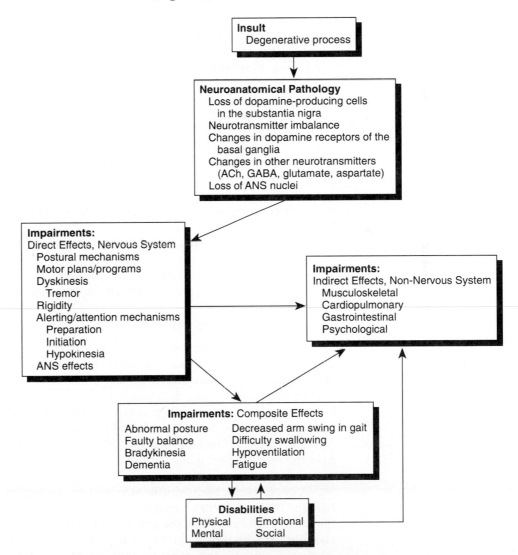

Figure 12–2. Overview of model for evaluation and treatment of patients with Parkinson's disease. ACh, acetylcholine, GABA, gamma-aminobutyric acid; ANS, autonomic nervous system. *(Reprinted with permission from Schenkman M, Butler R. A model for multisystem evaluation treatment for individuals with Parkinson's disease. Physical Therapy. 1989; 69(11):932–943.)*

This model can be used as a guideline for evaluating Parkinson patients. The therapist can begin by assessing the direct effects of the nervous system, such as tremor rigidity, hypokinesis, and autonomic nervous system (ANS) effects. While it is important to note these, it is also important to recognize that these impairments will respond less dramatically to physical therapy procedures than the indirect effect impairments.[9] The indirect effect impairments are changes in the musculoskeletal system, such as flexibility, strength, and vital capacity. The combined changes of these two areas makes up the major impairments listed in composite effects.

Evaluation Form

Figure 12–3 is an evaluation form that highlights and expands on the relevant impairments.

This form affords the therapist the ability to differentiate between the various types of impairment.

Under the impairment categories the therapist looks for the following:

1. Musculoskeletal impairments
   Trunk mobility— unilateral and then bilateral trunk limitation. Increased kyphosis, decreased lumbar extension.
   Pelvic mobility—Decreased rotation, decreased ability to tilt the pelvis.
   a. Range of motion limitations: Decreased motion in the plantar flexors, hip flexors, and neck rotators.
   b. Strength limitation: Weak hip extensors, dorsi/plantar flexors, and trunk extensors.
   c. Postural limitations: Forward head, rounded shoulders, kyphosis, increased hip and knee flexion.
2. Cardiopulmonary impairments: Decreased chest expansion and an increased heart rate and blood pressure.
   a. Slowed movements and difficulty breathing.
   b. Increased fatigue and orthostatic hypotension.
3. Neurological impairment: Increased rigidity, resting tremor, slowness of movement, difficulty initiating movement, and increased drooling and flushing.
   a. Balance impairment: Increased loss of balance.
   b. Gait impairment: Shuffling, festination, retropulsion, no arm swing, slow pace.
   c. Swallowing impairments: Increased difficulty swallowing.

Even with an extremely comprehensive form such as Figure 12–3, there are still areas that require special mention. Tremor, for example, may be overlooked because it is only present intermittently, minimally, or in one joint. Because tremor may be difficult to assess, the therapist should have the patient sit with arms resting on legs. The patient is then instructed to count backward by 2 from 100. This activity stresses the patient and brings out the resting tremor, which the therapist can then observe. Once the therapist has observed the tremor, placing the hands over the moving part will elicit the 4 to 7 second tremor and confirm the resting tremor.[10]

A good test for bradykinesia is to have the patient sit with both hands in his or her lap. The patient then supinates and pronates the forearms as rapidly as possible on one side and then the other. If the symptoms are unilateral the therapist should start with the uninvolved side. The patient must do this activity for at least 20 seconds with the therapist observing for quality of movement. There may be no noticeable impairment at first; however, after 3 to 4 seconds the patient will begin to substitute by shortening the arc, or will fail to flip hands over completely, and movement will generally slow. If this is noted, bradykinesia is confirmed.[10]

Name _____

History _____

FUNCTIONAL

Complaint _____
_____

MUSCULOSKELETAL IMPAIRMENTS

Trunk mobility _____
_____

Pelvic mobility _____
_____

Range of Motion Limitations _____
_____

Strength Limitations _____
_____

Limitations _____
_____

CARDIOPULMONARY IMPAIRMENTS

Chest Expansion _____

Pulmonary Limitations _____
_____

Heart rate, Blood Pressure _____

NEUROLOGICAL IMPAIRMENTS

Rigidity _____

Tremor _____

Motor Planning _____

ANS

Function _____

COMPOSITE IMPAIRMENTS

Balance _____

Gait _____

Swallowing _____

Bradykinesia _____
_____

Hypoventilation _____
_____

Fatigue _____
_____

Goals _____
_____
_____
_____
_____

Treatment Plan _____
_____
_____
_____
_____
_____
_____

Figure 12–3. Parkinson Evaluation Form. (© Carole B. Lewis)

Hand posture can be checked by standing above and behind the patient, grasping both wrists, and shaking both hands up and down. The therapist observes for looseness and thumb position. If the patient fails to show general looseness or opposition of the thumb while shaking this may be a sign of early stage involvement. As the disease progresses the patient will display finger adduction and flexion of the metacarpals, interphalangeal extension, and ulnar deviation. In the very advanced stages the wrist may be drawn into flexion and pronation.[10]

Rigidity should be assessed in the neck, trunk, and all the extremities. Assessment for rigidity simply involves moving the part through the range of motion, making sure the patient is relaxed and not tensing the muscles. The therapist then notes any resistance or tension. All normal muscle movements should float.[10]

Weindrich and associates[11] noted that limitations in the wrist and head in axial rotation related to the improvement of symptoms of Parkinson's disease. Therefore, this measure may be an important tool in assessment.

Gait Evaluation

Gait changes in Parkinson patients deserves special mention. According to the works of Murray and co-authors[12] there are significant changes in the Parkinson's gait as compared to the normal gait. These changes are

1. Decreased step length.
2. Wider stride width.
3. Increased knee flexion in the standing position. (Normally, 3° of hyperextension at the knee is observed in standing. Parkinson patients tend to stand in 3°, 6°, and 12° of flexion for mild, moderate, and severely disabled groups, respectively.
4. Decreased mean total amplitude for flexion–extension used during free walking (degrees respectively in disabled Parkinson patients).[12]
5. Simultaneous thoracic and pelvic rotation in free speed walking.
6. Decreased heel floor angle at heel strike (norms 21° and 16°, 11°, and 6°, respectively, for Parkinson patients).[12]

Functional Assessment

A final area of evaluation of the Parkinson patient is functional assessment. In a study Henderson and associates[13] functional or activities of daily living (ADL) assessments were shown to be good for assessing functional deficits. The study did find, however, that if a description of the disease was sought then an assessment of the actual signs of the disease would be better.[13]

Two ratings scales that incorporate both signs and ADL assessment are found in Table 12–1 and Figure 12–4.[10,14]

Once the therapist has conducted a thorough evaluation then the treatment can be initiated.

Treatment Considerations

When designing a treatment program for patients with Parkinson's disease the model of Schenkman and co-authors[9] can be useful. The therapist must keep in mind what deficits can be corrected and which respond minimally to physical therapy. Rigidity, for example, may be temporarily relaxed in order to facilitate muscle stretching. However, the permanent effects of relaxation training on muscle rigidity will be minimal.[15] Therefore, prior to initiating a program the therapist must prioritize the problems and interpret the goals in terms of what is efficacious. Table 12–2 is an example of this process.[16]

TABLE 12–1. PARKINSON'S DISEASE RATING SCALE

Directions: Apply a gross clinical rating to each of the ten listed items, assigning value ratings of 0–3 for each item, where (0) = no involvement and (1), (2), and (3) are equated to early, moderate, and severe disease, respectively. Refer to the discussions in the text for details of the examination and the ratings.

Bradykinesia of Hands—Including Handwriting
(0) No involvement.
(1) Detectable slowing of the supination–pronation rate evidenced by beginning difficulty in handling tools, buttoning clothes, and handwriting.
(2) Moderate slowing of supination–pronation rate, one or both sides, evidenced by moderate impairment of hand function. Handwriting is greatly impaired, micrographia present.
(3) Severe slowing of supination–pronation rate. Unable to write or button clothes. Marked difficulty in handling utensils.

Rigidity
(0) Nondetectable
(1) Detectable rigidity in neck and shoulders. Activation phenomenon is present. One or both arms show mild, negative, resting rigidity.
(2) Moderate rigidity in neck and shoulders. Resting rigidity is positive when patient is not on medication.
(3) Severe rigidity in neck and shoulders. Resting rigidity cannot be reversed by medication.

Posture
(0) Normal posture. Head flexed forward less than 4 inches.
(1) Beginning poker spine. Head flexed forward up to 5 inches.
(2) Beginning arm flexion. Head flexed forward up to 6 inches. One or both arms raised but still below waist.
(3) Onset of simian posture. Head flexed forward more than 6 inches. One or both hands elevated above waist. Sharp flexion of hand, beginning interphalangeal extension. Beginning flexion of knees.

Upper Extremity Swing
(1) One arm definitely decreased in amount of swing.
(2) One arm fails to swing.
(3) Both arms fail to swing.

Gait
(0) Steps out well with 18–30 inch stride. Turns about effortlessly.
(1) Gait shortened to 12–18 inch stride. Beginning to strike one heel. Turn around time slowing. Requires several steps.
(2) Stride moderately shortened—now 6–12 inches. Both heels beginning to strike floor forcefully.
(3) Onset of shuffling gait, steps less than 3 inches. Occasional stuttering-type or blocking gait. Walks on toes—turns around very slowly.

Tremor
(0) No detectable tremor found.
(1) Less than one inch of peak-to-peak tremor movement observed in limbs or head at rest or in either hand while walking or during finger to nose testing.
(2) Maximum tremor envelope fails to exceed 4 inches. Tremor is severe but not constant and patient retains some control of hands.
(3) Tremor envelope exceeds 4 inches. Tremor is constant and severe. Patient cannot get free of tremor while awake unless it is a pure cerebellar type. Writing and feeding are impossible.

(*continued*)

TABLE 12–1. PARKINSON'S DISEASE RATING SCALE (CONT.)

Facies

(1) Detectable immobility. Mouth remains closed. Beginning features of anxiety or depression.

(2) Moderate immobility. Emotion breaks through at markedly increased threshold. Lips parted some of the time. Moderate appearance of anxiety or depression. Drooling may be present.

(3) Frozen facies. Mouth open 1/4 inch or more. Drooling may be severe.

Seborrhea

(0) None.

(1) Increased perspiration, secretion remaining thin.

(2) Obvious oiliness present. Secretion much thicker.

(3) Marked seborrhea, entire face and head covered by thick secretion.

Speech

(0) Clear, loud, resonant, easily understood.

(1) Beginning of hoarseness with loss of inflection and resonance. Good volume and still easily understood.

(2) Moderate hoarseness and weakness. Constant monotone, unvaried pitch. Beginning of dysarthria, hesitancy, stuttering, difficult to understand.

(3) Marked harshness and weakness. Very difficult to hear and understand.

Self Care

(0) No impairment.

(1) Still provides full self-care but rate of dressing definitely impeded. Able to live alone and often still employable.

(2) Requires help in certain critical areas, such as turning in bed, rising from chairs, etc. Very slow in performing most activities but manages by taking much time.

(3) Continuously disabled. Unable to dress, feed him- or herself, or walk alone.

Reprinted with permission from Webster D. Critical analysis of the disability in Parkinson's disease. Mod Treat. 1969;5:257–282.

Schenkman's Approach

Schenkman suggests the following treatment progression

1. Relaxation.
2. Breathing exercises.
3. Passive muscle stretching and positioning.
4. Active range of motion and postural alignment.
5. Weight shifting.
6. Balance responses.
7. Gait activities.
8. Patient home exercises.[16]

As mentioned previously, relaxation can be used to temporarily decrease rigidity and increase flexibility. Relaxation of the muscles can be induced by slow rhythmic movements rotating beginning with very small motions and progressing to larger ones. Other techniques, such as biofeedback, contract- relax stretch, and deep breathing, can be helpful. The relaxation will be more effective if the approach begins supine and progresses to sitting and standing, and the more supported the individual is, the better will be their ability to relax. In addition, relaxation is better if it is begun passively and is progressed to active. Finally, the relaxation is more effective if the patient is taught to relax individual functional segments (for example, the head on the thorax, the shoulder on the thorax, and the lower extremity on the pelvis).

Parkinson Patient Disability Rating

PATIENT
  Name:
  Sex:
  Age:
  Ward:
Total score:

Note:
Use 0–4 for rating:

None		Never
Mild	or	Occasional % time
Moderate		Moderate % time
Severe		Considerable % time
Complete		Constant

Use 0.5 for readings that are not clearly categorized.

HEAD

1. *Ocular Movements* (consider rapidity of conjugate gaze in all directions, and the ability to open eyes after closure).
   Limitation of voluntary control.

complete	. . . .
severe	. . . .
moderate	. . . .
mild	. . . .
none	. . . .

2. *Blinking*
   (inability to blink)
   (1 min and over)
   (30–60 sec)
   (10–30 sec)
   (free)

complete	. . . .
severe	. . . .
moderate	. . . .
mild	. . . .
none	. . . .

3. *Emotional facial control*
   (Check degree of flattening of facial lines.
   Note facial expression with smiling.)

   Upper (forehead, eyes, nose)
   (absence of facial expression)

complete	. . . .
severe	. . . .
moderate	. . . .
mild	. . . .
none	. . . .

   Lower (mouth)
   (absence of facial expression)

complete	. . . .
severe	. . . .
moderate	. . . .
mild	. . . .
none	. . . .

— Continued —

─────── *Continued from previous page* ───────

4. *Voluntary facial control*
    (Ask patient to frown upward, inward; wrinkle nose; close eyes)

    Upper (forehead, eyes, nose)
    (absence of control)

complete	. . . .
severe	. . . .
moderate	. . . .
mild	. . . .
none	. . . .

    Lower (mouth). Ask patient to grimace and purse lips.
    (absence of control)

complete	. . . .
severe	. . . .
moderate	. . . .
mild	. . . .
none	. . . .

Note: If there is considerable difference between the two sides of
the face, please rate.

5. *Swallowing*
    (inability to swallow)
    (not voluntary and chokes reflexly)
    (slowed)
    (drooling, occasional choking)

complete	. . . .
severe	. . . .
moderate	. . . .
mild	. . . .
none	. . . .

6. *Motor speech*—degree to which speech is inaudible and
    unintelligible (inability to talk)

complete	. . . .
severe	. . . .
moderate	. . . .
mild	. . . .
none	. . . .

7. *Tongue movement*
    (inability to move)
    (can protrude tongue to lip margin)
    (can protrude tongue beyond lips but not full forward or in
       other directions)
    (full movement, but slowed)

complete	. . . .
severe	. . . .
moderate	. . . .
mild	. . . .
none	. . . .

NECK AND UPPER EXTREMITIES

8. *Head rotation* (sitting)
    (Best rating taken when patient decreases range with
    repetition—100% equivalent of 90°)

	Right		**Left**	
(inability to rotate)	complete	. . . . . .	complete	. . . .
(25–0%)	severe	. . . . . .	severe	. . . .
(50–25%)	moderate	. . . . . .	moderate	. . . .
(75–50%)	mild	. . . . . .	mild	. . . .
(100–75%)	none	. . . . . .	none	. . . .

Note: The head may be in an asymmetrical starting position, but where this is of a considerable degree,
marked limitation of head movement to right and left has been found and it has not interfered with rating.

─────── *Continued* ───────

Continued from previous page

9. *Shoulder elevation* (sitting)
    (Best rating taken when patient decreases range with repetition)

	Right		Left	
(inability to rotate)	complete	. . . . . .	complete	. . . . . .
(25–0%)	severe	. . . . . .	severe	. . . . . .
(50–25%)	moderate	. . . . . .	moderate	. . . . . .
(75–50%)	mild	. . . . . .	mild	. . . . . .
(100–75%)	none	. . . . . .	none	. . . . . .

10. *Lowering head to plinth* (supine position)

		Left	
(inability)		complete	. . . . . .
(can lower head to some extent)		severe	. . . . . .
(can lower head to plinth but slowly)		moderate	. . . . . .
(can lower head to plinth—moderate speed)		mild	. . . . . .
		none	. . . . . .

11. *Elevation of arms* (sitting)

	Right		Left	
(inability)	complete	. . . . . .	complete	. . . . . .
(below shoulder)	severe	. . . . . .	severe	. . . . . .
(shoulder level)	moderate	. . . . . .	moderate	. . . . . .
(partial hyperabduction)	mild	. . . . . .	mild	. . . . . .
(full hyperabduction)	none	. . . . . .	none	. . . . . .

12. *Handwriting* (depending on handedness—one score)

		Left	
(inability)		complete	. . . . . .
		severe	. . . . . .
		moderate	. . . . . .
		mild	. . . . . .
		none	. . . . . .

TRUNK AND LOWER EXTREMITIES

13. *Arising from standard chair with sidearms*

		Left	
(inability)		complete	. . . . . .
(can arise with examiner's support)		severe	. . . . . .
(can arise with maximal arm support by self)		moderate	. . . . . .
(can arise with moderate arm support by self)		mild	. . . . . .
(can arise with arms folded)		none	. . . . . .

14. *Walking*

		Left	
(cannot walk)		complete	. . . . . .
(can walk with observer's assistance)		severe	. . . . . .
(can walk with arm support by self)		moderate	. . . . . .
(can walk independently but slowly)		mild	. . . . . .
(can walk well)		none	. . . . . .

15. *Walking*

	Right		Left	
(cannot walk on heels and toes)	complete	. . . . . .	complete	. . . . . .
Can walk:				
(on heels or toes with maximal support)	severe	. . . . . .	severe	. . . . . .
(on heels or toes with moderate support)	moderate	. . . . . .	moderate	. . . . . .
(on heels and toes with moderate support)	mild	. . . . . .	mild	. . . . . .
(on heels and toes with no support)	none	. . . . . .	none	. . . . . .

16. *Climbing*

	Right		Left	
(cannot lift foot in walking and climbing)	complete	. . . . . .	complete	. . . . . .
(can lift foot in walking with observer's support but cannot climb)	severe	. . . . . .	severe	. . . . . .
(can lift foot in walking and climb with observer's support)	moderate	. . . . . .	moderate	. . . . . .

Continued

Continued from previous page

	Right		**Left**	
(can lift foot in walking and climb with own support)	mild	. . . . . .	mild	. . . . . .
(can lift foot in walking and climb 8 in. step without support)	none	. . . . . .	none	. . . . . .

17. *Trunk raising* (supine position)

(cannot lift head and shoulders off table)			complete	. . . . . .
Can lift head and shoulders:				
(off table with hands on side of plinth)			severe	. . . . . .
(off table with hands on abdomen or chest)			moderate	. . . . . .
(off table with hands on head)			mild	. . . . . .
(can arise to sitting position with hands on head)			none	. . . . . .

18. *Trunk turning* (supine position)

(cannot turn to right or left)			complete	. . . . . .
(can make some attempt to turn using arms)			severe	. . . . .
(can turn to one side using one arm but not other)			moderate	. . . . . .
(can turn to both sides using arms)			mild	. . . . . .
(can turn to both sides without using arms)			none	. . . . . .

19. *Straight leg raising*

	Right		**Left**	
(cannot flex thigh)	complete	. . . . . .	complete	. . . . . .
Can flex thigh:				
(with heel remaining on bed)	severe	. . . . .	severe	. . . . . .
(30° lifting partially extended lower extremity)	moderate	. . . . . .	moderate	. . . . . .
(60° lifting partially extended lower extremity)	mild	. . . . . .	mild	. . . . . .
(60° lifting fully extended lower extremity)	none	. . . . . .	none	. . . . . .

20. *Movement of ankles and toes*

	Right		**Left**	
(no spontaneous movement)	complete	. . . . . .	complete	. . . . . .
(slight movement)	severe	. . . . . .	severe	. . . . . .
(moderate movement)	moderate	. . . . . .	moderate	. . . . . .
(good, but slowed movement)	mild	. . . . . .	mild	. . . . . .
(free movement)	none	. . . . . .	none	. . . . . .

GENERAL

21. *General mobility*

(complete immobility at rest)			complete	. . . . . .
(mobility limited to head and neck)			severe	. . . . . .
(slight mobility in trunk and extremities)			moderate	. . . . . .
(moderate mobility in trunk and extremities)			mild	. . . . . .
(freely mobile)			none	. . . . . .

22. *Abnormal tone* (rigidity)

	Neck	**Back**
complete	. . . . . .	. . . . . .
severe	. . . . . .	. . . . . .
moderate	. . . . . .	. . . . . .
mild	. . . . . .	. . . . . .
none	. . . . . .	. . . . . .

RUE

	Shoulder	**Elbow**	**Wrist & Fingers**
complete	. . . . . .	. . . . . .	. . . . . .
severe	. . . . . .	. . . . . .	. . . . . .
moderate	. . . . . .	. . . . . .	. . . . . .
mild	. . . . . .	. . . . . .	. . . . . .
none	. . . . . .	. . . . . .	. . . . . .

Continued

Continued from previous page

LUE

	Shoulder	Elbow	Wrist & Fingers
complete	. . . .	. . . . . .	. . . .
severe	. . . . . .	. . . . .	. . . . . .
moderate	. . . . . .	. . . . .	. . . . . .
mild	. . . . . .	. . . . .	. . . . . .
none	. . . .	. . . . .	. . . .

RLE

	Hip	Knee	Ankle & Toes
complete	. . . . . .	. . . . .	. . . . . .
severe	. . . . . .	. . . . .	. . . . . .
moderate	. . . . . .	. . . . .	. . . . . .
mild	. . . .	. . . . .	. . . . . .
none	. . . .	. . . . .	. . . . . .

LLE

	Hip	Knee	Ankle & Toes
complete	. . . . . .	. . . . .	. . . . . .
severe	. . . . . .	. . . . .	. . . . . .
moderate	. . . . . .	. . . . . .	. . . . . .
mild	. . . . . .	. . . . .	. . . . . .
none	. . . .	. . . . . .	. . . . . .

Use finger or toe rating where wrist or ankle are immobile from fusion or contractures.

23. *Contractures and deformities*

	Neck	Back
complete	. . . . . .	. . . .
severe	. . . . .	. . . . . .
moderate	. . . . . .	. . . . . .
mild	. . . . . .	. . . . . .
none	. . . . . .	. . . .

RUE

	Shoulder	Elbow	Wrist & Fingers
complete	. . . .	. . . . .	. . . . . .
severe	. . . . . .	. . . . .	. . . . . .
moderate	. . . . . .	. . . . .	. . . . . .
mild	. . . . . .	. . . . .	. . . .
none	. . . . . .	. . . . .	. . . .

LUE

	Shoulder	Elbow	Wrist & Fingers
complete	. . . . . .	. . . . .	. . . . . .
severe	. . . . . .	. . . . .	. . . . . .
moderate	. . . . . .	. . . . .	. . . . . .
mild	. . . . . .	. . . . .	. . . . . .
none	. . . . . .	. . . . .	. . . . . .

Continued

Continued from previous page

RLE

	Hip	Knee	Ankle & Toes
complete	. . . .	. . . .	. . . . . .
severe	. . . . . .	. . . . . .	. . . . . .
moderate	. . . . . .	. . . .	. . . . . .
mild	. . . . . .	. . . .	. . . . . .
none	. . . .	. . . . . .	. . . .

LLE

	Hip	Knee	Ankle & Toes
complete	. . . . . .	. . . . . .	. . . . . .
severe	. . . . . .	. . . . . .	. . . . . .
moderate	. . . . . .	. . . . . .	. . . . . .
mild	. . . . . .	. . . . . .	. . . .
none	. . . .	. . . .	. . . .

24. Tremor

	Eyelids	Face	Jaw
constant	. . . . . .	. . . . . .	. . . . . .
considerable % time	. . . . . .	. . . . . .	. . . . . .
moderate % time	. . . . . .	. . . . . .	. . . . . .
occasional % time	. . . . . .	. . . . . .	. . . . . .
never	. . . .	. . . .	. . . .

	Tongue	Neck	RUE
constant	. . . . . .	. . . . . .	. . . . . .
considerable % time	. . . . . .	. . . . . .	. . . . . .
moderate % time	. . . . . .	. . . . . .	. . . . . .
occasional % time	. . . . . .	. . . . . .	. . . . . .
never	. . . .	. . . .	. . . .

	LUE	RLE	LLE
constant	. . . . . .	. . . . . .	. . . . . .
considerable % time	. . . . . .	. . . . . .	. . . . . .
moderate % time	. . . . . .	. . . . . .	. . . . . .
occasional % time	. . . . . .	. . . . . .	. . . . . .
never	. . . .	. . . .	. . . .

Figure 12–4. *(Reprinted with permission from Alba A, et al. A clinical disability rating for Parkinson's disease. Chron Dis 1968;21:507–522.)*

Breathing or breathing control should be encouraged throughout the various stages of treatment. The patient is taught to take deep relaxed breaths while doing the relaxation exercises. Once the patient has achieved some degree of relaxation in the thoracic area then deeper breathing combined with trunk stretching can help to increase chest expansion.

Passive muscle stretching is another commonly used modality for physical therapy. What is different for the patient with Parkinson's disease is the mode and area of application. As with relaxation the most effective stretch will be with the body in the most supported position due to the patient's decreased protective responses; therefore, begin with stretching in the supine or side-lying position. Areas requiring special stretching are

1. Lumbopelvic extensions are important for balance.
2. Rotation and lateral flexion of the pelvis.
3. Hamstring and plantar flexion.

TABLE 21–2. EXAMPLES OF PROBLEMS, INTERPRETATIONS, AND GOALS FOR PATIENTS WITH PARKINSON'S DISEASE

Problem[a]	Quantitative	Descriptive	Interpretation	Goal
Gait	Ambulates 25 ft[b] in 18 sec (18 steps)	Small steps; decreased left heel-strike; decreased trunk rotation; left knee in flexion from weight acceptance to push-off; no left arm swing	Problems attributable to limitations in left knee and ankle range of motion and decreased available trunk rotation combined with trunk and limb rigidity with motor programming and planning deficits	Ambulate 25 ft in 10 sec (12 steps); improved heel-strike, push-off, trunk rotation, and arm swing
Bed mobility (supine to sitting)	7 sec to complete task	Lacks trunk rotation and dissociation of pelvic complex from shoulder complex; appears fearful of losing balance	Problems attributable to combination of limited available trunk ROM, rigidity, and impaired balance	2 sec to complete task; improved trunk rotation with dissociation of shoulder complex from pelvic complex
Transfers (sitting to standing from low treatment table)	Sitting to standing from mat takes 10 sec	Lack of anterior pelvic tilt and of scooting forward on mat; excessive use of arms for push-off from mat	Problems attributable to lack of lumbopelvic mobility, rigidity, and difficulty motor planning and programming	Patient will accomplish task in 5 sec, use anterior tilt, scoot forward, and decrease need for use of arms
Decreased hip ROM	Straight leg raise (left leg: 0°–50°; right leg: 0°–45°); internal rotation (left leg: 0°–25°; right leg: 0°–30°)		Problems result from rigidity and improper posturing	Hip ROM within normal limits
Rigidity[c]		Moderate[d]	Attributable to primary impairments of disease	Patient will self-relax rigidity for increasing ROM

[a]Patient problems may relate to disabilities or impairments.
[b]1 ft = 0.3048 m.
[c]Rigidity is listed as a problem because of its causal role in most impairments of Parkinson's disease; however, objective measures of rigidity do not exist, and physical therapy does not appear to affect long-term changes.
[d]Feldman R, Lannon M. Parkinson's disease and related disturbances. In: Feldman R, ed. Neurology: The Physician's Guide. New York: Thieme Medical Publishers, 1984; 147–162.
Reprinted with permission from Schenkman M, et al. Management of individuals with Parkinson's disease: rationale and case studies. Phys Ther November 1989;69(11)944–955.

4. Cervical and thoracic extension, rotation, and lateral flexion.
5. Hip extension, external rotation, and abduction.
6. Elbow extension and supination.
7. Finger flexion and extension.

To achieve passive stretching, contract-relax stretching and passive stretching using Gustaffson's principle of 15 to 30 second stretches gives the best results.[17] Stretching is followed by active range of motion and postural alignment.

The key to achieving the best results in active range of motion and postural alignment is repetition. According to Nelson,[18] for a movement to become assimilated by the nervous system it needs millions of repetitions, which equates to hundreds to thousands of repetitions a day. Therefore, the patient should do the activity for 5 to 10 minutes instead of 5 to 10 times. Some of the most useful active motion activities for these areas are (1) pelvic clocks to enhance pelvic and lumbar motion, (2) isolated lateral and anterior pelvic tilts, and (3) clocks around any joint in the body. If the patient has limitation in the lumbar spine, the patient may substitute for lumbopelvic motion with pelvifemoral motion. Therefore, evaluate and treat any loss of mobility in the lumbar spine.

Once the patient is able to actively move the various body parts in a supine and then a standing position following stretching, then weight shifting in a standing position with the pelvis in a balanced position is practiced. Weight shifting, like the previous sequences, can be practiced from the supine to the standing positions.

Finally, balance activities and responses need to be stressed. Here the patient's balance can be challenged intrinsically and extrinsically. Methods of challenging the patient's intrinsic balance include having the patient reach overhead, from side to side, and backward in a rotational direction when sitting and standing. For extrinsic balance challenges, the therapist can apply an outside stress, such as a gentle shove, to disturb the patient's balance. Both are needed for everyday activity and should be practiced when sitting and standing.

Function is the final area of treatment and must always be kept in mind when designing the exercise program, because exercises are most effective if they relate to function. For example, trunk rotation should be followed by rolling in bed as an active functional activity that the patient can do on his or her own at home. Anterior pelvic tilting when standing is another useful home exercise employing a needed functional activity. When designing a home exercise program be sure to stress the functional carry-over. This way when the patient does daily activities, he or she is constantly doing the exercise program.

Flewitt-Handford Exercises

Another well-known program for Parkinson patients is the Flewitt-Handford exercises. These exercises were developed to help to improve the gait of Parkinson patients. The developers of the exercises believe that the gait seen is a result of adaption to gain control of forward progression and balance. Parkinson patients have plenty of propulsion, but they lack a braking mechanism. Flewitt-Handford exercises are directed to reteach heel strike, improve weight transference, increase motion of the hip and knee, and prevent stiffness of the lower extremity (Table 12–3).[19]

Patient education is an important component for the treatment of the Parkinson patient. The Parkinson's Disease Foundation is an excellent resource for information and assistance for the patient and the families. They have developed an exercise videotape for Parkinson patients called "Get up and Go," which is a useful tool for helping patients maintain the benefits of a rehabilitation program in a fun and interesting way.

Group Rehabilitation

Another treatment consideration is group rehabilitation.[20] Table 12–4 is a sample group evaluation and exercise progression.

TABLE 12–3. THE FLEWITT-HANDFORD EXERCISES

1. **Long sitting.** Alternate flexion/extension of toes, feet, and knees.
2. **Crook lying.** Rolling knees from side to side.
3. **Lying.** Alternate hip and knee flexion/extension, lift each foot off the plinth.
4. **Stand** facing and holding onto either parallel bars in a gym, or a heavy chair, table, or mantelpiece at home.
   a. High stepping.
   b. With straight knees and not leaning backward alternate feet dorsiflexion.
   c. Cross the left leg in front of the right and vice versa each time trying to touch the floor heel first.
   d. If in the gym, the patient should practice weight transference by walking sideways up and down the parallel bars. Then the same again, but crossing the legs over each other.
5. **Standing** at right angles to the parallel bars or chair, practice taking strides from toe off to heel-strike of first one leg, then the other. Pay attention to hip extension and proper heel-strike.
   When walking, patients must learn to put their heels down first with every step. Many patients become "stuck" while walking. They can easily unstick themselves by rocking backwards so their weight is going through their heels. Though taking a step backwards or sideways, they will find themselves able to move forwards again.

Reprinted with permission from Handford F. The Flewitt-Handford exercises for Parkinson's gait. Physiotherapy. August 1986; 72(8) 382.

TABLE 12–4. PARKINSONISM EVALUATION

Occupational Therapy

Upper Extremity Function	Activities of Daily Living

1. Drawing concentric circles
  a. number in 30 sec
  b. size of circles
  c. line quality
2. Alternating finger flexion/extension: number of complete repetitions in 10 sec
3. Grasp strength
4. Signature: time, legibility
	1. Dressing (in seconds)
	  a. put on shirt
	  b. fasten three buttons
	  c. put one shoe
	  d. tie one shoelace
	2. Transfers (in seconds)
	  a. standing to supine
	  b. supine to standing
	  c. standing to sitting
	  d. sitting to standing
	3. Mobility (in seconds)
	  a. rolling supine to prone
	  b. standing 360° turn
	  c. opening/entering doors
	  d. ascending/descending stairs

Physical Therapy

Muscle Tightness	Balance
1. Pectorals—active range 2. Hamstrings—passive range 3. Hip flexors—passive range 4. Hip adductors—passive range	1. Quadruped-balance on opposite arm and leg, 5 sec 2. Standing on one foot, 5 sec 3. Propulsion (push patient forward) 4. Retropulsion (push patient backward)

Reciprocation (repetitions in 30 sec)	Posture

1. Supine
2. Gait
3. Stop start walk: sec/15 m
	1. Standing
	  a. anterior–posterior
	  b. lateral
	2. Walking
	3 Supine

Phase I:

Warm-up exercises for range of motion, reciprocality, and mobility.
Mat exercises: bridging, trunk rotation, side leg raises, and reciprocal movements
Parallel bars: knee bends, side leg raises, balancing.
Bicycle/pulleys.

Phase II:

Activities for mobility and equilibrium.
Range of motion exercises for all major joints.
Facial exercises.
Static and dynamic balance: *Hokey Pokey, Alley Cat*

Phase III:

Activities for coordination and socialization:
Week 1: Special exercises for breathing   Special exercises for face, lips
    Alley Cat   Marching
    Shuffleboard   Hot potato
    Frisbee   Instrument playing
                                     Tic-Tac-Toe

(continued)

TABLE 12–4. PARKINSONISM EVALUATION (CONT.)

Phase III (*cont.*):	

Week 2: *Hokey Pokey*
    Ball: reciprocal bouncing, tossing, kicking,
        pass and reverse, beach ball
	Subgroup *a: Alley Cat*
	    cotton ball blow
	    hand-clapping patterns
	Subgroup *b:* individual tasks:
	    perceptual tasks, dexterity
	    boards, tracing

Week 3: Bean bag toss Sitting relay: overhead, sideways	Horseshoes Hot potato
Week 4: *Hokey Pokey* Bowling	Special exercises for arms, hands Wand passing Basketball

Reprinted with permission from Davis J. Team management of Parkinson's disease. Am J Occup Ther. May–June 1977;31(5):300–308.

STROKE

Even though stroke is not the major neurological problem of old age, it is significant because it is such a functionally devastating disease. In the United States alone between 250,000 and 300,000 persons have CVAs a year.[21] Most strokes occur late in life; 43% of stroke patients are over the age of 74.[22]

In absolute numbers, women and men over age 75 are almost equally afflicted with CVAs; however, because the ratio of women to men is so much greater (3 : 2), statistically men have a greater likelihood of developing stroke.[23] Blacks and Japanese Americans are more likely to have strokes than whites, and the geographic area with the highest percentage of strokes is the southern United States.[24]

Besides causing tremendous morbidity (it is estimated that 20% to 40% of stroke patients die within 30 days[25]), nearly 40% of people with this disease report limitations in their activities. Cerebral vascular disease results in an average of 36 days of restricted activity for stroke victims.[26]

There are three major types of strokes. The cerebral thrombosis occurs when an artery that supplies blood to the brain becomes narrowed by plaque and deposits. The blood may coagulate and form a clot that does not allow sufficient blood through to the area. A cerebral emboli is caused by a blockage of some foreign object in the bloodstream, such as a clot, that can become wedged where it obstructs blood flow to the brain. The final type of stroke is a cerebral hemorrhage, where the artery is not blocked but bursts and blood seeps into the surrounding brain tissue. Depending on the extent of the damage, a cerebral hemorrhage is usually the most severe type of stroke, followed by thrombosis, then emboli. The severity of the stroke also depends on what area of the brain is affected and the extent and duration of the blockage of blood. Table 12–5 shows the clinical symptoms of vascular lesions and neurovascular disease.[27]

Risk factors associated with stroke are similar for young and old. Spriggs and co-workers noted such factors as previous cerebral vascular disease, taking certain prescribed medicines, and regular cigarette smoking as high risk factors. Family history was also a factor but was not found to be significant in the older population.[28]

Perceptual deficits occur in varying degrees with a stroke. Table 12–6 is a chart of these deficits.

TABLE 12–5. CLINICAL SYMPTOMS OF CEREBRAL VASCULAR LESIONS AND NEUROVASCULAR DISEASE

Vessel	Clinical Symptoms	Structures Involved
CEREBRAL VASCULAR LESIONS		
Middle cerebral artery	Contralateral paralysis and sensory deficit	Somatic motor area
	Motor speech impairment	Broca's area (dominant hemisphere)
	"Central" aphasia, anomia, jargon speech	Parietoccipital cortex (dominant hemisphere)
	Unilateral neglect, apraxia, impaired ability to judge distance	Parietal lobe (nondominant hemisphere)
	Homonymous hemianopsia	Optic radiation deep to second temporal convolution
	Loss of conjugate gaze to opposite side	Frontal controversive field
	Avoidance reaction of opposite limbs	Parietal lobe
	Pure motor hemiplegia	Upper portion of posterior limb of internal capsule
	Limb-kinetic apraxia	Premotor or parietal cortex
Anterior cerebral artery	Paralysis—lower extremity	Motor area—leg
	Paresis in opposite arm	Arm area of cortex
	Cortical sensory loss	Sensory area
	Urinary incontinence	Posteromedial aspect of superior frontal gyrus
	Contralateral grasp reflex, sucking reflex	Medial surface of posterior frontal lobe
	Lack of spontaniety motor inaction, echolalia	Uncertain
	Perseveration and amnesia	Uncertain
Posterior cerebral artery		
Peripheral area	Homonymous hemianopsia	Calcarine cortex or optic radiation
	Bilateral homonymous hemianopsia, cortical blindness, inability to perceive objects not centrally located, ocular apraxia	Bilateral occipital lobe
	Memory defect	Inferomedial portions of temporal lobe
	Topographic disorientation	Nondominant calcarine and lingual gyri
Central area	Thalamic syndrome	Posteroventral nucleus ophthalmus
	Weber's syndrome	Cranial nerve III and cerebral peduncle
	Contralateral hemiplegia	Cerebral peduncle
	Paresis of vertical eye movements, sluggish pupillary response to light	Supranuclear fibers to Cranial nerve III
	Contralateral ataxia or postural tremor	Uncertain
Internal carotid artery	Variable signs according to degree and site of occlusion—middle cerebral, anterior cerebral, posterior cerebral territory	
Basilar artery		
Superior cerebellar	Ataxia	Middle and superior cerebellar peduncles
	Dizziness, nausea, vomiting, horizontal nystagmus	Vestibular nucleus
	Horner's syndrome on opposite side, decreased pain and thermal sensation	Decending sympathetic fibers / Spinal thalamic tract
	Decreased touch, vibration, position sense of lower extremity greater than upper extremity	Medial lemniscus
Anterior inferior cerebellar artery	Nystagmus, vertigo, nausea, vomiting	Vestibular nerve
	Facial paralysis on same side	Cranial nerve VII
	Tinnitus	Auditory nerve, lower coclear nucleus
	Ataxia	Middle cerebral peduncle
	Impaired facial sensation on same side	Fifth cranial nerve nucleus
	Decreased pain and thermal sensation on opposite side	Spinal thalamic tract
Hemorrhage		
Hypertensive hemorrhage	Severe headache	CT scan can detect hemorrhages greater than 1.5 cm in cerebral and cerebellar hemispheres; they are diagnostically superior to arteriography; they are especially helpful in diagnosing small hemorrhages that do not spill blood into cerebrospinal fluid; with massive
	Vomiting at onset	
	Blood pressure > 170/90; usually "essential" hypertension but can be from other types	
	Abrupt onset, usually during day, not in sleep	

(*continued*)

TABLE 12–5. CLINICAL SYMPTOMS OF CEREBRAL VASCULAR LESIONS AND NEUROVASCULAR DISEASE (CONT.)

Vessel	Clinical Symptoms	Structures Involved
Hemorrhage		
Hypersensitive hemorrhage (*cont.*)	Gradually evolves over hours or days according to speed of bleeding No recurrence of bleeding Frequency of blacks with hypertensive hemorrage is greater than frequency of whites Hemorrhaged blood absorbs slowly—rapid improvement of symptoms is not usual If massive hemorrhage occurs, client may survive a few hours or days secondary to brainstem compression	hemorrhage and increased pressure, cerebrospinal fluid is grossly bloody; lumbar puncture is necessary when CT scan is not available; radiographs occasionally show midline shift (this is not true with infarction); EEG shows no typical pattern, but high voltage and slow waves are most common with hemorrhage; urinary changes may reflect renal disease

Ruptured saccular aneurysm	Asymptomatic before rupture
	With rupture, blood spills under high pressure into subarachnoid space:
	  Excruciating headache with loss of consciousness
	  Headache without loss of consciousness
	  Sudden loss of consciousness
	Decerebrate rigidity with coma
	If severe—persistent deep coma with respiratory arrest, circulatory collapse leading to death; death can occur within 5 minutes
	If mild—consciousness regained within hours then confusion, amnesia, headache, stiff neck, drowsiness
	Hemiplegia, paresis, homonomus hemianopsia, or aphasia usually absent
		CT scan detects localized blood in hydrocephalus if present; cerebrospinal fluid is extremely bloody; radiographs are usually negative; carotid and vertebral arteriography are performed only if certain of diagnosis

Basilar artery Complete basilar syndrome	Bilateral long tract signs with cerebellar and cranial nerve abnormalities Coma Quadriplegia Pseudobulbar palsy Cranial nerve abnormalities	——— ——— ——— ——— ———
Vertebral artery	Decreased pain and temperature on opposite side Sensory loss from a tactile and proprioceptive Hemiparesis of arm and leg Facial pain and numbness on same side Horner's syndrome, ptosis, decreased sweating Ataxia Paralysis of tongue Weakness of vocal cord, decreased gag Hiccups	Spinal thalamic tract Medial lemniscus Pyramidal tract Descending tract and fifth cranial nucleus Descending sympathetic tract Spinal cerebellar tract Cranial nerve XII Cranial nerves IX and X Uncertain

(*continued*)

TABLE 12–5. CLINICAL SYMPTOMS OF CEREBRAL VASCULAR LESIONS AND NEUROVASCULAR DISEASE (CONT.)

Vesel	Clinical Symptoms	Structures Involved
NEUROVASCULAR DISEASE		
Thrombosis	*Extremely variable*	
	Proceeded by a prodromal episode	Cerebrospinal fluid pressure is normal
	Uneven progression	Cerebrospinnal fluid is clear
	Onset develops within minutes, hours, or over days	EEG: limited differential diagnostic value
	("thrombus in evolution")	Skull radiographs are not helpful
	60% occur during sleep—awaken unaware of problem,	Arteriography is the diffinitive procedure, it demonstrates
	rise, and fall to floor	site of collateral flow
	Usually no headache but may occur in mild form	CT scanning is helpful in chronic state when cavitation has
	Hypertension, diabetes, or vascular disease elsewhere	occurred
	in body	
TIAs	Linked to atherosclerotic thrombosis	Usually none
	Proceeded or accompanied by stroke	
	Occur by themselves	
	Last 2–30 minutes	
	Experience a few attacks or hundreds	
	Normal neurological examination between attacks	
	If transient symptoms are present on awakening, may	
	indicate future stroke	
Embolism	*Extremely variable*	
Cardiac	Occurs extremely rapidly—seconds or minutes	Generally same as thrombosis except for following:
Noncardiac	There are no warnings	If embolism causes a large hemorrhagic infarct, cerebro-
Atherosclerosis	Branches of middle cerebral artery are involved most	spinal fluid will be bloody
Pulmonary thrombosis	frequently, large embolus will block internal carotid	30% of embolic strokes produced small hemorrhagic
Fat, tumor, air	artery or stem of middle cerebral artery	infarct without bloody cerebrospinal fluid
	If in basilar system, deep coma and total paralysis may	
	result	
	Often a manifestation of heart disease, including atrial fibril-	
	slation and myocardial infarction	
	Headache	
	As embolis passes through artery, client may have neuro-	
	logical deficits that resolve as embolis breaks and passes	
	into small artery supplying small or silent brain area	

Reprinted with permission and adapted from Ryerson S. Hemiplegia resulting from vascular insult or disease. In: Umphred D, ed. Neurological Rehabilitation. St. Louis: Mosby: 1985: 476.

Before a therapist can begin evaluating and treating a stroke patient, a thorough understanding of the various stages of recovery of limb tone is essential. In the majority of cases the predominant abnormality on admission in both upper and lower extremity is flaccidity.[29] To the recover tone and go through the stages of progression occurred mainly in the first 7 to 14 days. By day 28, a total of 20% of the patients had normal upper limb tone and 28% of the patients had normal lower limb tone.[30]

Table 12–7 shows the recovery of limb tone at 28 days.[29]

Many of the following evaluative techniques are for assessing tone. It is imperative to realize that the greatest recovery occurs within the first 7 days, and many patients do regain spontaneous motor recovery within that time. Studies as of yet have not shown a difference in this early recovery stage between young and old.[29]

The efficacy of rehabilitation techniques for stroke patients has been questioned by legislature as well as administrative personnel. Nevertheless, there are several references that point to the efficacy of physical therapy.[30,31] Lehman, in the *Archives of Physical Medicine Rehabilitation*, showed that there are excellent statistics

TABLE 12–6. PERCEPTUAL DEFICITS IN CNS DYSFUNCTION

LEFT HEMIPARESIS: right hemisphere—general spatial-global deficits
Visual-perceptual deficits
    Hand-eye coordination
    Figure-ground discrimination
    Spatial relationships
    Position in space
    Form constancy
Behavioral and intellectual deficits
    Poor judgment, unrealistic behavior
    Denial of disability
    Inability to abstract
    Rigidity of thought
    Disturbances in body image and body scheme
    Impairment of ability to self-correct
    Difficulty retaining information
    Distortion of time concepts
    Tendency to see the whole and not individual steps
    Affect lability
    Feelings of persecution
    Irritability, confusion
    Distraction by verbalization
    Short attention span
    Appearance of lethargy
    Fluctuation in performance
    Disturbances in relative size and distance of objects
RIGHT HEMIPARESIS: left hemisphere—general language and temporal ordering deficits
Apraxia
    Motor
    Ideational
Behavioral and intellectual deficits
    Difficulty initiating tasks
    Sequencing deficits
    Processing delays
    Directionality deficits
    Low frustration levels
    Verbal and manual perseveration
    Rapid performance of movement or activity
    Compulsive behavior
    Extreme distractibility

Reprinted with permission from Ryerson S. Hemiplegia resulting from vascular insult or disease. In: Umphred D, ed. Neurological Rehabilitation. *St. Louis; Mosby; 1985, 476.*

for stroke patients over the age of 80 who are discharged to the home up to 2 years.[33] Older patients can improve on a stroke rehabilitation program if it is properly applied. Evaluation and treatment techniques for the older patient will be described next.

Evaluation

Several models for evaluating stroke patients can be used. As mentioned in the Parkinson's Disease section, Schenkman focuses on impairments and direct and indirect effects of the disease as well as on functional disability.[34] This model stresses that there are certain areas where physical therapy will be more beneficial.

Other authors have developed extensive forms and methods of evaluating stroke patients, and one interesting model developed by Tripp divides assessment into the following areas[35]:

TABLE 12–7. RECOVERY OF LIMB TONE AT 28 DAYS

Admission limb tone	Limb tone at 28 days					
	No.	Normal	Flexor	Extensor	Flaccid	Dead
Upper limb						
Normal	19	16	0	0	0	3
Flexor	43	10	14	1	4	14
Extensor	8	4	1	1	0	2
Flaccid	87	17	20	3	17	30
Lower limb						
Normal	47	38	0	2	0	7
Flexor	11	4	1	0	1	5
Extensor	45	15	5	9	3	13
Flaccid	54	15	4	4	7	24

Reprinted with permission from Gray C, French J, Bates D. Motor recovery following acute stroke. Age Ageing 1900;19:179–184.

1. Motor neuron response: Evaluates tone in terms of spasticity and ability to activate and relax muscle, and it describes associated reactions.
2. Fractionated movement: Evaluates the ability of the patient to move individual limb segments.
3. Movement consistency: Evaluates whether or not the patient's ability to perform gross motor activities is consistent with his or her ability to form isolated movements.
4. Mental status: Looks at ability to follow commands and ability to learn safety and judgment.
5. Functional assessment: Includes mobility and gross upper extremity function.[35]

Bobath Evaluation

Bobath,[36] one of the leaders in the area of stroke rehabilitation, provides one of the most in-depth assessments of stroke patients. The Bobath evaluation tool looks not only at range of motion and sensory deficits, but it also tests various movement patterns. The first test (Fig. 12–5) is for postural reactions in response to being moved. In addition, Bobath looks at tests for voluntary movements on request (Fig. 12–6) and at tests for balance and other automatic protective reactions (Fig. 12–7).

These tests are defined in detail in Bobath's text.[36] Looking at these assessment forms, a therapist can get an idea of some of the various movements and reactions being analyzed in the treatment setting. One of the strengths of Bobath's evaluative techniques is that they can not only be used to evaluate the patient, but the actual tests can be used as treatment techniques.[36]

Brunnstrom Evaluation

Brunnstrom[37] looks at the motor behavior of adults in terms of synergies. Brunnstrom discusses the flexor synergy of the various limbs of the body, describes them in detail, then asks the therapist to evaluate these synergy levels throughout the entire evaluation and treatment progression of the patient. The flexor synergy of the upper limb is

1. Flexion of the elbow to an acute angle.
2. Full range supination of the forearm.
3. Abduction of the shoulder to 90°.
4. External rotation of the shoulder.
5. Retraction or elevation of the shoulder girdle.

Tests for Postural Reactions in Response to Being Moved

Patterns to be tested:

Tests for shouldergirdle, arm, and hand to be tested separately in supine, sitting and standing as results are different.

At the end of each test, and at any one stage of each movement performed by the therapist, the normal reaction would be that the person tested should be able to maintain the position unaided when left unsupported.

	Abnormal resistance?	Abnormal assistance?	Uncontrolled full weight?
Grade 1			
a. Elevation of the extended arm in external rotation with supination. Wrist and fingers extended and fingers abducted. The arm is lifted forwards-upwards.			
b. Horizontal abduction, the arm and hand in the position described above.			
c. Placing the arm by the side of the patient's body, position of the arm and hand as above.			
Grade 2			
d. From any one of the above three positions the patient's arm is moved forward across body and palm placed on the opposite shoulder This is followed by lifting elbow so that forearm touches face, the hand remaining on the shoulder, with wrist extended.			
e. From the elevated extended position the patient's elbow is flexed, while upper arm is kept in elevation; palm is placed on the top of head. Then palm is placed to the back of head, while arm is abducted, and wrist extended.			

Supine Tests for Pelvis, Leg, and Foot

	Abnormal resistance?	Abnormal assistance?	Uncontrolled full weight?
Grade 1			
a. The patient's leg is fully flexed at all joints, so that the foot is off support. This is tested first with the sound leg fully flexed and held actively by the patient. Then with the sound leg extended on support.			
b. From the above flexed position the patient's foot is placed on the support; the leg remains flexed. Ankle and toes are dorsiflexed, foot everted, so that the heel only touches the support.			
c. From this position (b) the patient's foot is slowly and in stages moved downwards so that leg extends gradually. Dorsiflexion of the ankle and toes is maintained and tested at each stage, as well as testing for extensor thrust of the leg.			

Continued

Continued from previous page

	Abnormal resistance?	Abnormal assistance?	Uncontrolled full weight?

Grade 2

d. From the fully flexed position (a) the patient's leg is moved across the sound leg, and foot placed on the support on the opposite side. (Resistance to adduction of the leg and to rotation forward of the pelvis is tested.)

e. The patient lies near the edge of the plinth, the affected leg over the edge. Keeping hip extended the therapist bends knee, the foot and toes in dorsiflexion and eversion. (Resistance to flexion and to extensor thrust when extending the knee are tested.)

Prone Tests for the Leg and Hip

	Abnormal resistance?	Abnormal assistance?	Uncontrolled full weight?

Grade 1

a. The patient supports him- or herself on both forearms. The affected leg is externally rotated, foot dorsiflexed and everted and then bent at the knee to a right angle without hip being flexed. (Resistance to the movement is tested and whether there is extensor thrust when it is gradually extended.)

b. The patient's legs are extended with external rotation, feet dorsiflexed and everted so that heels touch each other. (Resistance is tested and whether the position can be kept.)

Grade 2

c. Test (b) is followed by the patient's knees being bent, heels kept together and feet dorsiflexed and everted. (Resistance to this movement is tested as above (a) and whether there is extensor thrust when the affected leg is extended.)

Sitting Tests for the Legs
(The patient is sitting on a chair, feet on the ground)

	Abnormal resistance?	Abnormal assistance?	Uncontrolled full weight?

Grade 2

a. Toes and ankles are dorsiflexed and foot placed backwards behind the sound one, knee being bent and heel kept on the ground. (Resistance to flexion of knee, ankle and to dorsiflexion of toes is being tested and whether there is downward pressure of the foot.)

b. The patient's leg is lifted, foot in dorsiflexion, and heel is placed on the edge of the chair, and from there it is placed on the knee of the sound leg. (Resistance to flexion is tested and whether patient can keep foot on the chair or on the sound knee.) The leg is then slowly lowered again until the foot reaches the ground. (Undue assistance to extension is tested when the leg is moved downwards.)

Continued

—— *Continued from previous page* ——

Grade 2 (continued)

c. The patient sits with knees adducted in midline. The therapist moves both knees as far as possible to either side, and feet remain in the original position. (Resistance to adduction of the affected leg and to rotation of the pelvis forward is tested when moving knees toward the sound side.)

Abnormal resistance?	Abnormal assistance?	Uncontrolled full weight?

Standing Tests for the Legs
Grade 2

a. The patient's affected leg is lifted, flexed at all joints and then slowly lowered into a step forward, toes and ankle held dorsiflexed and foot everted. (Resistance to flexion is tested and whether there is downward pressure of the leg and foot on lowering foot to the ground.)

b. The patient stands in step position, the affected leg behind. Knee is then bent, the foot supported in dorsiflexion and eversion, the hip to remain extended. (Resistance to flexion of knee and extension of hip is tested.)

c. The foot is then slowly lowered again to the initial position behind the sound leg, foot everted and dorsiflexed and the heel placed to the ground. (Undue assistance to lowering the foot with stiffening of the knee is tested.)

Abnormal resistance?	Abnormal assistance?	Uncontrolled full weight?

Figure 12–5. *(Reprinted with permission from Bobath B. Adult Hemiplegia: Evaluational Treatment. London: William Heineman Medical Books, 1970;18–71.)*

The extensor synergy of the upper limb shows

1. Extension of the elbow, complete range.
2. Full range of pronation–supination.
3. Abduction of the forearm in front of the body.
4. Internal rotation of the arm.
5. Fixation of the shoulder girdle in a somewhat protracted position.

The flexor synergy for the lower limb is

1. Dorsiflexion of the toe.
2. Dorsiflexion and inversion of the ankle.
3. Flexion of the knee to 90°.
4. Flexion of the hip.
5. Abduction and external rotation of the hip.

Finally, extensor synergy of the lower limb is

1. Plantarflexion of the toes (inconsistent).
2. Plantarflexion and inversion of the ankle.
3. Extension of the knee.
4. Extension of the hip.
5. Abduction and internal rotation of the hip.

Brunnstrom[37] suggests looking for the various synergies and patterns in patients who have sustained a stroke.

TESTS FOR VOLUNTARY MOVEMENTS ON REQUEST
Patterns to be tested
Tests for Arm and Shouldergirdle
To be tested separately in supine, sitting, and standing, so each will be different.

	Supine		Sitting		Standing	
	Yes	No	Yes	No	Yes	No

Grade 1

a. Can patient hold extended arm in elevation after having it placed there?
  With internal rotation?
  With external rotation?
b. Can patient lower the extended arm from the position of elevation to the horizontal plane and back again to elevation?
  Forward-downwards?
  Sideways-downwards?
  With internal rotation?
  With external rotation?
c. Can patient move the extended abducted arm from the horizontal plane to the side of body and back again to the horizontal plane?
  With internal rotation?
  With external rotation?

Grade 2

a. Can the patient lift arm to touch the opposite shoulder?
  With palm of hand?
  With back of hand?
b. Can patient bend elbow with upper arm in elevation to touch the top of head?
  With pronation?
  With supination?
c. Can patient fold hands behind head with both elbows in horizontal abduction?
  With wrist flexed?
  With wrist extended?

Grade 3

a. Can patient supinate forearm and wrist?
  Without side-flexion of trunk on the affected side?
  With flexed elbow and flexed fingers?
  With extended elbow and flexed fingers?
b. Can patient pronate forearm without adduction of arm at shoulder?
c. Can patient externally rotate the extended arm?
  (i) in a horizontal abduction?
  (ii) by the side of his body?
  (iii) in elevation?
d. Can patient bend and extend elbow in supination to touch the shoulder of the same? starting with:
  (i) arm by side of body?
  (ii) horizontal abduction of the arm?

Continued

Continued from previous page

Tests for Wrist and Fingers

Grade 1

	Yes?	No?
a. Can patient place the flat hand forward down on table in front?		
Can patient do this sideways when sitting on plinth?		
With fingers and thumb adducted?		
With fingers and thumb abducted?		

Grade 2

a. Can patient open hand to grasp?		
With flexed wrist?		
With extended wrist?		
With pronation?		
With supination?		
With adducted fingers and thumb?		
With abducted fingers and thumb?		

Grade 3

a. Can patient grasp and open fingers again?		
With flexed elbow?		
With extended elbow?		
With pronation?		
With supination		
b. Can patient move individual fingers?		
Thumb?		
Index finger?		
Little finger?		
Second and third finger?		
c. Can patient oppose fingers and thumb?		
Thumb and index finger?		
Thumb and second finger?		
Thumb and little finger		

Tests for Pelvis, Leg, and Foot: Prone Tests

Grade 1

	Yes?	No?
Can patient bend knee without bending hip?		
With foot in dorsiflexion?		
With foot in plantiflexion?		
Foot inverted?		
Foot everted?		

Grade 2

Can patient lie with both legs eternally rotated and extended, feet dorsiflexed and everted, heels touching?		
Hold position when placed?		
Turn affected leg out again to touch heel of sound leg after it has been internally rotated by therapist?		
Perform internal and external rotation unaided?		

Grade 3

a. Can patient keep heels together and touching while bending both knees to right angle?		
Affected foot inverted?		
Affected foot everted?		
b. Can patient hold knee of affected leg flexed at right angle and alternately dorsiflex and plantiflex ankle?		
Foot inverted?		
Foot everted?		
Without moving knee?		

Continued

Continued from previous page

Tests for Pelvis, Leg, and Foot: Supine

Grade 1

	Yes?	No?
a. Can patient bend affected leg?		
With sound leg flexed, foot off support?		
With sound leg extended?		
Without bending affected arm?		
b. Can patient bend hip and knee with foot remaining on the support from the beginning of extension until the foot is near pelvis?		
Can patient extend leg by degrees, with foot remaining on the support?		

Grade 2

	Yes?	No?
Can patient lift pelvis without extending affected leg, both feet on the support?		
Can patient keep pelvis up and lift sound leg?		
Without dropping pelvis on the affected side?		
Can patient keep pelvis up and adduct and abduct knees?		

Grade 3

	Yes?	No?
a. Can patient dorsiflex ankle?		
Dorsiflex toes?		
With flexed leg, foot on the support?		
With extended leg?		
With foot inverted?		
With foot everted?		
b. Can patient bend knee while lying near the edge of plinth, the leg over side of plinth?		

Sitting Tests on Chair

Grade 1

	Yes?	No?
a. Can patient adduct and abduct affected leg, foot on ground?		
b. Can patient adduct and abduct affected leg, foot placed on seat of chair?		

Grade 2

	Yes?	No?
a. Can patient lift affected leg and place foot on sound knee? (without use of hand to lift leg.)		
b. Can patient draw affected foot back under chair, heel on the floor?		
c. Can patient stand up with sound foot in front of affected one? (without use of hand?)		

Standing Tests

Grade 1

	Yes?	No?
Can patient stand with parallel feet, both feet touching?		

Grade 2

	Yes?	No?
a. Can patient stand on affected leg, lifting sound one?		
b. Can patient stand on affected leg, sound one lifted and bend and extend standing leg?		
c. Can patient stand in step position, weight forward on affected leg, sound leg behind on toes?		
d. Can patient stand in step position, sound leg forward with weight on it, affected leg behind and bend knee of affected leg without taking toes off ground?		

Grade 3

	Yes?	No?
a. Can patient stand in step postion, weight forward on sound leg, affected leg behind and lift foot without bending hip of affected leg?		
Foot in inversion?		
Foot in eversion?		

Continued

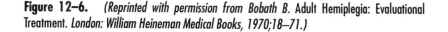

───── *Continued from previous page* ─────

Tests for Pelvis, Leg, and Foot: Supine (continued)
Standing Tests (continued)
Grade 3 (continued)

	Yes?	No?

b. Can patient stand on affected leg and transfer weight over it to make step with sound leg?
  Forward?
  Backward?		

c. Can patient stand on sound leg and make step forward with affected leg without hitching pelvis up?		
d. Can patient stand on sound leg and make step backward with affected leg without hitching pelvis up?		
e. Can patient stand on affected leg and lift toes?		

Figure 12–6. *(Reprinted with permission from Bobath B.* Adult Hemiplegia: Evaluational Treatment. *London: William Heineman Medical Books, 1970;18–71.)*

Figure 12–8 is the form used by Brunnstrom[37] for classification and recording of motion. The various synergies are noted as numbers in the chart. The synergy levels for flaccidity progressing to normal tone would be noted as:

1. No movement initiated or elicited.
2. Synergies or components first appearing.
3. Synergies or components initiated voluntarily.
4. Movements deviating from basic synergies.
5. Relative independence.
6. Coordinated movements.

The remainder of the forms are self-explanatory and can be found in Brunnstrom's *Movement Therapy in Hemiplegia.*[37]

Carr and Shepherd Evaluation

Carr and Shepherd,[38] physical therapists from Australia, have a different way of analyzing patients who have sustained strokes. These therapists have developed an entire strategy of motor relearning. The basic principle of their strategy is to eliminate unnecessary movements and to better organize the movement patterns. It is important to understand this principle when looking at their evaluation strategies. In evaluating upper limb function, for instance, instead of grading the function in terms of synergies or range of motion deficits, this approach outlines common problems and compensatory strategies. For example, in the arm, common problems are (1) poor scapular movement and persistent depression of the shoulder girdle; (2) poor muscular control of the glenohumeral joint caused by a lack of abduction, flexion, and inability to sustain position; and (3) excessive and unnecessary elbow flexion, internal rotation, shoulder, and forearm supination.

In looking at the hand, this approach would consider the following dysfunctional movement patterns:

1. Difficulty in grasping.
2. Difficulty in extending and flexing metacarpal phalangeal joints.
3. Difficulty with abduction and rotation of the thumb.
4. Difficulty cupping the hand.
5. Inability to hold different objects while moving the arm.
6. Tendency to pronate the forearm.
7. Excessive extension of the fingers and thumbs.
8. Inability to release objects.
9. Difficulty with abduction and rotation with the thumb in order to grasp.

TESTS FOR BALANCE AND OTHER AUTOMATIC PROTECTIVE REACTIONS

(N.B.) In order to test these reactions the patient must be able to assume and hold the test position. The patient should react with specific movements in order to regain balance or protect self against falling when being moved or pushed unexpectedly.

Balance Reactions   Yes?   No?

1. *Patient in prone lying, supporting body on forearms. State reaction.*
   a. Patient's shouldergirdle is pushed toward affected side. Does patient remain supported on affected forearm?   ☐   ☐
   b. Sound arm is lifted forward and up, as when reaching out with one hand. Does patient immediately transfer weight toward the affected arm?   ☐   ☐
   c. Sound arm is lifted and moved backward and patient is turned to side, support on affected arm. Does patient remain supported on affected arm?   ☐   ☐

These three tests can be done in slight cases with patient supporting self on extended arm instead of on forearm.

2. *Patient sitting on the plinth, feet unsupported. State reaction.*   Yes?   No?
   a. If patient is pushed toward the affected side, does he or she stay upright?   ☐   ☐
      Does patient laterally flex head toward the sound side?   ☐   ☐
      Abduct sound leg?   ☐   ☐
      Use the affected forearm for support?   ☐   ☐
      Use the affected hand for support?   ☐   ☐
   b. If patient is pushed forward, does he or she bend affected hip and knee?   ☐   ☐
      Extend spine?   ☐   ☐
      Lift head?   ☐   ☐
   c. Both legs are lifted up by the therapist, knees flexed. Does patient stay upright?   ☐   ☐
      Move affected arm forward?   ☐   ☐
      Support body backward with affected arm?   ☐   ☐
3. *Patient in four-foot kneeling. State reaction.*
   a. Body is pushed toward the affected side
      Does patient abduct the sound leg?   ☐   ☐
      Remain on all fours?   ☐   ☐
   b. Patient's sound arm is lifted and held up by the therapist
      Does patient keep affected arm extended?   ☐   ☐
   c. Sound leg is lifted.
      Does patient keep affected leg flexed and transfer weight on to it?   ☐   ☐
   d. Sound arm and affected leg are lifted
      Does patient keep affected arm extended?   ☐   ☐
   e. Affected arm and sound leg are lifted
      Does patient remain on affected flexed leg?   ☐   ☐
   f. Sound arm and leg are lifted
      Does patient transfer weight toward the affected side and maintain position?   ☐   ☐
4. *Patient in kneel-standing. State reaction.*
   a. Patient is pushed toward the affected side
      Does patient abduct the sound leg?   ☐   ☐
      Bend head laterally toward the sound side?   ☐   ☐
      Use affected hand for support?   ☐   ☐
   b. Patient is pushed toward the sound side
      Does patient abduct the affected leg?   ☐   ☐
      Extend the affected arm sideways?   ☐   ☐

Continued

Continued from previous page

	Yes?	No?

c. Patient is pushed backward and asked not to sit down
Does patient extend the affected arm forward? ☐ ☐

d. Patient is pushed gently forward, sound arm held backward by therapist
Does patient use affected arm and hand for support on the ground? ☐ ☐
Lift affected foot off the ground? ☐ ☐

5. *Patient half-kneeling, sound foot forward. (Patient should not use sound hand for support.) State reaction.*

a. Sound foot is lifted up by the therapist
Does patient remain upright? ☐ ☐
Keep affected hip extended? ☐ ☐

b. Sound foot is lifted by the therapist and placed sideways
Does patient remain upright? ☐ ☐
Show balance movements with affected arm? ☐ ☐

c. Sound foot is placed from the above position back to kneel-standing
Does patient keep upright? ☐ ☐
Keep affected hip extended? ☐ ☐

6. *Patient standing, feet parallel, standing base narrow. State reaction.*

a. Patient is tipped backward and not allowed to make step backward with sound leg. (Therapist puts foot on patients sound one to prevent step.)
Does patient step backward with affected leg? ☐ ☐

b. Patient is tipped backward and not allowed to make steps with either leg.
Does patient dorsiflex toes of affected leg? ☐ ☐
Big toe only? ☐ ☐
Dorsiflex ankle and toes of affected leg? ☐ ☐
Move affected arm forward? ☐ ☐

c. Patient is tipped toward sound side.
Does patient abduct affected leg? ☐ ☐
Abduct and extend affected arm? ☐ ☐
Make steps to follow with affected leg across sound leg? ☐ ☐

d. Patient is tipped toward the affected side
Does patient abduct the sound leg? ☐ ☐
Bend head laterally toward the sound side? ☐ ☐

7. *Patient standing on affected leg only. (Patient is not allowed to use sound hand for support.) State reactions.*

a. Sound foot is lifted by the therapist and moved forward as in making a step, extending knee.
Does patient keep the heel of affected leg on the ground? ☐ ☐
Keep the knee of the affected leg extended? ☐ ☐
Assist weight transfer forward over affected leg with extended hip? ☐ ☐

b. Sound foot is lifted by the therapist and moved backward as in making a step backward
Does patient keep the hip of affected leg extended? ☐ ☐
Assist weight transfer backward over affected leg? ☐ ☐

c. Sound foot is lifted by the therapist and held up while patient is pushed gently sideways toward the affected side.
Does patient follow and adjust balance, moving the foot of the affected leg sideways by inverting and everting foot alternately? ☐ ☐
The same maneuver is done pulling with patient toward the affected side.
Does patient follow and adjust balance by moving foot as above? ☐ ☐

Continued

Continued from previous page

	Yes?	No?
Tests for Protective Extension and Support of the Arm		

1. When testing these reactions the patient's sound arm should be held by hand, so that patient cannot use it. It is advisable to hold the sound arm in extension and external rotation because this facilitates the extension of the affected arm and hand. State reaction.
a. The patient stands in front of a table or plinth. Sound arm is held backward and patient is pushed forward toward the table.

	Yes?	No?
Does patient extend affected arm forward?	☐	☐
Support self on fist?	☐	☐
On the palm of hand?	☐	☐
Thumb adducted?	☐	☐
Thumb abducted?	☐	☐

b. The patient stands facing a wall, at a distance that allows patient to reach it with hand. Patient is pushed forward against the wall, sound arm held backward.

	Yes?	No?
Does patient lift affected arm and stretch it out against the wall?	☐	☐
Place hand against the wall, fingers flexed, thumb adducted?	☐	☐
Fingers open, thumb abducted?	☐	☐

2. *State reaction.*
c. The patient is sitting on the plinth, with sound arm held sideways by the therapist. Patient is pushed toward the affected side.

	Yes?	No?
Does patient abduct the affected arm and support self on forearm?	☐	☐
On extended arm?	☐	☐
Support self on fist?	☐	☐
On open palm?	☐	☐
Thumb and fingers adducted?	☐	☐
Thumb and fingers abducted?	☐	☐

d. The patient stands sideways to a wall, at a distance that allows patient to reach it with affected hand.

	Yes?	No?
Does patient abduct and lift the affected arm?	☐	☐
With flexed elbow?	☐	☐
Reach out for the wall with extended elbow?	☐	☐
Support self with fist against the wall?	☐	☐
With open hand?	☐	☐
With adducted thumb and fingers?	☐	☐
With abducted thumb and fingers?	☐	☐

3. *State reaction.*
e. The patient lies on the floor on back with sound hand placed under hip so that patient cannot use it. The therapist takes a pillow and pretends to throw it toward patient's head.

	Yes?	No?
Does patient move affected arm to protect face?	☐	☐
With flexed elbow?	☐	☐
With extended elbow?	☐	☐
With internal rotation?	☐	☐
With external rotation?	☐	☐
With fisted hand?	☐	☐
With open hand?	☐	☐
Can patient catch the pillow?	☐	☐

Figure 12–7. *(Reprinted with permission from Bobath B: Adult Hemiplegia: Evaluational Treatment. London: William Heineman Medical Books; 1970;18–71)*

HEMIPLEGIA—CLASSIFICATION AND PROGRESS RECORD (p. 1)
Upper Limb—Test Sitting

Name _____ Age _____ Date of onset _____ Side affected _____

Date

_____ Passive motion sense, shoulder _____ elbow _____

_____ pron.-supin. _____ wrist flex.-ext. _____

_____ 1. NO MOVEMENT INITIATED OR ELICITED _____

_____ 2. SYNERGIES OR COMPONENTS FIRST APPEARING. Spasticity developing _____

_____   Flexor synergy _____

_____   Extensor synergy _____

_____ 3. SYNERGIES OR COMPONENTS INITIATED VOLUNTARILY. Spasticity marked _____

FLEXOR SYNERGY   Active Joint Range   Remarks

_____	Shoulder girdle	Elevation _____	_____	_____	_____
_____		Retraction _____	_____	_____	_____
		Hyperextension			
_____	Shoulder joint	Abduction _____	_____	_____	_____
		Ext. rotation _____	_____	_____	_____
_____	Elbow	Flexion _____	_____	_____	_____
_____	Forearm	Supination _____	_____	_____	_____

EXTENSOR SYNERGY

_____	Shoulder	Pectoralis major	_____	_____	_____
_____	Elbow	Extension	_____	_____	_____
_____	Forearm	Pronation	_____	_____	_____
_____	4. MOVEMENTS DEVIATING FROM BASIC SYNERGIES Spasticity decreasing	Hand to sacral region	_____	_____	_____
_____		Raise arm forw.-horiz.	_____	_____	_____
_____		Pron.-supin. elbow at 90°	_____	_____	_____
_____	5. RELATIVE IN-DEPENDENCE OF BASIC SYNERGIES Spasticity waning	Raise arm side-horiz.	_____	_____	_____
		Raise arm over head	_____	_____	_____
_____		Pron.-supin. elbow extended	_____	_____	_____

6. MOVEMENT COORDINATION NEAR
   NORMAL. Spasticity minimal

———— *Continued* ————

Continued from previous page

Name _____
Date

_____ SPEED TESTS for classes 4, 5, 6   Strokes per 5 sec.

Hand from Normal	
lap to chin Affected	
Hand from lap Normal	
to opposite knee Affected	

_____ Passive motion sense, digits _____
_____ Fingertip recognition _____
_____ Wrist stabilization   1. Elbow extended _____
          for grasp   2. Elbow flexed _____
_____ Wrist flexion   1. Elbow extended _____
          and extension
_____ Fist closed   2. Elbow flexed _____
_____ Wrist circumduction _____

DIGITS

_____ Mass grasp _____ Dynamometer test   Normal _____ lb.
                                                                     Affected _____ lb.
_____ Mass extension _____
_____ Hook grasp (handbag, 2 lb.) _____
_____ Lateral prehension (card) _____
_____ Palmar prehension (pencil) _____
_____ Cylindrical grasp (small jar) _____
_____ Spherical grasp (ball) _____ catch _____ throw _____
_____ Indiv. thumb movements   1. Vertical movements _____
          hands in lap Ulnar side down   2. Horizontal movements _____
_____ Individual finger movements _____
_____ Button and unbutton shirt   Using both hands _____
                                   Using affected hand only _____
_____ Other skilled activities _____

Figure 12–8. *(Reprinted with permission from Brunnstrom S. Movement Therapy in Hemiplegia. New York: Harper & Row; 1970;8–12;38–41.)*

During assessment the therapist would look at these deficits, identify them, and treat them.

Carr and Shepherd's method[38] of assessing lower extremity and trunk deficits would be to describe them in terms of functional tasks, such as walking, balance, standing, standing from sitting, and sitting over the edge of the bed. In the analysis of sitting over the side of the bed, Carr and Shepherd identified two common problems: (1) Flexion of the hip and knee on the affected side; and (2) flexion of the shoulder and protraction of the shoulder girdle, which results in the patient's inability to use the appropriate body mechanics to get out of bed.

This analysis can then be easily transferred into the appropriate treatment strategies for working with these patients. More specific evaluative and treatment information is available in Carr and Shepherd's *A Motor Re-Learning Programme for*

Stroke.[38] In a subsequent section of this chapter, a specific form developed by Carr and Shepherd will be examined that goes over some of these points.[38]

In evaluating strength deficits, several studies have made a comparison between extension and torque in the knees, as well as various other joints of the body, and it can be a reliable and valid measure in stroke patients. Therefore, therapists can use manual muscle tests of dynamometry readings to assess strength in their elderly patients with a stroke.[39–41]

Olney and Colbourne's Gait Assessment

Another consideration that is extremely important in the area of stroke is the analysis of gait. One excellent article on this subject is "Assessment and Treatment of Gait Dysfunction in a Geriatric Stroke Patient" by Olney and Colbourne.[42] In this article, Olney and Colbourne describe some of the deficits in gait and discuss methods of treating the gait problem. They also divide the gait pattern into phases. The first phase, "late swing to foot flat," identifies three problems for stroke patients: (1) inability to attain full hip flexion during swing, (2) inability to extend the knee fully, and (3) inability to activate ankle dorsiflexor muscles. In addition, stroke patients may hyperextend the knee to avoid the problem of instability.

The next phase of gait that presents problems is "foot flat to heel off." Problems noted here are the decreased use of hip extensor muscles, limited hip extension motion, and that ankle plantar flexors contract inappropriately.

The next phase, "push off, pull off in early swing," causes residual weakness of ankle plantar flexors and hip flexors. It also results in the stance phase of the affected side being longer than normal, and the body's weight being transferred to the lower limb through push off.[42]

Rancho Los Amigos Gait Evaluation

Another interesting analysis of hemiplegic gait comes from Rancho Los Amigos. This method is called the Upright Control Evaluation.[43] Its purpose is to assess the patient's static ability to flex and then accept weight on the involved lower extremity. It is an intricate method of testing upright control and the criteria for this are given in specific detail in Table 12–8.[43]

Motor Assessment Scale

Specific compacted tests for the assessment of stroke patients are somewhat difficult to find, but they do exist. Carr and Shepherd have developed the Motor Assessment Scale in Figure 12–9A. All items on the form are constructed so that a score of six indicates optimal motor behavior. The criteria for scoring is listed in Figure 12–9B. These particular criteria are self-explanatory and give the examiner a six-point scale from which to assess the patient and show improvement in a very simple form.[44]

When evaluating a stroke patient, it is important to choose the tools that will appropriately reflect the patient's status and the methods to be used in the evaluation treatment progression. Several different types of tools have been provided and will be considered next.

Treatment Interventions

There are a number of treatment techniques commonly used by physical therapists ranging from the classic therapeutic exercise to the proprioceptive neuromuscular facilitation (PNF) to the Bobath and Brunnstrom techniques. A brief discussion of Bobath's, Brunnstrom's, and Carr and Shepherd's work will follow in the next section. Treatment considerations for gait will also be discussed, as will research on various types of ancillary modalities that can be used for the treatment of stroke deficits.

TABLE 12–8. UPRIGHT CONTROL (UC)

Criteria for UC Evaluation (Flexion and Extension)
1. Patient requires no more than one person to assist double or single limb stance.
2. Patient can understand instructions adequately to perform test

FLEXION

Number of Examiners

Two examiners required for testing; assisting examiner provides hand support, testing examiner demonstrates test to patient and determines grade.

Position for Test

Standing with use of assisting examiner's hand for support (balance only). Support should be sufficient for patient to maintain standing balance.

Technique for Administering Flexion Test for Each Segment
1. One demonstration by examiner.
2. One practice trial by patient (or two trials if needed to help patient understand test).
3. One test trial to determine grade.
4. If patient has bilateral lower extremity involvement, provide opposite lower extremity stabilization (manually, with AFO, KAFO) as needed to provide standing stability.

Pretest for Hip Flexion Test

Prior to the test for each segment:
1. Position the patient's limb that is to be tested in neutral or maximum available hip and knee extension.
2. The assisting examiner provides hand support in line with the greater trochanter of the femur on the side opposite the leg being tested.

Range of Motion

Measure and record the freely available range; do not stretch part through spasticity or soft tissue restriction. For the lower extremities, use standard range of motion evaluation and recording procedure (including beginning and ending range of motion), except evaluate dorsiflexion range with the knee extended using only two-finger pressure. For the trunk and upper extremities record WNL if range is within normal limits, record IF if limited range interferes with function.

Tone

Determine if muscle tone is normal or abnormal for the neck, trunk, and extremities by moving the part through a fast range of motion. Prior to evaluating muscle tone determine the available slow range of motion. If pain is present with passive movement of the part, defer fast motion assessment and note in comment section.

If spasticity (an exaggerated response to stretch) is present, evaluate its effect on the patient's overall function and record the grade based on the following key:

Slight (SL): Present but has no influence on patient's function.

Severe (SEV): Present to the degree that it interferes with or prevents function.

PROPRIOCEPTION

Evaluate proprioception of the upper extremity with the patient sitting; evaluate the lower extremity with the patient supine. Demonstrate the procedure to the patient before testing. Use either of the following methods.
1. Ask patient to close eyes or occlude vision. Move the part to any normal, pain-free position without putting the muscles on stretch, and ask patient to copy the position with uninvolved extremity.
2. Occlude patient's vision and move part. Ask patient to indicate if part is up, down, in, or out.

Use the following grading key:

Normal (N): Intact proprioception; characterized by rapid, correct response

Impaired (I): Responses are slow but correct the majority of the time.

Absent (0): Unable to duplicate or identify position of body part.

Instructions to Patient for Hip Flexion Test
1. "Stand as straight as you can."
2. "Bring your knee up toward your chest three times as high and as fast as you can."

Grading Hip Flexion

When observed range is borderline between Weak and Moderate, or Moderate and Strong give the lesser grade. If patient is unable to complete the three flexion efforts within 10 seconds, give Weak grade.

Weak (W): No motion or actively flexes less than 30°.

Moderate (M): Actively accomplishes an arc of hip flexion between 30° and 60°.

Strong (S): Actively accomplishes an arc of hip flexion more than 60°.

Base grade on true hip motion and not on substitutions, such as backward trunk lean or pelvic tilt.

Instructions to Patient for Knee Flexion Test
1. "Stand as straight as you can."
2. "Bring your knee up toward your chest three times as high and as fast as you can."

(continued)

TABLE 12–8. UPRIGHT CONTROL (UC) (CONT.)

Grading Knee Flexion

When observed range is borderline between Weak and Moderate, or Moderate and Strong give lesser grade. If the patient is unable to complete the three flexion efforts within 10 seconds, give the Weak grade.

Weak (W): No motion or knee-flexes less than 30°.

Moderate (M): Knee flexes between 30° and 60°.

Strong (S): Knee flexes more than 60°.

Instructions to Patient for Ankle Flexion Test

1. "Stand as straight as you can."
2. "Bring your knee and your foot up toward your chest three times as high and as fast as you can."

Grading Ankle Flexion

When observed range is borderline between Weak and Strong give the lesser grade. If the patient is unable to complete the three flexion efforts within 10 seconds, give Weak grade.

Weak (W): No motion or actively dorsiflexes to less than a right angle at the ankle joint.

Strong (S): Actively dorsiflexes to a right angle or greater at the ankle joint.

EXTENSION

Number of Examiners

Two examiners required for testing; testing examiner determines grade, assisting examiner assists in stabilizing or providing hand support as indicated under "Pretest Position and Stabilization."

Position for Test

Standing with the use of the examiner's hand for support (balance support adequate to maintain single limb stance).

Technique for Administering Test for Each Segment

1. One demonstration by examiner.
2. One practice trial by patient (or two trials if needed to help patient understand test).
3. One test trial to determine grade.
4. If patient has bilateral lower extremity involvement, assist opposite lower extremity flexion as needed to determine extension control of the stance limb.

Pretest Positioning and Stabilization for Hip Extension Test

1. Testing examiner positioned beside patient to provide hand support and to assure that patient begins from a position of neutral or maximum hip extension range.
2. Assisting examiner provides manual stabilization as demonstrated in diagram to maintain neutral knee extension and a stable ankle.
3. If there is a fixed equinus contracture greater than neutral, accommodate for the contracture by placing a 30° wedge under the patient's heel.
4. If unable to maintain a stable plantigrade platform for single limb stance either manually or with an AFO, record UT (Unable to test) for hip and knee extension. See "Grading Ankle Extension" for testinng and recording an appropriate ankle grade.

Instructions to Patient for Hip Extension Test

1. "Stand on both legs as straight as you can."
2. "Now stand as straight as you can on just your (R) (weaker) leg."—"Lift *this* leg up."—"Keep standing as straight as you can."

Grading Hip Extension

When patient is balanced on weaker leg, testing examiner gradually decreases amount of hand support to determine hip control.

Weak (W): Uncontrolled trunk flexion on hip (testing examiner must prevent continued forward motion of the trunk by providing additional hand support).

Moderate (M): Unable to maintain trunk completely erect or at end of available hip extension range but patient stops own forward trunk motion *or* trunk wobbles back and forth *or* patient hyperextends trunk on hip.

Strong (S): Maintains trunk erect on hip or at end of available hip extension range.

Pretest Positioning and Stabilization for Knee Extension Test

1. Assisting examiner positioned behind patient. Assisting examiner provides hand support and maintains trunk erect on hip.
2. Testing examiner positions patient's knees in 30° of flexion bilaterally.
3. If unable to maintain feet flat with approximately 30° knee flexion, use a 30° wedge.

Instructions to Patient for Knee Extension Test

1. "Stand on both feet with your knees bent" (approximately 20° to 30°; use a wedge to accommodate for limited ankle dorsiflexion range if necessary).
2. "Keep your knees bent and lift your (L) (R) (stronger) leg."

Demonstrate and give instruction number 3 only if patient can support body weight on a flexed knee during single limb support without further collapse into flexion.

3. "Now, straighten your knee as much as you can."

(continued)

TABLE 12–8. UPRIGHT CONTROL (UC) (CONT.)

Grading Knee Extension Control

If knee flexion contracture present, grade cannot exceed "moderate."

Weak (W): Unable to maintain body weight on a flexed knee (knee continues to collapse into flexion or heel rises).

Moderate (M): Supports body weight on a flexed knee without further collapse into flexion or without heel rise.

Strong (S): Supports body weight on a flexed knee and, on request, straightens knee to end of available knee extension range (hyperextension allowed).

Excessive (E): Unable to position knee in flexion secondary to severe extensor thrust or extensor tone.

Pretest Positioning and Stabilization for Ankle Extension Test

If patient has knee flexion contracture, record UT (unable to test) for ankle extension control.

1. Assisting examiner positioned behind patient to maintain trunk erect on hip.
2. Testing examiner positioned to prevent knee hyperextension (i.e., plantar flexion of ankle).
3. Assess passive ankle range with knee extended and accommodate for neutral or less than neutral ankle range with a 30° wedge.

Instructions to Patient for Ankle Extension Test

1. "Stand on both legs as straight as you can."
2. "Lift and hold up your (L) (R) (stronger) leg."

Demonstrate and give instructions for number **3 only** if patient can control the knee at neutral.

3. "Keep your knee straight and go up on your toes as high as you can."

Grading Ankle Extension

Weak (W): Unable to maintain knee at neutral (knee collapses into flexion or wobbles back and forth between flexion and extension or hyperextension/extensor thrust cannot be controlled by examiner).

Moderate (M): Maintains knee at neutral.

Strong (S): Maintains knee at neutral and lifts heel off floor on command (any degree of heel lift while maintaining neutral knee).

Excessive (E): Equinus or varus so severe patient is unable to maintain stable plantigrade platform.

Reprinted with permission from Parker K, Zablotny C, Jordan C. Analysis and management of hemiplegic gait dysfunction. Stroke Rehabilitation State of the Art. Downey, Calif: 1984. Rancho Los Amigos Medical Center.

MOTOR ASSESSMENT SCALE

NAME _____

MOVEMENT SCORING SHEET

DATE _____	0	1	2	3	4	5	6
1. Supine to side lying							
2. Supine to sitting over side of bed							
3. Balanced sitting							
4. Sitting to standing							
5. Walking							
6. Upper-arm function							
7. Hand movements							
8. Advanced hand activities							
9. General tonus							

Figure 12–9A. *(Reprinted with permission from Carr J, Shepherd R, et al. Investigation of a new motor assessment scale for stroke patients . Phys Ther. February1985;65(2).)*

Criteria for Scoring Figure 12–9A.

I. Supine to Side Lying onto Intact Side

1. Pulls self into side lying. (Starting position must be supine lying, not knees flexed. Patient pulls self into side lying with intact arm, moves affected leg with intact leg.)
2. Moves leg across actively and the lower half of the body follows. (Starting position as above. Arm is left behind.)
3. Arm is lifted across body with other arm. Leg is moved actively and body follows in a block. (Starting position as above.)
4. Moves arm across body actively and the rest of the body follows in a block. (Starting position as above.)
5. Moves arm and leg and rolls to side but overbalances. (Starting position as above. Shoulder protracts and arm flexes forward.)
6. Rolls to side in 3 seconds. (Starting position as above. Must not use hands.)

II. Supine to Sitting over Side of Bed

1. Side lying, lifts head sideways but cannot sit up. (Patient assisted to side lying.)
2. Side lying to sitting over side of bed. (Therapist assists patient with movement. Patient controls head position throughout.)
3. Side lying to sitting over side of bed. (Therapist gives stand-by-help by assisting legs over side of bed.)
4. Side lying to sitting over side of bed. (With no stand-by help.)
5. Supine to sitting over side of bed. (With no stand-by help.)
6. Supine to sitting over side of bed within 10 seconds. (With no stand-by help.)

III. Balanced Sitting

1. Sits only with support. (Therapist should assist patient into sitting.)
2. Sits unsupported for 10 seconds. (Without holding on, knees and feet together, feet can be supported on floor.)
3. Sits unsupported with weight well forward and evenly distributed. (Weight should be well forward at the hips, head and thoracic spine extended, weight evenly distributed on both sides.)
4. Sits unsupported, turns head and trunk to look behind. (Feet supported and together on floor. Do not allow legs to abduct or feet to move. Have hands resting on thighs, do not allow hands to move onto plinth.)
5. Sits unsupported, reaches forward to touch floor, and returns to starting position. (Feet supported on floor. Do not allow patient to hold on. Do not allow legs and feet to move, support affected arm if necessary. Hand must touch floor at least 10 cm [4 in] in front of feet.)
6. Sits on stool unsupported, reaches sideways to touch floor, and returns to starting position. (Feet supported on floor. Do not allow patient to hold on. Do not allow legs and feet to move, support affected arm if necessary. Patient must reach sideways not forward.)

IV. Sitting to Standing

1. Gets to standing with help from therapist. (Any method.)
2. Gets to standing with stand-by help. (Weight unevenly distributed, uses hands for support.)
3. Gets to standing. (Do not allow uneven weight distribution or help from hands.)
4. Gets to standing and stands for 5 seconds with hips and knees extended. (Do not allow uneven weight distribution.)
5. Sitting to standing to sitting with no stand-by help. (Do not allow uneven weight distribution. Full extension of hips and knees.)
6. Sitting to standing to sitting with no stand-by help three times in 10 seconds. (Do not allow uneven weight distribution.)

V. Walking

1. Stands on affected leg and steps forward with other leg. (Weight-bearing hip must be extended. Therapist may give stand-by help.)
2. Walks with stand-by help from one person.
3. Walks 3 m (10 ft) alone or uses any aid but no stand-by help.
4. Walks 5 m (16 ft) with no aid in 15 seconds.
5. Walks 10 m (33 ft) with no aid, turns around, picks up a small sandbag from floor, and walks back in 25 seconds. (May use either hand.)
6. Walks up and down four steps with or without an aid but without holding on to the rail three times in 35 seconds.

Continued

Continued from previous page

VI. Upper-Arm Function
1. Lying, protract shoulder girdle with arm in elevation. (Therapist places arm in position and supports it with elbow in extension.)
2. Lying, hold extended arm in elevation for 2 seconds. (Physical therapist should place arm in position and patient must maintain position with some external rotation. Elbow must be held within 20° of full extension.)
3. Flexion and extension of elbow to take palm to forehead with arm as in step 2. (Therapist may assist supination of forearm.)
4. Sitting, hold extended arm in forward flexion at 90° to body for 2 seconds. (Therapist should place arm in position, and patient must maintain position with some external rotation and elbow extension. Do not allow excess shoulder elevation.)
5. Sitting, patient lifts arm to above position, holds it there for 10 seconds, and then lowers it. (Patient must maintain position with some external rotation. Do not allow pronation.)
6. Standing, hand against wall. Maintain arm position while turning body toward wall. (Have arm abducted to 90° with palm flat against the wall.)

VII. Hand Movements
1. Sitting, extension of wrist. (Therapist should have patient sitting at a table with forearm resting on the table. Therapist places cylindrical object in palm of patient's hand. Patient is asked to lift object off the table by extending the wrist. Do not allow elbow flexion.)
2. Sitting, radial deviation of wrist. (Therapist should place forearm in midpronation-supination, that is, resting on ulnar side, thumb in line with forearm and wrist in extension, fingers around a cylindrical object. Patient is asked to lift hand off table. Do not allow elbow flexion or pronation.)
3. Sitting, elbow into side, pronation and supination. (Elbow unsupported and at a right angle. Three-quarter range is acceptable.)
4. Reach forward, pick up large ball 14 cm (5 in.) in diameter with both hands and put it down. (Ball should be on table so far in front of patient that he or she has to extend arms fully to reach it. Shoulders must be protracted, elbows extended, wrist neutral or extended. Palms should be kept in contact with the ball.)
5. Pick up a polystyrene cup from table and put it on table across other side of body. (Do not allow alteration in shape of cup.)
6. Continuous opposition of thumb and each finger more than 14 times in 10 seconds. (Each finger in turn taps the thumb, starting with index finger. Do not allow thumb to slide from one finger to the other or to go backwards.)

VIII. Advanced Hand Activities
1. Picking up the top of a pen and putting it down again. (Patient stretches arm forward, picks up pen top, releases it on table close to body.)
2. Picking up one jellybean from a cup and placing it in another cup. (Teacup contains eight jellybeans. Both cups must be at arms' length. Left hand takes jellybean from cup on right and releases it in cup on left.)
3. Drawing horizontal lines to stop at a vertical line 10 times in 20 seconds. (At least five lines must touch and stop at the vertical line.)
4. Holding a pencil, making rapid consecutive dots on a sheet of paper. (Patient must do at least two dots a second for 5 seconds. Patient picks pencil up and positions it without assistance. Patient must hold pen as for writing. Patient must make a dot not a stroke.)
5. Taking a dessert spoon of liquid to the mouth. (Do not allow head to lower toward spoon. Do not allow liquid to spill.)
6. Holding a comb and combing hair at back of head.

IX. General Tonus
1. Flaccid, limp, no resistance when body parts are handled.
2. Some response felt as body parts are moved.
3. Variable, sometimes flaccid, sometimes good tone, sometimes hypertonic.
4. Consistently normal response.
5. Hypertonic 50% of the time.
6. Hypertonic at all times.

Figure 12–9B.

Bobath's Treatments

Bobath's principles for treating stroke patients with deficits revolve around the idea that their problem is not their lack of power; rather it is that they cannot perform normal movements. Therefore, strengthening techniques such as PNF, therapeutic exercise, and even Brunnstrom's techniques are in sharp contrast to her beliefs.[36] The aim of Bobath's approach is to change the abnormal movement patterns of the stroke patient into normal movement patterns. Bobath's theory revolves around reflex-inhibiting movement patterns as a means of facilitating more normal movement patterns. The patients in the program learn to know what normal movement feels like. Using this assessment tool, the therapist develops a treatment plan based on the following:

1. Whether the patient needs to increase or decrease body tone.
2. What type of movement patterns should be taught and which patterns should be facilitated and which inhibited.
3. What functional skills the patient needs to work on.

With this in mind, Bobath pursues various stages of recovery and designs a treatment program.

The first stage is the initial flaccid stage, during which the treatment must be coordinated with the nursing staff and with family members. The patient's sleeping and sitting positions must be designed to facilitate proper tone. For example, when the patient is supine, the extensor tone will be accentuated and, therefore, the patient must be positioned with some flexion in the lower extremity, possibly on the side or on the back, with pillows to accentuate that flexion.

An example of movement patterns would be having the patient lie on his or her side with knees bent and the involved extremity on top. The therapist provides active and passive movement to the shoulder girdle with the arm in extension and external rotation while extending and abducting the thumb. This can be followed by providing resistance and distraction to stimulate active movement in the upper extremity. The patient can also be encouraged to have the arm placed in a outward position by a family member while he or she is lying on the side in bed and holding on to the headboard while reaching overhead. Bobath does a lot of work with mobilizing the shoulder, and when the patient is able to sit, she also stresses the importance of weight bearing on the arm in a sitting position.

The next stage of recovery is spasticity. It is extremely important for the therapist to work on decreasing the spastic patterning and on facilitating the person's use of the arm in functional positions. The patient is encouraged to move the arm in the supine position. For example, with the elbow pointing toward the ceiling, the patient is encouraged to straighten the elbow and touch the head, or the patient is told to bring the arm across the body toward the mouth, which encourages a functional position. In the lower extremity, the patient may be asked to lie prone and bend the knee. Bobath also uses quite a bit of quadruped and biped training, which encourages weight transfer onto the affected side to encourage more normal tone and weight bearing.[36]

The final stage of relative recovery focuses on placing the patient in the proper positions and challenging proper movement. An example of a technique used in this stage is patterning to break up some of the associated reactions. For example, to facilitate ankle dorsiflexion–plantar flexion while walking, the therapist may push the patient unexpectedly backward to facilitate the ankle dorsiflexion reaction. Bobath's techniques are extremely practical and a detailed analysis of these are given in her book.[36]

Brunnstrom's Treatment

Brunnstrom's approach to the treatment of hemiplegic patients is first to facilitate the stages of the spasticity development and then to eventually facilitate the patient's ability to overcome the tone. For example, in the flaccid first stage, the therapist attempts to stimulate muscle activity and to elicit movement. Brunnstrom uses primitive reflexes to stimulate increased tone at this point. The therapist can get the asymmetrical tonic neck reflex by having the patient turn the head, which elicits associated movements in the upper extremity.

In the second stage, when the synergies first appear, the therapist should attempt to strengthen the synergies by working with the patient on associated reactions and on muscle strengthening programs using repetition.

The third stage of recovery is synergy, and isolated muscle components are initiated voluntarily. During this phase, the therapist is attempting to decrease the spastic pattern by using techniques that can break this pattern. The person then progresses to the next phase, and becomes relatively independent. In this phase, the therapist begins to work with normal strengthening patterns. The last phase involves the area of coordination and normal movement, and the therapist works with coordination exercises to facilitate normal movement.[37]

Carr and Shepherd's Approach

Other well-accepted physical therapy interventions are the Carr and Shepherd techniques. Their treatment revolves around five principles:

1. Elimination of unnecessary muscle activity.
2. Any human activity becomes better organized and more effective when it is practiced.
3. A muscle response depends on the condition of the muscle at the moment with the following perimeters: length, velocity, temperature, and joint ankle.
4. The body must have the ability to adjust to gravity and change segmental alignment for all motor activities. Therefore, the person must be trained to preserve balance.
5. A learned task is not just doing the task in front of a therapist. A learned task is when a person can do it in a situation without actually thinking.

In their treatment approach, Carr and Shepherd go through four steps: (1) analyze the task, (2) practice the missing component, (3) practice the task as a whole, and (4) transference of training.

An example of this would be a patient who has difficulty standing. First, analyze the difficulty (i.e., hip position). Second, practice the missing component. For instance, the difficulty in standing comes from the patient's hip position (i.e., work with the hip). Third, practice this task (i.e., standing with proper hip position). Fourth, transfer to another activity with the same problem (i.e., standing in the proper position with a slight bend on a stool or a wedge under the foot).

During treatment, motor tasks are practiced in their entirety. There is not a real technique. The person is just instructed and manually guided through various deficits. The person may first be passively placed in the proper position, and then the patient takes over active control. As the patient develops more control, the therapist does less.

The most important component of Carr and Shepherd's approach is the patient's contribution to the effort. Patients are encouraged to do the exercises as often as possible and to keep a notebook of their efforts and responses. In the notebook, the patient is encouraged to write down their actual program progression.[44]

Shoulder Problems in Hemiplegia

Shoulder pain in hemiplegia has always been a concern and several clinicians have suggested that excessive distraction on the shoulder may lead to pain.[27,36,44]

In an article by Kumar,[45] the use of overhead pulleys was found to cause the highest risk of developing shoulder pain for patients with hemiplegia, and it was suggested that this should be strongly discouraged with these types of patients.[45]

In training upper extremity problems, it is preferred to provide increased weight training through the upper extremity, as well as facilitating proper positioning.[36,44]

Bohannon and associates[46] found that it is not necessarily the position that explained the "synergistic" increased force of the elbow strength, but possibly the length of the muscle in various positions. Therefore, in working with the upper extremity, it is important not only to look at the neurological factors, such as tone, but also at the length tension relationship of the muscles. Therapists should facilitate range of motion and proper posture, as well as encourage weight bearing through the upper extremity in the proper position.

Gait Treatment Suggestions

The upright control evaluation mentioned earlier differentiated different gait variations. In addition, in the same study, the authors outlined a specific program for lower extremity problems.[43] Their treatment techniques revolve around the use of ankle-foot orthotics with various types of dorsiflexion stops, as well as electrical stimulation to the weak areas. For example, if a therapist notices stance deviation of inadequate hip and knee extension, he or she can suggest ankle-foot orthotics with dorsiflexion stops and electrical stimulation to the quadriceps or gluteus maximus for strengthening and facilitation. Inhibitive casting is used for excessive plantar flexion or with increased tone. Prolonged icing is suggested to inhibit tone. The treatment approach is to divide the various phases of gait and treat each separately according to deficit.

In the area of gait, it appears that weight shifting is one of the biggest problems. Patients must be taught the concept of proper weight shifting, and this can be done using bicycle ergonometry or EMG for proper muscle use.[46,47]

CONCLUSION

Despite the various techniques suggested for stroke intervention (ranging from therapeutic exercise to biofeedback), the therapist must be careful to check the efficacy of the various treatment programs.[48] For example, Sackley[49] showed that symmetry and weight shifting strongly correlated with motor function. These components appear to be very important and should be treated vigorously with weight shifting exercises. In contrast, Trueblood and co-workers[50] showed that pelvic positioning exercises were helpful while the patient did the exercise. However, after the exercise session, stroke patients did not carry the pelvic position into daily activities.[50]

Finally, Logigian and associates[51] showed that both facilitation and traditional exercise improved functional and motor performances and that there was no difference between the two exercises.[51] This study provides quite a bit of food for thought, especially for those working with a geriatric patient. Finding the most appropriate program, working within the patient's tolerance, and reviewing the results that accompany the treatment progression are extremely important for achieving the optimal outcomes.

PEARLS

- Parkinson's disease is the number one neurological disease in the elderly.

- The most common symptoms of Parkinson's disease are slowness with ADLs, shuffling, tremor, difficulty with speech, and erratic movements.

- When assessing and treating Parkinson patients, it is imperative to thoroughly assess and discriminate between direct, indirect, and composite impairments when designing treatment interventions.

- Parkinson patients may respond to a specific evaluation and treatment progression as outlined by Schenkman, the well-known Flewitt-Handford exercises, or group classes.

- Numerous methods exist for assessing older stroke patients. Schenkman, Bobath, Brunnstrom, Olney and Coulbourne, Rancho Los Amigos, and Carr and Shepherd have the greatest functional emphasis and applicability to geriatric rehabilitation.

- Treatment strategies for stroke range from Bobath to Brunnstrom to Carr and Shepherd, and, when modified for the aged, stress the most functional aspects of each.

- The hemiplegic shoulder can respond to modalities, proper sling use, and appropriate exercise.

- Exercise and rehabilitation can help the older patient to improve in function. To date, no specific technique has been statistically shown to have superior results, however.

REFERENCES

1. Schenkman M, Butler R. A model for multisystem evaluation, interpretation and treatment of individuals with neurologic dysfunction. *Phys Ther.* July 1989; 69(7):538–547.
2. Topp B. Towards a better understanding of Parkinson's disease. *Ger Nurs.* July/August 1987; 180–182.
3. Mutch W, Strudwick A, Sisare R, et al. Parkinson's disease: disability, review and management. *Br Med J.* September 3, 1986; 293:675–677.
4. Wilson J, Smith R. The prevalence and aeitology of long- term L dopa side effects in elderly Parkinson's patients. *Age Ageing.* 1989; 18:11–16.
5. Amenoff MJ. Parkinson's disease in the elderly: current management strategies. *Geriatrics.* July 1987; 42(7):31–37.
6. Hoehn M, Yahr M. Parkinsonism: onset, progression and mortality. *Neurology.* May 1967; 17(5):427–442.
7. Greer M. Recent developments in the treatment of Parkinson's disease. *Geriatrics.* February 1985; 40(2):34–41.
8. Banks M. Physiotherapy benefits patients with Parkinson's disease. *Clin Rehab.* 1989; 3:11–16.
9. Schenkman M, Butler R. A model for multisystem evaluation treatment for individuals with Parkinson's disease. *Phys Ther.* November 1989; 69(11):932–943.
10. Webster D. Critical analysis of the disability in Parkinson's disease. *Mod Treat.* 1968; 5:257–282.
11. Weinrich M, Koch K, Garcia F, et al. Axial versus distal motor impairment in Parkinson's disease. *Neurology.* April 1988; 38:540–545.
12. Murray MP, Sepic S, Gardner G, et al. Walking patterns of men with parkinsonism. *Am J Phys Med.* 1978; 57(6):278–294.
13. Henderson C, Kennard C, Crawford S, et al. Scales for rating motor impairment in Parkinson's disease: studies of reliability and convergent validity. *J Neur Psych.* 1991; 54:18–24.
14. Alba A, Trainor F, Ritter W, et al. A clinical disability rating for Parkinson's disease. *J Chron Dis.* 1968; 21:507–522.
15. Hallet M. Physiology and pathophysiology of voluntary movement. In: Tyler K, Dawson D, eds. *Current Neurology.* Boston: Houghton-Mifflin; 1979; 351–376.
16. Schenkman M, Donovan J, Tsubota J. Management of individuals with Parkinson's disease: rationale and case studies. *Phys Ther.* November 1989; 69(11):944–955.
17. Saal JS, ed. *Flexibility Training and Rehabilitation of Sports Training.* Philadelphia; Hanley & Belfus; 1987.
18. Nelson A. Lecture Notes. New York: Hospital for Special Surgery; September 1988.
19. Handford F. The Flewitt-Handford exercises for Parkinson's gait. *Physiotherapy.* August 1986; 72(8):382.
20. Davis J. Team management of Parkinson's disease. *Am J Occup Ther.* May–June 1977; 31(5):300–308.
21. Rusin M. Stroke rehabilitation: a geropsychological perspective. *Arch Phys Med Rehab.* October 1990; 71:914–920.

22. Robins M, Baum H. Incidents. *Stroke*. 1981; 12(suppl 1):45–57.
23. Kelley R. Cerebral vascular disease. In: Weiner W, Goetz C, eds. *Neurology for the Non-Neurologists*. 2nd ed. Philadelphia: Lippincott; 1989:52–66.
24. Gillum R. Stroke in blacks. *Stroke*. 1988; 19:1–9.
25. Baxter D. Clinical syndromes associated with stroke. In: Brandstater M, Basmajian JV, eds. *Stroke Rehabilitation*. Baltimore: Williams and Wilkins; 1987:36–54.
26. Dawson D, Adams P. Current estimates from the National Health Interview Survey. United States 1986 National Center for Health Statistics. *Vital Health Statistics* 1987; 10:164.
27. Ryerson S. Hemiplegia resulting from vascular insult or disease. In Umphred D, ed. *Neurological Rehabilitation*. St Louis: Mosby; 1985.
28. Spriggs D, French J, Murdy J, et al. Historical risk factors for stroke—a case controlled study. *Age Ageing*. 1990; 19:280–287.
29. Gray C, French J, Bates D. Motor recovery following acute stroke. *Age Ageing*. 1990; 19:179–194.
30. Feigenson JS. Stroke rehabilitation: effectiveness, benefits, and costs. Some practical considerations. *Stroke*. January/February 1979; 10(1):1–4.
31. Anderson TP, McClure WJ, Athelstan G, et al. Stroke rehabilitation: evaluation of its quality by assessing patient outcomes. *Arch Phys Med Rehab*. April 1978; 79(4):170–175.
32. Anderson TP, Baldridge M, Ettinger MG. Quality of care for completed stroke without rehabilitation: evaluation by assessing patient outcomes. *Arch Phys Med Rehab*. March 1979; 60(3):103–107.
33. Lehman JF, Delateur BJ, Fowler RS, et al. Stroke: does rehabilitation affect outcome? *Arch Phys Med Rehab*. September 1975; 56(9):375–382.
34. Schenkman M, Butler RB. A model for multisystem evaluation interpretation and treatment of individuals with neurologic dysfunction. *Phys Ther*. 1989; 69:538–547.
35. Tripp N, Boudoures K, Dalum A, et al. Initiation of a systemic evaluation to categorize the hemiplegic patient. *Phys Ther*. June 1991; 71(suppl 6):57.
36. Bobath B. *Adult Hemiplegia: Evaluational Treatment*. London: William Heinemann Medical Books; 1970:18–71.
37. Brunnstrom S. *Movement Therapy in Hemiplegia*. New York: Harper & Row; 1970:8–12, 34–41.
38. Carr J, Shepherd R. *A Motor Re-Learning Programme for Stroke*. Rockville, Md: Aspen; 1986.
39. Bohannon R. Knee extension torque in stroke patients: comparison of measurements obtained with a hand-held and a Cybex Dynamometer. *Physiotherapy Canada*. November/December 1990; 42(6).
40. Bohannon R. Consistency of muscle strength measurements in patient with stroke: examination from a different perspective. *J Phys Ther Sci*. 1990; 2:1–7.
41. Bohannon R. Is the measurement of muscle strength appropriate in patients with brain lesions? A special communication. *Phys Ther*. March 1989; 69(3).
42. Olney S, Colbourne GR. Assessment and treatment of gait dysfunction in the geriatric stroke patient. *Top Ger Rehab*. 1991;6(3).
43. Parker K, Zablotny C, Jordan C. Analysis and management of hemiplegic gait dysfunction. In: *Stroke Rehabilitation State of the Art*. Rancho Los Amigos Medical Center, Downey Medical Center, Downey, CA; 1984.
44. Carr J, Shepherd R, Nordholm L, Lynne D. Investigation of a new motor assessment scale for stroke patients. *Phys Ther*. February 1985; 65(2).
45. Kumar R, Metter EJ, Mehta AJ, et al. Shoulder pain in hemiplegia. *Am J Phys Med*. August 1990; 69(4):205–208.
46. Bohannon R, Warren M, Cogman K. Influence of shoulder position on maximum voluntary elbow flexion force in stroke patients. *Occup Ther J of Research*. March/April 1991; 11(2):73–79.
47. Brown DA, DeBacher GA. Bicycle ergometer and electromyographic feedback for treatment of muscle imbalance in patients with spastic hemiparesis. *Phys Ther*. November 1987; 67(11):1715–1719.
48. Wissel J, Ebersbach G, Gutjahr PDL, et al. Treating chronic hemiparesis with modified biofeedback. *Arch Phys Med Rehab*. August 1989; 70:612–617.
49. Sackley CM. The relationship between weight-bearing asymmetry after stroke, motor function and activities of daily living. *Physiotherapy Theory and Practice*. 1990; 6:179–185.
50. Trueblood PR, Walker JM, Perry J, et al. Pelvic exercise and gait in hemiplegia. *Phys Ther*. January 1989; 69(1).
51. Logigian MK, Samuels MA, Falconer J. Clinical exercise trial for stroke patients. *Arch Phys Med Rehab*. August 1983; 64:364–367.

Cardiopulmonary Treatment Considerations

Cardiopulmonary considerations are particularly important when treating the elderly population. Diseases of the heart, lungs, and blood vessels are by far the most prominent causes of morbidity and mortality among elderly individuals, and they rise logarithmically with age.[1] Eventually, the process of aging will compromise an individual's cardiovascular and cardiopulmonary systems and his or her ability to supply the amount of oxygen needed for any activities beyond the resting state.[2]

There are over 25 million people in the United States who are 65 years of age and older, and of these, 50% have some cardiopulmonary or cardiovascular disorders. Indeed, cardiovascular disease is the major cause of death after the age of 65 and accounts for more than 40% of deaths in this age group as a whole. Elderly people, who constitute 68% of all deaths in the United States annually, account for 78% of all deaths attributed to cardiovascular disease. In the most rapidly growing segment of the US population (those 85 years of age and older), cardiovascular and cardiopulmonary diseases account for more than 76% of all deaths.[3] Morbidity is similarly prevalent in the population over the age of 65. In this age group, 28% reported significant health impairments that are related to heart and lung conditions, including angina, congestive heart failure, rhythm disturbances, and chronic obstructive pulmonary disease (COPD).[4]

The most frequently occurring problem is atherosclerotic heart disease, and it is common to find hypertension coexisting with atherosclerotic heart disease. Congestive heart failure, arrhythmias, and electrocardiographic abnormalities also have an increased incidence with aging.[5] Cardiac disease in the elderly is complicated because it rarely occurs in isolation. Pulmonary problems, such as COPD and emphysema, usually result in death not from the pulmonary problem but rather from the cardiac complications they impose. Vascular diseases generally accompany cardiac disease or predispose an individual to the development of cardiovascular and cardiopulmonary pathologies (see Chapter 5). Chronic inactivity resulting from musculoskeletal or neuromuscular causes or systemic diseases further exacerbate aging's effects on the cardiovascular system.

Cardiac rehabilitation is a means of improving one's cardiopulmonary response to increased oxygen demands during increased activity through endurance and conditioning exercises. The progression of the aging process eventually evolves into diseases of the cardiovascular and cardiopulmonary systems. Any of the pathologies already mentioned will lead to an inhibition of the cardiopulmonary responses to increased oxygen demands. The functional level of activity decreases because a vicious cycle of inactivity and deconditioning, imposed by a variety of medical problems in the musculoskeletal, neuromuscular, and sensory systems, may cause cardiovascular disability or exacerbate an underlying cardiac disease.

Prolonged inactivity and bed rest quickly and markedly impair cardiovascular functional capacity.[6] And, all too often, deconditioning of the cardiopulmonary system is potentiated by the prescription of excessive bed rest and the overmedication of the elderly cardiac patient. Even prior to illness, many elderly patients decrease their activity level due to a combination of musculoskeletal and neuromuscular problems. Additionally, because of the decreased aerobic capacity with aging, any submaximal task is perceived as requiring increased work because of its increased relative energy cost and resulting fatigue. Relative inactivity thus potentiates the decreased physical work capacity in the elderly, often threatening their independent life-style. This can be avoided, and indeed, functional capacity can be improved with conditioning and endurance exercises and the reinstitution of the elder's participation in functional activities of daily living (ADL).

There has been an increased interest in research about the effects of exercise on the aged cardiac patient,[2,6] perhaps because of their growing numbers and the changing demographic and sociological patterns.[3] Individuals are living relatively healthy lives well beyond the socially imposed demarcation line that defines old age.[7,8] The expectations of acceptable functional levels for the elderly segment of the population have changed. Research studies have demonstrated that exercise is not only beneficial for maintaining a functional baseline condition in the unimpaired elderly individual, but it is also therapeutic for reversing the effects of impairment and for improving baseline condition in diseased individuals who have become deconditioned as a result of their symptoms' limitations (e.g., angina and dyspnea).[3]

Elderly people, because of society's increased focus on exercise and the elderly population's expectation of an active life-style, have increased their participation in physical activity programs. As a result, it is important that physical therapists be involved with the development of clinical procedures that are safe and effective in exercise assessment and prescription for the elderly. Therapeutic evaluation and program planning have reached the point where the elderly individual (who was once confined to bed because of angina and dyspnea resulting from cardiopulmonary disease) can be evaluated and treated with a total rehabilitation program, including an individualized exercise prescription that considers the severity of disease, attempts symptom reversal, and has functional improvement as its primary goal. Cardiopulmonary considerations are important in the geriatric population for the prescription of any activity, as cardiopulmonary pathological manifestations are most likely to accompany increasing age in close to 100% of the elderly population seen in clinical practice.

PHYSIOLOGICAL ASPECTS OF EXERCISE

Human performance is a remarkable integration of all of the systems of the body. Practically no tissue or organ escapes involvement when increasing activity levels. While the muscles perform the work, the heart and peripheral vascular systems deliver the nutrients and, with the assistance of the pulmonary system, provide oxygen to and remove carbon dioxide from the working tissues. The nervous and endocrine systems integrate all of this activity into a meaningful performance. At the cellular level, the mitochondria and numerous enzymes are activated and energy is generated that enables the muscle to contract. Skin acts as the heating and cooling system as activity is prolonged, and the kidneys assist in maintaining a homeostatic fluid balance. It is apparent that any pathological manifestation involving any of the body systems will negatively influence the physiological response to exercise.[6]

The heart is an amazing organ. Despite its decreased power and ability to contract, slower rate of recovery, diminished cardiac reserve, and other changes from aging and disease, the human heart continues to function well as long as it is not overwhelmed by disease. By the time a person is 80 to 90 years of age, the heart has outperformed the best mechanical pumps devised by man. By the age of 100, the human heart has beat more than 3.6 billion times and pumped more than 288 billion cubic centimeters of blood. The ability of the cardiovascular and cardiopulmonary systems to respond to stress admittedly decreases with advancing age, but many elderly people, even with heart disease, can continue normal routine activities well into old age.

During the normal life span, the cardiovascular and cardiopulmonary systems are subject to a variety of normal physiological stimuli and processes that may create pathological consequences. In addition, the biological changes of aging, beginning after the process of growth and development and the evolution of maturity and adulthood, and proceeding into the phases of senescence and old age, modify the anatomical, physiological, and functional capabilities of the heart, lungs, and vascular systems.

CARDIOPULMONARY CHANGES WITH AGING AND DISEASE

The changes in the cardiopulmonary system related to aging and disease have been discussed in Chapters 3 and 5, and will only be summarized here as a foundation for cardiopulmonary treatment considerations in the elderly.

There is some controversy over the degree of physiological change that is expressly age related as opposed to disease related. Most investigators agree, however, that certain changes in muscle strength and in cardiac and pulmonary function are so common that they may be thought of as universal. Because rehabilitation exercise programs increase the level of activity above resting states, these changes are likely to affect the older person. Aerobic capacity ($\dot{V}O_2$ max) decreases with advancing age, and declines in aerobic capacity are probably greater in the patient who has become deconditioned during a recent hospital stay or who had poor exercise habits prior to developing a disability. Exercise capacity may be further affected by decreases in vital capacity and minute volume.[9] Additional cardiopulmonary changes related to aging include increased blood pressure and decreased maximum cardiac output.[10] Maximal obtainable heart rate and stroke volume decline in relation to decreases in maximal oxygen consumption ($\dot{V}O_2$ max).[9] With age, lean muscle mass decreases as does muscle strength,[11] and these decreases will be discussed in this chapter as they relate to the cardiopulmonary systems need to meet the working muscles energy demands. Orthostatic hypotension is frequently seen, particularly in those recently bedridden. Peripheral vascular resistance rises with age and increases the risk of developing hypertensive episodes with exercise programs.

The heart demonstrates little change in the size of its chambers, but the left ventricular wall thickens and becomes less compliant.[12] There is a thickening of or a development of nodular ridges along the attachments of the aortic cusps.[13] The conduction system displays relatively little change in the atrioventricular (AV) node or the bundle of His, though the number of proximal bundle fascicles connecting the left to the main bundle may become less.[14]

Coronary artery or ischemic heart disease is the most prevalent disease in individuals over the age of 60.[8] In 90% to 95% of the cases, the reduction of blood flow to the heart is the result of atherosclerotic narrowing of the coronary lumen.[12] This reduction in flow causes angina, myocardial infarction, and sudden death. Angina and infarction impair function by decreasing the maximum cardiac output and maximum oxygen consumption. Infarction or necrosis of the heart muscle limits the distensibility of the heart and reduces the stroke volume. Collectively, these pathological changes produce a self-limiting impediment to cardiac function. Increased systemic demands for oxygen necessitate an increase in cardiac output or myocardial work. Increased work requires an increase supply of oxygen to the myocardial muscle. The restricted coronary blood flow results in ischemia, which increases the left end-diastolic pressure, prolongs systole as the heart is unable to relax, and stiffens the ventricle wall. A destructive cycle is instituted as these physiological changes reduce the perfusion of the myocardium and increase the degree of ischemia further damaging cardiac tissue.[3] The result of this vicious circle is a progressive deconditioning of the heart as angina and dyspnea self-limit and impair functional activity and exercise capacity.

Lung changes are characterized by an increase in residual volume accompanied by a decrease in vital capacity. Declines are seen in maximal voluntary ventilation, the surface area for gas exchange, the rate of diffusion, and the arteriovenous oxygen differential.[15] Both the lung tissue and chest wall lose elasticity. Cardiopulmonary demands can usually be met, but when disease or deconditioning are present the demands may exceed the available reserve. All of these changes result in a reduced tolerance for physical activity and are important to consider with regard to rate and intensity of activities for the older person. Due to the wide variety in life-styles of older people, the rate and magnitude of changes cannot be predicted and may not be apparent until they impact ADLs.

The anatomical and functional changes seen in COPD mimic those seen in normal aging. Both are characterized by microtraumas that occur over time, which do not interfere with resting or low-level ventilatory function.[16] The pathological tissue changes seen with emphysema and chronic bronchitis are also similar to the tissue changes of advancing age. The degree of impairment is the distinguishing factor between what is considered normal aging and what is considered pathological. In emphysema, there is an abnormal enlargement of the terminal airspaces as a result of a loss in tissue elasticity of the lung. This results in an expiratory collapse of the larger airways. Expiration is difficult for the patient with emphysema. Chronic bronchitis is accompanied by a persistent productive cough on a daily basis. The result of these respiratory conditions is an increase in the work of breathing and an inability to meet the energy demands required for functional activities of living, exercise, or both.

Maximal Oxygen Consumption (VO₂ max)

The major function of the cardiovascular and cardiopulmonary systems during exercise is to deliver blood to the active tissues, which supplies oxygen and nutrients and removes metabolic waste products. If exercise is prolonged, the cardiovascular system also assists in maintaining body temperature.

The cardiac and pulmonary systems integrate a number of component functions in order to adequately acquire and distribute oxygen to the working muscles. The muscles of the thorax contract to initiate an increase in thoracic volume and lower the intrathoracic pressure. A decrease in the intrathoracic pressure creates gas flow from the higher pressured atmosphere into the conducting tubules, where the gas is warmed, filtered, humidified, and mixed with existing gasses to produce an alveolar oxygen tension of 90 to 100 mm Hg.[6] Alveolar oxygen is diffused across the 70 m^2 blood–gas interface into pulmonary capillaries via an approximate 40 mm Hg pressure gradient where it combines with hemoglobin and then enters the left atrium. The heart, through rhythmic contraction, delivers the oxygenated blood to the myocardial muscle first, then to the peripheral tissues. The pressure created by the contraction of the heart (systolic) overcomes systemic pressure and generates blood flow through the arterial vascular system.

Maximal oxygen consumption (VO_2 max) is the best measure of cardiopulmonary fitness. It can be derived by a simple equation: $VO2 = Q \times (aO_2 - vO_2)$. VO_2 is the amount of oxygen the system absorbs and is equal to cardiac output (Q) multiplied by the arterial oxygen content (aO_2) minus the central venous oxygen content (vO_2). Each link of this multistaged process needs to be functioning adequately in order for the system to efficiently acquire, transport, and deliver oxygen. An impairment at any phase as a result of disease, age, or deconditioning limits the oxygen uptake and competent delivery to the working tissues.

Heart Rate

The resting heart rate is influenced by age, body position, the level of cardiopulmonary fitness, and various environmental factors (e.g., temperature, humidity, or altitude). Resting heart rate remains relatively constant with age, though in advanced age it may show a decline. Better cardiopulmonary fitness results in a decreased resting heart rate, whereas the resting heart rate will be increased at higher environmental temperatures or increased altitudes.

Before exercise, the heart rate may be increased by an anticipatory response, which is a reflection of a sympathetic neurohumoral effect. As exercise begins, the heart rate increases, but during low levels of exercise at a constant work load, the heart rate will reach a plateau or steady state. As the work load increases, the heart rate increases in roughly a linear manner. At higher work loads, the heart rate takes longer to plateau. For two persons doing the same work load, the fitter individual will have a lower steady state value.

The older individual shows a lower response than a younger given the same work load, but at progressively higher work loads, there will eventually be a level that totally exhausts the individual. Prior to this, however, the heart rate will reach a plateau at its maximum.

The maximum heart rate declines with age, and each individual has a definable maximum heart rate. The equation for maximum achievable heart rate is 200 minus age. This provides an approximation of the mean maximal heart rate for any one age category with a standard deviation of 10, so this equation should be used cautiously. The decline in the maximum heart rate with age has been attributed mainly to changes in the myocardial oxygen supply but additional factors include pathological impairment of blood flow to the sinus node that produces a lower heart rate during maximal exercise (sick sinus syndrome) and a greater stiffness (reduced compliance) of the heart wall that increases the time required for filling of the ventricles and interferes with the "feedback" of information on venous filling to the cardioregulatory center.

Heart rate responses will vary at rest and submaximal exercise levels according to the degree of cardiovascular impairment, whereas the maximum achievable heart rate shows a progressive decline with age.[6] Heart rate responses to physiological stimuli, such as postural change and cough, have also been shown to decrease as age increases.[13]

Stroke Volume

The difference between the end-diastolic and end-systolic blood volumes is the stroke volume, and the stroke volume response is highly dependent on hydrostatic pressure effects. When sitting or standing (without exercise), the stroke volume is reduced relative to the supine position due to blood pooling in the extremities. The maximum stroke volume attained during exercise in the supine or sitting positions is only slightly higher. The increase is sufficient to overcome the effect of venous pooling. Stroke volume at rest in the erect position varies between 50 mL and 80 mL. In a highly trained athlete, this volume can be as high as 200 mL. The stroke volume increases linearly with the work load until it reaches its maximum at approximately 50% of the individual's capacity for exercise.[6]

There is some controversy as to whether there is a change in stroke volume with age or if the changes are a result of a decline in $\dot{V}O_2$ max, a slower maximum heart rate response, and increased peripheral resistance that diminishes the ejection fraction.[17] Understanding the significance of stroke volume changes has been hampered to some extent by the inability to accurately measure absolute left ventricular dimensions (i.e., end-diastolic and end-systolic volumes).[18] Studies have suggested that there is no age related change in stroke volume at rest[19] and that the ejection fraction remains unchanged with age at rest.[20] During exercise, end-diastolic volume and end-systolic volume showed marked age related increases as higher levels of exercise were achieved according to Rodeheffer and associates.[21] Elderly subjects showed an increase in the end-diastolic volume at low levels of exercise and continued to show progressive increases with increasing exercise intensity. End-systolic volume in elderly subjects also increased with exercise, though less dramatically. Younger subjects at high levels of exercise showed no change in the end-diastolic volume from resting levels while end-systolic volume decreased significantly. The implication of these volume changes is that the young population maintains cardiac output by achieving a high heart rate and that healthy older individuals maintain cardiac output by dilating the ventricle and using the Frank-Starling mechanism to increase stroke volume.[21]

Cardiac Output

The cardiac output at rest is 4 to 6 L/min, and it increases linearly with work load. At exercise levels of 40% to 60%, the increase in cardiac output is accomplished through an increase in both the heart rate and the stroke volume. At higher levels of exercise, the increase in cardiac output results solely from the continued increase in heart rate. Maximal values of cardiac output during exercise are dependent on many factors, but body size and the degree of physical fitness appear to have the most prominent influence on it. For instance, in a small, deconditioned individual maximum cardiac output during exercise could be as little as 20 L/min, whereas in a large well-conditioned individual cardiac output can reach 40 L/min.[2]

Physiological changes in the cardiovascular system primarily involve the determinants of cardiac output. Cardiac output is affected by preload and afterload conditions, which are altered by aging. Early diastolic filling is decreased as a result of mitral valve thickening, the decrease in the compliance of the left ventricle, or both.[14] There is an increase in afterload with aging as well, which is possibly produced by an increase in the rigidity of the ascending aorta and a general decrease in the diameter of the peripheral vascular system. This combination of factors increases the overall load on the myocardium and is responsible for an age associated decrease in cardiac output.

Blood Pressure

The normal response of the blood pressure to aging is a linear increase in systolic pressure with increasing work (200 mm Hg or higher). Blood pressure changes in aged individuals are dependent on many factors, including extracellular fluid volume, vascular tone and reactivity, the autonomic nervous system, and the arterial baroreceptor reflexes. Each component factor can affect responsiveness in the aged individual somewhat differently. Resting systolic and diastolic blood pressures tend to rise with age, however, the range is quite variable.[14] Diastolic blood pressure changes little in healthy elderly individuals. An increase in systemic blood pressure with age is related to the loss of elasticity in the walls of the larger arteries, which raises systolic and depresses diastolic pressures. There is also the increased liability of vasopressor control that tends to raise both systolic and diastolic pressures. As a result, the systolic arterial blood pressure rises progressively up to the age of 75 years; and the diastolic pressure rises slightly to the age of 60 and then gradually declines.[22]

Arteriovenous Oxygen Differential

The arteriovenous oxygen differential is the difference between the oxygen in the arteries compared to the oxygen content in the veins, and it reflects the amount of oxygen that the peripheral tissues extract. The maximum arteriovenous oxygen difference tends to decrease with age.[23] Shepard[2] suggests that factors contributing to this decline with age include lower levels of physical fitness, a reduction of arterial oxygen saturation, a decreased hemoglobin level, poor peripheral blood distribution, a loss of activity in tissue enzyme systems, and a greater relative blood flow to the skin.

The arteriovenous oxygen difference tends to be larger in the elderly compared to young adults both at rest and at submaximal exercise levels, indicating that there is a decrease in the amount of oxygen extracted in older subjects.[24] Some increase in the stroke volume in combination with a decrease in mechanical efficiency of the cardiopulmonary and cardiovascular systems could explain this. Horvath and Borgia[25] report that there is no reduction in the amount of oxygen saturation/transport capacity of arterial blood. The metabolic potential of skeletal muscle does not decline,[26] however, there is a decrease in the capillary/fiber ratio in the aged muscle[27] and a reduction in the amount of blood that flows to the periphery.[28]

Peripheral Vascular Resistance

Blood flow from the heart varies with tissue needs. During exercise, blood is shunted from areas of little or no metabolic activity (i.e., the gut) to those tissues that are involved in the exercise. Blood to the heart increases proportionately to the increase in metabolic activity.[6] Blood to the skin and muscles is increased, and blood to the stomach and intestines is decreased. The effective blood volume decreases from maximal levels with prolonged work and in a hot and humid environment, because of the increased blood flow to the periphery that promotes both metabolic and environmental heat loss.[2]

Vascular age changes affect each tissue layer differently. The cells of the intima become irregularly aligned instead of orienting themselves along the longitudinal axis of the vessel.[14] The subendothelial layer becomes thickened due to lipid deposition, calcification, and increased cross-linking of the connective tissue. The media demonstrates increased calcification and fraying of the elastic fibers. These changes all lead to regional differences in vessel diameter and an increase in the resistance to blood flow.

The peripheral vascular resistance may be increased by atheromatous plaques in the lumina and, with a loss in vessel elasticity, a failure to vasodialate in response to increasing activity. Regular exercise can reduce the resting systemic pressure by about 5 mm Hg, but it has little influence on the peripheral pressure during maximum effort.[28a]

Neurohumoral Factors

There is a decline in the neurohumoral controls with aging that reduces the ability to adjust to external and internal stresses.[2] The body's hormones contribute to the regulation of circulating fluid volumes and cardiovascular performance, and they mobilize blood glucose, liberate fat, and break down protein to provide energy for increasing activity levels. Neurohumeral factors are important in tissue repair as they are involved with the synthesis of new proteins (anabolism), which is important in the healing process at the cellular level.

Fluid loss during prolonged exercise results in a decrease in plasma volume and hemoconcentration of red blood cells (RBC) and plasma proteins. This hemoconcentration results in an increase in RBC by 20% to 25%, and there is a shift of fluid from the plasma to the interstitial fluid.[2]

The blood pH shows little change up to approximately 50% intensity of exercise. Past 50% the pH decreases, and the blood becomes more acidic. This decrease in pH is primarily the result of an increase in anaerobic muscle metabolism and corresponds to an increase in blood lactate.

Neurohumeral regulatory changes affect the physiological response of the elderly individual. Catecholamines function to maintain the systemic pressure, mobilize muscle glycogen to sustain plasma glucose, liberate fatty acids, stimulate gluconeogenesis in the liver, stimulate glucagon secretion, and inhibit insulin secretion.[2] Although there may be an increase in the plasma-catecholamine levels with advancing age,[29] there is a decrease in the end-organ responsiveness to β-adrenergic stimulation.[14] This variation in circulating catecholamines or decrease neuroresponsiveness may partially account for the decreased heart rate and blood pressure response to activities such as a cough or Valsalva's maneuver. This attenuated responsiveness is also partly attributed to decreased baroreceptor sensitivity.[29]

PULMONARY RESPONSE TO EXERCISE

Pulmonary ventilation or minute volume increases from approximately 6 L/min at rest to over 100 L/min during maximal exercise, and in a well-conditioned individual, this can exceed 200 L/min. This is accomplished by an increase in both the tidal volume and respiratory frequency. Tidal volume at rest is about 0.5 L/min and can increase to 2.5 to 3.0 L/min during maximal exercise efforts. Resting respiratory frequency ranges from 12 to 16 breaths/min and increases to 40 to 50 breaths/min during maximal exercise.[6]

The respiratory system is responsible for ventilation through the coordinated contraction of the diaphragm and associated ventilatory muscles, the displacement of the rib cage, and the expansion of the lungs by the negative pressure created by the contraction of these muscles. The resting length and strength of the ventilatory muscles, thoracic cage compliance, and compliance of the lungs are important factors in generating adequate gas flow. Aging produces a progressive decrease in the thoracic wall and bronchiolar compliance.[30] Because of the structural changes in the bone, cartilage, and elastic structures with age, the chest wall becomes stiff. There is an increase in cross-linking of collagen fibers, a decrease in the resiliency of elastic and cartilaginous tissue, and a decrease in collagen and the annulus fibrosis.[2,28a] The elastic fibers within the lung change so that there is an increase in compliance of the lung but a decrease in its elastic recoil.[31] Superimposed on a decreased compliance of the thoracic wall this results in a decrease in total lung compliance with age and an increase in the size and number of alveolar fenestrae[32] that, in combination with the change in elastic features at the alveolar levels and the loss of tissue from the alveolar walls and septa, result in a decrease in the surface area available for gas exchange. The conducting tubules become more rigid, decrease their radius, and increase the resistance to gas flow.[28a] The result is an increased mechanical work load for breathing and a decrease in the efficiency of gas exchange.

The pulmonary systemic changes produced by pathological lung changes like those seen in COPD, emphysema, and chronic bronchitis increase the work of breathing and decrease the energy supply available to working muscles. There is a reduction in vital capacity due to an increased residual volume, decreased forced expiratory volume, and a reduced arterial oxygen tension with an increase in the carbon dioxide tension.[2] In combination with a decrease in thoracic compliance and a progressive narrowing of the airways, the force required for the ventilatory muscles to create airflow severely stresses the cardiopulmonary system and compromises its ability to efficiently supply oxygen to peripheral tissues.[33]

BENEFITS OF EXERCISE TRAINING IN THE ELDERLY

Cardiac and pulmonary diseases need not be a barrier to better fitness. Too many health care professionals working with the elderly have set their sights too low by accepting that the reduced physical abilities of aging people, who are inactive, sedentary, or incapacitated by subclinical or clinical disease, are normal. For instance, a decline in cardiac output is considered a normal aging process, however, according to noninvasive, radioactive thallium nuclear and echocardiographic studies[21] the decline in cardiac output is absent in physically fit older people without occult coronary artery disease. Most studies dealing with changes in cardiopulmonary response to exercise are done on more sedentary and less physically fit elderly individuals who may well have subclinical cardiopulmonary or cardiovascular disease.

There are few studies on the role of exercise in the prevention of coronary and pulmonary problems in the elderly population, however, epidemiological studies suggest a clear role exists for increased activities (i.e., exercise, occupational, and leisure) for decreasing the risk of developing cardiovascular and cardiopulmonary diseases.[6,34,35] Lack of exercise becomes a progressively more important risk factor in the development of cardiopulmonary and cardiovascular pathologies.[36] Even the relative body weight has less influence on the chance of having a fatal heart attack.[37] Shepard[2] suggests that this may reflect the confounding influence of the increasing loss of lean tissue.

Regularly performed aerobic exercise results in an increase in $\dot{V}O_2$ max in young adults. The magnitude of the change is determined by the intensity, frequency, and duration of exercise.[2] Sidney and Shepard[38] have reported that elderly men and women respond to endurance exercise training with similar relative increases in $\dot{V}O_2$ max. They demonstrated that the frequency, intensity, and duration of the exercise also impacted the beneficial exercise outcomes in older subjects. Cross-sectional studies have shown that older endurance athletes have a higher $\dot{V}O_2$ max than age-matched sedentary controls.[39,40] This difference ranged between 44% and 62% when $\dot{V}O_2$ max was expressed in L/min and between 62% to 100% when it was corrected for body weight (mL/kg/min). In master athletes (65+ years of age), the VO_2 max was only 9% lower compared to younger runners with whom they were matched in terms of performance, training, body weight, and body composition.[41] This means that regular exercise could positively influence the integrated response to an external (e.g., environmental) or internal (e.g., pneumonia) stress, and it could play a role in putting up a barrier to these internal accentuations.

Endurance exercise results in a significant increase in $\dot{V}O_2$ max in older men and women.[39] Verg and co-workers[39] observed a 25% increase in $\dot{V}O_2$ max after 1 year of training in a group of subjects aged 60 to 66 years of age. With low-intensity training, male and female subjects aged 61 to 65 years increased their $\dot{V}O_2$ max by 12%.[42] An additional 6 months of high-intensity training produced a further substantial effect and increased the $\dot{V}O_2$ max gains to 18%. Thomas and associates[43] found that the best predictor of what an elderly subject's VO_2 max will be after 1 year of training is the initial VO_2 max. These findings support the hypothesis that the age related decline in aerobic capacity is in part due to modifiable factors, such as inactivity.

Cross-sectional comparisons of master athletes between the ages of 61 and 65 years and similarly aged sedentary subjects that endurance exercise training protects against the decline in ventilatory function with age.[39] When the minute volume was compared to controls at the same absolute submaximal exercise intensity, it was 12% lower in the study group of exercising individuals, which indicates a decrease in the actual work of breathing in the trained elderly. The master athletes also had a higher maximum voluntary ventilation and used a significantly higher percentage of their maximum voluntary ventilation capacities at maximal exercise than sedentary controls. Frontera and Evans[44] evaluated sedentary, healthy men and women aged 61 to 65 and found that endurance training for 1 year increased their $\dot{V}O_2$ max by 25%. There were no significant changes in the maximum voluntary ventilation, however, at the same submaximal $\dot{V}O_2$, the minute volume was 9% lower after training—a reflection of a more efficient ventilation. In addition, the maximal minute ventilation and the percentage of the maximum voluntary ventilation used at maximal exercise increased significantly. This study made it apparent that the older, sedentary individual can expect to achieve the same efficient level of ventilation during submaximal exercise and use the same percentage of maximum voluntary ventilation during maximal effort as the master athlete. The age related changes in the ventilatory apparatus do not preclude improvements in function with endurance exercise training.

Prolonged endurance exercise training results in significant adaptations in cardiovascular function. Heath and co-workers[40] compared endurance athletes aged 53 to 65 to a group of 20- to 24-year-old athletes of similar body weight and training habits. All of the athletes were compared with similar age-matched, healthy, untrained men. Both young and master athletes in the study groups had significantly greater left ventricular volume and mass when compared to the untrained group, and all of the athletes in both age groups had higher values for posterior wall thickness and septal thickness when normalized for body surface area. The master athletes had a significantly larger end-diastolic volume index as compared to the younger athletes. The difference in ventricular mass was not statistically significant in either athletic group. Also of significance in this study was that no differences among the three groups were noted in indicators of myocardial contractile function measured by echocardiography (i.e., percentage of fiber shortening and mean velocity of fiber shortening at rest). Both groups of athletes had significantly slower heart rates at rest and during three levels of submaximal exercise than did the group of untrained subjects. This suggests that regular exercise for men is likely to maintain cardiovascular function above that of deconditioned younger men.

According to Sals and associates[45] endurance training for 1 year resulted in a significant increase in the functional aerobic capacity. There was a small but significant rise in maximal stroke volume, though changes in maximal cardiac output were not significant. An increase in the arteriovenous oxygen difference suggests that there is a more efficient oxygen extraction at the muscular level, which indicates that peripheral adaptations are more important than central changes.

Skeletal muscle increases its oxidative capacities with endurance training. Endurance exercise increases the muscle mitochondrial–protein content and improves its oxidative capacity, even if it does not reduce the skeletal muscle atrophy associated with aging in rats.[46] Beyer and associates[47] substantiated this finding and concluded that the capacity to oxidize fats and carbohydrates can be maintained in aging animals with increased physical activity.

Endurance training for 8 weeks also has a positive effect on skeletal muscle metabolism in sedentary men aged 56 to 70.[48] Suominen and associates[48] found that there was an increased level of enzyme activity with endurance training, which represents aerobic muscle metabolism. These metabolic alterations in skeletal muscle are associated with lower blood lactate levels during submaximal exercise.[45,48] This suggests that the lower blood levels are due to a decreased lactate production and a greater aerobic contribution to energy production.

Extremes in cardiovascular fitness in the elderly exist. John E Kelley of East Dennis, Massachusetts, who ran the Boston Marathon for the 27th time in 1992 at the age of 84, is a good example. Hazel Wolf, who is 95, kayaks extensively, portaging her own kayak and camping gear. Wolf, a Seattle resident, founded most of Washington State's Audubon Society chapters. These are clearly exceptions to the rule. They are individuals whose self-discipline and ability to achieve and perform great physical activity has been a way of life since very early in their lives. By contrast, most individuals who reach the age of 65 years have slowed down considerably, and inactivity is one of the major predisposers to cardiovascular and cardiopulmonary pathologies.

EVALUATION/EXERCISE TESTING

In an elderly person's routine cardiopulmonary and vascular physical evaluation, particular attention must be paid to the neuromuscular, musculoskeletal, and sensory examinations, because results of these tests will yield valuable information on the person's residual abilities and potential for improvement. Goals of the examination include observation of deviations from the normal structure or function, evidence of secondary complications from cardiopulmonary and cardiovascular diseases, and assessment of residual strengths.

Skin should be closely inspected, particularly over bony prominences, for evidence of excessive pressure, friction, or maceration that may lead to breakdown. With the high prevalence of diabetic and arteriosclerotic peripheral vascular disease in the elderly, it is also prudent to inspect the skin of the feet, particularly between the toes.

A musculoskeletal exam should include an evaluation for posture, joint range of motion, flexibility, tenderness, and muscle strength with an emphasis on existing imbalances or asymmetry. An assessment for complaints of pain should also be incorporated. Ambulatory status and gait pattern assessment are crucial in developing a reconditioning program.

In a neurological examination, mental status should be routinely evaluated. A routine check on appearance, affect, orientation, and communication is helpful when determining an elderly individual's level of functioning and safety. Other areas of importance in the neurological examination include the testing of sensation (particularly vibration and proprioception), deep tendon reflexes, balance (sitting and standing), and coordination.

In the cardiopulmonary examination, a check for orthostatic hypotension may prove valuable, particularly if the individual complains of lightheadedness, dizziness, or episodes of blacking out with falling. This is particularly important in patients on hypertensive medications with orthostatic side effects. Checking the resting heart rate with comparison to a postactivity heart rate may yield valuable clues as to the person's level of endurance and tolerance of exercise. Identifying arrhythmias, murmurs, rales, or evidence of COPD may help to explain exercise intolerance with easy fatiguability or dyspnea. Evaluating the respiratory pattern, posture, strength of cough, segmental lung expansion, and diaphragmatic excursion should be a routine part of evaluation, especially in an individual with known pulmonary disease. Cardiopulmonary patients often present with chronic musculoskeletal problems or peripheral adaptations, such as clubbing of the fingers and toes, discoloration of the nail beds, or edema in the feet and ankles.

Checking extremity pulses is important, especially if the patient presents with complaints of claudication or peripheral sensory changes. The amount of activity needed to induce claudicant pain should be determined. As objective measures, local blood pressures and the time it takes for claudication to occur are helpful measures for establishing a baseline with which treatment effects can be compared. For instance, in a normal individual, treadmill or walking exercise tends to increase the systolic pressure at the ankle, but in the claudicant individual, the ankle pressure falls to a very low level and is slow to recover.[49]

Stress testing to determine an elderly individual's cardiopulmonary response to exercise is a crucial component of evaluation. (Several means of acquiring a baseline exercise level will be discussed in a subsequent section.) The appropriate stress test protocol and method for exercise testing employed will be determined by the older person's ambulatory and functional status, level of physical fitness, medical status, motivation, mentation, and safety of the test chosen. Many elderly individuals will not tolerate maximal test levels and submaximal testing needs to be used to determine a safe level for prescribing and starting endurance training protocols. The importance of stress testing can not be overstated.

Another important consideration for determining the protocol that best tests an individual's exercise capacity is the method of exercise that will be used in the endurance training.

Step Tests

Steps are among the least expensive devices available for the administration of an exercise stress test. The most commonly employed step test is the Master's Step Test. It requires a platform of 2 steps, each 9 inches high. The individual walks up and down the steps at a given rate determined by age and sex using a metronome to keep pace. This diagnostic test lasts only 3 minutes. Step testing is usually inadequate for the measuring of aerobic work capacity, and it has its limitations in the elderly, especially in those of advanced age. Quadriceps strength and endurance may not be adequate to maintain stepping for the full 3 minute period, and the test is too strenuous for some cardiac patients, yet it does not induce enough stress to adequately determine exercise capacity in the elderly without occult cardiopulmonary problems.

Another step test, which uses a single platform that can be raised vertically to increase the external work load, determines cardiovascular response to progressive exercise. This graduated, multilevel step test parallels the principles used in the design of treadmill tests.[50] A stepping rate of 24 steps/min is maintained while the platform is raised vertically at periodic intervals (generally 2 cm every minute). The second phase of the step increases the cadence to 30 steps/min, again gradually increasing the height of the platform at the same time.

Modified Chair-Step Test for the Elderly

A particularly helpful modification of the step test is employed more commonly in the nursing home setting or with the frail elderly who can not maintain their balance during a step, bicycle, or treadmill test.[51] This test is done with the patient sitting with a bar or platform of adjustable height placed in front of the seated individual. The feet are alternately lifted and placed on the bar as in stepping at a cadence of 24 to 30 steps/min. The height of the bar or platform is gradually increased, depending on the physical capabilities of the elder, in 3 to 6 inch increments every 1 to 3 minutes up to the height of 18 inches. If the person is able to reach the 18 inch height, he or she can continue with the final phase of the testing protocol, which employs upper extremity reaching over the head each time a foot is raised. This has been found to be an effective means of evaluating cardiovascular and cardiopulmonary response to gradually increasing levels of work in the deconditioned elderly.

Walking Test

A test that is applicable to the elderly without balance problems or ambulatory deficits is the walking test. A 12-minute walk[52] is employed in the elderly with cardiac or respiratory problems. The walk is accomplished on a level surface at a pace as brisk as the individual can manage, and the distance is recorded at the end of the 12 minute period. This test is particularly useful for establishing a baseline walking level for those elderly who cannot walk on a treadmill or ride a bicycle because of angina or dyspnea.

For the more physically fit elderly, the use of a 1-mile walk is a good measure of cardiopulmonary capabilities. The 1-mile walk test[53] is conducted on a level surface. A brisk pace is established by the individual, and the amount of time it takes the individual to cover the last quarter mile is recorded. The VO_2 max is determined by a formula that incorporates the heart rate during the 1st quarter mile, the distance covered in the last quarter mile, and the age, sex, and weight of the individual exercising regressed against a constant (see Kline and associates[53] for details).

Treadmill Tests

The most commonly used treadmill test for the determination of maximal oxygen intake is the Bruce or Modified Bruce protocol.[9] In elderly individuals, the modified test, which incorporates a much more gradual increase in the speed and incline of the treadmill, is most frequently employed. Initially the speed is set at 1.7 mph at a grade of 10% (though in some protocols the initial grade is set at 5% and increased to 10% during the first 3 minutes of the test for the more impaired elderly). Every 3 minutes the speed and the percentage of incline is increased in a specified manner until a speed of 5 mph at a grade of 18% is reached. This stress test protocol can be used with relatively fit elderly individuals to accurately measure the cardiopulmonary response to exercise.

The Modified Balke Test is an alternative to treadmill stress testing. The rationale of the test is the same, but the speed of the treadmill is held constant (as determined by the individual's perceived capabilities) and every 2 minutes the grade is increased from 0% by 3.5% increments.[54]

In both of these protocols, assessment parameters include expired air analysis,

ECG, heart rate, blood pressure and respiratory rate monitoring. The test is terminated using the following criteria: a decrease in blood pressure, ischemic drop of the ST segment or arrhythmias on the ECG, tachycardia, bradycardia, severe shortness of breath, angina, dizziness, or leg pain. Often the elderly individual's perceived limit of exertion will be the ending point of the stress test.

A low level functional treadmill walking test is an intermittent walking test used with patients with moderate to severe cardiac or respiratory involvement. It is divided into three stages and monitors ECG, blood pressure, respiratory rate, heart rate, oxygen saturation, and pulmonary function. Stage I is a 6 minute walk on a level surface at a pace of approximately 1.5 to 2.0 mph. The objective of this phase of the assessment is to determine the cardiopulmonary response at this intensity of walking. At the end of 6 minutes the patient is allowed to return to baseline heart rate, respiratory rate, and oxygen saturation.

Stage II is a functional ambulation assessment. The treadmill is set at a speed and incline equal to the functional work capacity based on the individual's physiological and symptomatic response during Stage I. This phase is also 6 minutes long, and the patient is allowed to return to baseline before proceeding to Stage III.

Stage III is the maximum exercise tolerance component of the test, and it is also 6 minutes. The treadmill is set to produce a heart rate of 70% to 85% max or a preestablished ventilatory max. Termination of the test is based on: (1) reaching 85% of the predicted heart rate maximum, (2) oxygen saturation of 85% or below, (3) reaching the predicted ventilatory maximum, (4) the development of significant cardiac arrhythmias, or (5) the development of significant symptoms. This modified stress test elicits a safe exercise response that produces an actual exercise limit and enables accurate measurement of maximal levels in elderly individuals with severe pulmonary, coronary, or both impairment. It also allows flexibility in establishing the work load by allowing modification of the test according to the person's physiological and symptomatic response. It also establishes an accurate baseline for exercise prescription.

Cycle Ergometer Test

The bicycle ergometer test provides another alternative to exercise testing. Its advantages are that the individual is supported by the bike and can maintain balance by using the handlebars. A tractor seat may be used in place of a regular bike seat to further facilitate the patient's stability and comfort while on the bike. For screening an older person for exercise prescription, a continuous test of 6 to 9 minutes of cycling with gradual incremental increases in intensity and speed is employed.[51] The individual should work up to 70% to 85% of the predicted maximum heart rate. The same parameters are monitored during the bike stress test as during the treadmill tests.

EXERCISE PRESCRIPTION

Intensity, duration, and frequency are the three major components of exercise prescription. These three elements are used when formulating an appropriate exercise level based on the results of exercise stress testing. Evidence suggests that the best prescription to improve cardiovascular training effects should incorporate an intensity of 60% or greater of the maximum heart rate and it should be done for a duration of 20 minutes or more with a frequency of three or more times per week.[9,44] In the absence of cardiopulmonary impairment, the elderly can achieve a cardiovascular training effect with aerobic exercise. As a result of the decline in maximum heart rate with age, a training effect is obtained at smaller relative heart rate increases as compared to younger subjects.[2]

Elderly individuals with cardiopulmonary impairment may be restricted in the amount of aerobic activity they can do because of dyspnea or angina. As Irwin and Zadai[16] so aptly put it,

> At the present time, the question remains of whether patients with COPD ever achieve the hallmark "anaerobic threshold" even at the higher heart rates they demonstrate with lower levels of exercise. The improvements seen in COPD patients after exercise training are not consistent with the changes demonstrated by exercising normals (central cardiovascular training effect).

Intensity of exercise is a significant factor in determining the successful improvement of aerobic capacity with exercise.[39,56] In healthy elderly, the heart rate is usually used as a reliable indicator of exercise intensity. Heart rate can be a useful indicator for those people who can palpate their own pulse (or have access to a wrist monitoring device). When prescribing exercise for the elderly, it is important to establish a target heart rate that is 60% plus that achieved during exercise testing in order to obtain the desirable VO_2 max. Once an exercise prescription has been determined that provides the time and the distance necessary to improve endurance, a safe heart rate (usually between 60% to 70% max initially) must be maintained by the patient throughout the exercise session.

In the elderly individual with cardiopulmonary disease, however, heart rate may be an inadequate reflection of oxygen consumption as the oxygen cost of an ineffective breathing pattern and an inefficient cardiac pump can shift the amount of oxygen supply away from the working peripheral muscles. In addition, heart rates are often modified by the medications prescribed for cardiac conditions. It is important to instruct the individual in heart rate monitoring as the heart rate is correlated with the oxygen demand that produced significant symptoms during the stress test. The elderly individual is instructed not to exceed that heart rate during an exercise session. Given the unreliability of the heart rate as an indicator of oxygen consumption during exercise, rather than having these individuals rely on heart rate as an indicator of exercise intensity, the intensity is prescribed by recommending a certain amount of work to be accomplished over a given period of time. For instance, a person who was able to walk 1 mile in the 12 minute walking test should continue to walk for endurance with the goal of 1 mile in 30 minutes. Gradually the distance can be extended as determined by the patient's cardiopulmonary tolerance, self-perceived endurance, and motivation. In endurance terms, the intensity of the exercise is determined by the distance covered in a specific amount of time.

The primary goal of endurance training is to increase the elderly individual's functional activity level by improving the exercise capacity. In order to improve endurance the duration of exercise needs to be a part of the prescription. If an elderly individual is only able to accomplish Stage I (6 minutes) of the low level functional test, intermittent exercise periods would be one way to incorporate the principle of duration. The initial prescription has a duration time (e.g., 20 minutes) that equals the eventual goal, however, the exercise is performed in 4 to 5 minute segments with 2 to 3 minute rest periods in between. As the exercise progresses, the rest periods are gradually decreased until the individual is able to walk the entire 20 minute period continuously. In the nursing home environment, it is not uncommon to have an elderly exercise for 2 to 3 short sessions a day at first before progressing to one long session. The same principle is applicable for those elderly exercising in the community on their own. Gradually the time of the exercise session can be increased as endurance improves.

Frequency is another consideration in exercise prescription. Initially, especially with the intermittent exercise program, it is recommended that exercise session be done daily unless the individual is limited by symptoms or the weather. Once the person is able to exercise for 20 to 30 consecutive minutes, four to five times per week will maintain and improve the training effects of exercise.

As previously discussed, recovery times are frequently longer in the elderly due to their increased oxygen demands. Warm-up and cool-down sessions are essential as part of the exercise prescription, because individualized warm-up and cool-down sessions can address muscle imbalances, postural problems, flexibility exercises, and overall strength. Stretching and flexibility exercises can also incorporate breathing exercises to facilitate the mobilization of the thorax and improve ventilation. Balance and coordination are often facilitated with rhythmic exercises as well.

SPECIAL CONSIDERATIONS WHEN PRESCRIBING EXERCISE

Obesity

Obesity is related to an increased risk for cardiovascular disease in the elderly. In fact, Jarret[56] found an increased risk for the development of cardiovascular problems at both extremes of the weight distribution curve. The evidence suggests that obesity heightens other atherogenic risk factors (e.g., smoking or coexisting disease) and thereby contributes to increased risk.[57] Data from the Framingham study at the 30-year follow-up demonstrate a continuous relationship between obesity and coronary morbidity and mortality that was stronger in men than in women. Obesity is associated with both increased blood pressure and increased serum lipoprotein levels.[58] In the Framingham study,[59] correlation between relative weight and either systolic or diastolic pressure declined steadily over adult life. Havlik and associates,[60] using the body mass index (BMI) ([weight/height^2] $\times$ BMI and blood pressure), reported similar declines in men over the age range 30 to 70 years. Harlan and co-workers[61] showed a reduction in association between BMI and systolic blood pressure in older women. The weaker association at older ages remains significant for men but not for women.

In the Framingham study, the correlation between relative body weight and total plasma cholesterol is not significant over age 50 years for men; for women, it is significant only among 35 to 39 year olds.[62] Further analyses showed that, over age 50 years, BMI is no longer significantly associated with low-density lipoproteins (LDL) cholesterol in either sex. However, the strong inverse relationship between HDL cholesterol and BMI remains statistically significant, even among subjects aged 70 to 79 years.[62,63] Therefore, the benefits of maintaining optimal weight for height are associated with a positive effect on high-density lipoproteins (HDL) cholesterol levels.[64]

The effects of weight change on blood lipid profiles are considerable. In the Framingham study, the investigators found that a 10-unit change in weight relative to height was associates with a change in serum total cholesterol of 11 mg/dL in men and 6.3 mg/dL in women. There was no diminution in these relationships among older age groups.[59] Both Wolf and Grundy[65] and Zimmerman and associates[66] found modest increases in HDL cholesterol with weight reduction.

Both blood lipids and blood pressure are sensitive to the degree of obesity.[64] A significant drop in age-specific blood pressure indicates that effective control of obesity, especially the prevention of weight gain in middle adult life, is potentially of great value for reducing cardiovascular mortality.[67] Few studies compare the relative risks associated with weight fluctuation and sustained obesity. In the Framingham study, weight at younger ages has been found to be an important predictor of cardiovascular disease.[68,69] Weight reduction through exercise and diet has been shown to confer substantial improvement in the cardiovascular risk profile; therefore, it is recommended for elderly individuals who are 20% or more above desirable weight as defined by BMIs of 27.2 for men and 26.9 for women.[70] In individuals with diabetes, hypertension, dyslipidemia, and gout, lesser degrees of overweight should be reversed.[71]

Medications

Almost all patients who have cardiac problems are on medications such as β-blockers or calcium channel blockers. β-Blockers are cardioselective adrenoreceptor blocking agents that usually result in a reduction in both the resting and exercise heart rate and cardiac output. Calcium channel blockers inhibit the influx of calcium, thereby reducing the heart rate and blood pressure for any given load. In other words, these medications reduce the cardiac responsiveness to increasing activity levels, and heart rate is not, therefore, a good measure of exercise stress.

Recovery rates appear to be a good practical indicator of stress levels in these individuals. If a return to the resting heart rate occurs within 2 minutes following cessation of exercise, it is considered a safe level of activity. If the individual returns to a resting heart rate within 1 minute or less, they may increase the exercise level. A period of recovery 3 minutes or greater is considered to be an indication that the individual is exercising at a level that is too stressful to the cardiopulmonary system, and the intensity of exercise needs to be decreased.

Medications used for patients with pulmonary diseases include oxygen, systemic and inhaled bronchodilators, steroids, and antibiotics. Most of these drugs are used to increase the oxygen supply and decrease the oxygen demand through a decrease in the work of breathing. Antibiotics are used to combat infection.

Diabetes Mellitus

Cross-sectional studies have shown that the impaired glucose tolerance of aging is significantly related to the level of physical fitness or activity.[72] Few studies have been done specifically on those 60 years of age and older. One prospective trial of the effects of exercise on glucose tolerance was carried out on men 60 years of age and older. It was found that, while glucose levels did not change, both insulin and C peptide levels were lower.[45] In addition, HDL cholesterol levels increased, and triglyceride levels decreased. Exercise trials in patients with type II diabetes mellitus have failed to show a major advantage of short-term exercise programs over diet alone.[37] However, trials that last 5 or more months did find improvements in glucose tolerance.[73,75]

Besides the possible beneficial effects of exercise on glucose tolerance, exercise training may also improve cardiovascular fitness, lipid profiles, hypertension, osteopenia, and psychological function in diabetic patients. Risks of exercise in diabetics include hypoglycemia, ketosis, dehydration, myocardial ischemia, arrhythmias, acceleration of proliferative retinopathy, increased proteinurian, and trauma (particularly in patients with neuropathy). The National Institutes of Health (NIH) consensus panel concluded that the effects of exercise on metabolic control in non-insulin-dependent diabetes mellitus is often variable and of small magnitude.[76] Pacini and co-workers[77] demonstrated that normal weight, physically active older subjects have a normal insulin-binding capacity, insulin sensitivity, and insulin secretory capacity in response to glucose stimulus. Helmrich and associates[75] showed that increased activity levels actually decreased the incidence of diabetes mellitus. Studies of long-term exercise programs need to be undertaken before a formal recommendation for an exercise prescription can be given; however, the benefits of exercise for cardiovascular conditioning and the potential for modifying glucose intolerance in the diabetic clearly outweigh the risks.

Osteoporosis

Osteoporosis in the elderly population must be considered when prescribing cardiovascular reconditioning exercise programs. The estimated loss of bone from its peak in young adulthood to age 80 is comparable to the reported 35% to 45% decline in muscle strength during the life span.[78] Since a clear relationship between muscle strength and bone mass has been established,[79–82] physical activity has gained attention as a method for improving bone mass. The mechanisms by which the skeleton responds to activity are yet to be defined, but the evidence suggests that bone mass increases in response to application of mechanical stress.[83-85] Bone density appears to be higher in physically active people, and the literature suggests that exercise reduces the rate of age related bone loss.[86-88]

It is not known which type of exercise is best for improving bone mass, however, all the recommended exercises involve aerobic, weight bearing activities, such as walking and jogging, that directly impact the cardiopulmonary system. It is important to evaluate the elderly patient with osteoporosis for cardiovascular and cardiopulmonary involvement and likewise to determine if the individual with cardiac, pulmonary, vascular, or a combination of these problems is at a higher risk for stress fractures as a result of osteoporosis.

CONCLUSION

It would be impossible to overlook the great therapeutic potential of physical exercise in the elderly. As Ernst Jokl[89] has noted,

> The theoretical basis for understanding the unimpaired adaptability to exercise with aging was provided more than 100 years ago by the great pathologist, Julius Cohnheim, who pointed out that irrespective of age, physiological challenges of all kinds are reliable in that they invariably result in an enhanced functional status. Training for strength increases strength; training for endurance increases endurance; training for skill increases skill.

Physical exercise and nutrition provide a solid foundation for a sound and healthy old age and can delay the inevitable deterioration of the aging process. The body's adaptability to exercise remains unimpaired with age, although adaptation to exercise is less reliable when pathological processes are present. Reports in the medical literature and clinical experience provide numerous instances in which physical exercise and activity benefitted patients with coronary artery disease, diabetes mellitus, hypertension, pulmonary disorders, and other chronic illnesses. Physical exercise and training not only improves the physical capacities and skills of older people, it also affects the body's adjustability to physiological stresses.

Several physiological mechanisms maintain homeostasis during an acute bout of external or internal stress. Age related changes affect each of these responses and limit exercise performance and VO_2 max. Exercise has been shown to alter and reverse some of these changes and slow the decline in functional aerobic capacity. In doing so, an elderly individual's ability to perform ADLs are improved and the quality of life enhanced. Exercise and functional mobility exercises should be considered an integral part of a rehabilitation program for the elderly.

PEARLS

- Cardiovascular disease is the major cause of death after age 65, accounting for more than 40% of this population's deaths.

- Cardiopulmonary changes related to aging include a decrease in aerobic capacity, vital capacity, minute volume, maximum cardiac output, maximal obtainable heart rate, stroke volume, maximal oxygen consumption and an increase in blood pressure.

- The outcomes of aging on the pulmonary system result in an increased mechanical work load for breathing, a decrease in the efficiency of gas exchange, and a compromise in the ability to efficiently supply oxygen to peripheral tissues.

- A decline in cardiac output is absent in physically fit older persons without heart disease.

- The components of a thorough cardiopulmonary evaluation include assessment of the neuromusculoskeletal system, sensory system, and cardiopulmonary screening along with appropriate stress testing.

- Submaximal stress testing can be done safely for older persons. The various types of tests (step test, modified chair-step test, walking test, treadmill testing, and cycle ergometer testing) are all of use for testing the elderly.

- Intensity, duration, and frequency, the three major components of exercise prescription, are different for the elderly. Intensity is safe at 60%, duration, which is usually 20 minutes, may need to be cut to 4 to 5 minutes initially, and frequency should be daily.

- When prescribing exercise for an older person, special consideration and modifications should be made for obese, diabetic, and osteoporotic patients, and those on cardiopulmonary medications.

REFERENCES

1. National Center for Health Statistics. *Advance Report of Final Mortality Statistics. Monthly Vital Statistics Report.* Hyattsville, Md; US Public Health Service. US Dept of Health and Human Services, publication PHS 88–1120; 37–6(suppl), 1988.
2. Shepard RJ. *Physical Activity and Aging*, 2nd ed. Gaithersburg; Md: Aspen; 1987.
3. Verbrugge L. Recent, present, and future health of American adults. In: Breslow L, Fielding JE, Lave LB, eds: *Annual Review of Public Health.* Annual Reviews; Palo Alto, Calif: 1989; 10.
4. *Technology and Aging in America.* US Congress, Office of Technology Assessment, OTA-NS-264. Washington DC; US Office of Technological Assessment; 1985.
5. Palmore EB. Trends in the health of the aged. *Gerontologist.* 1986; 26:298–302.
6. Astrand PO. Exercise physiology and its role in disease prevention and in rehabilitation. *Arch Phys Med Rehabil.* 1987; 68;305.
7. Rowe JW, Besdine RW. *Health and Disease in Old Age.* Boston; Little, Brown; 1982.
8. Crimmins EM, Saito Y, Ingegneri D. Changes in life expectancy and disability-free life expectancy in the United States. *Pop Dev Rev.* June 1989; 15(2):235–267.
9. Bruce RA. Functional aerobic capacity, exercise and aging. In: Adres R, Bierman EL, Hazzard WR, eds. *Principles of Geriatric Medicine.* New York: McGraw-Hill; 1985:87–103.
10. Shepard RJ. The cardiovascular benefits of exercise in the elderly. *Top Ger Rehab.* 1985; 1(1):1–10.
11. Cress ME, Schultz E. Aging muscle: functional, morphologic, biochemical, and regenerative capacity. *Top Ger Rehab.*1985; 1(1):11–19.
12. Gerstenblith G, Weisfeldt ML, Lakatta EG. Disorders of the heart. In: Andres R, Bierman EL, Hazzard WR, eds. *Principles of Geriatric Medicine.* New York: McGraw-Hill; 1985; 515–526.
13. Wei JY. Heart disease in the elderly. *Cardiovasc Med.* 1984; 9:971–998.
14. Wei JY. Cardiovascular anatomic and physiologic changes with age. *Top Ger Rehab.* 1986; 2(1):10–16.
15. Redden WG. Respiratory system and aging. In: Smith EL, Serfass RC, eds. *Exercise and Aging: The Scientific Basis.* Hillside, NJ: Enslow Publishers; 1981; 89–108.
16. Irwin SC, Zadai CC. Cardiopulmonary rehabilitation of the geriatric patient. In: Lewis CB, ed. *Aging: The Health Care Challenge.* 2nd ed. Philadelphia: Davis; 1990; 181–211.
17. Mann DL, Deneberg BS, Gash AK, et al. Effects of age on ventricular performance during graded supine exercise. *Am Heart J.* 1986; 111:108–115.
18. Rodeheffer RJ, Gerstenblith G. Effect of age on cardiovascular function. In: Johnson HA, ed. *Relations Between Normal Aging and Disease.* Aging Series. 1985; 28:85–99.
19. Gerstenblith G, Lakatta EG, Weisfeldt ML. Age changes in myocardial function and exercise response. *Progr Cardiovasc Dis.* 1976; 19:1–21.
20. Port S, Cobb FR, Coleman RE, et al. Cardiac ejection fraction in aging. *New Eng J Med.* 1980; 303:1133–1137.
21. Rodeheffer RJ, Gerstenblith G, Becker LC, et al. Exercise cardiac output is maintained

with advancing age in healthy human subjects: cardiac dilatation and increased stroke volume compensate for a diminished heart rate. *Circulation.* 1984; 69:203–213.

22. Harris R. *Clinical Geriatric Cardiology: management of the Elderly Patient.* Philadelphia: Lippincott; 1986; 29–42.

23. Weisfeldt ML, Gerstenblith ML, Lakatta EG. Alterations in circulatory function. In: Andres R, Bierman EL, Hazzard WR, eds. *Principles of Geriatric Medicine.* New York: McGraw-Hill; 1985; 248–279.

24. Niinimaa V, Shepard RJ. Training and oxygen conductance in the elderly. *J Gerontol.* 1978; 33:354–367.

25. Horvath SM, Borgia JF. Cardiopulmonary gas transport and aging. *Am Rev Respir Dis.* 1984; 129 (suppl):569–571.

26. Aniansson A, Hedberg M, Henning GB, et al. Muscle morphology, enzymatic activity, and muscle strength in elderly men: a follow-up study. *Muscle Nerve.* 1986; 9: 585–591.

27. Coggan AR, Spina RJ, King DS, et al. Skeletal muscle adaptations to endurance training in 60–69 year old men and women. *J Appl Physiol.* 1992; 72:1780–1786.

28. Martin WH III, Kohrt WM, Malley MT, et al. Exercise training enhances leg vasodilatory capacity of 65-year-old men and women. *J Appl Physiol.* 1990; 69:1804–1809.

28a. Smith EL, Serfass RC, eds. *Exercise and Aging: The Scientific Basis.* Hillside, NJ: Enslow; 1981.

29. Shimada K, Kitazumi T, Sadakne N, et al. Age-related changes of baroreflex function, plasma, norepinephrine, and blood pressure. *Hypertension.* 1985; 7:113–118.

30. Irwin SC. Cardiac rehabilitation for the geriatric patient. *Top Ger Rehab.* 1986; 2:44–54.

31. Turner JM, Mead J, Wohl ME. Elasticity of human lungs in relation to age. *J Appl Physiol.* 1968; 25(6):664–683.

32. Pump KK. Fenestrae in the alveolar membrane of the human lung. *Chest.* 1974; 65:799–802.

33. Loke J, Mahler DA, Paul-Man SF, et al. Exercise impairment in chronic obstructive pulmonary disease. Symposium on exercise: physiology and clinical applications. *Clin Chest Med.* 1984; 5(1):121–129.

34. Paffenbarger RS, Wing AL, Hyde RT, Jung DL. Physical activity and incidence of hypertension in college alumni. *Am J Epidemiol.* 1983; 117:245–256.

35. Paffenbarger RS, Hyde RT, Wing AL, Hsieh CC. Physical activity, all-cause mortality and longevity of college alumni. *New Eng J Med.* 1986; 314:605–613.

36. Baker PB, Arn AR, Unverferth DV. Hypertrophic and degenerative changes in human hearts with aging. *J Coll Cardiol.*1985; 5:536A.

37. Krotkiewski M, Lonroth P, Mandroukas K, et al. The effects of physical training on glucose metabolism in obesity and type II (noninsulin-dependent) diabetes mellitus. *Diabetologia.* 1985; 28:881–890.

38. Sidney KH, Shepard RJ. Frequency and intensity of exercise training for elderly subjects. *Med Sci Sports.* 1978; 10:125–131.

39. Verg JE, Seals DR, Hagberg JM, et al. Effects of endurance exercise training on ventilatory function in older individuals. *J Appl Physiol.* 1985; 58:791–794.

40. Heath GW, Hagberg JM, Ehsani AA, et al. A physiological comparison of young and older endurance athletes. *J Appl Physiol.* 1981; 51:634–640.

41. Allen WK, Seals DR, Hurley BF, et al. Lactate threshold and distance running performance in young and older athletes. *J Appl Physiol.* 1985; 58:1281–1284.

42. Seals DR, Hagberg JM, Hurley BF, et al. Effects of endurance training on glucose tolerance and plasma lipid levels in older men and women. *JAMA.* 1984; 252:645–649.

43. Thomas SG, Cunningham DA, Rechnitzer PA, et al. Determinants of the training response in elderly men. *Med Sci Sports Exerc.* 1985; 17:667–672.

44. Frontera WR, Evans WJ. Exercise performance and endurance training in the elderly. *Top Ger Rehab.* 1986; 2(1):17–32.

45. Seals DR, Hagberg JM, Hurley BF, et al. Endurance training in older men and women. I. Cardiovascular responses to exercise. *J Appl Physiol.* 1984; 57:1024–1029.

46. Farrar RP, Martin TP, Murray Ardies C. The interaction of aging and endurance exercise upon the mitochondrial function of skeletal muscle. *J Gerontol.* 1981; 36:642–647.

47. Beyer RE, Stames JW, Edington DW, et al. Exercise-induced reversal of age-related declines of oxidative reactions, mitochondrial yield and flavins in skeletal muscle of the rat. *Mech Ageing Dev.* 1983; 24:309–323.

48. Suominen H, Heikkinen E, Liesen H, et al. Effects of 8 weeks' endurance training on

skeletal muscle metabolism in 56–70-year-old sedentary men. *Eur J Applied Physiol.* 1977; 37:173–180.

49. Thiele BL, Strandness DE. Disorders of the vascular system: peripheral vascular disease. In: Andres R, Bierman EL, Hazzard WR, eds. *Principles in Geriatric Medicine.* New York: McGraw-Hill; 1985:527–535.

50. Nagle FJ, Balke B, Naughton JP. Gradual step tests for assessing work capacity. *J Appl Physiol.* 1965; 20:745–752.

51. Smith EL, Gilligan C. Physical activity prescription for the elderly. *Phys Sports Med.* 1983; 11:91–101.

52. McGavin CR, Cupta SP, McHardy GJR; Twelve-minute walking test for assessing disability in chronic bronchitis. *Br Med J.* 1976; 1:822–826.

53. Kline G, Parcari JP, Hintermeister R, et al. Estimated VO_2 max from a one-mile track walk, gender, age, and body weight. *Med Sci Sports Exerc.* 1987; 19:253–259.

54. Ellestad NH. *Stress Testing: Principles and Practice.* Philadelphia: Davis; 1979.

55. Bruce RA. Exercise, functional aerobic capacity, and aging—another viewpoint. *Med Sci Sports Exerc.* 1984; 16:8–15.

56. Jarret RJ. Is there an ideal body weight? *Br Med J.* 1986; 293:493–495.

57. Stallones R. Epidemiologic studies of obesity. In: Foster WR, Burton BT, eds. Health implications of obesity. *Ann Intern Med.* 1985; 103 (6, pt 2):1003–1005.

58. Kannel WB, Gordon T. *An Epidemiologic Investigation of Cardiovascular Disease.* Section 5. Washington, DC: US Public Health Service. US Dept of Health, Education, and Welfare publication; 1968.

59. Ashley FW Jr, Kannel WB. Relation of weight change to changes in atherogenic traits: the Framingham study. *J Chronic Dis.* 1974; 27:103–114.

60. Havlik RJ, Hubert HB, Fabsitz RR, et al. Weight and hypertension. *Ann Intern Med.* 1983; 98(2, pt 5):855–859.

61. Harlan WR, Hull AL, Schmouder RL, et al. High blood pressure in older Americans: the first national health and nutrition examination survey. *Hypertension.* 1984; 6(1):802–809.

62. Jannel WB, Gordon T, Castelli WP. Obesity, lipids, and glucose intolerance: the Framingham study. *Am J Clin Nutr.* 1979; 32:1238–1245.

63. Wilson PWF, Garrison RJ, Abbott RD, et al. Factors associated with lipoprotein cholesterol levels: the Framingham study. *Arteriosclerosis.* 1983; 3:273–281.

64. McGandy RB. Nutrition and the aging cardiovascular system. In: Hutchinson ML, Munro HN, eds. *Nutrition and Aging.* Orlando, Fl: Academic Press; 1986.

65. Wolf RN, Grundy SM. Influence of weight reduction on plasma lipoproteins in obese patients. *Arteriosclerosis.* 1983; 3:160–169.

66. Zimmerman J, Kaufman NA, Fainaru M, et al. Effective weight loss in moderate obesity on plasma lipoprotein and apolipoprotein levels and on high density lipoprotein composition. *Arteriosclerosis.* 1984; 4:115–123.

67. Drizd T, Dannenberg AL, Engel A. Blood pressure levels in persons 18–74 years of age in 1976–80, and trends in blood pressure from 1960 to 1980 in the United States. *Vital Health Stat.* 1986; 234(11): 1–68.

68. Dannenberg A, Drizd T, Horan, et al. Cardiovascular disease. *Epidemiology Newsletter.* 1985; 68(abstract).

69. Higgins M, Kannel WB, Garrison R, et al. Hazards of obesity: the Framingham experience. *Acta Med Scand.* 1987; 723 (suppl):23–26.

70. Chernoff R. *Geriatric Nutrition: The Health Professional's Handbook.* Rockville, Md: Aspen Publishers; 1991.

71. Kannel WB. Nutrition and the occurrence and prevention of cardiovascular disease in the elderly. *Nutr Rev.* 1988; 46:68–78.

72. Rosenthal MJ, Hartnell JM, Morley JE, et al. UCLA geriatric grand rounds: diabetes in the elderly. *J Am Ger Soc.* 1987; 35:435–447.

73. Saltin B, Lindgarde F, Houston M, et al. Physical training and glucose tolerance in middle-aged men with chemical diabetes. *Diabetes.* 1979; 28 (suppl 1):30–32.

74. Bogardus C, Ravussin E, Robbins DC, et al. Effects of physical training and diet therapy on carbohydrate metabolism in patients with glucose intolerance and noninsulin-dependent diabetes mellitus. *Diabetes.* 1984; 33:311–318.

75. Helmrich SP, Ragland DR, Leung RW, et al. Physical activity and reduced occurrence of noninsulin-dependent diabetes mellitus. *N Eng J Med.* 1991; 325:147–152.

76. Karam JH. Therapeutic dilemmas in type II diabetes mellitus: improving and maintaining B cell and insulin sensitivity. *West J Med.* 1988; 148:685–690

77. Pacini G, Valerio A, Beccaro R, et al. Insulin sensitivity and beta-cell responsivity are not decreased in elderly subjects with normal OGTT. *J Am Ger Soc.* 1988; 36:317–323.

78. Johnson T. Age-related differences in isometric and dynamic strength and endurance. *Phys Ther.* 1982; 62:985–989.

79. Doyle F, Brown J, LaChance C: Relation between bone mass and muscle weight. *Lancet.* 1970; 1:391–393.

80. Aloia JF, Cohn SH, Babu T, et al. Skeletal mass and body composition in marathon runners. *Metabolism.* 1978; 27:1793–1796.

81. Sinaki M, Offord K. Physical activity in postmenopausal women: effect on back muscle strength and bone mineral density of the spine. *Arch Phys Med Rehab.* 1988; 69:277–280.

82. Sinaki M, McPhee MC, Hodgson SF. Relation between bone mineral density of spine and strength of back extensors in healthy postmenopausal women. *Mayo Clin Proc.* 1986; 61:116–122.

83. Rubin CT, Lanyon LE. Regulation of bone mass by mechanical strain magnitude. *Calcif Tissue Int.* 1985; 37:411–417.

84. Rubin CT, Lanyon LE. Regulation of bone formation by applied dynamic loads. *J Bone Joint Surg.* 1984; 66:397–402.

85. Carter DR, Fyrie DP, Whalen RT. Trabecular bone density and loading history: regulation of connective tissue biology by mechanical energy. *J Biomech.* 1987; 20:785–794.

86. Talmadge RV, Stinnett SS, Landwehr JT, et al. Age-related loss of bone mineral density in non-athletic and athletic women. *Bone Miner.* 1986; 1:115–125.

87. Brewer V, Meyer BM, Keele MS, et al. Role of exercise in prevention of involutional bone loss. *Med Sci Sports Exer.* 1983; 15:445–449.

88. Smith EL, Redden W, Smith PE. Physical activity and calcium modalities for bone mineral increase in aged women. *Med Sci Sports Exerc.* 1981; 13:60–64.

89. Jokl E. Abstract: XII International Congress of Gerontology. Hamberg, Germany. July 12–17, 1981.

CHAPTER *14* FOURTEEN

Establishing Community Based Screening Programs

The prevention of disease or mitigation of disability can improve a person's quality of life at any age. Anyone can benefit from gains in function, fewer periods of acute illness, more days free of disability, and less need for long-term care.[1] Prevention strategies can also conserve health resources. In 1988, those over age 65 years represented 12% of the population, but they accounted for more than 30% ($175 billion) of public health care costs.[2] Health care expenditures by older people totaled $73 billion, an average of $2394 per person.[2,3] Expenditures for health care grew from 13% in 1977 to an average of more than 18% of an elderly individual's 1988 personal income. Since the older age group is the fastest growing segment of the population, these health care cost estimates signal the need to examine strategies that might lower expenditures, such as health promotion and disease prevention, for those over age 65 years. In the next 25 years, the number of people over the age of 60 years will double; and those over 85 years are projected to increase more than any other age group.[5]

Nearly $1 of every $4 spent on health care each year can be attributed to behavioral factors, including crime, drug abuse, and the use of alcohol and tobacco; therefore behavior accounts for $171 billion of the $666 billion Americans spend on health care.[2] The health care crisis cannot be successfully resolved unless damaging patterns of behavior are altered. Twenty-two billion dollars in annual health care costs are attributable to cigarette smoking and other forms of tobacco use, and alcohol abuse may add another $85 billion a year. Other behavioral cost factors include failure to use technology like seat belts and smoke detectors, failure to have routine medical check-ups that could expose cancer and other treatable conditions, and participating in dangerous recreational activities.

There are many factors that contribute to the concept of "successful aging,"[6] the most important of which is optimal health. The human being's resiliency is incredible. It allows many elderly individuals to function adequately with considerable degrees of disability because of their unconceivably large amount of reserve. A person's ability to function independently is closely associated with optimum health status because it impacts the ability of the elderly person to successfully reside in the community at the highest possible level of independence rather than being institutionalized. Other factors that directly impact an individual's ability to maintain independence in the community are adequate financing and the individual's support system (e.g., significant others such as family, kin, friends, or church).[7] In a report published by the Department of Health and Human Services, this conclusion was reached:

> Many analysts of the Medicaid program argue that one of the major problems of both Medicare and Medicaid is the total reliance on institutional care, acute hospital care, and long-term nursing home care. Presently under Medicaid, approximately 70 percent of total program dollars are spent on institutional care: 33 percent in hospitals, 37 percent in long-term care facilities. According to these analysts, both forms of institutional care are some of the more expensive available options. The critics of Medicaid's heavy reliance on institutional care argue that Medicaid incorrectly emphasizes curing the ills of the elderly as opposed to preserving the health of the elderly. They state that in order to increase the preventive aspects of Medicaid, both the federal and state government should encourage the growth of community-based alternatives to institutional care. They argue that in many cases people who could live on their own with very little help with shopping, cooking, or medical care are inappropriately placed in nursing homes.[8]

The allocation of resources focuses on long-term care in an institutional setting like nursing homes rather than on preventative care, a costly alternative. There is a gap in the system between the income support provided to the "well" elderly and the intense health care provided to the "sick" elderly. There is nothing in between. Physical therapists have a unique opportunity to demonstrate innovation and leadership in the development of community screening programs that combine health care, personal care, and social maintenance; maximizes effective preventive approaches; uses the special knowledge of physical rehabilitation potentials to reduce unnecessary institutionalization; and ensures proper use of limited resources. This chapter focuses on screening programs that are community based and enhance the elderly individual's ability to maintain the highest level of physical functioning and independence.

Physical problems affecting the older adult are often undetected until they cause a debilitating loss in the person's capability to independently maintain activities of daily living (ADLs) and functional ambulation. The complications of many chronic diseases can be minimized or prevented by early detection through community based screening programs, regular medical care, environmental adaptations to facilitate function, and fitness programs that promote independence and the overall well being of the elderly. Few elders have annual physical checkups, and rarely, if ever, are functional limitations directly addressed. In light of this, preventive screening programs have the triple benefit of identifying high-risk individuals, detecting medical and physical problems, and preventing them from progressing into a loss of functional independence.

PREVENTION/HEALTH PROMOTION

Every day clinical experiences in working with the elderly reveal that prevention is probably the single most effective strategy for any significant gains in their functional and health status. Even the policymakers and third-party payers, in their efforts at cost containment, are showing particular interest and greater acceptance of the role that prevention and health promotion can play in decreasing the overall costs of medical care for the aged[9] and improving the quality of life by the avoidance of institutionalization. Many chronic illnesses that affect health and functional status are not merely part of the aging process. The elderly understand and appreciate the impact that life-style, behavior, and environment have on the development of some possibly preventable diseases, such as heart disease, cancer, and lung disease.[10] Interventions, such as exercise, diet, stress reduction, and smoking cessation, have been shown to positively affect the cardiovascular, cardiopulmonary, musculoskeletal, sensory, and neuromuscular systems (see Chapters 11, 12, and 13). These preventive modalities can lead to corrective and ameliorative changes that have the potential of delaying the onset of pathologies, as well as preventing the disabling effects of existing chronic disease(s).[11] Even in the oldest old population, those 85 years of age and older, research reveals that improvements can be made in every system of the body through exercise.[12] Proper attention to diet significantly modifies the onset of certain disease processes,[13] and the implementation of dietary control in combination with exercise has the potential of reversing, if not avoiding, some pathological manifestations, such as diabetes[14,15] and coronary artery disease.[16] Stress reduction and exercise also have positive effects on hypertension.[17] It is never too late to stop smoking. For example, a study by Rogers and associates[18] showed a significant improvement in cerebral blood flow in elderly subjects who stopped smoking and this improvement happened in a matter of 3 to 5 days. In a relatively short period of time, the abstinence from cigarettes also significantly improves cardiovascular and cardiopulmonary circulation and perfusion.[19] In terms of the quality of life for the elderly, preventive interventions can have a substantial impact on health care needs and days free of disability.

Types of Prevention

There are three levels in preventive health care: primary, secondary, and tertiary. Primary aging is the maturation of an organism exclusively attributable to the passage of time. Primary prevention is the prevention of any ill effects that may occur as a result of microtrauma during that maturation process. The goal of primary prevention is to avoid or delay the onset of debilitating pathologies and functional disabilities. An example would be a fitness program for the well elderly that included aerobic as well as stretching and strengthening exercises to enhance the cardiovascular, musculoskeletal, and neuromuscular systems. Primary prevention is synonymous with health promotion and seeks to prevent disease in susceptible individuals by reducing the exposure to risk factors. The basic interventions include better diet, more exercise, smoking cessation, better sanitation, and accident prevention. Primary prevention uses education to encourage individuals to modify behaviors.

Secondary aging relates to systemic or organ-specific changes associated with either acute or chronic disease. Secondary prevention is the implementation of therapeutic interventions at the earliest possible time within the acute phase of an illness. For instance, with pneumonia, the early intervention with chest physical therapy and the early resumption of ambulation and exercise clearly avoids the debilitating effects of bed rest and increases the individual's ability to ward off the infection.[20] Secondary prevention in chronic illness deals with the earliest possible intervention to reverse or maintain existing impairments and prevent further deficits from impeding the maximal functional capabilities of the elderly individual. Screening programs are the hallmark of secondary prevention at the community level.

Tertiary aging refers to functional impairments that have already progressed to the level of disability (see Chapter 9) and impede ADLs. Tertiary prevention attempts to minimize the ill effects of diseases once they have occurred and to rehabilitate the elderly individual's residual capacities. Functional activities and therapeutic interventions, such as proprioceptive neuromuscular facilitation (PNF) and Bobath techniques, in addition to strength and endurance training, are all important elements in restoring function and preventing further decline in chronic illnesses.

Webster[21] states, "It is increasingly clear that what was previously accepted as normal primary aging actually relates much more to unappreciated secondary or tertiary influences." Preventive measures that address the most prevalent diseases, such as heart disease, cancer, and cerebral vascular accidents, are particularly applicable in the elderly population. There is a correlation between healthful interventions like diet and exercise and the development of disease, and there is compelling evidence that suggests that the control of risks, such as smoking, an unhealthy diet, high blood pressure, physical inactivity, and exposure to toxic substances in the environment, could significantly diminish the prevalence of the three leading causes of death in the United States.[10]

HEALTH PROBLEMS IN THE ELDERLY/SYMPTOM PREVALENCE

Studies estimate that of the US population who are 65 years of age and older, 86% have at least one chronic disease that limits their functional activities and decreases the number of "disability-free" days progressively with advancing age.[22] Chronic diseases that affect older adults are sometimes misidentified as normal age changes and can go untreated for years.

Heart disease, cancer, and cerebral vascular disease cause almost 70% of deaths in the United States.[10] According to the National Center for Health Statistics, the elderly population is afflicted (in decreasing order of frequency) by arthritis (48%), heart disease (40%), hypertension (39%), cataracts (36%), diabetes (28%), cancer (26%), osteoporosis/hip fracture (16%), and stroke (9%). Comorbidities are common, and the frequency of these disorders increases with advancing age.[23]

The major causes of frailty and disability in the elderly relate to the broad functional problems of immobility and instability. Intellectual impairment is also a major component of functional decline. Confounding factors with the elderly include depression and transient dementias, isolation, urinary and bowel incontinence, sexual dysfunction, immune deficiency and infections, malnutrition, sleep disorders, impairment of sensory abilities, and iatrogenesis. Many of the health problems of the elderly are especially well suited for preventive efforts. For instance, impaired mobility, injuries, sensory loss, adverse drug reactions, deconditioning due to lack of exercise, depression, malnutrition, alcohol abuse, hypertension and cardiovascular disease, cancers, osteoporosis, urinary incontinence, and abuse and neglect are all preventable or can be postponed as a result of screening programs that identify these problems and follow-up intervention to address each individual's risk factors.

SCREENING CONCERNS IN THE ELDERLY

Planning preventive care packages and counseling approaches for older people requires special considerations. Most older people suffer from one or more chronic diseases or syndromes and total risk increases as a function of the number of individual risk factors.[24]

Screening tests and lab standards have not been developed or adapted specifically for the elderly.[25] "Aging, even without disease, changes physiology, which can alter lab test results."[26] Most of the normal lab values are based on 20- to 40-year-old subjects. This makes it difficult to determine what is abnormal in terms of a test result in the elderly. Aside from lab values, normal physiological changes of aging and the use of medications to treat chronic diseases may mask the symptoms of other physical problems.

Some diseases and conditions, such as coronary heart disease, may manifest themselves differently in older patients than in younger.[27] For example, an elevated serum cholesterol level becomes less predictive of heart related morbidity in an older individual. In fact, a low serum cholesterol level is a predictor of mortality in people of advanced age,[28] because they are associated with an increased risk of cancer and hemorrhagic stroke.

Some chronic conditions common in old age have competing risk factors. For example, obesity is a major risk factor for heart disease, diabetes, and other chronic diseases, but modest obesity is protective for osteoporosis.[29] Conversely, low body weight is a significant risk factor for hip fracture.[30]

In older individuals, functional disabilities associated with chronic diseases become as important as preventing the onset of disease.[31] Of the population aged 65 years who live independently, 24% have some degree of functional impairment, 15% are unable to perform major activities, and 11% are less impaired. Of those who are dependent on others for daily care, 6% are in nursing homes and 14% are homebound.[22]

What to Screen for

Many diseases can be prevented or forestalled by identifying and avoiding high-risk behaviors, while others can be treated in the early stages, thereby reducing the risk of disability or death. Yearly physical assessments are the preferred method for identifying problems, however, the majority of people 65 years of age and over do not seek medical attention on an annual basis. As a result of initiatives implemented by the surgeon general in the early 1980s, many agencies now offer preventive health programs, including screening for high-risk behaviors and the presence of disease. The costs associated with the treatment of chronic disease are clearly not desirable in today's malnourished economy. Health screening and early detection of disease processes can reduce costs substantially.

Screening programs for the elderly need to address behavior patterns, such as smoking, level of activity, dietary habits, living environment, health care needs such as dental and foot care, and immunization history. These programs aim at determining what the problems are and addressing them from an educational perspective. Ideally, screening programs should have a follow-up mechanism or referral sources for evaluating and treating physical or medical problems identified during the screening. Screening programs for the elderly can be holistic, and screen all systems of the body, or they can be system or disease specific (e.g., blood pressure screening, diabetes screening, cholesterol screening, or dental screening).

Primary prevention screening programs include immunizations, accident prevention, exercise programs, posture and flexibility assessment, nutritional modifications, and smoking and alcohol cessation. Secondary prevention screening focuses on early detection and treatment and is particularly applicable in disorders such as hypertension, vision and hearing impairments, musculoskeletal problems, neuromuscular involvement, depression, and iatrogenic adverse drug affects. Tertiary preventive screening focuses on functional assessment and maximizing physical potential and environmental efficiency to prevent the progression of functional decline.

The United States Preventive Services Task Force[32,33] has identified screening interventions that successfully alter the outcomes of various diseases, and it emphasizes the importance of educating the elderly population in high-risk behavior modification. For instance, the Task Force advised that elderly individuals be provided with educational material regarding the benefits of physical activity in disease prevention and that guidance in establishing appropriate exercise levels and selected modes of exercise be provided on an individual basis to each person screened. Other components in the Task Forces recommendations include smoking cessation programs; dietary modification to prevent diseases associated with dietary excesses or imbalances (e.g., osteoporosis, heart disease, some cancers, cerebral vascular accidents, or dental diseases); alcohol cessation programs when abuse is identified; home modification screening to reduce the potential for accidental injuries; vaccination programs for pneumococcal, influenza, and tetanus immunization; and screening for preventive "chemoprophylaxis" programs, such as low-dose aspirin therapy (325 mg every other day) for those at risk for cardiovascular diseases and estrogen replacement therapy for women who are at increased risk of developing osteoporosis.

Prescreening for High-Risk Populations

Before a comprehensive community based screening program is initiated, it is valuable to prescreen the community served to identify groups within the older population that would benefit from specific health screening procedures. Health questionnaires or interviews are helpful tools in identifying subgroups within the elderly population that may require special attention (e.g., diabetes mellitus, cardiovascular or pulmonary problems, a decrease in functional ADLs, or foot problems). There are some particularly valuable prescreening tools available. For instance, the Self-Evaluation of Life Function questionnaire developed by Linn and Linn[34] includes questions about health behaviors, existing diseases, symptoms, level of basic and instrumental ADLs, medication use, cognitive status, and socioeconomic well-being.

Another useful tool for prescreening the community elderly is the Health Hazard Appraisal (HHA), which is used in many preventive health care programs in both the United States and Canada[35] to determine high-risk populations for screening in community based settings. Safer[35] demonstrated that through the use of the HHA prescreening tool, Milwaukee residents reduced their health risk by 32% as a result of the health screening, follow-up counseling, and interventions that were employed to address the health care needs determined by the prescreening. The HHA prescreening is based on the assumption that "an individual's response to health threats depends on how he or she feels physically rather than on a rational calculation of health benefits and risks." The HHA is a valuable educational tool. By questioning elderly individuals and generating a "health hazard score," it informs people about how their health habits and life-styles affect their probability of dying within 10 years from potentially preventable causes. The HHA also helps to target the populations that are most likely to benefit from health screening and follow-up counseling and intervention programs.

Secondary Prevention Screening Tests

Screening and assessments necessary for health promotion in the elderly should include the evaluation of the presence of chronic diseases; symptoms that may suggest the presence of disease; health habits including nutrition, exercise and activity levels, smoking, medication use, and substance abuse; the evaluation of musculoskeletal, neuromuscular, and sensory deficits; safety; and mental status.

Cardiovascular Disease

Routine monitoring of blood pressure is an important component in controlling and reducing high blood pressure. Individuals with diagnosed high blood pressure need to be counseled regarding appropriate exercise levels, weight reduction, dietary sodium reduction and alcohol consumption. Periodic screening with the finding of persistent high blood pressure (e.g., greater than 140/90 mm Hg) may direct the health care professional to refer the individual for possible drug therapy to control excessively high blood pressure. Routine monitoring of the ECG is recommended in individuals who are symptomatic (e.g., had a previously positive ECG, angina, or dyspnea on exertion), but it is not recommended for those elderly who are asymptomatic. Though somewhat controversial, total serum cholesterol measurements are often employed to determine the presence of elevated blood cholesterol levels that have also been shown to place an individual at a higher risk for the development of cardiovascular diseases.

Cardiovascular screening should also include weight monitoring, and in those individuals who are 20% overweight by the height/weight standards, appropriate dietary and exercise counseling should be implemented as a preventive measure. Additionally, information on transient ischemic attacks, the presence of diabetes mellitus, cardiac arrhythmias, claudication, and any musculoskeletal limitations that place the individual at a high risk of developing problems associated with inactivity should be recorded and monitored. Peripheral vascular status and skin condition are important to evaluate, especially in the diabetic or someone with known peripheral vascular disease.

Cancer

There is little agreement as to the efficacy of screening for cancer in the elderly, and there is conflicting data regarding the accuracy and efficiency of the screening strategies in all ages (e.g., breast exams, mammography, and Papanicolaou [Pap] testing). Because certain cancers are more easily treated if diagnosed early, the consensus is that regular screening for cancer is recommended until more substantial evidence is presented that negates the value of the screening strategies in question. According to a 1988 pamphlet published by the American Cancer Society entitled *Summary of Current Guidelines for the Cancer-Related Checkup: Recommendations,*[36] the recommendations for cancer screening are:

- Annual Pap smears and pelvic examinations for all women who are sexually active or are 18 years of age or older. After three consecutive normal annual examinations, Pap tests may be performed less frequently or at the discretion of the physician.
- Endometrial tissue samples at menopause for women who are at high risk.
- Baseline mammogram between 35 and 39 years of age. Repeat every 2 years from age 40 to 49 and annually thereafter.

- Breast physical examination every 3 years for women between 20 and 40 years of age and yearly thereafter.
- Breast self-examination monthly for all women 20 years and older.
- Stool guaiac slide test every year for men and women over 50.
- A sigmoidoscopic examination every 3 to 5 years for men and women over age 50.
- Yearly digital/rectal examination for men and women over age 40 to screen for prostate and rectal cancer.
- Cancer examination and health counseling every 3 years after age 20 and yearly after age 40.

The second most common neoplasm in the United States is colorectal cancer, and it also has the second highest mortality rate.[36] Sigmoidoscopy and fecal occult blood testing are important in the early detection of this disease, especially in a known high-risk population (e.g., family or personal history of cancer, colonic polyps, or inflammatory bowel disease). High-risk patients include those with ulcerative colitis involving the entire colon with a duration of 7 or more years, a past history of an adenoma of the colon, or a past history of colon cancer or female genital cancer.[37] Early detection is particularly important in colorectal cancer as the survival rate in asymptomatic patients is 90% compared to 43% in those with more advanced disease.[37] Once symptoms of colorectal cancer occur, the disease is usually in an advanced and nonlocalized stage, which decreases the likelihood of successful surgical removal. There are home screening tests for occult blood that are reliable and available through a pharmacist, however, the tests require several stool smears over a 3 day period with dietary restrictions and are difficult to accurately accomplish when elders have physical or cognitive deficits. Cost effectiveness studies clearly indicate that the early detection of colorectal cancer significantly reduces the overall medical costs and improves survival.[38]

Breast cancer is the second leading cause of cancer deaths in women, and of those deaths 50% occur in women over the age of 65 years[39] and 75% of all breast cancers occur in women over the age of 50 years.[40] There is some controversy regarding the accuracy of both self-breast exams and mammography, however, it is recommended that breast examination be taught to all women, especially to those over the age of 50, and that a breast self-examination be done monthly. After the age of 40, the American Cancer Society recommends that women have a breast examination by a physician and a mammogram annually.[36]

Cervical cancer is accurately detected by a Pap test, however, many older women do not have Pap smears on a regular basis. For the most part, women diagnosed with cervical cancer after the age of 65 years are usually in the advanced stages of the disease, and 41% of all deaths from cervical cancer occur in women over the age of 65 years. Yearly screening using the Pap smear for 3 consecutive years is recommended by the American Cancer Society,[36] and if the test is negative for 3 years it is recommended that Pap tests be done at the discretion of the physician or at least once every 5 years thereafter.

Digital rectal examination is the best way to screen for prostate cancer in men. The American Cancer Society recommends that men receive a yearly screening for prostate cancer after the age of 40, and every 3 to 5 years after the age of 50 as the greatest incidence of this form of cancer occurs in the age range of 40 to 50 years.

A total skin examination is an important part of the routine physical examination. Inspection of the mouth is also recommended for those who are known smokers and for those who use excessive amounts of alcohol. Seventy-five percent of deaths from oral cancers occur in individuals 55 years of age and older.[41] Screening for oral cancer can be done routinely during periodic dental care, however, many elderly individuals do not go to the dentist on a regular basis, and it is recommended that oral screening be done by the physician or other health care personnel at community based screening clinics and health fairs since it is a noninvasive assessment.

Diabetes Mellitus

Over 4.5 million people in the United States over the age of 65 have diabetes mellitus.[41a] Diabetes has been found to contribute to cardiovascular diseases, end-stage renal failure, amputations, blindness, and peripheral neuropathies.[42] The American Diabetes Association[42] recommends that periodic serum glucose measurements be taken in the elderly population as the incidence of diabetes mellitus increases exponentially with increasing age. In known diabetics, the recommendations include periodic testing for asymptomatic bacteriuria, hematuria, and proteinuria by urinalysis screening.

Osteoporosis

The elderly population, particularly white females over the age of 60, have the highest risk for developing osteoporosis. Subtle changes in posture related to the breakdown of vertebral body height directly affect the individual's flexibility and strength. The person may report that he or she is "shrinking," or that he or she has pain in the cervical, thoracic, or lumbar region(s) of the back. Because height changes are frequently the first clinical indication of osteoporosis, regular screening should include height measurement. Reed and Birge[43] found that 75% of the elderly that they screened who had a 2 inch loss in height had osteoporotic changes on x-ray. Measuring height is a reliable, inexpensive, and noninvasive screening tool for osteoporosis.

Other valuable screening information for the evaluation for osteoporosis include nutritional information and dietary habits (e.g., calcium intake, excessive caffeine or soda consumption, or excessive protein intake), level of activity or inactivity, family history of osteoporosis, and alcohol and tobacco consumption. All of these factors have been found to have a contributory effect toward the development of osteoporosis. Low estrogen levels in women have also been found to influence the integrity of bone.[44] It is particularly important in postmenopausal women that height measurements be taken periodically to screen for osteoporotic changes. Since osteoporosis contributes to more than 1 million fractures in people over the age of 65 years annually,[44] screening becomes a vital component in the identification of risk factors and the prevention of accidental injury.

Health Habits

Nutrition, exercise levels, smoking, substance abuse, and medication use need to be considered when screening the elderly. Optimal health is the key factor in maintaining an independent and productive life. Health promotion and disease prevention activities have the potential of interrupting or slowing the progression of aging and disease before pathological changes become irreversible. The expected outcome of health promotion must reach beyond longevity toward an acceptable quality of life without debilitating physical or mental disabilities.[23,45] Preventive measures seek to detect the precursors that allow for early intervention and risk factors for disease that can be modified,[45a] because modification of personal health habits could have a potential impact on disease outcomes. For instance, smoking cessation improves physical stamina and lessens susceptibility to infections, while it reduces the risk of lung cancer and heart disease.[10]

To meet the needs of the elderly population, health care practitioners involved in screening strategies should educate individuals on ways to promote good health by adopting better life-style habits and a safer local environment, assist people to identify their own genetic/familial predispositions and risk factors for specific diseases, and promote public awareness of the myths, as well as the realities, pertaining to good health.[29]

One of the most significant advances in the past decade has been the convergence of opinion on what constitutes a "proper diet." Two documents, the 1988 *Surgeon General's Report on Nutrition and Health*[46] and the 1989 National Research

Council's *Report on Diet and Health,*[47] summarize the consensus of the scientific community and make dietary and health recommendations for the general public,[48] including reducing dietary fats and cholesterol; limiting salt intakes; limiting the use of alcohol; maintaining adequate but not excessive protein intakes; eating more fruits, vegetables, and complex carbohydrates; balancing caloric intake with expenditure to maintain a healthy weight; and avoiding the use of dietary supplements in excess of the NRC's recommended dietary allowances (RDAs). Both documents caution against unsafe dietary practices, health fads, and outright health fraud, much of which is directed at older persons.[46] Screening for nutritional problems is best accomplished by a registered dietitian, however, if this is not feasible, the collection of information on socioeconomic status, food supply, eating patterns, and self-perceived nutritional and dietary status is valuable in establishing the need for further counseling and education.

The effects of inactivity mimic the effects of aging.[49] Almost 50% of the functional decline attributed to aging may, in fact, be related to inactivity.[50] Increasing energy expenditure through exercise appears to influence mortality and morbidity through a number of complex physiological mechanisms (see Chapter 13).

Despite these benefits, there has been some reluctance in recommending fitness programs for elderly because exercising too intensely may injure muscles or joints, provoke heart attacks and irregular heart rhythms, increase blood pressure, and increase fall-related fractures.[51] Regular exercise training can increase protein turnover (37% higher muscle catabolism) in the elderly. As a result, elderly individuals prescribed an exercise program should be advised to increase their protein intake.[52] Some elderly are unable to maintain high-intensity training programs because of the weight reductions associated with the loss of lean muscle mass.[53] Therefore special attention to the dietary needs of the exercising elder need to be considered when prescribing a fitness program. It is important to determine the intensity, duration, and frequency of physical training to delay declines in functional capacity. These variables vary from one elderly individual to the next.

Combined with a calorie-appropriate diet, regular physical activity maintains a reasonable body weight, delays loss of lean muscle mass, and promotes good physical performance. A high activity level can predict survival for both institutionalized and people living in the community aged 60 to 90.[54,55] High-intensity training appears to decrease fat cell hypertension, increase insulin resistance, and slow the rate of decline of VO_2 max in older persons.[56–58]

Exercise programs designed for the elderly can reduce bone loss and strengthen skeletal muscle in both men and women of very advanced age,[56,59] thus decreasing the risk of falls and fractures.[60,61] For example, a group of sedentary men and women aged 86 to 96 years, including those with a past history of falling, increased the strength in the knee extensors by as much as 167% to 180% after an 8 week course in weight-lifting exercise.

It is never too late to quit smoking. At any age, cigarette smoking imposes higher risks of coronary heart disease, lung and mouth cancers, stroke, and osteoporosis.[62] Smoking cessation results in a decline of body nicotine within 6 months, a reduced risk of sudden heart attack in 1 to 2 years, and a lowered risk of cancer in about 15 years. Smoking combined with low calorie intakes can also compromise vitamin C status, which is essential in wound healing, infection, and maintenance of the connective tissue health. Smokers take two to three times longer to heal wounds, require longer to recover from acute illnesses such as pneumonia, and are twice as likely to die prematurely of coronary artery disease.[62]

The use of medications is another risk factor to look for when screening an elderly population. The 1991 National Disease and Therapeutic Index indicates that 42.7% of all prescription drugs are doled out to people 60 years of age and older in the United States. The average number of prescriptions per elderly American is 15.7, and there are over 9 million adverse drug reactions in people over the age of 65 years each year.[63] Normal aging results in changes in the way older adults absorb, metabolize, distribute, and excrete medications. The half-life of drugs is longer in the elderly and the cumulative effects of drugs last longer. Because the elderly are often existing on polypharmacy, they are more likely to overdose and experience adverse effects when medication combinations are inappropriate. Falls and fractures can be related to drug effects, for instance, β-blockers often induce an orthostatic hypotensive response on standing. Certain drugs actually induce neurological symptoms, such as tardive dyskinesia and parkinsonism, and many drugs create mental impairment. These drugs are discussed more thoroughly in Chapter 8. Additionally, noncompliance has been found to be a problem in close to 50% of the elderly.[63] Wolf and co-workers[63] found that the factors related to older persons not taking their medications were financial difficulties, language barriers, sensory deficits, accidental overdoses, and cognitive impairments.

Pharmacists often evaluate and monitor medication problems that may occur, but the elderly do not always go to the same pharmacy. Over 13% of all expenditures for medications by the elderly are for over-the-counter medications, which makes monitoring that much more difficult.[64] Screening and education for medication use often takes the form of health education programs (see Chapter 21) combined with a review of current medications by a pharmacist or nurse in a community screening program.

According to Maddox[65] over 5% of the elderly population abuse alcohol. "Late-onset" alcohol related problems occur in less than 1% of the elderly, however, because most were abusers before reaching the age of 65 years.[65] In addition, as an individual ages the alcohol tolerance diminishes: Less alcohol is required to produce intoxication in the elderly, so dependency may develop at a level of drinking that would not cause addiction in a younger individual. Willenbrig and Spring[66] have developed a screening tool that contains four questions and is accurate for identifying alcohol abuse 95% of the time. One question is designed to elicit subtle defensiveness while the other three directly ask about drinking habits and patterns. While individual screening by health care professionals is recommended, mass screening is not because of the low incidence of late-onset alcoholism and the fact that the screening has not been shown to lead to a decrease in morbidity or mortality.[28]

Drug abuse is not an issue in the elderly population. It can be expected, however, that as those individuals who use substances, such as cocaine, heroin, marijuana, and so forth, age, drug abuse may become a significant problem.

Sensory Deficits

Visual acuity testing in asymptomatic older adults should be done routinely. Although many older persons maintain nearly normal vision, their eyesight is subject to various changes and disabilities as discussed in Chapters 3 and 5. Yearly eye exams are recommended to detect the presence or progression of presbyopia, as well as the presence of disease. Three disorders—cataracts, glaucoma, and senile macular degeneration—are commonly found through screening.[28]

Anyone with impaired hearing should receive an otoscopic examination and audiometric testing. Between 30% and 60% of people over age 65 and up to 90% of nursing home residents in that age group are estimated to suffer from some degree of hearing loss.[67] Screening for hearing loss can range from a thorough history and interview of family members to testing by a clinical audiologist. A tuning fork is a wonderful screening tool. According to Alpert,[68] if the health care provider can hear the fork's hum when the client can no longer hear it and visual inspection of the ear shows no gross pathology (e.g., cerumen, serous otitis), then there is a hearing deficit. With a suspected hearing deficit, a more definitive audiometric screening by a trained individual can be easily employed in a community setting.

Psychological Problems

Elderly individuals should be specifically screened for depression and the potential for suicide. This screening needs to include a family history of depression/suicide, the presence of a chronic illness, recent loss (real or perceived), problems with sleep disorders, the presence of multiple somatic complaints, recent divorce or separation, unemployment, alcohol abuse, living alone, and the presence of prolonged bereavement. Depression is more prevalent in the older population than any other age group. White men, in particular, are at the highest risk for suicide. Alpert[68] recommended the Beck Depression Inventory as a reliable test in elderly populations.

Dementia

The Mental Status Questionnaire, Fact-Hand Test, and Dementia Rating Scale are frequently used along with screening for other mental, neurological, and physical deficits to determine if patients are suffering from dementia. In the early stages, however, it is difficult to distinguish true dementia from depression, the adverse effects of medication, and other mental and physical illnesses. Screening can only determine whether or not a problem exists, not what the underlying cause is. Magaziner and associates[69] were able to show that a shortened version of the Mini-Mental Status Examination could be used as a reliable predictor of scores on the longer version of the test. The shortened version makes screening easier and more cost effective.

Urinary Incontinence

Urinary incontinence affects a significant number of elderly persons. In fact, urinary incontinence contributes to nursing home admission in nearly half of those elderly admitted to long-term care facilities. Women have a weakening of the muscles of the pelvic floor and abdomen following pregnancy, which can be treated with Kegel exercises. In addition, birth injuries, hormonal changes, infections, tumors, or side effects of medications may cause urinary incontinence. Men develope urinary incontinence most often because of bladder or prostate disease. Causes of urinary incontinence need to be determined to prevent the need for institutionalization.

Safety

Elderly individuals account for almost 30% of all accidental deaths and about 15% of all hospitalized accident victims. Baker and Harvey[70] report that for every fall that results in a hip fracture, the incidence of mortality is higher. Decreased mobility, reduced independence, and a higher incidence of illness are common after a hip fracture. Impaired hearing and eyesight, slower physical reactions, poor balance and coordination, circulatory changes, orthostatic hypotension, and decreased physical stamina are among the reasons for the high accident rate in elders. For these reasons it is important to assess the older adult's risk for falls as well as the presence of fall hazards in the home. The US Consumer Product Safety Commission has developed a "Home Safety Checklist for Older Consumers" to help spot possible safety problems in the home. These were distributed through Area Agencies on Aging (AAAs) in 1986 to senior centers, public health departments, and other community groups. Copies may be obtained from the US Consumer Safety Commission, Washington, DC, 20207.

PRIMARY PREVENTION

Advancing primary prevention for those over the age of 65 requires a change in attitude that accepts the growing proof that individuals of any age may benefit from adopting health-promoting behaviors.[27] The attitude that diseases of old age are irreversible and inevitable needs to be dismissed. Life expectancy has been extended, accounting for the growth in population of those over the age of 85. In fact, those who are presently age 65 years can expect to live an average additional 17 years (19 years for women and 14.5 years for men).[22]

Primary preventive efforts directed at personal health practices are among the most effective interventions available to health care practitioners caring for older adults. Traditional clinical activities, such as routine unfocused testing, are generally of less value in preventing disease than counseling. Although demonstrated advantages of preventive services for older people are limited, emerging research is quite convincing. For instance, research on cancer etiology suggests that a 10- to 20-year latent period exists between events that may induce some cancers and the clinical expression of disease. Based on an average 15-year latency period, cancer detected after age 70 could have begun between ages 55 and 60 years. Therefore, many of the quarter of a million cancers induced in people after age 60 might have been prevented by primary prevention measures, such as smoking cessation and dietary changes.[71] Comprehensive screening strategies should be tailored to the individual risk profile of each elderly person.

Older individuals are more susceptible to acute diseases and episodes, such as infections, pneumonia, food poisoning, and orthostatic hypotension with resulting falls and injury.[72] Most of these conditions are preventable with proper intervention to maintain optimum health, thereby warding off these acute episodes. The growth of community "wellness" services or activities for older people signals a growing commitment to postponing disease and disabilities in older persons. Using Title IIIB grants from the federal government in response to Surgeon General Koop's efforts, 37 states had initiated community wellness programs for the elderly by 1985.[72]

Over the past 20 years, some of the major causes of morbidity and mortality in old age have declined, although the extent to which health promotion efforts are responsible has not been determined. Over these two decades, stroke deaths declined 55%, heart attacks decreased by 40%, and substantial progress had been made in hypertension control.[1] Evidence indicates that those who reach old age in good health tend to stay healthy until shortly before death, often well into the seventh or eighth decade of life.[73]

A COMMUNITY BASED SCREENING PROGRAM/MODEL PROJECT

Screening for Foot Problems

Many systemic diseases manifest themselves in the lower extremity, including diabetes, peripheral vascular disease, heart and kidney disease, arthritis, and nutritional deficiencies.[74-76] Many orthopedic conditions, arising from long-standing biomechanical imbalances, ill-fitting shoes, or both, plague the elderly patient and interfere with functional mobility. The most common foot disorders in individuals over the age of 65 years include pes planus (flat feet), excessive calluses, hallux abducto valgus, painful bunions, and toe deformities.[76,77] With advancing age the plantar fat pads atrophy,[78] resulting in increased stress on and microtrauma to the underlying soft tissue and osseous structures. Degenerative joint diseases compromise the articular surfaces of the joints of the foot, interfering with weight bearing and leading to decreased mobility. Circulatory changes further compromise the integrity of the tissues of the foot. Elders may not even be aware of losses in sensation to pain, pressure, and temperature. The loss of "protective sensation" to shoe pressures, wrinkles in the socks, or foreign objects in the shoe may be the beginning of a pressure point that may quickly become a callus or an open sore, which, if left untreated, may develop ulceration, infection, or gangrene, and lead to eventual amputation.[77-80] Routine foot screenings can help eliminate small problems and keep them from becoming larger.

Foot problems are the fourth leading cause of complaint in institutionalized elderly individuals.[75] Lack of ambulation and the ability to independently get to the bathroom are often reasons for admission to nursing homes. Individuals who are mobile and ambulatory in their own homes and community retain their dignity and generally live longer than those who are immobilized or institutionalized.[74,79]

Low-income elders are particularly at risk for poor foot care, because podiatric services are not covered by insurance companies. Elders who are on a fixed pension or receive a small social security check cannot afford out-of-pocket visits to have toe nails cut. Medicare will not cover the cost of protective shoe gear for the diabetic person at risk for amputation, but it will cover the cost of shoes following an amputation (as part of the prosthetic costs). Complications from foot problems are the cause of 20% of all diabetic admissions to hospitals, and 50% of all nontraumatic amputations in the United States occur in diabetics.[81] The financial burden of an amputation is enormous. Inpatient hospitalization, surgical procedures, and rehabilitation programs including prostheses, result in costs of $10,000 to $30,000. Both the personal and financial impacts of foot problems in diabetic patients are of serious magnitude. Preliminary findings from the Medicare Shoe Demonstration Project currently underway by Mathmatica (a research group contracted by the Health Care Financing Administration [HCFA]) in the states of New York, California, and Florida strongly supports the cost benefits of providing protective foot gear to diabetic patients.[80,82]

Low-income elders often wear shoes that are inadequate, ill-fitting, and therefore, dangerous. Ill-fitting shoes may create excessive pressure to the foot or repetitive pressures leading to foot lesions that are difficult to heal in the diabetic. Ill-fitting shoes increase the likelihood of falling and hip fractures are a major factor in the morbidity of elders.[83]

Medicare's lack of reimbursement for routine foot care forces elders to attempt self-care of the feet. Limited limb mobility, decreased eyesight, diminished sensation, and unsteady hands may lead to wounds that fail to heal and result in eventual amputation.

Foot care is a unique medical specialty that contributes to the physical, psychological, and social health of the elderly individual. Delivery of a comprehensive foot care program reduces the problems associated with foot pain and discomfort, lower extremity fatigue, and the secondary problems associated with lack of ambulation.

The "Community Foot Care Project" servicing low income elders in 14 communities in Central Massachusetts was inspired by the nonambulatory status of patients that were being admitted to hospitals and nursing homes. In one nursing home, 72% (based on an unpublished clinical data collection at Cushing Hospital in Framingham, Massachusetts) of the patients returned to an ambulatory status after receiving foot care, shoes, and orthotics. Preventing foot problems was key to keeping the community elders from becoming institutionalized elders. The foot care program was developed to screen low-income elders in the community for foot and medical problems, provide education on foot care, and dispense orthotics and free shoes.

The Foot Care Project uses an interdisciplinary team of a community coordinator, social worker, podiatrist, and physical therapist who work together to provide 18 community clinics held yearly in 14 different communities. The community coordinator schedules the clinics at community senior centers, and the social worker takes a detailed medical history on the 18 to 20 patients seen at each clinic. A podiatrist renders free nail cutting and debridement of excessive calluses, and the physical therapist evaluates the elder person for lower extremity problems and specific foot dsyfunction using the screening tool shown in Figure 14–1. After the initial evaluation in the community setting, if the screening reveals foot dysfunc-

Foot Screening Tool

Date _____

Name _____

Address _____

Phone (   ) _____

Sex _____ DOB _____

Language or Communication problems: ☐ No

☐ Yes   (describe) _____

Primary Doctor/Podiatrist _____

Address _____

Phone (   ) _____

SUBJECTIVE DATA

Medical History: _____

_____

1. Do you have:
   - ☐ Arthritis _____
   - ☐ Circulatory Problems_____
   - ☐ Heart Disease _____
   - ☐ Diabetes Mellitus _____
   - ☐ Kidney Problems _____
   - ☐ High Blood Pressure _____
   - ☐ Foot Problems _____
   - ☐ Eye Problems _____
   - ☐ Thyroid Problems _____
   - ☐ Hearing Problems _____
   - ☐ Vertigo _____
   - ☐ Dizziness _____
   - ☐ Fx hip _____

2. Did you have an injury in the:

	Left Leg		Right Leg	
	Sprain	Fx	Sprain	Fx
No				
Yes hip				
knee				
ankle				
foot				
back				

3. Are you experiencing any leg pain?

	Left Leg	Right Leg
No		
Yes Hip		
Knee		

If yes, describe:

	Left Leg	Right Leg
Night cramps		
Claudications		
Radiating		

Continued

Continued from previous page

4. Are you experiencing any foot pain?

	Left Leg	Right Leg
No		
Yes Aching		
Burning		
Stabbing		
Nail pain		
Shoe pain		
Met heads		
Toes		

Pain increased:	Left Leg	Right Leg
When standing		
When walking		
When wearing shoes		
In the morning		
In the afternoon		
At other times (describe)		

OBJECTIVE DATA

1. Ambulates without assistance?   ☐ No   ☐ Yes

2. Ambulates with assistive devices?   ☐ No   ☐ Yes

cane	
walker	
crutches	
other	

3. Falls?   ☐ No   ☐ Yes   describe _____

4. Distance ambulated?   ☐ Home   ☐ 1 block   ☐ 2 blocks   ☐ 5 blocks
   ☐ 1 mile   ☐ Unlimited

5. Regular exercise?   ☐ No   ☐ Yes

Continued

Continued from previous page

6. Examination of Feet (Removing shoes and stockings)

	Left Foot		Right Foot	
	Unacceptable	Acceptable	Unacceptable	Acceptable
Cleanliness of foot?				
Socks/stockings a good fit?				
Proper fitting shoes?	☐ Short		☐ Short	
	☐ Long		☐ Long	
	☐ Narrow		☐ Narrow	
	☐ Worn down		☐ Worn down	
Shoe Wear: Heel				
Sole				
Lateral Counter				

7. Problems

☐ Bunions

	Left Foot	Right Foot
HAV		
Taylor		

		Left Foot					Right Foot				
		I	II	III	IV	V	I	II	III	IV	V
☐ Calluses	Spin										
	Pinch										
	IPK										
	Sub										
	Shear										
☐ Corns	Met Heads										
	Heloma Molle										
	Heloma Durum										
☐ Involuted Nails											
☐ Ingrown Toenails											
☐ Nail Trophic Changes											

Continued

Continued from previous page

	Left Foot					Right Foot				
	I	II	III	IV	V	I	II	III	IV	V
☐ Circulatory Problems										

	Left Foot	Right Foot
	DPP: ☐ 0 PTP: ☐ 0	DPP: ☐ 0 PTP: ☐ 0
	☐ 1+ ☐ 1+	☐ 1+ ☐ 1+
	☐ 2+ ☐ 2+	☐ 2+ ☐ 2+
	☐ 3+ ☐ 3+	☐ 3+ ☐ 3+

		I	II	III	IV	V	I	II	III	IV	V
☐ Toe Clubbing											
☐ Toe Deformities	Hammer										
	Claw										
	Mallet										
	Crossing										
	Hallux										
		I	II	III	IV	V	I	II	III	IV	V

		Left Leg	Right Leg
☐ Foot/Ankle Deformities			
☐ Dermatitis/[PI]Fungus Infection			
☐ Dry, Scaly Skin			
☐ Edema	Foot		
	Ankle		
	Extremity		

☐ Infection (Describe) _____

☐ Other _____

ASSESSMENT

_____
_____
_____
_____
_____
_____
_____
_____

Continued

Continued from previous page

Recommend: ☐ None
                 ☐ Refer to orthotics clinic   Date: _____   Time: _____
                 ☐ Refer for shoes _____
                 ☐ Refer to pediatrist
                 ☐ Refer to podiatrist
                 ☐ Educated in _____
                 ☐ Orthotics fabricated   Date: _____ Time: _____

                   _____

                   2-month follow-up: Date: _____ Time: _____
                   6-month follow-up: Date: _____ Time: _____

Comments:

_____
_____
_____
_____
_____
_____
_____
_____
_____
_____
_____
_____
_____
_____
_____
_____
_____
_____
_____
_____
_____
_____
_____
_____
_____
_____
_____
_____
_____
_____
_____
_____

Figure 14–1.

tion or biomechanical problems leading to functional losses, the patient is scheduled for an outpatient clinic visit for orthotic fabrication and shoe distribution by the physical therapist and physical therapy intervention as needed for musculoskeletal/biomechanical problems. Patients return to the outpatient clinic for 2- and 6-month reassessments. Foot care is taught to family members when patients are unable to care for themselves. Knowledge of foot care (Fig. 14–2) is assessed by a questionnaire before and after treatment. Guidelines for foot care by the patient and family are provided and explained at the first visit (Fig. 14–3). This project is funded by a Federal III B grant from the Massachusetts Baypath Area Agency on Aging. Matched funds and resources are provided by Medicare and Rehabilitation Specialists, a geriatric rehabilitation service based in Norwood, Massachusetts. The Cushing Hospital physical therapy department in Framingham, Massachusetts was resourceful in securing the free shoes given to patients. Over 100 letters were drafted and sent to area stores and manufacturers of shoes asking for donations, which yielded 1500 pairs of shoes. Research projects were also established, with area shoe manufacturers donating 36 to 50 pairs of shoes for each of these projects. Shoe drives among hospital employees also yield numerous pairs of adequate shoes.

Goals for any community foot care program should be to promote pain-free ambulation, restore maximum function, maximize foot care knowledge and safety awareness and decrease hospitalizations related to foot problems.

To meet these goals the following methods are proposed

1. Offer foot care at community centers close to home for the greatest possible participation. (Greater participation was seen when the foot care team went to the patients rather than having them attend a hospital or outpatient-based clinic. For many, lack of transportation was a major deterrent to seeking help and needed foot care.)
2. Establish an easy screening tool that is reliable and highly reproducible.
3. Determine whether the foot dysfunctions are complications associated with tissue changes, biomechanical abnormalities, or chronic disease processes.
4. Provide easy to read literature and offer corrective treatment so that the elders can participate in community and personal activities.
5. Arrange the details for getting the patient to the outpatient clinic for orthotic fabrication and treatment.
6. Have local radio or newspaper spots explaining the service.
7. Team up with agencies conducting screening clinics (i.e., the American Diabetic Association) so that patients can be identified and treated within the same clinic appointment.

Resources for meeting these objectives are provided in Figure 14–4. It is evident from the remarkable response to the program that a desire for foot care and a willingness to participate in order to remain an active and useful member of the community was enhanced.

SPECIAL CONSIDERATIONS IN SCREENING PROGRAMS

The majority of elderly adults are highly motivated to seek out strategies for improving their health. Annual physical examinations provide screening for problems in the older adult, however, screening procedures are often not paid for by third-party payers, and regular check-ups become an out-of-pocket expense for the elderly. In many cases they are abandoned. Older adults seek acute care much more frequently than younger people.[22] This may be the result of incidious symptoms left unchecked by the lack of annual physical examinations. Additionally,

Foot Care Knowledge Questionnaire

Name: _____

Date: _____

1. Do you inspect your feet
   - A. Once a month
   - B. Once a week
   - C. Once a day

2. Do you wash your feet
   - A. Daily
   - B. Two times a week
   - C. Weekly

3. When you wash your feet do you use
   - A. Cool water
   - B. Lukewarm water
   - C. Hot water

4. At night do you walk around barefoot
   - A. Never
   - B. Sometimes
   - C. Always

5. Daytime, do you walk around barefoot
   - A. Never
   - B. Sometimes
   - C. Always

6. How often do you change your socks
   - A. Every day
   - B. Twice a day
   - C. Less than three times a week

7. Do you buy shoes that
   - A. Are tight and need to be broken in
   - B. Just fit
   - C. Are a little big

8. Do you
   - A. Trim your toenails straight across
   - B. Trim your toenails in a curve
   - C. Never trim your toenails

9. Do you treat your own corns/calluses
   - A. With a razor blade
   - B. With medicine to dissolve them
   - C. Wait for the podiatrist or other doctor

10. If you have a blister, do you
    - A. Open it up
    - B. Keep it covered so it does not pop open
    - C. Ignore it

Figure 14–2.

Self-Care Guidelines: Recommended Foot Care

1. Inspect feet daily for swelling, sores, cracks, reddened areas or cuts. Observation of bottom of feet can be done with a mirror.

2. Wash feet daily. Use mild soap and lukewarm water. Rinse thoroughly. Dry carefully and gently with clean, soft towel, especially between the toes.

3. If skin is dry, apply lanolin or other lubricating lotions or creams. Do not put lanoline or other preparations between toes or around the toenails. Avoid excess of lanolin or other preparations. Polysorb Hydrate, Carmol, or Nivea can be used.

4. Powder or cornstarch can be used when feet tend to perspire.

5. Do not go barefoot. Always protect feet, especially when on the beach or in swimming. Sharp stones, glass, cans, ringworm, ticks, chiggers, staples, pins are hazardous for feet.

6. Wear clean stockings or socks at all times. Avoid socks or elastics that constrict legs (i.e., knee socks with tight tops).

7. Break in new shoes gradually (wear for a few hours each day). Recommended heel height: 1/2″ for men, 3/4″ for women. No tapered or pointed shoes.

8. Check shoes before putting them on. Shake them to make sure nothing is in them.

9. Do not use hot water bottles or heating pads on feet.

10. Do not soak feet.

11. Never perform bathroom surgery. Go to your doctor or podiatrist about corns, calluses, ingrown toenails, bacterial and fungal infections, abscess, and lacerations.

12. Trim your toenails frequently. Cut them straight across and not too short.

13. Care of your feet should include doing exercise several minutes a day to speed up blood flow. Bend feet up and down and side to side, and move feet in circles at the ankle. When sitting, place your feet as high as your chair and NEVER CROSS YOUR LEGS!

14. When buying shoes you should have 1/2″ space in front of your longest toe and shoe shape should fit the contour of your foot. The best shoe is a tie shoe with a wide and deep toe box and strong heel counter.

15. Smoking constricts the blood vessels. Smoking is discouraged.

Figure 14–3. *(Courtesy of Jennifer M. Bottomley, M.S., P.T. and Hollis Herman, M.S., P.T. Department of Physical Therapy, Cushing Hospital)*

many older adults, especially the groups at highest risk, such as minorities (who make up 10% of the total elderly population) and those living at or below the poverty level (who make up 20% of the elderly population),[84] do not have their own physicians and are treated only on an acute-care basis through clinics and emergency rooms.

These problems need to be addressed through an interdisciplinary approach using a variety of community service settings. Groups, such as public health and

Patient Educational Resources

Krames Communications
312 90TH Street
Daly City, CA 94015-1898

Pamphlets:
1. The Foot Book (#1078)
2. Foot Owner's Manual (#1005)
3. Ankle Owner's Manual (#1073)
4. Foot Surgery (#1119)
5. Laser Foot Surgery (#1321)
6. Walking For Fitness (#1263)
7. Running (#1117)
8. Diabetes and Your Feet (#1372)

Thermal-Moldable Shoes, Inc
100 DeVille
Williamsville, NY 14221-4408

Pamphlet:
1. For Diabetics On the Go
2. For Arthritics On the Go
Thermold Shoes

P.W. Minor and Son, Inc
3 Treadeasy Avenue
P.O. Box 678
Batavia, NY 14021-0678

Extra Depth Shoes

The Langer Foundation
1011 Grand Blvd
Deer Park, NY 11729

Pamphlets:
1. Walking As an Exercise
2. "Facts for Runners and Other Athletes"
3. When Your Feet Hurt You Hurt All Over

Channing L. Bete Co., Inc
Scriptographic Booklet
South Deerfield, MA 01373

Pamphlet:
1. About Foot Care
2. Fun, Fitness and Your Feet

The Arthritis Foundation
Massachusetts Chapter
Parker Building
124 Watertown, MA 02172

Pamphlet:
1. Arthritis Surgery Information to Consider
2. Arthritis Basic Facts
3. Arthritis—Exercise and Your Arthritis
4. Arthritis—A Serious Look At the facts

Fund for Podiatry Education and Research
9312 Old Georgetown Road
Bethesda, MD 20814

Newsletter
"Foot News"

US Department of Health, Education, and Welfare
US Government Printing Office
Washington, DC 20402

Pamphlet:
Feet First—A Booklet About Foot Care

PAL Health Technologies, Inc
293 Herman Street
Perkin, IL 61554

Pamphlets:
1. Maybe You Need Orthotics
2. What Is Pronation?
3. Oh My Aching Feet!
4. Foot Surgery
5. Walking—Make It Easy On Yourself
6. Running . . . and Jogging
7. Skiing—Your Feet . . .
8. Ice Skating/Roller Skating

Department of Public Health
Center for Health Promotion
150 Tremont Street
Boston, MA 02111

Pamphlet:
Walking—A Lifetime Activity

Figure 14–4.

social services departments, senior centers, and area agencies of aging (AAAs), need to come together to identify potential barriers to the provision of health promotion, screening, and assessment programs. The collaborated effort will enable health care practitioners to pool information and resources and provide the most successful and well-attended programs for screening in the elderly.

CONCLUSION

Much emphasis has been placed on prevention. "We must protect what we can't replace," as some wise old gentleman once said. Helfand states, "Ambulation is many times the key or the catalyst between an individual remaining in a community living environment or being institutionalized."[79] The remarkable response to screening programs in the community setting demonstrates that elderly individuals desire preventive care and wish to remain active and useful members of the community.

PEARLS

- Prevention strategies can improve the quality of life and conserve health resources.

- "Successful aging" is a combination of good life-style and behavioral habits, including exercise, diet, and socioeconomic well-being.

- Resiliency of the human being is incredible.

- There is a need to change the health care approach from curative to preventive interventions. It is important to convince third-party payers through research efforts of the efficacy of preventive approaches.

- Primary, secondary, and tertiary prevention are the three levels of health intervention.

- Eighty-six percent of those aged 65 and older have at least one chronic disease.

- "We must protect what we can't replace."

REFERENCES

1. McGinnis JM. Year 2000 health objectives for the nation. In: *Surgeon General's Workshop on Health Promotion and Aging.* Washington, DC: US Dept of Health and Human Services, 1988:20–25.
2. Roybal ER. Elderly health care costs likely to rise to one-fifth of income. *Congressional Record.* March 23, 1989; E978–E980.
3. NCHS Health Statistics on Older Persons. *United States, 1986: Analytical and Epidemiological Studies.* Series 3. NCHS: Washington, DC: US Dept of Health and Human Services; Publication No. 25 (PHS):87–1409.
4. Sundwall D. Health promotion and Surgeon General's workshop. *Surgeon General's Workshop on Health Promotion and Aging.* Washington, DC: US Dept of Health and Human Services;1988.
5. Fisk CF. *Address, Opening Plenary Session.* Surgeon General's Workshop on Health Promotion and Aging. Washington, DC: US Dept of Health and Human Services; March, 1988.
6. Rowe JW, Kahn RL. Human aging—usual and successful. *Science.* 1987; 237:143–149.
7. Shore H. Therapeutic strategies and institutional care. In: Lesnoff-Caravaglia G, ed. *Handbook of Applied Gerontology.* New York: Human Sciences Press, Inc.; 1987; 447–452.

8. Department of Health and Human Services. *Recent Medicaid Cutbacks: Shocking Impacts on the Elderly*. HHS Pub. 148; 1992.

9. Wallack SS, Tompkins CP, Gruenberg L. A plan for rewarding efficient HMOs. *Health Affairs*. Summer, 1988; 80–96.

10. Havas S. Prevention of heart disease, cancer and stroke: the scientific basis. *World Health Forum*. 1987; 8:344–351.

11. Frame PS. Clinical prevention in primary care: the time is now! *J Fam Pract*. 1989; 29:150–156.

12. Liarson EG, Bruce RA. Exercise and aging. *Ann Intern Med*. 1986; 105:783–785.

13. Chernoff R. *Geriatric Nutrition: The Health Professional's Handbook*. Rockville, Md: Aspen Publishers; 1991.

14. Bogardus C, Ravussin E, Robbins DC, et al. Effects of physical training and diet therapy on carbohydrate metabolism in patients with glucose intolerance and noninsulin-dependent diabetes mellitus. *Diabetes*. 1984; 33:311–318.

15. Helmrich SP, Ragland Dr, Leung RW, et al. Physical activity and reduced occurrence of non-insulin-dependent diabetes mellitus. *N Engl J Med*. 1991; 325:147–152.

16. Astrand, PO. Exercise physiology and its role in disease prevention and in rehabilitation. *Arch Phys Med Rehabil*. 1987: 68:305–311.

17. Paffenbarger RS, Hyde RT, Wing AL, Hsieh CC. Physical activity, all-cause mortality and longevity of college alumni. *New Engl J Med*. 1986; 314:605–613.

18. Rogers R, Meyer J, Judd B, et al. Abstention from cigarette smoking improves cerebral perfusion among elderly chronic smokers. *JAMA*. 1985; 253(20):2:970–974.

19. McGinnis JM, Nestle N. The Surgeon General's report on nutrition and health: policy implications and implementation strategies. *Am J Clin Nutr*. 1989; 49(1):23–28.

20. Gladman JRF, Barer D, Venkatesan P, et al. The outcome of pneumonia in the elderly: a hospital survey. *Clin Rehab*. 1991; 5:201–205.

21. Webster JR. Prevention, technology, and aging in the decade ahead. *Top Ger Rehab*. 1992; 7(4):1–8.

22. Crimmins EM, Saito Y, Ingegneri D. Changes in life expectancy and disability-free life expectancy in the United States. *Pop Develop Rev*. June, 1989; 15(2):235–267.

23. Center for Disease Control. Comorbidity of chronic conditions and disabilities among older persons—United States, 1984. *MMWR*. 1989; 38:788–791.

24. Tinetti ME, Speechley M, Ginter SF. Risk factors for falls among elderly persons living in the community. *N Engl J Med*. 1988; 319(26):1701–1707.

25. Celentano D, Klassen A, Weisman C, et al. Cervical cancer screening practices among older women; results from the Maryland Cervical Cancer Case-Control Study. *Clin Epidemiology*. 1988; 41(6):531–541.

26. Garner B. Guide to changing lab values in elders. *Ger Nurs*. 1989; 10(3):144–145.

27. Ory MG. Considerations in the development of age-sensitive indicators for assessing health promotion. *Health Promotion*. 1988; 3(2):139–149.

28. Frame PS. A critical review of adult health maintenance: part 4. Prevention of metabolic behavioral and miscellaneous conditions. *J Fam Pract*. 1986; 23(1):29–39.

29. Koop CE. *Keynote Address, March 20–23, 1988: Surgeon General's Workshop on Health Promotion and Aging*. Washington, DC: US Dept of Health and Human Services; 1–4, 1988.

30. Pruzansky ME, Turano M, Luckey M, et al. Low body weight as a risk factor for hip fracture in both black and white women. *J Orthop Res*. 1989; 7(2):192–197.

31. Fried LP, Bush TL. Morbidity as a focus of preventive health care in the elderly. *Epidemiol Rev*. 1988; 10:48–64.

32. Woolf SH, Kamerow DB, Lawrence RS, et al. The periodic health examination of older adults: the recommendations of the US Preventive Service Task Force. *J Am Ger Soc*. 1990; 38:817–823.

33. Woolf SH, Kamerow DB, Lawrence RS, et al. The periodic health examination of older adults: the recommendations of the US Preventive Service Task Force. *J Am Ger Soc*. 1990; 38 (part II):933–942.

34. Linn M, Linn B. Self-Evaluation of Life Function (SELF) scale: a short, comprehensive self-report of health for elderly adults. *J Gerontol*. 1984; 39(5):603–612.

35. Safer M. An evaluation of the Health Hazard Appraisal based on survey data from a randomly selected population. *Pub Health Rep*. 1982; 97(1):31–37.

36. American Cancer Society. *Summary of Current Guidelines for the Cancer-related Checkup: Recommendations*. Atlanta, Ga: American Cancer Society; 1988. Pamphlet No. 334701-PE.

37. Winawer S. Screening for colorectal cancer: an overview. *Cancer.* 1980; 45(5 suppl):1093–1098.

38. Allison J, Feldman R. Cost benefits of hemoccult screening for colorectal carcinoma. *Dig Dis Sci.* 1985; 30(9):860–865.

39. Verbrugge LM. Long life but worsening health? Trends in health and morbidity of middle-aged and older persons. *Milbank Memorial Fund Quarterly/Health and Society.* 1989; 82:475–519.

40. Hayward R, Shapiro M, Freemen A, et al. Who gets screened for cervical and breast cancer? Results from a new national survey. *Arch Intern Med.* 1988; 148(5):1, 177–181.

41. American Cancer Society. *Cancer Facts and Figures.* New York: American Cancer Society; 1985.

41a. National Center for Health Statistics. Advance report of final mortality statistics. *Monthly Vital Statistics Report.* Hyattsville, Md: US Public Health Service; 1988. US Dept of Health and Human Services, publication PHS 88–1120;37:6(suppl).

42. American Diabetes Association. Position statement: office guide to diagnosis and classification of diabetes mellitus and other categories of glucose intolerance. *Diabetes Care.* 1992;15(suppl 2):4.

43. Reed A, Birge S. Screening for osteoporosis. *J Gerontol.* 1988; 14(7):18–20.

44. Dowd T. The female climacteric. *Nat OB-GYN Group.* 1990; 6:1:32–54.

45. Walker SN. Health promotion for older adults: direction for research. *Am J Health Promotion.* Spring 1989; 3(4):47–52.

45a. National Institutes of Health. Nutrition Coordinating Committee, Program in Biomedical and Behavioral Research and Training, 11th Annual Report of the National Institutes of Health. Washington, DC: US Dept of Health and Human Services; 1987: 111.

46. Surgeon General's Report on Nutrition and Health. *Dietary Fads and Frauds.* US Public Health Service. Washington DC: US Government Printing Office; 1988. US Dept of Health and Human Services publication No. 88–50210; Stock No. 017–001–00465–1.

47. Commission on Life Sciences, National Research Council. *Report on Diet and Health.* Washington, DC: National Academy Press; 1989.

48. McGinnis JM. *Promoting Health/Preventing Disease: Year 2000 Objectives for the Nation.* Office of the Assistant Secretary for Health, Office of Disease Prevention and Health Promotion. Washington DC: US Government Printing Office; 1989.

49. Drinkwater BL. *The Role of Nutrition and Exercise in Health. Continuing Dental Education.* Seattle, Wash: University of Washington; 1985.

50. Nieman DC. *The Sports Medicine Fitness Course.* Palo Alto, Calif: Bull Publishing, Co.; 1986.

51. Peck WA, Avioli LV. Physical exercise and bone health. In: *Osteoporosis the Silent Thief.* Washington, DC; American Association of Retired Persons; 1988.

52. Suominen H, Heikkinen E, Liesen H. Effect of 8 weeks endurance training on skeletal muscle metabolism in 56–70 year old men. *Eur J Appl Physiol.* 1987; 37:173–180.

53. Shepard RJ. *Physical Activity and Aging.* 2nd ed. Rockville, Md: Aspen Publishers, Inc.; 1987.

54. Kaplin GA, Seeman TE, Cohen RD, et al. Mortality among the elderly in the Alameda County study: behavioral and demographic risk factors. *Am J Pub Health.* 1987; 77(3):307–312.

55. Stones MJ, Dornan B, Kozma A. The prediction of mortality in elderly institution residents. *J Ger Psychol Sci.* 1989; 44(3):72–79.

56. Evans W. Exercise and muscle metabolism in the elderly. In: Hutchinson ML, Munro HN, eds. *Nutrition and Aging.* Orlando, Fl: Academic Press; 1986.

57. Craig BW, Garthwaite SM, Holloszy JO. Adipocyte insulin resistance: effects of aging, obesity, exercise, and food restriction. *Am Physiol Soc.* 1987; 62(1):95.

58. Wang JT, Ho LT, Tang KT, et al. Effect of habitual physical activity on age-related glucose tolerance. *J Am Ger Soc.* 1989; 37(3):203–209.

59. Smith EL, Gilligan C, Smith PE, et al. Calcium supplementation and bone loss in middle-aged women. *Am J Clin Nutr.* 1989; 50:833–842.

60. Tinette ME, Speechley M. Prevention of falls among the elderly. *N Engl J Med.* 1989; 320(16):1055–1059.

61. Blake AJ, Morgan K, Bendall MJ, et al. Falls by elderly people at home: prevalence and associated factors. *Age Ageing.* 1988; 17(6):365–372.

62. Hemenway D, Coldtz GA, Willet WC, et al. Fractures and lifestyle: effects of cigarette smoking, alcohol intake and weight on risk of hip fracture in middle-aged women. *Am J Pub Health.* 1988; 78:1554–1558.

63. Wolf S, Fugate L, Halstrand E, et al. *Worst Pills Best Pills.* Washington, DC: Public Citizen Health Research Group; 1988.
64. Gibson R, Waldo D. National health expenditures. *1980 Health Care Financing Rev.* 1981; 3:1–54.
65. Maddox G. Aging, drinking, and alcohol abuse. *Generations.* 1988; 12(4):14–16.
66. Willenbrig M, Spring W. Evaluating alcohol use in elders. *Generations.* 1988; 12(4):27–31.
67. Kart C, Metress E, Metress S. *Aging, Health and Society.* Boston: Jones & Bartlett; 1988.
68. Alpert M. Health screening to promote health for the elderly. *Nurse Pract.* 1987; 12(5):42–44,48–51,54–58.
69. Magaziner J, Bassett S, Hebel J. Predicting performance on the Mini-Mental Status Exam: use of age and education specific equations. *J Am Ger Soc.* 1987; 35(11):996–1000.
70. Baker S, Harvey A. Fall injuries in the elderly. *Clin Ger Med.* 1985;1(3):501–512.
71. Sorenson AW, Seltser R, Sundwall D. Primary cancer prevention as an attainable objective for the elderly. In: Yancik R, ed. *Perspectives on Prevention and Treatment of Cancer in the Elderly.* New York: Raven Press; Raven Press Aging Series: 1983:24.
72. Maloney S. Healthy older people. In: *Surgeon General's Workshop on Health Promotion and Aging.* Washington, DC: US Dept of Health and Human Services; March, 1988.
73. Munro HN. Aging and nutrition: a multifaceted problem. In: Hutchinson ML, Munro HN, eds. *Nutrition and Aging.* Orlando, Fl: Academic Press; 1986.
74. Collet BS. Podiatry and public health: a systematic approach. *Cur Podiatry.* 1979; 28:32–37.
75. Collet BS, Katzew AB, Helfand AE. Podiatry for the geriatric patient, *Annual Review of Gerontology/Geriatrics.* 1984; 4:221–234.
76. Evanski PM. The geriatric foot. In: Jahss M, ed. *Disorders of the Foot.* Philadelphia: WB Saunders; 1982:964–978.
77. Gould N, Schneider W, Ashikaga T. Epidemiological survey of foot problems in the continental United States: 1978–1979. *Foot Ankle.* 1980; 1:8–10.
78. Helfand AE. *Clinical Podogeriatrics.* Baltimore: Williams and Wilkins; 1981.
79. Helfand AE. Common foot problems in the aged and rehabilitative management. In: Williams TF, ed. *Rehabilitation in the Aging.* New York: Raven Press; 1984:291–303.
80. Soulier SM. The use of running shoes in the prevention of plantar diabetic ulcers. *J of Am Podiatric Med Assoc.* 1986;76(7):395–400.
81. Bessman AN. Foot problems in the diabetic. *Comprehensive Ther.* 1991; 8(1):32–38.
82. Mathmatica. *The Medicare Shoe Demonstration Project: Preliminary Findings.* Summary for HCFA, Unpublished document; October, 1990.
83. Jette AM, Harris BA, Cleary PD. Functional recovery after hip fracture. *Arch Phys Med Rehab.* 1987; 68:735–740.
84. American Association of Retired Persons (AARP). *A Profile of Older Americans.* Washington, DC; 1988. AARP pamphlet No. PF3049 (1228)-D996.

Communication

Normal Changes with Age Affecting Communication	Ethnicity
	The Team
Hearing	Writing
Vision and the Other Senses	Compliance and Motivation
Voice Changes with Age	Conclusion

A patient gets better, a child graduates from college, a pain is felt, a new idea comes to mind, and yet this information is unable to be communicated. Why? Is it old age? Is it because the recipients of the information do not understand? Is there some pathological process that is going on that is impairing the communication process?

This chapter will attempt to answer some of these questions. The first section will explore the older individual in terms of normal and pathological changes with age that impact communication. A special section discusses the ethnic influences on aging and communication. Impediments and enhancements to communication with the health professional will also be examined. The final sections of this chapter will explore writing skills and the important topic of compliance and motivation.

NORMAL CHANGES WITH AGE AFFECTING COMMUNICATION

Hearing

Normal Changes with Age Affecting Hearing

Hearing loss is second only to arthritis as the most common physical complaint of the aged.[1] Statistics show that approximately 24 million persons over the age of 65 suffer from hearing loss.[1] In addition, with each consecutive decade after 70, the prevalence of those affected increases dramatically.[1]

Changes in the major structures of the ear establish the three main types of hearing loss: conductive, sensorineural, and mixed. Conductive hearing loss is a result of changes in the outer or middle ear that blocks the acoustic energy. The changes in the external and middle ear follow.

Changes in the external ear

1. Decreased sensation that causes the patient to be unaware of a build-up of wax.
2. Excess hair growth in the outer ear, especially in men, that can aid in the accumulation of wax.
3. A decrease in the wax-producing glands and a subsequent tendency for the wax to become drier.

Changes in the middle ear

1. The tympanic membrane becomes more rigid and translucent with age.
2. Negative pressure in the middle ear as a result of a decrease in the elasticity and displacement of tissue in the nasopharynx causes the eustachian tube to resist opening.[2]

Sensorineural hearing loss occurs because of changes in the inner ear. These changes follow.

Changes in the inner ear

1. Death of hair cells in the cochlea.
2. Damage to the basilar membrane within the cochlea.[3]

Mixed disorders are a combination of sensorineural and conductive. In general, conductive hearing disorders may be reversed, sensorineural disorders cannot, and mixed disorders can be partially reversed.

A common term used to describe the hearing loss of old age is presbycusis. This general type of hearing loss is sensorineural and, therefore, not reversible. The characteristics of presbycusis are

1. A reduced sensitivity to high-pitched sounds, such as sh, s, t, z, v, f, ch, and g.
2. Bilaterally the hearing loss is equal.
3. Men are more affected than women.
4. A decreased hearing of pure tones.

The hearing loss often associated with old age is usually insidious. It gradually appears, and often patients do not realize that they are misinterpreting communications. For example, when an older person with presbycusis is asked, "How old are you?" The answer may be "fine." This inappropriate response may lead to frustration on the part of the patient, family, and health professional. In addition, the older person with hearing loss may feel depressed, isolated, and angry.[4]

Pathological Changes with Age Affecting Hearing

The classification, manifestation, and approach to the pathological changes with age affecting hearing are similar to the normal changes already listed. In conductive hearing loss, some of the common causes might be infection and otosclerosis.[2] In the area of sensorineural changes, some causes may be drug toxicity, brain tumor, or Meniere's disease.[2] Finally, in mixed disorders, a foreign body or an infection can cause the problem.

Evaluation

For both normal and pathological changes in hearing with aging, thorough screening is imperative to delineate the cause and type of hearing loss. Table 15–1 lists several signs of hearing impairment.

In addition, once a person is suspected of having a hearing loss, the "Hearing

TABLE 15–1. CLUES TO DETECTING HEARING IMPAIRMENT

The person states that words are difficult to understand.

The person is unable to hear high-pitched sounds (a faucet dripping, high notes of a violin).

The patient may complain of a continuous hissing or ringing background noise.

The person ceases to enjoy concerts, TV programs, and social get-togethers because he or she is unable to understand much of what is being said.

The person understands a conversation that takes place in a quiet room, but misunderstands most of the conversation when the room is noisy.

The person can participate in a conversation with one other person but has difficulty if two or more conversations are going on.

You may need to get the person's attention before speaking to him or her.

The person understands you when you are speaking face to face but is confused when your back is turned or your mouth isn't clearly visible. This person may be "speech-reading" (watching lips, facial expressions, and gestures) to understand the message.

The person becomes angry and frustrated when he or she misunderstands something.

The person may attempt to blame hearing loss on outside factors. He or she may accuse you of talking too fast or of mumbling or they may say, "It's too noisy in here."

The person becomes irritable and tires easily during conversation, because listening is hard work.

The person may become annoyed when spoken to loudly (recruitment). This occurs commonly with presbycusis.

Reprinted with permission from Dwyer B. Detecting hearing loss and improving communication in elderly persons. In: Focus on Geriatric Care & Rehabilitation. Rockville, Md: Aspen Publishers; 1987;1(16)3–4.

Handicap Inventory" can be administered. This test evaluates the person's response to the hearing loss emotionally and socially. Figure 15–1 is a sample hearing handicap test.

After the hearing-impaired person completes this test, the care giver totals the numerical value of the responses for a total score and two subscores delineating values for the emotional and social/situational areas. Patients who avoid social encounters and are becoming emotionally isolated are identified by a high "S" score value. Persons whose emotional supports are weak would score high points in the "E" category.

A rough estimate of total scores is as follows[2]:

- 0–16   The individual does not have a perceived handicap due to hearing loss. These persons either have little objective hearing loss or enjoy adequate coping skills.

- 17–42   The person has a mild-to-moderate self-perceived handicap. This person requires evaluation for other stressors and may need help with realistic goal setting, defining needs, and following through with care.

- 43+   The person's coping skills are extremely limited. This person requires concrete direction in terms of self-care and seeking proper assistance for the hearing loss.

Interventions

Interventions for hearing loss range from specific rehabilitation programs to appropriate assisstive devices (i.e., hearing aides). In addition, the health team can keep in mind measures and aides to communication (Tables 15–2 and 15–3).

The Hearing Handicap Inventory for the Elderly

The purpose of this scale is to identify the problems your hearing loss may be causing you. Answer YES, SOMETIMES, or NO for each question. *Do not skip a question if you avoid a situation because of your hearing problem.* If you use a hearing aid, please answer the way you hear *without* the aid.

		YES (4)	SOME-TIMES (2)	NO (0)			YES (4)	SOME-TIMES (2)	NO (0)
S-1.	Does a hearing problem cause you to use the phone less often than you would like?	☐	☐	☐	E-14.	Does a hearing problem cause you to have arguments with family members?	☐	☐	☐
E-2.	Does a hearing problem cause you to feel embarrassed when meeting new people?	☐	☐	☐	S-15.	Does a hearing problem cause you difficulty when listening to TV or radio?	☐	☐	☐
S-3.	Does a hearing problem cause you to avoid groups of people?	☐	☐	☐	S-16.	Does a hearing problem cause you to go shopping less often than you would like?	☐	☐	☐
E-4.	Does a hearing problem make you irritable?	☐	☐	☐	E-17.	Does any problem or difficulty with your hearing upset you at all?	☐	☐	☐
E-5.	Does a hearing problem cause you to feel frustrated when talking to members of your family?	☐	☐	☐	E-18.	Does a hearing problem cause you to want to be by yourself?	☐	☐	☐
S-6.	Does a hearing problem cause you difficulty when attending a party?	☐	☐	☐	S-19.	Does a hearing problem cause you to talk to family members less often than you would like?	☐	☐	☐
E-7.	Does a hearing problem cause you to feel "stupid" or "dumb"?	☐	☐	☐	E-20.	Do you feel that any difficulty with your hearing limits or hampers your personal or social life?	☐	☐	☐
S-8.	Do you have difficulty hearing when someone speaks in a whisper?	☐	☐	☐	S-21.	Does a hearing problem cause you difficulty when in a restaurant with relatives of friends?	☐	☐	☐
E-9.	Do you feel handicapped by a hearing problem?	☐	☐	☐	E-22.	Does a hearing problem cause you to feel depressed?	☐	☐	☐
S-10.	Does a hearing problem cause you difficulty when visiting friends, relatives, or neighbors?	☐	☐	☐	S-23.	Does a hearing problem cause you to listen to TV or radio less often than you would like?	☐	☐	☐
S-11.	Does a hearing problem cause you to attend religious services less often than you would like?	☐	☐	☐	E-24.	Does a hearing problem cause you to feel uncomfortable when talking to friends?	☐	☐	☐
E-12.	Does a hearing problem cause you to be nervous?	☐	☐	☐	E-25.	Does a hearing problem cause you to feel left out when you are with a group of people?	☐	☐	☐
S-13.	Does a hearing problem cause you to visit friends, relatives, or neighbors less often than you would like?	☐	☐	☐					

FOR CLINICIAN'S USE ONLY: Total Score: _____
Subtotal E: _____
Subtotal S: _____

Figure 15–1. *(Reprinted with permission from Ventry I, Weinstein B. The hearing handicap inventory for the elderly: a new tool. In: Ear Hear. Baltimore: Williams & Wilkins; 1982; 128–134.)*

TABLE 15–2. COMMUNICATING WITH THE HEARING IMPAIRED

Keep the following measures in mind

Get the person's attention by calling his or her name but do not shout or touch the person first, since this may startle him or her.

Keep your conversation focused and introduce the topic (for example, "Mr A, I'd like to talk with you about your family"). The person then can focus on ideas and key words. Let the person know when you are going to change topics.

If the person does not understand you, phrase your thought differently rather than repeating the same statement over and over. Repetition only leads to frustration.

Face the person directly during conversations. A distance of 3 to 6 feet is ideal. In group situations, no speaker and listener should be more than 6 feet apart.

Your face should be visible to the listener. Do not eat, chew gum, or smoke while talking to hearing-impaired persons.

Do not speak to hearing-impaired persons from another room or while they are concentrating on an activity, such as reading or watching television.

Speak at a slightly greater than normal loudness and at a normal rate.

Do not overarticulate. This distorts the sounds of speech and the speaker's face, thus limiting the use of cues from facial expression.

Reduce the amount of background noise when carrying on conversations. Turn off the radio or TV. If there are other conversation nearby, move to a quieter area.

Be certain that hearing-impaired persons wear their eyeglasses and hearing aids, if they have these devices.

Use body language, facial expressions, and gestures to help convey what you have to say.

Never speak directly into the person's ear. Although this amplifies the sound of your voice, it decreases clarity, and the listener is unable to make use of visual cues.

Provide a public address system for group situations or meetings. Many elderly persons complain that they enjoy meetings, but for various reasons the speaker avoids using a microphone.

Reprinted with permission from Dwyer B. Detecting Hearing Loss and Improving Communication in Elderly Persons. In: Focus on Geriatric Care & Rehabilitation. Rockville, Md: Aspen Publishers, 1987;1(6):6.

TABLE 15–3. AIDS TO COMMUNICATION

The following tips are for hearing-impaired individuals, who by definition experience difficulty communicating.

Do not strain to hear or to read lips. A combination of hearing and seeing enables you to understand most speakers better.

Watch the speaker carefully so that you can observe the lips, as well as other body language.

Look for ideas rather than isolated words. As you become familiar with the rhythm of a person's speech, you will pick up key words that will help you put together what the speaker is trying to communicate.

Position yourself directly across from the speaker. Avoid facing a bright light.

Try to determine the subject under discussion as quickly as possible. Ask your friends to give you a lead, such as, "We are talking about the housing situation."

Remember that conversation is a two-way affair. Do not monopolize it in an attempt to control it. Listening takes more energy, but you learn more.

Don't be afraid that people will think you are staring at them while you are trying to understand what they are saying. It is always polite to look at the person who is talking to you.

Tell the speaker what part of what he or she said that you don't understand. Merely saying, "I didn't understand," does not provide the necessary information to correct your problem. Let speakers know that they are talking too softly, that their hand is in front of their mouth, and so on.

If you don't understand something, ask the speaker to rephrase the statement. If you have understood some part of what has been said, use those words in your question, asking the speaker to supply the words you have missed.

Don't get into the habit of allowing anyone else, such as your spouse of friends, to speak or listen for you.

Everyone needs time to relax. At such times, a person simply does not listen. Allow yourself the luxury of withdrawing at times, but do not confuse this with your hearing loss.

Reprinted with permission from Dwyer B. Detecting hearing loss and improving communication in elderly persons. In: Focus on Geriatric Care & Rehabilitation. Rockville, Md: Aspen Publishers, 1987;1(6):6.

Vision and the Other Senses

Hearing obviously impacts communication. Nevertheless, changes in the other senses also impact communication. The major, but normal, change with age in vision, called presbyopia, begins as early as the fourth decade. (For specific information on presbyopia and vision changes, see Chapter 3.) Most vision deficits normally caused by aging can be managed by changes in lenses.[5] In addition, environmental modifications can enhance communication as well as ensure safety.[6]

The literature also notes a decline in the senses of touch, taste, and smell.[7] Lack of information in these areas can alter normal communication. Suggestions for health professionals in this area are

1. Try to use touch as much as possible to enhance communications.
2. Bring in the other senses as much as possible. For example, describe the smell of the bread the patient is making or the roses they just received.
3. Instruct the family or staff in methods of seasoning food to enhance the sense of taste (i.e., different healthy seasonings).
4. Make a mental checklist to include the other senses in a treatment session (for example, show the patient the menu for the day, and discuss the taste and smell of the food).

Voice Changes with Age

A person's ability to vocalize is another important variable in communication. Studies on voice cues alone have shown that older speakers tend to be negatively rated as compared to younger speakers.[8,9] There are normal changes that occur with age in the voices of men and women, however, they do not cause significant problems with communication. Men, according to Honjo and Isshiki,[10] experience a higher fundamental frequency due to "vocal fold atrophy." Women, on the other hand, experience a lower frequency due to a slight hoarseness and vocal fold edema.[10]

Normal aging changes can affect voice production. A list of the changes with age in the human body that can affect speech follows.

1. Reduced respiratory efficiency caused by
   a. Degeneration of vertebral discs (senile kyphosis).[11]
   b. Decreased elasticity of the rib cartilages, as well as ossification, and calcification of these cartilages.[12]
   c. Reduced recoil and elasticity of the lungs[13] resulting in lower frequencies, decreased loudness, and shortening of the length of utterances per breath.[14]
2. Changes in the oral cavity caused by
   a. Changes in the structure of the lower jaw.
   b. Loss of dentition.
   c. Weakening and loss of sensitivity of the pharyngeal muscles.
   d. Reduced activity of the salivary glands.[15]
   e. Atrophy of the lips and tongue[16] resulting in an alteration in resonance, increased nasality, and reduced articulatory accuracy.
3. Changes in the laryngeal cavity caused by
   a. The laryngeal cartilages undergoing ossification and calcification.
   b. Drying out of the laryngeal mucosa.
   c. Reduced vascular supply to the mucosa.
   d. Progressive thinning and shortening of the vocal folds resulting in vocal tremors, roughness, breathiness, and hoarseness.[17]

As mentioned earlier, the changes listed essentially have minimal effect on communication; however, pathological causes, such as dysarthria, apraxia, aphasia, dementia, laryngectomy, and chronic obstructive pulmonary disease (COPD), can cause significant impairment in communication (Table 15–4).

TABLE 15–4. PATHOLOGICAL CAUSES OF IMPAIRED COMMUNICATION

Name	Characterized By	Disease Associated	Speech Muscles	Communication
Flaccid dysarthria	Damage to the peripheral nervous system Cranial nerve Motor muscle Spinal or cranial nerve axons Myoneural junctions	Bulbar palsy Myasthenia gravis Muscular dystrophy Polymyositis	Weak Hypotonic	Slurred Slow Breathy Weak Hypernasality
Spastic dysarthria	Damage to central nervous system Bilateral upper motor neuron lesions	Multiple cerebrovascular accidents (CVA) Multiple sclerosis (MS) Traumatic brain injury	Hypertonicity Disintegration of movement	Slow Labored Low pitch Imprecise consonants Monopitch Hypernasality
Ataxic dysarthria	Damage to cerebellum or its tracts	CVAs Tumors MS Toxic or metabolic disorders Encephalitis	Uncoordination of force, speed, timing, range, and direction	Imprecise consonants Inconsistent nasality Scanning speech Vocal tremor Loudness variation
Dyskinetic dysarthria	Damage to extrapyramidal motor system Hypokinetic Hyperkinetic	Parkinson's disease Epilepsy Tics Chorea Ballism Encephalitis	Rigidity Reduced range of force Tremor at rest Abnormal Interrupted	Monopitch loudness Breathy or hoarse Short rushes of speech Difficulty initiating speech Erratic changes in pitch and loudness Intermittent hypernasality Harshness
Mixed dysarthria	Damage to multiple lesions in the central nervous system	Multiple strokes Tumors Head trauma Degenerative disease—ALS or MS	Combination of hypokinetic and hyperkinetic depending on motor system affected	Combination of hypokinetic and hyperkinetic depending on motor system affected
Wernicke's aphasia	Damage to the left cerebral hemisphere (posterior lesion of temporal lobe)	CVA Brain tumor Cerebral trauma Cerebral infection Intracranial surgical procedures		Impaired auditory comprehension Fluent, flowing verbal output, low in information Word substitution
Broca's aphasia	Damage to the left cerebral hemisphere (anterior lesion of frontal lobe)			Restricted vocabulary and grammar Word retrieval difficulties Slow, labored, halting
Verbal apraxia	Same—coexists with Broca's aphasia			Impairment in motor programming, not muscle function Difficulty initiating speech Inconsistent articulation errors
Right hemisphere	Damage to right hemisphere (nondominant side of brain)	CVA		Attention and perceptual deficits Unable to comprehend emotional and perceptual tone Flat effect, monotone

(continued)

TABLE 15–4. PATHOLOGICAL CAUSES OF IMPAIRED COMMUNICATION (CONT.)

Name	Characterized By	Disease Associated	Speech Muscles	Communication
Dementia	Progressive degeneration to central nervous system	Hydrocephalus Alzheimer's Vitamin deficiency Multi-infarct dementia Endocrine disorders Pick's disease (See Chapter 4 for further listing)		**Initial stage** Fluent conversation with elaborate detail Reduced attention and memory Disorientation Repetition and blame **Mid stages** As above plus word-finding deficits Perservative responses Self-correction absent **Advanced** Unable to communicate or understand Echolalia
Laryngec-tomy	Surgical removal of larynx due to cancer	Cancer	No muscles of speech in larynx	No voice—person communicates with facial expression and writing Uses esophagal muscles to speak
COPD	Chronic airflow obstruction with reversible or irreversible components	Emphysema Bronchitis Asthma		Restricted loudness and pitch range Chronic hoarseness Difficulty with energy expenditure of talking

Evaluation of pathologies of the voice should be done by a trained speech and language professional. The treatment, however, cannot be done solely by these professionals. To maximize the benefits of treatment, the family, staff, and rehabilitation team must become involved. Table 15–5 provides a list of strategies for improving communication for the various pathologies already noted.[3]

ETHNICITY

How can a person's origins, rules, and contrasts affect communication between the person, family, and health professional? Is cultural diversity a major concern when looking at the demographics in the United States? To answer the latter question first, by the year 2000, 30% of the US population will be Asian, Hispanic, Native American, and African-American.[18] Often, people tend to overgeneralize or overemphasize cultural differences and therefore miscommunicate. Table 15–6 provides a list of possible verbal and nonverbal miscommunication sources between cultural groups.[19]

So how does one work most effectively with cultural differences? Like other areas of human intervention, the therapist must make an appropriate evaluation of the situation. Table 15–7 provides examples of assessment categories for ethnic behavior.[20]

The therapist should consider this checklist when working with older adults; however, prior to implementing any intervention the therapist should rank its importance. In a study done by Chee and Kane,[21] the priority of ethnic factors was addressed. They discovered that Japanese-Americans highly rated ethnic factors in a nursing home, such as similar ethnic background of staff, ethnic foods, program-

TABLE 15–5. STRATEGIES FOR IMPROVING COMMUNICATION

Aphasia

1. Be familiar with the person's level of comprehension and adjust rate, length, and complexity of language to a level at which the person can respond with success.
2. Use concrete, familiar vocabulary in short, clear sentences.
3. Use gesture and facial expression to augment what is said, or demonstrate the information you are trying to convey.
4. Provide written and visual cues.
5. Phrase questions for short responses, multiple choice, or yes/no responses.
6. Rephrase a message if not understood initially.
7. Give the person adequate time to respond.
8. Encourage the aphasic person to use gestures, facial expressions, and writing, if appropriate, to augment what is said.
9. Let the person know that you have understood the message by repeating it back conversationally.
10. Be patient and supportive to reduce any stress associated with communicating.
11. Treat the person as an adult at all times.

Right Hemisphere Dysfunction

1. Minimize external distractions in the environment.
2. Position yourself and any materials within the person's visual field if he or she has a left visual field defect.
3. Establish eye contact to ensure attention to the conversation.
4. Provide orienting materials like clocks and calendars.
5. Provide structured activities.
6. Help the person structure responses by cueing with relevant details; if the person goes off on a tangent, cue him or her back to the topic at hand.
7. Be concrete and direct in language use; avoid figurative language and sarcasm.
8. This person may not understand lengthy, complex directions, so repeat and rephrase to assure understanding of important details.

Dementia

1. Establish eye contact prior to addressing the person to ensure attention.
2. Use short, grammatically simple, and concrete input. Avoid the use of pronouns.
3. Keep to one topic at a time. Be redundant; repeat and rephrase critical information.
4. Provide multisensory input, both visual and tactile, to enhance comprehension. For example, provide illustrations or photographs, write down key words, or use gesture and demonstration.
5. Ask yes/no and either/or questions.
6. Provide external orientation and memory aids, such as name bracelets, reminder signs, and calendars.
7. Share successful communication techniques with the patient's care givers.

Dysarthria

1. Communicate in a quiet, nondistracting environment.
2. Encourage the person to speak at a slower rate.
3. Have the person exaggerate production of consonants and separate syllables within words.
4. Encourage the use of shorter utterances compatible with breath support and meaning.
5. Provide honest feedback about the intelligibility of the message.
6. Provide appropriate feedback about loudness level.
7. Become familiar with the person's alternate or augmentative communication methods, such as language boards and gestures.

Laryngectomy

1. Talk in a quiet environment.
2. Consider facial expressions, gestures, speech-reading cues, and situational and linguistic context, if you have difficulty understanding the person.
3. Ask the person to repeat a message if it is not understood.
4. Provide support and encouragement for the use of the new voice.

Chronic Obstructive Pulmonary Disease

1. Encourage short utterances compatible with breath supply.
2. Encourage a reduced rate of speech.
3. Do not engage in conversation while the person is involved in physical activity.

Reprinted with permission from Cherney L. Aging and communication. In: Lewis C, ed. Aging: The Health Care Challenge. Philadelphia: Davis; 1989.

TABLE 15–6. SOME POSSIBLE VERBAL AND NONVERBAL SOURCES OF MISCOMMUNICATION BETWEEN CULTURAL GROUPS

Blacks	Opposing View	Hispanics	Opposing View
• Touching of one's hair by another person is often considered offensive.	• Touching of one's hair by another person is a sign of affection.	• Hissing to gain attention is acceptable.	• Hissing is considered impolite and indicates contempt.
• Preference for indirect eye contact during listening, direct eye contact during speaking as signs of attentiveness and respect.	• Preference for direct eye contact during listening and indirect eye contact during speaking as signs of attentiveness and respect.	• Touching is often observed between two people in conversation.	• Touching is usually unacceptable and usually carries a sexual overtone.
• Public behavior may be emotionally intense, dynamic, and demonstrative.	• Public behavior is expected to be modest and emotionally restrained. Emotional displays are seen as irresponsible or in bad taste.	• Avoidance of direct eye contact is sometimes a sign of attentiveness and respect; sustained direct eye contact may be interpreted as a challenge to authority.	• Direct eye contact is a sign of attentiveness and respect.
• Clear distinction between "argument" and "fight." Verbal abuse is not necessarily a precursor to violence.	• Heated arguments are viewed as suggesting that violence is imminent.	• Relative distance between two speakers in conversation is close.	• Relative distance between two speakers in conversation is farther apart.
• Asking "personal questions" of someone one has met for the first time is seen as improper and intrusive.	• Inquiring about jobs, family, and so forth of someone one has met for the first time is seen as friendly.	• Official or business conversations are preceded by lengthy greetings, pleasantries, and other talk unrelated to the point to business.	• Getting to the point quickly is valued.
• Use of direct questions is sometimes seen as harassment (e.g., asking when something will be finished is seen as rushing that person to finish).	• Use of direct questions for personal information is permissable.		

Asians	Opposing View
• Touching or hand-holding between members of the same sex is acceptable.	• Touching or hand-holding between members of the same sex is considered as a sign of homosexuality.
• Hand-holding/hugging/kissing between men and women in public looks ridiculous.	• Hand-holding/hugging/kissing between men and women in public is acceptable.
• A slap on the back is insulting.	• A slap on the back denotes friendliness.
• It is not customary to shake hands with persons of the opposite sex.	• It is customary to shake hands with persons of the opposite sex.
• Finger beckoning is only used by adults to call little children and not vice-versa.	• Finger beckoning is often used to call people.

Blacks (continued):
Blacks	Opposing View
• Interruption during conversation is usually tolerated. Access to the floor is granted to the person who is most assertive.	• Rules of turn-taking in conversation dictate that one person has the floor at a time until all points are made.
• Conversations are regarded as private between the recognized participants. "Butting in" is seen as eavesdropping and is not tolerated.	• Adding points of information or insights to a conversation in which one is not engaged is seen as being helpful.
• Use of expression "you people" is seen as pejorative and racist.	• Use of expression "you people" tolerated.
• Accusations or allegations are general rather than categorical and are not intended to be all-inclusive. Refutation is the responsibility of the accused.	• Stereotypical accusations or allegations are all-inclusive. Refutation or making exception is the responsibility of the person making the accusation.
• Silence denotes refutation of accusation. To state that you feel accused is regarded as an admission of guilt.	• Silence denotes acceptance of an accusation. Guilt is verbally denied.

American Indians	Opposing View
• Personal questions may be considered prying.	• Personal questions are acceptable particularly when establishing case history information.
• Gushing over babies may endanger the child.	• Gushing over babies shows admiration of the child.
• A bowed head is a sign of respect.	• Lack of eye contact is sign of shyness, guilt, or lying.
• It is acceptable to ask the same question several times, if you doubt the truth of the person.	• It is a sign of inattention if the same question is asked several times.

Reprinted with permission from Cole L. E Pluribus Unum: Multicultural Imperatives for the 1990s and Beyond. Rockville, Md: American Speech–Language–Hearing Association; September 1989; 69.

TABLE 15–7. ASSESSMENT CATEGORIES WITH WHICH TO ELICIT RITUALS, BELIEFS, AND SYMBOLS OF CARE ACTIVITIES

Sleep

Condition of room/environment: Occupancy of rooms and bed/sleeping surface, kind of bed/sleeping surface and other furniture, condition of room (temperature, lights, doors and windows open or closed, other artifacts/symbols in room).

Kinds of covering, comforting materials: Pillow/head support (height/number of supports used, type, positioning); covering (blanket type, sheet type, other).

Sleepwear: Covering on head, body, legs, feet (type and variation by season or event).

Care of bed linen: Kind of cleaning, frequency, how, by whom.

Bedtime ritual: Time, tasks, others involved, food or liquid consumed, sensory stimulation, symbols/icons used.

Rules for sleeping: When, with whom, how, in what positions, where, beliefs related to rules.

Rules for awakening: By whom/what, how, mechanisms used.

Awakening rituals: Time, tasks, others involved, food or liquid consumed, sensory stimulation, symbols/icons used.

Personal Hygiene

Tending one's body: Rituals for mouth care (tools and substances used, time, who can assist); rituals for body and hair care (how, when, where, how often, substances used, taboos, gender rules, symbols, beliefs associated with aspects of ritual).

Associations with health/illness: Care associated with body fluids/excretions, symbolism, body temperature, activities of tending one's body, substances used in rituals, seasonal/climate taboos, kinds of activities, time of day/year, gender rules, beliefs.

Eating

Kinds of foods: Preferences, dislikes, specific to an event, ritual, specific to time of day/week/month/year, seasonal, rules or taboos for hot foods, cold foods, rules for amount, type, composition, beliefs, and symbolism associated with specific foods.

Schedule of foods: Rules for when/when not to eat; amount related to time of day; healthy/ill status; associated with certain rituals, beliefs, symbols; before/after meal rituals, symbols/icons used/present.

Environment for eating: Place, people, position, taboos/rules, symbols/icons used/present.

Implements/utensils: Kind, number, rules for use of each, taboos, utensils as symbols.

Reprinted with permission from Rempusheski V. The role of ethnicity in elder care. Nursing Clinics of N Am. September 1989;24(3).

ming, activities, and community involvement.[21] The blacks in this study placed more emphasis on access to family than on the ethnic considerations.[21]

The key to ethnic considerations in communications with older persons is to evaluate effectively the needs of the patient, become more sensitive to their concerns, and to provide modifications in the environment commensurate with the needs identified.

THE TEAM

Why place the team in the middle of a chapter on communication? There are two reasons: First, to explore the method in which the team interacts with itself and its effectiveness in this effort; and second, to examine the team or the individual on the team's ability to communicate with the older patient.

What is the role of the team in geriatric rehabilitation? There is no definitive answer to this question. In the studies to follow, the team is a constantly changing variable. It can simply be a doctor and a nurse, or it can be expanded to include a social worker, dietitian, occupational therapist, speech-language pathologist, physical therapist, leisure services professional, psychologist, or dentist.[22]

Is the team more effective in delivering care to the older person? The results of several studies on this subject follow.

1. The use of a geriatric consultation team resulted in a comprehensive view of the elderly and reduced early recurrent readmissions.[23]
2. The geriatric consultation service improves awareness of functional problems, and increases use of rehabilitative services, but does not decrease the rate of readmission.[24]
3. The geriatric consultation team was unable to alter the degree of functional decline.[25]
4. The geriatric consultation team in the acute care hospital caused a 21% decline in the census of older patients.[26]
5. The patients who received consultation from the geriatric team fared similarly to the control group.[27]

It appears from these results that the efficacy of the geriatric team is not completely proven in controlled studies. Some of the negative outcomes may be a direct result of poor communication among the team. To improve this communication, Lee, Pappius, and Goldman[28] suggest

1. Direct communication (preferably face-to-face or by phone).
2. Frequent follow-up notes.
3. Agreement on the reason and roles of the team's intervention.
4. Limited suggestions to other team members.[28]

Finally, Blumfield and associates[29] suggest providing a complete educational program prior to implementing the geriatric team in an acute hospital.[29]

The most important member of the team, and one that is classically left out of studies of the type listed, is the patient. Patients desire information. However, they do not engage in information seeking behavior when communicating with doctors.[30] Beisecker and Beisecker's study[30] in this area provides five important points to consider when working with patients (Table 15–8).

In addition, health professionals tend to spend less time with older patients as is evidenced by the startling results of Radecki and co-authors' study[31] on the amount of time physicians spent with older patients. In this study, the authors found that internists and cardiologists spend more time with patients (approximately 18 minutes), as compared to general practitioners (approximately 12 minutes). All types of physicians studied spent less time with the older patient (2 to 3 minutes less).[31]

Finally, in communicating with this valuable member of the team, what is an appropriate label to use? According to Barbato and Feezel,[32] the only terms rated positively by both young and old were, retired person, mature American, and senior citizen. All other terms were rated negatively.[32]

The key to communicating effectively with the older patient is best described by Purtillo in *The Allied Health Professional and the Patient: Techniques of Effective Interaction.*[33]

TABLE 15–8. PATIENT INFORMATION-SEEKING BEHAVIOR WHEN COMMUNICATING WITH DOCTORS

1. Patients express a uniformly strong desire for medical information.
2. Patients are much less willing to assume responsibility for medical decision making, preferring to delegate that responsibility to doctors.
3. Patients, on the average, exhibit relatively low rates of information-seeking behavior when interacting with doctors.
4. Situational variables explain information-seeking communication behavior for all types of patients better than do patient attitudes and sociodemographic characteristics.
5. Patient attitudes toward medical decision making are related to patient information-seeking communication behaviors only for patients with long interactions with physicians.

Reprinted with permission from Beisecker A, Beisecker B. Patient information-seeking behaviors when communicating with doctors. Medical Care January 1990;28(1):19–28.

TABLE 15–9. SIMPLE STEPS TO MORE EFFECTIVE LISTENING

- Be selective in what you listen to.
- Realize that words are only symbols—we impose our meanings on others' words.
- Concentrate on central themes rather than isolated statements.
- Judge content rather than style or delivery.
- Listen with an open mind—do not focus on emotionally charged words.
- The average person can listen four times faster than he or she can speak—use extra time to summarize.

Reprinted with permission from Walker R. Effective listening. Am J Med Technol. 1969;35:8–10.

The success of verbal communications depends on (1) the way material is presented—the vocabulary used, the clarity of voice and the organization; (2) the attitude of the speaker; (3) the tone and volume of his voice; (4) the degree to which both speaker and receiver are able to listen effectively.[33]

WRITING

The topic of writing is adequately covered in numerous books and articles.[34–41] This section will define the different types of writing and give suggestions for the specialist to improve them.

The first major type of writing for communication is clinical documentation, which is composed of initial, progress, daily, and discharge note writing. For both legal and reimbursement purposes, the keys to effective note writing are

1. Accuracy: State exactly what you plan to do and did.
2. Completeness: Provide all necessary information and avoid extraneous comments.
3. Timeliness: Chart as close to the time of interaction as possible.
4. Honesty: Tell exactly what happened, do not assume, appear, or seem.

Appendix A provides samples of initial, discharge, progress, daily, and plan of care notes. Table 15–10 provides a list of Dos and Don'ts for charting.[42]

Another important area of writing is professional writing. Professional writing includes articles for publication and business letters. One of the best reference sources for writing business letters is by Piotrowski.[35] One of the best reference sources for the health professional in the area of article writing is by Lynch.[34] Appendix B contains two excellent articles on starting to write, and an outline from a series done by Dr Lynch for the *PT Forum*.

COMPLIANCE AND MOTIVATION

The final areas to be discussed in this chapter are compliance and motivation. Motivation is an inner urge that moves a person to action.[43] Compliance is following orders and doing what is instructed.[44] As important as all the skills used in evaluation and treatment are in the rehabilitation realm, a person's drive and ability to follow through with a program may be just as important as the actual program itself.

Motivation may be broken up into internal and external motivations. Internal motivation is made up of the person's past values and experiences (desire, fear, thirst, and hunger).[43] The therapist can gain insight into a person's internal motivation by learning as much as possible about them. Table 15–11 provides a checklist to assist the therapist in gathering this information.

External motivation is characterized by the factors in the person's physical and social environment. Some of these factors are privacy, rewards, expectations from others, lighting, and temperature.[43] It is obvious that the therapist can influ-

TABLE 15–10. THE DOS AND DON'TS OF CHARTING

Do

Chart concisely, completely, and accurately.
Be objective and avoid tentative or vague statements.
Chart promptly.
Be neat and legible.
Make entries in sequence, beginning with the most important data.
Use standard abbreviations and those approved by the agency.
Sign all timed entries with written signature and credentials.
On flow sheets, include as much routine data as possible.
Record problem-focused client information.
Make corrections appropriately.
Omit unnecessary words like "client" when the meaning is clear.
Include refusals of or omissions in care with the reason for the refusal or omission.

Don't

"Block" time on the chart.
Skip lines or leave white space.
Use ditto marks to repeat information.
Erase or use correction fluid over a notation.
Chart before the fact.
Use pencil or colored pens other than black or dark blue.
Make personal comments, argue, or complain on the medical record.

Reprinted with permission from Ignatevicius D. Documentation. Focus on Geriatric Care and Rehabilitation. Rockville, Md: Aspen Publishers, 1988;2(4).

ence external factors with a well designed environment and appropriate interaction with the patient.

Additional compliance and motivation factors can be described by various models. One of the most widely accepted models for health behavior is the Health Belief Model by Becker,[45] which is illustrated in Figure 15–2. Its main benefit in understanding patient behavior is isolating factors in individual patient compliance.

Orem's Self-Care Model is a particularly useful model for the rehabilitation of

TABLE 15–11. HINTS TO GAINING INSIGHT INTO PATIENTS' INTERNAL MOTIVATING FACTORS

- Read the case history with care.
- Talk with the client about his/her history.
- Ask the client about his/her current and past expectations about performing activities of daily living.
- Ask family members about their performance expectations for the client.

Stay alert for past experiences and values that could affect motivation. Listen and look for
- Successful past motivators
- Cultural factors that could influence behaviors.
- Past experiences of pain.
- Need for approval.
- Need for independence.
- Need for control.
- Fear.
- Depression.

Reprinted with permission from Duchene P. Motivation of older adults. Focus on Geriatric Care and Rehabilitation. Rockville, Md: Aspen Publishers; 1990;3(8):2.

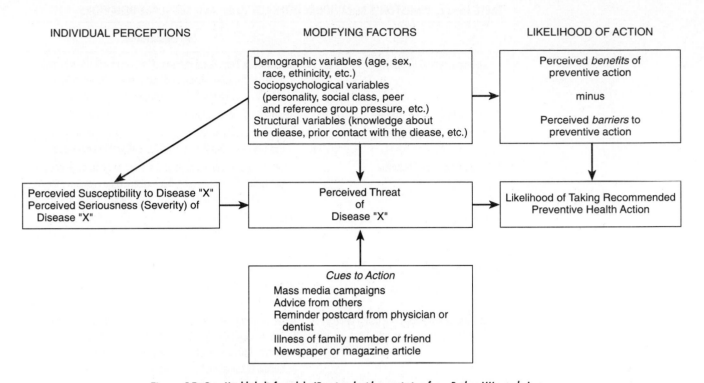

INDIVIDUAL PERCEPTIONS   MODIFYING FACTORS   LIKELIHOOD OF ACTION

Figure 15–2. Health belief model. *(Reprinted with permission from Becker MH, et al. A new approach to explaining sick-role behavior in low-income populations. AJPH. March 1974;64(3):206.)*

older patients. It differentiates between self-care (a patient's choice to act in a way that promotes health) and compliance (the patient's choice to follow instruction).[46] Figure 15–3 is a visual representation of the Orem model.[47] To use this model, the therapist must assess and contrast the person's assets and liabilities along the following dimensions: cognitive, psychological, and physical, and they must design a strategy based on these findings.[46]

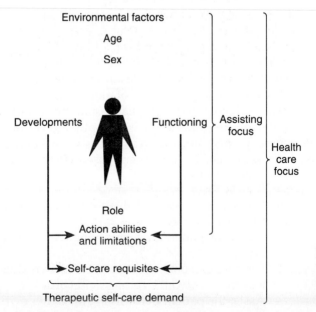

Figure 15–3. Orem's self-care model. *(Reprinted with permission from Orem DE. Nursing: Concepts of Practice. 3rd ed. New York: McGraw-Hill; 1985.*

TABLE 15–12. PINKSTON'S BEHAVIORAL INTERVENTIONS INTO SELF-CARE BEHAVIORS

Step	Implementation
1. Defining desired behavior	Select specific behavioral outcome (i.e., client will dress in underwear, slacks, shirt, shoes, and socks; client will wash face 3 times a day; client will use washroom 4 times a day).
2. Setting and using a schedule	Designate a time to begin and end each occurrence of self-care.
3. Providing response opportunity	Arrange or ask client to arrange materials (e.g., clothing, soap, and towel) so that they are usable and within easy reach.
4. Prompting correct behavior	Have the support person prompt the client to go through each step of the task in the correct order. If there is no response, the prompt is repeated once or twice, then 2 minutes later if necessary.
5. Allowing time for behavior to occur	If the client is attempting to complete a self-care task, instruct the care giver to wait until the task is completed. This should occur within 5 minutes.
6. Praise appropriate behavior	If the client is able to complete the task, the care giver offers praise or touching (food, token, or point on the recording form may also be used) and then prompts the client to go on to the next step.
7. Assistance if the behavior does not occur	If the client does not respond to the prompt within 30 seconds, the care giver guides the older person through the various steps required. The care giver provides help with any items the client is unable to complete because of physical impairment or pain.
8. Ignoring inappropriate behavior	If the client engages in inappropriate behavior, such as complaining, arguing, or any behaviors that serve to bring about an unnecessary delay in the process, the care giver should remove his or her attention from the client until the behavior ceases. Care giver then returns to step 4.
9. Recording	Behavior is recorded on recording form.

Reprinted with permission from Pinkston EM, Linsk NL. Behavioral family intervention with the impaired elderly. Gerontologist. 1984;24:576–583.

The Pinkston Behavioral Model is another useful model for geriatric rehabilitation, especially for patients with cognitive impairments. It requires mutual participation of care giver and patient, the use of behavioral reinforcement, and continued care giver involvement.[46] Table 15–12 lists Pinkston's behavioral interventions for self-care behaviors, and Figure 15–4 provides an example of Pinkston's behavioral record. Besides models, various lists have been generated to help the practitioner in the area of motivation (Tables 15–13 and 15–14).

The final concept in compliance and motivation, and a thoughtful end to this discussion of communication, is an exploration of the Advocacy Model as it relates to compliance and motivation as discussed by Guccione.[48] In this model, the therapist acts on behalf of the patient based on the patient's desires. Getting to this point, however, takes five steps.

1. Provide the patient with all the information, so he or she is able to fully exercise free choice.
2. Assist the patient in determining which information is relevant to the decision.
3. Disclose personal views, so the patient realizes that the clinician may have a personal as well as professional bias.
4. Assist the patient in clarifying his or her own values.
5. Ascertain how patients comprehend their individuality.[48]

An Example of Pinkston's Behavioral Record

Name: Mr. Green   Date: Wednesday, November 3

Behavior: *Conversation—Communication or talking where Mr. G says at least three words in response to questions or statements by another family member.*

Please note when the behavior occurs and what happens before and after.

TIME		BEFORE	DURING	Describe what others did AFTER the behavior occurred. Check box.					
start	stop	What happened before the behavior occurred?	What happened when the behavior occurred?	Did not notice	Ignored	Criticized	Asked to do something else	Praised or rewarded	Other
9:00	9:03	Sitting at table	Asked for more breakfast ☐	☐	☐	☐		X	Gave more eggs
9:05	9:07	Asked what will do today	Said he would like to go for a walk ☐	☐	☐	☐		X	☐
10:30	10:33	Returned from walk	Complained about cold ☐ ☐ ☐ ☐ ☐	☐ ☐ ☐ ☐ ☐	☐ ☐ ☐ ☐ ☐	X ☐ ☐ ☐ ☐		☐ ☐ ☐ ☐ ☐	☐ ☐ ☐ ☐ ☐
TOTAL			3				1	2	

Figure 15–4. *(Reprinted with permission from Pinkston EM, Linsk NL. Care of the Elderly: A Family Approach. Elmhurst, NJ: Pergamon Press; 1984;30.)*

TABLE 15–13. MOTIVATION LIST

The following is a list suggested by Dr. Raymond Harris to assist a leader (or therapist) to motivate an older individual to participate in the physical exercise program.

1. Recognition that the approach requires mental, emotional, and physical engagement.
2. Individualization of the program to the group or to the person.
3. Satisfaction of some of the participant's basic psychic needs.
4. Provision of choice elements and alternatives.
5. Social support and reinforcement.
6. Continuous productive measurement certifications from the beginning by assessment devices.
7. Incorporation of creative opportunities, such as novelty, change of pace, or improvisations.
8. Engagement of recreational elements, such as play and game qualities.
9. Personal projections of the leader as a concerned, interested, competent, and helpful person.
10. Attention to the aesthetics of the environment and the propitious atmosphere.
11. Counseling to some degree as an adjunct.

Reprinted with permission from Harris R, Frankel L. A Guide to Fitness After Fifty. New York: Plenum Press; 1977.

TABLE 15–14. YOUR CLIENT AND MOTIVATION FOR SELF-CARE

- Learn what the client believes is important and identify the client's priorities.
- Set mutual goals together.
- Recognize that your client's goals are more important than the staff's or institution's goals.
- Incorporate the individual's past experiences in the goal determination process.
- Help your client to have realistic expectations by discussing program goals.
- Stress that increasing independence in self-care is often a long, slow process.
- Reinforce positive and independent behaviors by giving concrete feedback on goal attainment.
- Use concrete, visible, and personally significant rewards.
- Involve the family in the goal-setting process whenever possible.

Use contracts as motivators
- Establish a contract with the client emphasizing choices based on realistic short-term goals.
- Include a realistic plan and time frame for goal accomplishment.
- Be certain to include reinforcers for goal attainment.
- Encourage the individual to agree verbally or consent to the contract.
- Have the contract signed by the individual and the health care providers.

Reprinted with permission from FOCUS on your client and motivation for self-care. In: Focus on Geriatric Care and Rehabilitation. Rockville, Md: Aspen Publishers; 1990.

CONCLUSION

To truly be an advocate for and with the patient requires open communication. This chapter provides a means of understanding the normal and pathological changes that occur with age that affect communication, the senses, and the voice. This chapter also explored communication across cultures and among the team. In addition, writing as a means of communication was investigated. Finally, compliance and motivation were described as a possible outcome of adequate communication.

PEARLS

- Changes in the major structures of the ear establish three main types of hearing loss: conductive (which can be reversed), sensorineural (which cannot be reversed) and mixed (which can be partially reversed).

- Detecting hearing loss in a physical therapy setting can range from the use of cues to screenings to more formal tests, such as the Hearing Handicap Inventory.

- Simple interventions, such as changes in the mode of communication and environment (i.e., speaking slowly in a noncompeting environment), will enhance communication.

- All five major senses tend to decline with old age, and yet they are needed to enhance communication; therefore, physical therapists should bring in the other senses as much as possible.

- The voice of an older person changes with age because of reduced respiratory efficiency and changes in the oral and laryngeal cavities. Nevertheless, these changes have little impact on the older person's ability to communicate.

- Understanding the effectiveness of all the team members, especially the patient, will help to enhance communication.

- Accuracy, completeness, timeliness, and honesty are the keys to effective note writing.

- To motivate older persons, the therapist must first assess the person's internal motivation (i.e., values and experience) and then assess and appropriately modify the external factors of motivation (i.e., the physical and social environment).

REFERENCES

1. Kelly LS. Are we ready for the year 2000? *Hear J.* 1985; 38:15–17.
2. Dwyer B. Detecting hearing loss and improving communication in elderly persons. *Focus Ger Care & Rehab.* Nov/Dec 1987; 1(6).
3. Cherney L. Aging and communication. In: Lewis C, ed. *Aging: The Health Care Challenge.* Philadelphia; Davis; 1989.
4. Heller B, Gaynor E. Hearing loss and aural rehabilitation of the elderly. *Clin Nurs.* 1981; 3:1.
5. Boone D, Bayles K, Koopmann C. Communicative aspects of aging. *Otolaryngol Clin N Am.* May 1982; 15(2).
6. Cullinan TR, Silver JH, Gould ES, et al. *Lancet.* 1979; 24:1642–1644.
7. Maguire G. The changing realm of the senses. In Lewis C, ed. *Aging: The Health Care Challenge.* Philadelphia; Davis; 1989.
8. Ryan EB, Capadano HL. Age perceptions and evaluative reactions toward adult speakers. *J Ger.* 1978; 33:98–102.
9. Stewart MA, Ryan EB. Attitudes toward younger and older adult speakers: effects of varying speech rates. *J Language and Social Psych.* 1982; 1:91–109.
10. Honjo I, Isshiki N. Laryngoscopic and voice characteristics of aged persons. *Arch Otolaryngol.* 1980; 106:149–150.
11. Kahane JC. Anatomic and physiologic changes in the aging peripheral speech mechanism. In: Beasley DS, Davis GA, eds. *Aging: Communication Processes and Disorders.* New York; Grune & Stratton; 1981:21–46.
12. Noback GJ. Correlation of stages of ossification of the laryngeal cartilages and morphologic age changes in other tissues and organs. *J Gerontol.* 1949; 4(abstract):329.
13. Lynne-Davies P. Influence of age on the respiratory system. *Geriatrics.* August 1977; 57–60.
14. Meto M. Aging and motor speech production. *Top Ger Rehab.* July 1986; 1(4).
15. Massler M. Oral aspects of aging. *Postgrad Med.* 1971; 49:179–183.
16. Cohen T, Gitman L. Oral complaints and taste perception in the aged. *J Ger.* 1959; 14:294–298.
17. Mysak E, Hanley T. Aging processes in speech: pitch and duration characteristics. *J Ger.* 1958; 13:309–313.
18. Meadows J. Cultural diversity. *Community Health Section Newsletter.*
19. Cole L. E Pluribus Unum: multicultural imperatives for the 1990s and beyond. *ASHA.* September 1989; 69.
20. Rempusheski V. The role of ethnicity in elder care. *Nurs Clin N Am.* September 1989; 24(3).
21. Chee P, Kane R. Cultural factors affecting nursing home care for minorities. *J Am Ger Soc.* February 1983; 31(2).
22. Maguire G. *Care of the Elderly: A Health Team Approach.* Boston; Little Brown & Co; 1985.
23. Berkman B, Campion E, Swagerty E. Geriatric consultation team: alternate approach to social work discharge planning. *J Ger Social Work.* Spring 1983; 5(3):77–87.
24. Campion E, Jette A, Berkman B. An interdisciplinary geriatric consultation service: a controlled trial. *J Am Ger Soc.* December 1983; 31(12):792–796.
25. McVey L, Becker P, Saltz C, et al. Effect of a geriatric consultation team on functional status of elderly hospitalized patients. *Annals of Intern Med.* January 1989; 110(1):79–84.
26. Barker W, Williams F, Zimmer J, et al. Geriatric consultation teams in acute hospitals: impact on back-up of elderly patients. *J Am Ger Soc.* June 1985; 33(6):422–427.
27. Gayton D, Wood-Dauphinee S, deLorimer M, et al. Trial of a geriatric consultation team in an acute care hospital. *J Am Ger Soc.* August 1987; 35(8):726–736.
28. Lee T, Pappius E, Goldman L. Impact of inter-physician communication on the effectiveness of medical consultation. *Am J Med* January 1983; 74:106–112.
29. Blumenfield S, Morris J, Sherman F. The geriatric team in the acute care hospital. *J Am Ger Soc.* October 1982; 30(10):660–664.
30. Beisecker A, Beisecker B. Patient information-seeking behaviors when communicating with doctors. *Medical Care.* January 1990; 28(1):19–28.
31. Radecki S, Kane R, Solomon D. Do physicians spend less time with older patients? *J Am Ger Soc.* August 1988; 36(8):713–718.
32. Barbato C, Feezel J. The language of aging in different age groups. *Gerontologist.* 1987; 27(4):527–532.
33. Purtillo R. *The Allied Health Professional and the Patient: Techniques of Effective Interaction.* Philadelphia; Saunders; 1973.

34. Lynch B, Chapman C. *Writing for Communication in Science and Medicine.* New York; Van Nostrand Reinhold Co.; 1980.

35. Piotrowski M. *Rewriting Strategies and Suggestions for Improving Your Business Writing.* New York; Harper & Row; 1989.

36. Aslanian M, Manalio G, Taylor C. The joys of paperwork: care plans really can work. *Caring.* October 1986; 92–94.

37. Austin MJ, Skelding AH, Smith PL. Managing information. In: *Delivering Human Services.* New York; Harper & Row; 1977:360–371.

38. Bouchard MM, Shane HC. Use of the problem-oriented medical record in the speech and hearing profession: Special Reports. *ASHA.* March 1977; 157–159.

39. Griffith J, Ignatavicius D. *The Writer's Handbook.* Baltimore; Resources Applications, Inc.; 1986.

40. Lampe S. Focus charting: streamlining documentation. *Nurs Man.* 1985; 16–7,43.

41. Murphy J, Beglinger JE, Johnson B. Charting by exception: meeting the challenge of cost containment. *Nurs Man.* 1988; 19:2,56–72.

42. Ignatavicius D. *Documentation. Focus on Geriatric Care and Rehabilitation.* September 1988; 2(4):1–8.

43. Duchene P. *Motivation of older adults. Focus on Geriatric Care and Rehabilitation.* February 1990; 3(8):1–8.

44. Ransdem E. Compliance and motivation. *Top Ger Rehab.* April 1988; 3(3):1–15.

45. Becker MH, McVey LJ, Saltz CC, et al. A new approach to explaining sick-role behavior in low-income populations. *AJPH.* March 1974; 64(3):206.

46. Thibodaux L, Shewchuk R. Strategies for compliance in the elderly. *Top Ger Rehab.* April 1988; 3(3):21–34.

47. Orem D. *Nursing: Concepts of Practice.* 3rd ed. New York; McGraw-Hill; 1985.

48. Guccione A. Compliance and patient autonomy: ethical and legal limits to professional dominance. *Top Ger Rehab.* April 1988; 3(3):62–74.

Appendix A   Sample Notes

Initial Note

Initial Evaluation

Initial Discharge

Initial Plan of Care

Daily Note

Initial Note

PHYSICAL THERAPY SERVICES OF WASHINGTON, D.C., INC.

1150 18th Street, N.W.
Suite 4
Washington, D.C. 20036

June 19

Dear Dr.

Thank you for referring _____ to Physical Therapy Services for treatment of her left shoulder adhesive capsulitis. She was evaluated on 6/19 and at that time revealed a history of having had a frozen shoulder for approximately one year. Functionally, _____ is unable to perform routine ADLs, such as overhead dressing, lifting objects of more than 2 pounds, and washing her hair, secondary to pain and weakness. The pain is in the deltoid area and at night radiates into the arm and wrist.

On objective evaluation, _____ is extremely limited in range of motion with active shoulder abduction to 68° and flexion to 85° with reports of pain at end range of both movements. Internal rotation is limited to 42°, external rotation to 11°. The patient presents with 3+/5 strength in external rotation, 4/5 strength in internal rotation, 4/5 strength in flexion and abduction. Patient reports extreme pain on resistance to all these movements. Right grip strength is 53 pounds, left grip strength is 42 pounds. On a postural evaluation, _____ presents with 8/10 forward head as well as 8/10 rounded shoulders.

The program we would like to pursue with _____ is one of heat, electrical stimulation, ultrasound, exercise, and ice, and a strong home exercise program. We will continue to see _____ twice a week for 2 months depending on patient's progress with goals being normal range of motion, normal strength, and ability to perform ADLs without pain.

If you have any questions or comments please don't hesitate to contact me. For billing and insurance purposes please sign and return the enclosed treatment plan.

Sincerely,

Carole Lewis, P.T., G.C.S., Ph.D.

Figure 15A-1.

Initial Evaluation

Date: _____

Patient's Name: _____ Phone: _____

Address: _____

Attending Physician's Name: _____

Diagnosis for which treatment has been prescribed: _____

_____

_____

Patient's Program: _____

_____

_____

Goals: _____

_____

History: _____

_____

_____

Function: _____

_____

Pain Where: _____

     When: _____

ROM: _____

_____

Strength: _____

_____

Gait: _____

_____

Posture: _____

_____

Sensation: _____

Figure 15A–2.

Initial Discharge

PHYSICAL THERAPY SERVICES OF WASHINGTON, D.C., INC.

1150 18th Street, N.W.
Suite 4
Washington, D.C. 20036

September 19

Dear Dr.

Thank you for referring _____ to Physical Therapy Services. She received her last treatment on 8/19 and at that time had made significant improvements. Her shoulder flexion has increased from 85° to 171°. Her abduction is now 167°, external rotation has improved from 11° to 79°, internal rotation has improved from 42° to 79°. _____ now has presented with 4+/5 strength in all motions, although she still reports pain at end range. She is independent with all her ADLs at this time. She is also independent on a very comprehensive exercise program of strengthening and stretching that she will perform on a daily basis. She will contact us in 1 month as to her status.

If you have any questions or comments please don't hesitate to contact me.

Sincerely,

Carole Lewis, P.T., G.C.S., Ph.D

Figure 15A–3.

Initial Plan of Care

PHYSICAL THERAPY SERVICES

OF
WASHINGTON, D.C., INC.

1150 18th Street, N.W.,
Suite No. 4
Washington, D.C. 20036

Patient _____ Physician _____

Age _____ Diagnosis _____

Treatment received during the total course of therapy:

___ Hot Packs	___ Ultrasound	___ Taping	___ Therapeutic Exercise
___ Cold Packs	___ Electrical Stim.	___ TENS	___ Act. Range of Motion
___ Cervical Traction	___ Phonophoresis	___ Soft Tissue Mob.	___ Act. Assistive ROM
___ Pelvic Traction	___ Joint Mobilization	___ Massage	___ Pas. Range of Motion
___ Back School	___ Myofascial Release	___ Paraffin	___ Spray and Stretch
___ Posture Evaluation	___ Functional Electrical Stim.	___ Iontophoresis	___ Medcosonolator
___ Functional Activities	___ Neuromuscular Reeducation	___ Gait Training	___ Whirlpool
___ Home Visit	___ Office Assessment	___ Other (_____)	

Admission Goals

1. _____
2. _____
3. _____
4. _____
5. _____

Frequency _____ times per week   Duration for _____ weeks

Notes _____

_____

_____

_____

Therapist _____ Date _____ Physician _____ Date _____

Therapist _____ Date _____ Physician _____ Date _____

Therapist _____ Date _____ Physician _____ Date _____

Please sign and return to Physical Therapy Services. Thank you.

Figure 15A–4.

Daily Note

PHYSICAL THERAPY SERVICES

OF
WASHINGTON, D.C., INC.

MODALITIES

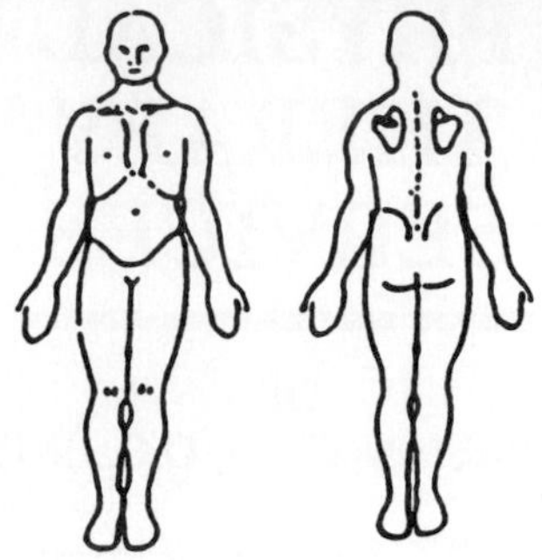

Date: _____

Patient Name: _____

Notes: _____

_____

_____

_____

_____

_____

_____

_____

_____

_____

_____

_____

_____

_____

_____

_____

_____

_____

_____

_____

Figure 15A–5.

Appendix B   Selected Portions of Workshops by B. Lynch

SESSION I: WANTED: THE PT WRITER*

Do you at moments think that you have an important observation to share with others? Or maybe a helpful hint, a solution to a management problem, a strong opinion, the results of a study? Perhaps you have mentioned your idea to a colleague, who responded with an enthusiastic suggestion to write about it in an article for a professional journal, such as *Physical Therapy Forum* or *Topics in Geriatric Rehabilitation*. Which of the following was your response to the suggestion?

1. Your mouth felt dry and your chest tightened.
2. You scoffed, commenting that your idea was not so important.
3. You reddened, saying that the idea was too personal and not significant to anyone else.
4. You felt satisfied with the praise of your colleague and friend, but feared that anyone else would think, "So what?"
5. You said that you didn't have time to write.
6. You sighed: "I did that once and my article was rejected."
7. You said: "I can't write well, and writing is laborious, even painful."

None of the above? or most of the above? especially Number 7?

The PT: Predisposed to Be a Writer

The responses are common, but they are not logical for the physical therapist. Having seen first hand the remarkable results physical therapists achieve with their patients, and the skills and observations required of the PT in working with patients, I know that PTs not only have important information to communicate to one another, but also have a special predisposition, by virtue of their training and practice, to develop and improve writing skills. The PT is already trained to:

- Observe each patient critically and note overt and subtle diagnostic signals.
- Perceive small increments of progress.
- Expect specific outcomes, not immediately but down the line.
- Communicate carefully and explain thoroughly.
- Practice patience.

These are precisely the characteristics a developing writer must have.

How can you best develop professional writing skills? Ordinarily I would recommend participating in an interactive program, such as a workshop or seminar. However, given the above characteristics you have already cultivated as a PT, and given your professional motivation, I believe that you can advance considerably through this series of articles, which will guide you incrementally through the basics of writing well and of identifying the symptoms of faulty writing. This Wordshop series offers instruction and programmatic exercises that you may patiently apply in improving your own writing. To get the most benefit from the "therapy," you should participate in *all* the exercises, because they build progressively, each honing some aspect of writing ability necessary for later exercises.

*Reproduced with permission from Lynch B, Chapman C. *Writing for Communication in Science & Medicine.* New York: Van Nostrand Reinhold Company; 1980.

Record each exercise in a singular-to-purpose notebook so that you will have a permanent record of your responses and can review your writing progress. The notebook, henceforth referred to as a *journal,* should be bound (not loose-leaf or spiral). Number and date each exercise as you enter it into your journal.

Although you may do this program alone, consider sharing it with one or two colleagues. In working with others, meet once a week and review the exercises. By interacting with others, you will learn more and will probably have more fun.

Motivation

The first step in becoming a writer is to think of yourself as a writer and to understand your motives for writing. Writing can be pleasurable, satisfying, and even fulfilling. A writer may have published 1 article or 200 articles; but, as in biomedical research and clinical practice, fulfillment comes as much through the habit of writing as with the product itself. With the habit comes the identity of self as writer. I hope to lead you not only to the habit of but also to an addiction to writing.

Meanwhile, other rewards are possible—fame, for example, or at least professional recognition. In writing a piece, you become the *author;* in having it read, you become an *authority.* Please be encouraged by the knowledge that authority begins with *author.*

Among the great wonders of professional and academic life is a syndrome known as *publish-or-perish.* Lamentations have been voiced about the demand by universities and medical institutions that faculty members and even staff write, submit, and publish research, clinical, and observational information. Health professionals may see themselves as pressured to pursue an artificial goal of publication rather than that of satisfying specific needs, obligations, and services. Nonetheless, an alternative view is that publication overtly proves one's professional competence and fulfills one's responsibility to inform colleagues of new ideas—and even opinions. Furthermore, the number of publications generally seems to correlate directly with professional promotion and institutional reputation. Finally, a reputation built through publications means grant money for more programs, in turn leading to more publications about the results. Publish-or-perish may seem a poor motive for writing, but it is decidedly evolutionary in the survival of the fittest. If this is your stimulus for writing, you are eager, if not anxious, to get articles written and published. With luck, as you struggle for publishing success, you will strive for excellence and satisfaction in writing as well.

I hope that you want not only to be published but also to be *read.* If so, you must write *well.* If all clinical articles were clearly written, imagine how much more would be read and how many more patients and practitioners would benefit.

Standards, Audience, and Opportunity

Coincident with a writer's idealistic or altruistic motive to write well so that his or her message will serve humanity is the countering fear of rejection. Such fear is soundly based. Journals are becoming more and more particular about what they accept. They do not lack materials; to the contrary, most publishers of professional journals are swamped with submissions. And printing costs are much higher today than they were just a few years ago. So publishers can afford to be choosy. While you may be perishing, they are enjoying the benefit of publishing. They must be strict about both the content and the style of writing; after all, the prestige of their journals depends on both.

A frequent occurrence, however, is not out-and-out rejection, but the acceptance of an article "contingent on editing." What do you do then? Chances are that when you wrote and submitted the paper, you thought it was reasonably coherent and lucid. Or, possibly you knew it had problems, but you could not figure out what they were or how to correct them when you did spot them. Could you edit a manuscript that an author returned? Do you know how to spot and correct the problems of syntax, organizational structure, or content? Publication of the paper depends on your editing and rewriting skills—but I expect that as you complete this writing program you will be able to edit and rewrite credibly.

Also, remember that editors and reviewers are human. Besides stacks of work, they have moods. If your writing is confusing, muddled, boring, or abstruse, no matter how important the content, the editor might become annoyed and impatient and, consequently, overly critical of your manuscript; or he or she might ignore it altogether, except, of course, for the brief moment taken to reject it. But, with all these human variables, the challenge of writing becomes that much more intriguing because the writing hypothesis is communication—whether or not you are able to make others comprehend ideas from your own mind as represented in your writing.

The first step toward success in writing is to understand who your audience is and what publications are available to you as a PT writer. The focus in this program is on the physical therapist as the primary audience, and on physicians and other professionals who work with PTs as the secondary audience. The available publications are weekly newspapers, professional journals, research journals, books, and book chapters. Each publication has its range of subjects, types of articles, and standards for writing. The subjects covered in the publications range from announcements and reports of special meetings to accounts of personal professional experiences, helpful tips for the practitioner, case reports, research reports, and suggestions for improving business administration and professional skills (including those involved in writing).

The first program of exercises will help you understand the opportunities and standards for publishing in the PT field, and to perceive yourself as a potential conveyor of information within the profession. Remember to enter every exercise in your writing journal; record all related observations and thoughts.

Program 1

Exercise 1

In the next 2 weeks, look at the available physical therapy journals and newspapers with the points of view of writer/editor, rather than simply as reader. Analyze each publication for:

1. Types of articles.
2. Lengths and numbers of each type of article.
3. Format for each type, that is, the order in which the information is organized.

Exercise 2

List or photocopy pertinent information from the "Instructions for Authors" page of each publication, noting specifically the types of materials called for, the name and address of the publisher, and all particulars relating to manuscript preparation and submission.

Exercise 3

Identify all of your own motives for writing, and record those motives in your journal.

Exercise 4

Think about your own work experiences, case encounters, techniques for client management, and what might be said that is worth saying. Write a list of these ideas. Also, list the publications in which your subject matter would be most appropriate. Note the format that would suit your topics best.

SESSION II—OUTLINING

Many writing courses begin with the teacher expecting the students to write a complete outline of the articles they will write. Unfortunately, and realistically, for the novice writer the very thought of being able to have a complete plan at the start paralyzes minds and fingers. The reaction is similar to focusing on the mountain you intend to climb and thinking that you will never make it. I find it easier to look up the trail a few hundred yards to an agreeable spot that will offer an encouraging view of what I have, in fact, so effortlessly (!) managed to traverse. Soon enough, I am on top of the mountain and have a complete overview.

Composing an article can proceed similarly—idea to idea, section to section. Sometimes when you begin writing, you do not really know where the trail of thoughts will lead you, and it is a good practice to keep your mind open to forks in the trail. An opportunity to explore an unexpected line of thought may lead you to an important discovery.

So, view the overall article as a series of steps. You use individual words to construct phrases, phrases to construct clauses, clauses to construct sentences. Each piece, considered separately, is easy to write. Composing the larger part is just another step—a matter of putting together what you have already written so clearly. Remember, because you have edited each word so carefully, and have made your sentences so logical, constructing paragraphs will be a simple matter of organization. That organization relates to the overall composition (or idea movement) of the entire article; therefore, we will now look at how to conceptualize the article, and in a subsequent session we will look at the internal organization of paragraphs.

Go Back to the Beginning

In the first few sessions of this Workshop, we considered the three steps you should take before beginning your article. You may have now written 12–16 paragraphs of the article, so now is a good time to return to your original intention (you noted this in your journal) and consider whether or not you should revise those steps. Or, perhaps you were not sure at that time and now can complete the steps. The three steps are

1. Decide on the audience you want to read your article: physical therapists; all allied health professionals; specialists; subspecialists; technicians; lay public; students; adults/children, etc.
2. Pick the publication you will submit your article to. Consider the type of publication suitable to your purposes: professional journal; professional newspaper; popular magazine. Consider several that may be appropriate for your article. Carefully review each candidate publication for *content* (Does it seem to match what you have to offer?); *audience appeal* (the same audience as your target audience?); *use of figures and tables; the average length of the articles.*
3. Carefully review the "Information for Authors" page from the journal you have chosen. Note any particular details pertinent to your article: photos, tables, figures, bibliography, etc.

Try an Outline

Although some writers can dictate an entire article without the benefit of a definitive outline, most writers find outlines helpful at some draft stage. In fact, outlines are helpful in many ways—in organizing the writing of the first draft; in preparing the abstract or summary; in preparing spinoff works such as professional lectures, class notes, and even letters to colleagues and friends; and in preparing experimental protocol.

An outline is by no means required before or while you write your article.

Indeed, some authors are stymied and stifled by outlines. However, it is a good idea to try working with an outline at least once to find out if the mode suits you.

Outlining the Research Article

If you are doing experimental or clinical research, the outline tends to evolve by itself in your lab notes—with the hypothesis stated at the beginning of the research project, the steps of the method briefly described, and results listed as data are analyzed. When your research is finished, complete the outline, keeping in mind the journal you have selected. The clearest example of an outline is that for an IMRAD article. IMRAD is an acronym for introduction, materials and methods, results, and discussion.

The first marks you should make on paper are rather skeletal and simple: just write the name of each formal section of the IMRAD used by the journal. To leave plenty of space between each heading, write each heading on a separate sheet of paper. Assign a roman numeral to those headings.

I. Introduction
II. Method and Materials
III. Results
IV. Discussion
V. Summary/Conclusion/Abstract

That was simple, but you are not yet finished with this step. Each of those headings represents a sizable body of words, some more than others, but each sizable enough to warrant the assumption that there is a succinct theme to each, that is, a major idea you are expressing. Everything you will say in a given section should relate to that major idea. Formulate the theme of each section in a single sentence and write it after the appropriate heading in the outline.

I. Introduction: (thematic statement)
II. Method and materials: (name method)
III. . . . etc.

If you have already done some scribbling and scratching in your lab book, the next activity will be easier than if you are thinking about your article for the first time. Take your outline and, section by section, reflect on each thematic statement. On scratch paper, scribble down the main points you think should be made about that theme. Remember, these are only main ideas, not the supporting details or the supporting reasons that prove or illustrate the ideas. These main ideas are the topics of the section's theme and, as such, warrant a full paragraph of explanation in your article. The one-sentence statement of the topic should be assigned a capital letter, beginning the list with "A."

I. Introduction: (thematic statement)
  A. (Topic statement)
  B. (Topic statement)
II. Method: (state method)
  A. (Description of patients or materials)
  B. (Description of method in study)
III. Results:
  A. (Topic sentence—results, category 1)
  B. (Topic sentence—results, category 2)
IV. Discussion
  A. (Conclusion 1)
  B. (Conclusion ?)
  C. (Implications)

If you have done that much, that is, if you have thought through all the main ideas in topic form, you have done a lot. In fact, the crisis is over and what follows is the fun of developing each topic by dissecting it into its various components. Those components may be dissected by logic (inductive or deductive), by cause-and-effect relationships, by physical description, by chronological directions, or by syntheses. (You will learn how to do this in the session on paragraphs.)

Whether or not you develop your outline into components or even into further detail (a, b, c, etc.) is a matter of personal style. Some writers like to itemize so thoroughly in outline form that they need only supply transitional and connecting phrases to actually write the article. Others prefer to let thoughts flow more randomly on paper at the outline stage. Some find it best not to write full sentences in an outline and instead use phrases, producing what is called a topic outline.

Whichever, when you have completed the outline, study it for overall flow of thesis. Does each topic sentence lead in some order, whether logical, chronological, or spatial, to the next topic sentence? If not, you probably have some rearranging to do, or maybe you have left out an important thought-step. If two topic sentences within a single section seem redundant, maybe combining them is in order.

You probably remember the rule that if there is an A there must be a B, if a 1, a 2. The reason is that the divisions of an outline *divide* thoughts into components. With only one component, only one idea is given; thus, there is no division. The component should be represented, therefore, as a single idea. Conceivably, for example, the Introduction might in one, short succinct paragraph state the central thesis of the entire article. In that event, the thematic sentence accompanying roman numeral I should suffice. However, if the Introduction has at least two components, those should be specified.

Outlining the Essay-Type Article

Now let's outline an article that does not have a predetermined format. An essay is a short article on one subject usually presenting the personal views of the author. The essay may argue for or against an idea, or present an objective discussion or description of the subject. Physical therapists find the essay a useful form for describing and encouraging the use of a therapeutic technique. The essay's structure is not formalized, but several sections are typical: an introduction, idea development or argument, and conclusion.

The following is an outline of an article by Rebecca A. Davidson that appeared in the *PT Forum*, January 14, 1991. If you have that issue, follow the article's developments as you read through the outline. I will use a full-sentence outline.

> *Outline of "The Art of Listening—The Heart of a Caring Profession"*
> Introduction: Health professionals tend not to listen to patients.
>   A. During a physical therapy session, a patient reveals that his last therapist was not very good because the therapist "didn't listen."
>   B. Diagnostic and therapy machinery and a lack of time tend to preempt the essential listening skill.
> I. PTs should carefully listen to patients for several reasons.
>   A. To confirm a diagnosis or to discover a different reason for the patient's problem, the therapist must listen to the patient's account of his symptoms and behaviors.
>   B. To develop appropriate treatment plans and goals, health care providers must take into account the patient's goals and cares.
>   C. To engender trust and gratitude in the patient relationship, the therapist must show interest—by listening.
>   D. To demonstrate to the patient that you care about him and his progress you must show that you are open to him—by listening.

II. Here's how you can become a good listener.
   A. Make eye contact.
   B. Focus your attention exclusively on the patient.
   C. Express compassion.
Conclusion: By listening, you can help the patient to restore a sense of self-worth and improve your quality of care.

The above outline is broad, not detailed. It's the sort of outline you might be able to construct from your basic ideas even before beginning to write. As you write, you "flesh out" the subcomponent and begin to discover what you know and think about each topic. As you complete a section or subsection, go back and fill in more details in your outline. For example, Part I.C. might develop with the following details:

I.

   C. To engender trust and gratitude in the patient relationship, the therapist must show interest—by listening.
      1. People need to be heard.
      2. Patients expect you to be interested in hearing about their ailments.
      3. A person feels better physically after speaking and feels better emotionally.
      4. Refusing to listen will produce resentment and magnify physiological problems.

The actual paragraph is written as follows:

A less practical, but no less important motive for listening is patient gratification. People feel the need to be heard. Patients assume that you are interested in their bodies; they expect you, of all people, to listen to their ailments. We cannot deny psychosomatic realities—when a person feels emotionally relieved after speaking, he/she is likely to feel better physically as well. Likewise, if a person is denied a listening ear, feelings of hostility, resentment, or disappointment tend to magnify physiological and functional problems. Listen, and make someone's day.

Outlining with a Gimmick

Occasionally, use of a gimmick might be an original and appropriate way to develop an article. For example, in the article "Early Intervention—Bedside PT" in *PT Forum* (March 15, 1991), Mary Russell uses the word "bedside" as the title, the subject, and the sectional development gimmick of her article. To give suggestions on maximizing your bedside care of patients, she instructs: "Think B.E.D.S.I.D.E.!," then develops a topic for each letter of the word. A topic outline of her article would look like the following:

Introduction:	My experience as bedside PT		
	I.	B:	Body Mechanics
	II.	E:	Equipment
	III.	D:	Document!
	IV.	S:	Scheduling
	V.	I:	Initiative
	VI.	D:	Demonstrate
	VII.	E:	Encourage!
Conclusion:	You can make a difference.		

The proper form of the outline is not so important as the flow of development, and you should not let formalities block your writing process early in the article's development. At this stage, just get your thoughts in order and under control. As you write the sections you can refer back to the outline, altering its structure with the flashes of perception that come from the illuminating (!) writing process itself. To make your outline even more useful, you might leave an oversized margin on the left or right, in which you can make notes concerning ideas, figures, tables, and references corresponding to appropriate topics.

Program

Exercise One

Make a broad outline of any three published articles.

Exercise Two

Make a broad outline (roman numerals and capital letters) of the article you are writing. Remember first to review the first three steps.

Exercise Three

Add another level of detail to your outline (1, 2, 3, etc.)

(Dr Lynch, author of the book Writing for Communication in Science and Medicine, *is a freelance writer in the Washington, DC, area and a former university professor. She welcomes your comments and questions about writing. She may be contacted at: 815 Bowie Road, Rockville, MD 20852.)*

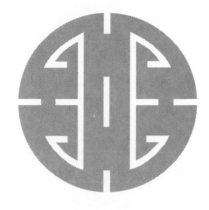

PART III

Administration and Management

CHAPTER *16* SIXTEEN

Attitudes and Ethics

HOW MEDICAL CARE IS CHANGING

In today's world, the growing elderly population, advances in technology, and philosophical attitudes are changing the way we think ethically. In the past, the medical treatment of a patient was primarily humanistic due to the paucity of scientific knowledge. Patients were treated spiritually rather than the disease being treated. Given the rapid advances in medical science, there is a great concern that spiritual treatment or meeting the patient's emotional needs will take a back seat to more technologically oriented treatments.[1] As this concern grows, the ability to meet the emotional needs of the elderly has also diminished, which has been a natural consequence of the increased specialization in medical technology.[1] An older person with multiple problems may have several different physicians and therapists to care for his or her different needs. With the demise of the general practitioner, the intimate relationship between clinician and patient likewise ceases.

In addition to technological changes, attitudes are changing and a concern for the patient's "rights" is growing. The Miranda decision,[2] which required that people accused of a crime be informed of their rights under the law, has dramatically changed the legal institution. Likewise, an analogous development is occurring in

485

the health care system with more of an emphasis placed on informing the patient of his or her rights. Medicine is shifting away from a paternalistic role to giving the patient more responsibility in decision making, and this may be threatening, especially to the elderly who are more comfortable with traditional roles.[3] Clinicians in the past have used paternalism to express compassion and minimize the patient's fear and pain, but patients have often taken this role to mean, "They will decide and do what is necessary for me." The shift away from this relationship requires patients—with proper guidance and information—to determine their own medical care.

PERSONAL ATTITUDES

How the aged are dealt with depends on how they are viewed. When negative stereotypes exist and therapists have a negative view of the elderly, the health care the individual receives is compromised.

Most studies of attitudes toward the elderly have focused on gender, contact, race, and socioeconomic status. Even though labels are an important descriptive tool, attitudes may develop toward a group as a whole that ignores individual differences.[4] Increased contact with the elderly allows people to view them on a more personal level rather than generalizing or stereotyping about the meaning of being old. Harris and Fiedler[5] demonstrated that the more contact preadolescents had with the elderly, the more positive their attitude was to that population. Preadolescent attitudes are important to examine since according to Piaget, preadolescence is a transitional stage between concrete and formal operations, as well as the beginning of attitude judgments and stereotyping.[5]

At a very young age, people learn that all old people must be looked after and attribute personality traits to them, such as childishness, irritability, incapability of reasoning or of learning new information, and inability to make important decisions about their lives. If the physical therapist makes these generalizations regarding the elderly, he or she may fail to notice or investigate personality changes that have recently occurred, such as confusion. It may be assumed that the patient has been confused for a long time because he or she is old, when in reality the onset of confusion was a week prior to contact and due to physiological or pharmaceutical causes.[6]

Society also tends to believe that body image is not important to an older person and does not view the elderly as sexual beings. It is easy, therefore, to overlook the emotional needs of an 85-year-old woman who has just had a mastectomy and fail to explain the prosthetic options that are available.[6]

MEDICAL DECISION MAKING

One of the basic ethical principles that guides health care providers in making decisions is called *beneficence*. This involves providing benefits to the patient, including preserving life. When a clear medical picture is present, the clinician and patient usually agree on the decisions that must be made, however, when it is not present, "defensive medicine," which does not necessarily benefit the patient but instead builds evidence against malpractice, is often practiced.[7]

The paradigm of good decision making is properly informing competent patients of their care options, and the possible outcomes and risks of treatments so they can decide the course of treatment, which should be limited only by the clinician's availability and willingness to provide the treatment.[8] The clinician should not be a neutral party and should take an active role in encouraging acceptance of an appropriate treatment, but the patient must not be coerced or deceived.[9]

An important consideration in medical decision making is the individual's value system. What constitutes quality of life to the patient may be very different from the clinician's philosophical beliefs, and when making decisions, the *self-determination* or *autonomy* of the patient should always prevail.[7] Decisions in physical therapy treatment, which have usually been based on scientific knowledge and professional experience, can be deficient since the moral aspect of the treatment may have been ignored. The value system of the patient must be considered, especially with regard to goal setting. What may be considered functional by the therapist may not meet the goals the patient has set.[10]

Decisional capacity must be assessed by the health provider before intervention is implemented and should be based on the individual's mental status, judgment, and short-term memory. The greater the risk of the treatment, the more carefully the decisional capacity must be evaluated. Many elderly people who are not capable of making their own decisions are treated as if they are, because they nod their head and agree with everything the clinician says. Elderly patients are denied the right to choose proper medical care if they are not properly evaluated by the health care team.[9]

If it is determined that an elderly patient is no longer able to make his or her own decisions, the first appeal should be to any specific documents of empowerments executed while the patient was capable. These empowerments or advanced directives, which include power of attorney and living wills, make it possible for health care professionals to determine the wishes and values of the patient and will be covered in depth later.

If the patient is unable to make medical decisions and advanced directives are not present, a surrogate decision maker must be chosen. This surrogate is usually a spouse or, as is often the case with the elderly, a son or daughter. For the elderly who have outlived all family and friends, the only alternative may be a court appointed guardian. In special cases where the court feels the patient is unable to make medical decisions but the clinician and family feel the patient is capable, both the patient and the court appointed surrogate must agree on a course of treatment.[9]

Conflicts regarding medical decisions may exist within the elderly patient, such as retaining a normal appearance versus attaining the best cure possible, or deciding whether to spend one's life savings on a costly treatment knowing it will be a financial burden on the rest of the family. In these cases, the patient should be the one to resolve the dilemma with the help and support of the clinician. The responsibility of the clinician is to present the facts regarding the treatment choices, but it may be more helpful to supply information about others who have been through similar experiences.[8]

Professional conflicts may be present that affect decision making by placing the patient's needs in competition with the clinician's interests. For example, a physical therapist may want a patient to reach a normal, functional status but also hopes the patient will need his or her services for a long period of time to financially support the practice. In this case, the clinician must obviously serve the needs of the patient and disregard his or her own incentives.[8]

Other difficult situations arise when a competent patient has poor judgment regarding his or her ability to function at home or in society (such as driving a car) in which case the clinician is responsible for weighing the risks of performing these activities and must act to preserve the safety of the patient and others. In such cases, the therapist must not act in ways that would be only moderately beneficial to the patient but would also be detrimental to society or the patient's overall safety.[8]

Insufficient legal focus has been placed on discharge planning, which has become more of an issue with the formation of diagnostic related groups (DRGs). It was determined, however, that if a patient is capable of making decisions, it is illegal to place that patient in a residential facility against his or her will. The family would have to petition the court for guardianship in order to override the patient's discharge preference.[9]

ALLOCATION
OF RESOURCES

The growth of the elderly population, especially of that over the age of 85, poses economic and ethical dilemmas due to the rapid increase in the demand for health care services at a time when resources are scarce. Some important questions are (1) how should these resources be rationed, (2) who should be responsible for allocating these resources and (3) how should the scarcity of these resources affect medical policy decisions.

Allocation of resources is commonly based on need and the belief that society should take care of its members. The disproportionate amount of medical care the elderly needs makes this group particularly vulnerable when it comes to rationing resources. Critics of Medicare view the program as "overgenerous and unwarranted" for people who do not have the need for this special help. Some feel that the dispensing of Medicare funds should be based on financial need rather than on medical need. Public opinion on this topic is indicated in a state poll showing moderate support (36%) for age criteria in health care, and the feeling that resources should be given to people who will receive the most long-term benefit from the treatment, which can exclude the elderly.[2,11]

Clinicians have always felt age is an important consideration when making medical decisions, but they are unclear about the ethical and moral implications of their actions. Sometimes it is felt that it is better to allocate resources to the young, who have their whole life ahead of them rather than the elderly who have already experienced life, since the young are more capable of adjusting to handicaps and will be able to repay the costs with future contributions. Productivity has always been a criteria of need, which is ironic because elderly people are forced out of the workplace due to mandatory retirement and are, therefore, considered less productive. However, one must also consider that the elderly have contributed to society and that society has a responsibility to take care of them.[4,11,12]

One difficulty in basing medical decisions on age is the uncertainty of the prognosis in determining how long a person will live, particularly for an older person who is suffering from multiple illnesses. Another important factor that age criteria fails to recognize is that each person's life is important to him or her, and a longer life is not more valuable than a shorter one. Society must be careful not to devalue the life of an older individual, particularly one who is dependent, since this may lead to abusive discrimination of the elderly. Each person has an equal right to life no matter how old the individual is, and the quality of life should be evaluated by the patient only and not the clinician.[9,11]

When limited resources exist obviously not everyone will be entitled to every possible medical benefit, but the question remains of how rationing should be implemented. Should health care be distributed according to ability to pay or is it a social obligation to supply care regardless of financial ability? Ideally everyone should have the right to proper health care, which should not be considered a luxury but a basic need. Conflicts arise when people use resources without replenishing them by either paying personally or having insurance that will pay. When this occurs, society is harmed because other people, in addition to not receiving the services, will have to replenish the funds.[13,14]

Who should be responsible for distributing these scarce resources? If the physical therapist is given the chore of making funding decisions the trust between the patient and the practitioner may be jeopardized. Patients trust that the physical therapist will provide the treatment needed regardless of financial concerns. Controlling expenditures are counterbalanced by the ethical obligations of the practitioner and negligence laws that demand that maximum effort should be made to cure the patient.[9]

With the growth of the Health Maintenance Organization (HMO) industry, clinicians are given the new role of "gatekeeper" and, given the limited resources, must face the situation where resources spent on one patient will mean fewer resources for another. When a patient's health provider or insurance policy does not provide payment for health care services, the clinician should respect the right of the patient to limit treatment he or she does not value if it involves using personal funds. Conflicts for the clinician arise when the patient wants the treatment more than the provider and will pay for the care with personal funds. In this scenario, the clinician must consider that even though financial resources will not be compromised, access to resources (space and equipment) may hinder other patients from receiving care who need it more.[3]

In the past the patient had to be cautious because reimbursement policies encouraged clinicians to provide unnecessary treatment. Today with the change in public policy and the addition of DRGs the patient's rights are in danger of being violated due to incentives to limit treatment, decreasing the role of the clinician as the patient's advocate. The presence of these DRGs will affect the elderly the most since treatment will be discontinued prematurely for individuals with long-term illnesses. When economic incentives provided to clinicians lead them to deny beneficial care, there is a direct threat to the requirement that clinical decisions be competent and respect the patient's decision-making autonomy. For example, one cost control method is rewarding an institution for offering a treatment at a lower cost. Hospitals that deliver treatment for less than the DRG rate can keep the difference. As a result hospital administrators are examining the decisions of the clinicians to use resources and are applying pressure to physicians to deny beneficial treatment and the patient's right to choose that treatment.[4,13]

Another new medical policy that creates a conflict of interest is the addition of case managers to insurance companies because the managers' dominant measure of success is keeping costs low even though they want the patients to be satisfied with their care. If the patient's interests were always served, obviously the cost-saving goal would not be achieved. Therefore, formal ethics do not provide the answer. One suggestion is to give the balancing responsibility to the direct-care provider who is given incentives to conserve costs, but also possesses the moral and professional desire to meet the needs of the patient. This, however, creates a conflict of interest for the clinician, who is left with a situation in which the balance between the benefit for the patient and the cost to the system is unclear: to deny the patient the resource without informing him or her about the denial is ethically wrong. Providers have an obligation to inform patients regarding care options, even though they are denied these options by the system.[8]

Because of all these conflicts regarding allocation of resources, one can see that health care professionals will become frustrated with not being able to supply quality treatment unless they become more directly involved with health care policy formation and evaluation. The true challenge for the medical care system in the future will be learning how to balance the increasing medical needs of the elderly with the financial limitations of the system.[4,8]

CARE GIVER STRESS

Contrary to what many people believe, a majority of elderly people are being cared for at home by family members. In the United States, it was estimated that 1 million people suffering from dementia reside in nursing homes, while 1.5 to 2.5 million people are living at home. Studies show that family members who provide care to disabled relatives experience emotional, physical, and social strain. They also suffer from higher rates of depression, perceived burden, social isolation, family discord, and poor physical health than people who do not have this responsibility. A study done by Rabins and associates[15] of a small sample of elderly chronically ill individuals revealed family care givers underwent some adaptations over a 2-year period. It was found that anger and anxiety toward their situation decreased but guilt and depression persisted.[15]

Two reasons physical therapists would naturally involve the family of an elderly patient is that they are a valuable source of information and they will provide care for the patient. However, the practitioner should be aware that the plan of care worked out by the patient and the clinician may be a burden on family members, and there are limits to the burdens of care that should be placed on the family. This creates a conflict of interest between the patient and the family.[3]

If the care of the elderly patient places a financial burden on the family, there is an ethical obligation to allow the family to participate in decision making. Conflicts arise when the decisions of the family and the patient differ, putting pressure on the two parties and possibly compromising the autonomy of the patient. Problems also occur when the family underestimates the difficulty or cost to them of the proposed patient care, which may lead to harm to all parties. Caring for an elderly relative at home impairs the freedom, independence, and satisfaction of others in the home, and responsibilities fall more on the functional family members, which causes resentment. In this case, it is the moral obligation of the clinician as well to help the family evaluate the responsibility they are undertaking.[3]

PATIENT DIGNITY

Elderly people should be able to live the rest of their lives with dignity, security, and independence. The tendency in American society is to place the elderly in nursing homes where they lose their identity, self-esteem, and individuality instead of encouraging and helping them to spend their remaining years in the dignity of their own homes. The readiness to place the elderly in these institutions stems from a negative basic attitude toward the elderly in this country. In Scandinavia, there is a system called "open care" where the elderly are not dependent on the charity and patience of relatives: Older people in this system retain their independence through programs that allow them to live in their own homes safely with outside help. The cost of this expensive program is paid for by the Scandinavian people through extremely high taxes. This basic attitude—that it is the responsibility of society to take care of its elderly—differs from the United States, which tends to be motivated by politics and would not consider advocating the costly care the Scandinavians have chosen.[16]

Principle I of the American Physical Therapy Association (APTA) Code of Ethics states that physical therapists must respect the rights and dignity of all individuals. This must be considered when implementing medical intervention because to ignore this principle is to treat the individual as less than human. When the physical therapist is not able to see the older person as an individual, treating the patient with dignity is compromised.[4]

One way the clinician can maintain the dignity of patients is to respect their autonomy and right to make decisions regarding their care. The health care professional must remember that even though elderly persons may be in a dependent state, the individuals have had a whole lifetime of self-determination that should not cease because they are temporarily or permanently disabled. This includes their right of confidentiality with respect to family members at the onset of treatment. This does not preclude the clinician from exploring the reasons the patient desires this confidentiality, especially when bad feelings are present, but ultimately the desires of the patient should prevail.[3]

There is also a tendency for health care professionals to treat the elderly, given their dependent state, like children, which is an assault on the individual's self-esteem and dignity. Because of this view, the clinician may assume that sons and daughters of the elderly should assume a parenting role, and important decisions will be discussed with the patient's children rather than with the patient. The health care provider may treat the older patient like a child on a smaller scale, such as assume the patient may be addressed by his or her first name, placing bows in an elderly woman's hair, or referring to an elderly man or woman as "cute," all of which compromise the patient's dignity.[6]

The main way to promote self-esteem and dignity in the elderly population is to change the attitude that society has toward growing old. Given the difficulty of changing this global problem it may be a start to at least change the way physical therapists feel toward the elderly.[6]

PATIENT RIGHTS

The physical therapist is responsible for the maintenance of the basic rights of human beings during their illnesses, such as independence of expression, decision, and action. The APTA House of Delegates has adopted rights* for the individual referred or admitted to the physical therapy service that include but are not necessarily limited to:

1. The selection of a physical therapist of one's own choosing to the extent that it is reasonable and possible.
2. Access to information regarding practice policies and charges for services.
3. Knowledge of the identity of the physical and other personnel providing or participating in the program of care.
4. Expectation that the referral source has no financial involvement in the service. If this is not the case, knowledge of the extent of any financial involvement in the service by the referring source must be explained.
5. Awareness of the physical therapy goals, desired outcomes, and procedures that are being rendered.
6. Receipt of information necessary to give informed consent prior to the initiation of services.
7. Participation in decisions involving the physical therapy plan of care to the extent reasonable and possible.
8. Access to information concerning his or her condition.
9. Expectation that any discussion or consultation involving the case will be conducted discreetly and that all communications and other records pertaining to the care, including the source of payment for treatment, will be treated as confidential.
10. Expectation of safety in the provision of services and safety in regard to the equipment and the physical environment.
11. Timely information about impending discharge and continuing care requirements.
12. Refusal of physical therapy services.
13. Information regarding the practice's mechanism for the initiation, review, and resolution of patient complaints.[17]

There is a particular need to safeguard the rights of elderly individuals in nursing homes. Ombudsman funded by Medicare are available to provide information regarding patient rights and protection in long-term care facilities.[9] Task forces have also been formed consisting of nursing home staff members and administrators, government officials, and medical, legal, and social service professionals to help protect the rights of elderly people in long-term care facilities. One accomplishment of the task force was to determine when it is appropriate for a patient to receive "supportive care" in a facility by setting up recommendations and guidelines. In the past, nursing homes abused patients by placing them on

*Patients' Rights reprinted with permission of the American Physical Therapy Association.

supportive care orders regardless of their health status. Sometimes supportive care is taken to mean "no care necessary," leading to neglect of the elderly patient's basic needs. The task force defines supportive care as care that is intended not to prolong life but to promote the dignity of the patient, minimize pain, preserve hygiene, and support the psychological, social, emotional, and spiritual needs of the patient and family.[18,19]

The Right to Refuse

One right that has the interest of lawyers and ethicists but has not been focused on by health professionals is the right to refuse. One may wonder if a refusal is due to the patient's denial of his or her illness or even to suicidal desires, or if it is a result of a well-thought out balancing of the risks and benefits of a particular treatment. The courts have distinguished between a suicide and refusal of care that may or may not prolong life and protects the rights of the individual to refuse treatment. When dealing with the elderly where chronic irreversible and debilitating conditions are present for which there is often no cure, limited treatment may be desired by the patient. One reason for this is that although the care is meant to prolong life, it is actually prolonging death. The American Medical Association's (AMA) Council on Ethical and Judicial Affairs states that competent patients have the moral and legal right to refuse treatment whether it is life sustaining or not. This may be overridden in the case where the refusal of treatment affects another person, particularly minor children.[3,9,19]

One important fact the clinician must remember is a refusal does not mean the patient is incompetent or crazy, and it has been suggested that for some groups of chronically ill patients, refusal should be offered as an option before treatment is initiated. The single greatest reason for refusal of care is misunderstanding or miscommunication of the treatment involved. A study by Applebaum and Roth[19] concluded many patients refuse treatment as a way to find out more information regarding their care. When psychological factors were implicated in reasons for refusal it was usually due to the distinctive way that individual deals with stress; the denial of illness was not commonly a direct cause.[9,19]

Often the clinician does not investigate the reason the patient is refusing and, therefore, does not respond accordingly. For example, if a patient is refusing because he or she misunderstood the treatment plan, the response of the clinician would not be to offer clearer information since the reason for the refusal was not sought. Forced treatment by health professionals as a response to refusal was not uncommon but was usually limited to patients who were incompetent and unable to make their own decisions. Substitute consent was not usually obtained in these cases before treatment was started. When dealing with competent patients, there were responses of what was termed "forceful persuasion," where patients were told they had no choice if the treatment was considered essential by the clinician.[19]

In physical therapy, refusal of care can be as obvious as refusing treatment or as subtle as not performing the prescribed home exercise program. These patients are typically labeled noncompliant, and it is usually assumed that this problem exclusively lies with the patient, and the only solution is their compliance. The patient's right to autonomy over his or her body is not recognized, and the right of the patient not to comply with the advise of the physical therapist is not acknowledged. In a long-term care facility, noncompliance is often the only way a patient can exert control over his or her life, particularly in a rehabilitation setting. Reasons for the patient's noncompliance should be sought with the intention of understanding the rationale for nonparticipation. When a clinician places the problem of noncompliance totally on the patient, it is easy for therapists to avoid examining their own behavior or the influence of the health care setting on the patient's nonparticipation. The physical therapist can enhance compliance by taking the time to explain routine procedures, listening to the patient's concerns and fears, and involving the patient in goal setting. Although persuading the patient with clear and accurate information is encouraged, the autonomy of the patient must always be respected, even when the patient continues to not comply.[20]

The physical therapist must also be wary of patients who unquestioningly follow every directive of the clinician and should not assume these patients understand the treatment being implemented. Often, this behavior is motivated out of fear of the health professional or fear of a bad medical outcome. The need to evaluate the decision-making capacity of a compliant patient is easy to miss because it is the patients who refuse care that are usually having their competency challenged. From a moral point of view, therefore, unquestioned compliance may be as much of a problem as noncompliance.[20]

Rights of Demented Patients

In order to respect the rights of demented patients, their wishes regarding medical intervention must be documented when they are still in a competent state. Often family understanding of the patient's wishes or prior values without specific documentation is not sufficient to make decisions about life-sustaining treatment. Given the difficulty of determining what best serves the interests of a severely demented patient, the court system recommends that the individual state specific preferences before the onset of disability. Discontinuing treatment that would prolong severe pain in the patient is clearly permissible according to the courts, because it is universally accepted that death is preferable to living with unrelenting pain. The clinician must also consider the pain and suffering that is present when treatment is forced on the incompetent patient against his or her wishes. An incompetent patient often can have strong preferences regarding treatment even though these preferences are not based in reality, and forcing unwanted treatment may cause the patient to experience a painful and humiliating violation.[21]

As previously mentioned, when it has been determined by careful evaluation that a patient is unable to make his or her own decisions regarding medical care, a surrogate decision maker must be chosen. It is believed that to the extent possible the rights of the incompetent patient should be an extension of the rights of the competent, and respect, self-determination, and promotion of well-being should be observed.[12]

For the clinician, it is clear that one must yield to the wishes of a competent patient, but dealing with a surrogate who may be acting in bad faith or have conflicts of interest is more complicated. For example, if the surrogate demands treatment that the clinician deems unnecessary, the clinician must make it clear that treatment is not indicated. If the family member still insists on the treatment, a court order must be obtained. This is an expensive and time-consuming process and tends to discourage a family member acting out of guilt or self-serving motives. Only the court can authorize a plan of care that is opposed by an incompetent patient's next of kin. If the health care professional has concerns regarding the decision made by the surrogate, the surrogate appointment should be reviewed by an ethics committee or consultant but can be legally changed only by the court system. Even though the surrogate should be more limited in his or her decision-making power than a competent patient, the family members should have some range of discretion so that they are not just carrying out the desires of the clinician.[7]

When considering the ability of the mentally impaired to make medical decisions, a precise mental evaluation is critical since the legal system has customarily taken an all or nothing approach to this decision. Either an individual is capable of making all decisions or he or she is declared incompetent and denied the right to make any decisions at all.[22] Elderly patients with fluctuating mental abilities need to be carefully evaluated before they are judged incapable of making medical decisions. "Windows of lucidity" may exist in patients where, in their more lucid moments, they are able to understand information that is given to them and consequently make clear decisions. An elderly person may experience what is called "sundowning" in which he or she experiences increased confusion at night and may need to be evaluated at different times of day in order to evaluate his or her ability to understand information.[9]

General mental status exams may be a good assessment for impairments when cognition is already severely compromised, but they are not adequate in assessing gradations of decision-making capacity.[23] In assessing competence, the most important part of the formal evaluation should be testing of the patient's ability to understand his or her medical situation. For example, the patient may not know what day it is but appears to understand the benefits of physical therapy and, therefore, is capable of making decisions even though disorientation is present.[7]

It is often assumed that preconceived beliefs about the elderly, as well as the paternalistic patterns of medical practice, may lead clinicians to underestimate the decisive capabilities of the older patient. However, in a study done by Fitten and associates,[23] it was found that when clinicians rely on brief medical evaluations, test of recall, and their own judgment, they are most likely to assume incorrectly that the decision-making capacity of the patient is intact. The outcome of this research stresses the importance of a systematic evaluation that directly probes the patient's understanding of the issues involved and the reasoning underlying his or her treatment decisions.[23]

INFORMED CONSENT

The legal and ethical foundation of informed consent is self-determination and autonomy, or, in other words, the right to decide what is done to one's body. Medical professionals are obligated to provide information regarding the risks and benefits of the recommended treatment plan in a language and style that the patient can understand, as well as to inform the patient about alternate treatment options. By giving the patient proper and clear information the health professional is allowing the patient to execute his or her right to choose.[9]

All states have a combination of statutes, common laws, and regulations that require that the informed consent of a competent patient must be obtained before treatment is started. Some states do recognize *therapeutic privilege*, which is an exception to the informed consent process and allows a physician to withhold information if, in the opinion of the physician, the patient would suffer direct harm as a result of the knowledge. This doctrine is not usually appropriate.[9]

The perception of the elderly as being too old to learn new information can compromise their right to be informed. The health professional must remember that learning is a lifelong process, even though age related changes can affect learning and comprehension. Some variables that may affect learning in the older patient are alterations in sensory perception, motivation, response time, memory, and sleep–wake cycles, all of which require modified teaching strategies in order to enhance the comprehension of information. One of the major factors in the learning process is sensory perception, such as sight and hearing, and because this is often compromised in the elderly, it should be evaluated and compensated for, if needed, before the clinician begins to present information. One can compensate for the increased response time that may be present in an older person by decreasing the rate and amount of information presented. Creating a relaxed, private atmosphere may be necessary to decrease anxiety and increase the client's capacity to comprehend.[24] The clinician must take responsibility to implement these strategies in order to ensure that elderly patients can understand what medical treatments are being considered and can exercise their right to be informed.

Informed consent is generally recognized as necessary when providing potentially dangerous treatment, such as chemotherapy, blood transfusions, and surgery. However, in treatments like physical therapy, which is considered noninvasive, the necessity of consent is often overlooked. From a moral point of view obtaining consent to perform "harmless" treatment is just as important as hazardous treatment. Physical therapy may be considered routine, however, rehabilitation can be considered extremely invasive considering the amount of time patients need to dedicate to it and the impact it has on their lives.[20]

It is felt that it is the therapist's responsibility to ensure that information presented to the patient is understood and to be sensitive to cues regarding the patient's level of understanding. Purtilo feels it is better to give the patient too much rather than too little information.[4] Those who do not believe informed consent is appropriate feel patients cannot possibly understand the complexity of the medical situation and are, therefore, incapable of making decisions. However, what these individuals fail to recognize is that it is not necessary for the patient to understand every detail but only the major issues.[25]

Physical therapists are also in a special situation regarding informed consent since their main focus is management of disability and pain control. Patients who are experiencing pain, changes in life-style, and anxiety may agree to anything that could possibly make their situation better. The clinician should not take this eagerness for granted and should always properly explain what is being implemented.[25] Informed consent should not simply be obtained for legal or malpractice reasons but to protect the patient's right to know and preserve patient autonomy.

DEATH ISSUES

Advances in medical technology that tend to prolong the dying process have created a new group of ethical issues regarding patient autonomy and death. Dying at home has become rare; it now occurs most frequently in hospitals and long-term care settings that are dominated by professionals and their use of technology. Medical management is usually geared toward promoting life at all costs, which often can overlook the value systems and desires of the individuals involved.

Advanced directives, which are documented desires of medical management, can be used to ward off unwarranted care and promote death with dignity. Specificity is important in order for advanced directives to be as effective as possible. The documents should include a statement that the person has presence of mind and is able to make decisions regarding specific possible medical events of the future. A list of interventions that is undesired in the event of certain illnesses should also be included. A competent individual can delegate decision rights to someone else by giving that person power of attorney. Legally, in order for that power to continue after the onset of incompetence, a durable power of attorney must be obtained.[9]

Living Wills

A living will is one example of an advanced directive in which a competent adult expresses his or her wishes regarding medical management in the event of incapacitation. In November 1990, President Bush signed the Patient Self-Determination Act, which was created to increase patient involvement regarding decisions involving life-sustaining equipment and encourage more patients to prepare documents, such as living wills, in advance by providing them with the proper information. The Patient Self-Determination Act requires hospitals and skilled nursing facilities to develop written policies regarding advanced directives as a condition of Medicare and Medicaid payment. These facilities are required to ask all new patients whether or not they have prepared these documents, as well as to provide written information regarding facility policy and patient rights under the law. In December 1991, requirements went into effect that provide immunity to physicians and other health professionals when they are carrying out the wishes of the patient.[26]

The importance of clear, advanced directives was demonstrated in the US Supreme Court decision of *Cruzan* v. *Director of Missouri Department of Health*, the first case in which a high court considered termination of lifeprolonging measures for an incompetent patient. The court upheld the Missouri decision not to remove the feeding tube of Nancy Cruzan, who was in a vegetative state, at the request of her parents since there was no "clear and convincing" evidence that the patient, if competent, would want it removed.[27]

There are many shortcomings regarding living wills that can make the document ineffective. For example, a living will is only applicable for the terminally ill, and there are limitations on the types of treatments that can be refused by the patient. There is also no penalty for the health provider who refuses to honor the document, and there is a tendency for physicians to make medical decisions based on their interpretation of the living will. For this reason it is important to accompany the document with a durable power of attorney to make it mandatory for the clinician to discuss treatment options with an individual selected by the patient.[28]

Durable power of attorney is present in every state and was primarily developed in order to manage financial matters of incapacitated individuals. Additional proxy laws are being developed state to state that specifically deal with health care. These laws would give an agent named by the patient the same authority for decision making as the patient would have if competent. The decision of the agent prevails when disagreements among family members are present regarding medical management. Since the physician may have difficulty honoring a living will over the objections of the family, the presence of this agent is essential to ensure that the wishes of the patient are respected.[28]

Euthanasia

According to *Webster's Dictionary*, euthanasia is defined as the action of inducing the painless death of a person for reasons assumed to be merciful. A moral distinction is made, which is accepted by most physicians, between passive and active euthanasia in which it is considered acceptable to remove life-sustaining treatment but it is unacceptable to actively terminate another person's life. A statement adopted by the House of Delegates of the AMA in 1973 considered "mercy killing" to be contrary to the medical profession's ethical position. On the other hand, the opinion of the AMA was that ceasing extraordinary treatment that prolongs the life of a body when death is imminent is the decision of the patient, family, or both, with the aiding advice of the physician.[29]

Controversy is centered around active voluntary euthanasia that, for instance, would allow the physician at the request of the patient to administer a lethal medication. The concept that killing someone is morally worse than letting them die is one reason why people believe there is a moral difference between active and passive euthanasia. However, this belief does not account for the patient who is in severe unrelieved pain with days to live and who desires to terminate his or her own life. According to the AMA doctrine, the physician is permitted to stop treatment that prolongs the pain thereby causing the patient to suffer more than if direct action were taken.[29,30]

The American Geriatric Society (AGS) opposes active euthanasia and feels that while lethal injections may be appropriate for the few patients suffering from unrelenting pain, there is too much of a risk for abuse of frail, disabled, and economically disadvantaged members of society. The AGS is also concerned that legalized active euthanasia would weaken the motivation of society to develop solutions for proper care of the dying, such as hospice programs and that, given our fiscally obsessed society, active euthanasia may be viewed as a way to contain medical costs.[30]

The mental anguish caused by having to face another day waiting to die may be a growing reason for requests for voluntary active euthanasia. The presence of intractable pain is no longer as widely used as a justification for active euthanasia given the presence of anesthetic levels of pain-relieving medications. The psychological suffering of the patient would be minimized if the individual were able to legally choose the time and place of their death. It has also been argued that making these choices regarding death is fundamental and honors the autonomy of the patient.[31]

If patients were legally given the choice of active euthanasia, the question is how many patients would pursue it. Hospice physicians report that although the topic of active euthanasia frequently arises in passing conversation, only a few patients seriously and persistently pursue its implementation.[31]

The debate regarding legalizing voluntary active euthanasia is far from over, and the degree to which supportive services for the dying should be made available must be addressed. Society must develop policies for the dying that will benefit the patient and enhance autonomy but not lead to potential abuses of the weaker members of society.

Cardiopulmonary Resuscitation

In the health care setting cardiopulmonary resuscitation (CPR) is considered a routine procedure administered to patients suffering cardiopulmonary arrest. It has always been assumed that consent to perform CPR is present since the patient is incapacitated and inaction will lead to death. The practice of performing CPR on any patient experiencing cardiac arrest regardless of the state of their illness and chances for survival is a cause of concern.[32] The right of the patient to refuse treatment also applies to the use of resuscitation, and a patient may express in advance that this procedure be withheld.[33]

The right of the patient to have do not resuscitate (DNR) orders placed in his or her medical chart is established but the question is how involved is the patient in the decision making? One study revealed that 95% of a group of physicians believed that patients should be involved in resuscitation decisions but only 10% discussed this issue with their patients. Another study showed that only 20% of the patients with DNR orders in their chart discussed their preferences with their physician prior to the initiation of the orders.[33] Even though decreased mental capacity may be one reason preferences were not discussed, the difficulty both physicians and patients have with discussing death may be another reason for inadequate patient participation. However, the need for this discussion is essential in order for the patient to participate in the decision-making process. In order to assist physicians in managing patients who are not appropriate for CPR, guidelines have been established by the Council on Ethical and Judicial Affairs.[33]

Another concern is that the presence of DNR orders will affect other therapeutic care given to the patient. A study done by Zimmerman and co-authors[34] showed that within 1.7 days of placement of a DNR order in the chart the patient either died or was discharged from the ICU. These results suggest that even though DNR orders only specify withholding of CPR, other therapeutic limits may accompany the order.[34]

A difficult situation arises when the patient, family, or both insists on CPR orders even when the procedure would clearly be futile. Inappropriate resuscitation may even cause harm by producing a chronic vegetative state. Patients and their families may insist on resuscitation out of guilt or fear, as well as out of unrealistic hopes for a cure. In this situation patient autonomy cannot be the only guide and does not allow a patient to demand treatment that is nonbeneficial and potentially harmful.

However, in this scenario, the question arises as to what is the point of offering the patient the choice in an attempt to preserve his or her rights of autonomy if these wishes are later denied. For this reason some physicians believe CPR should not be offered to this type of patient since the choice represents a potential for benefit when there is none.[32]

The issue of CPR in the nursing home setting is a complex one. The benefits are difficult to assess given the degree of debilitation in individuals present in a skilled nursing facility. Furthermore, the violence of the procedure and its small likelihood of success argue against it. However, to withhold life-saving therapy from a certain population just because they are dependent can be construed as discriminatory. A limited study done by Finucane and co-workers[35] demonstrated that there is an implicit policy by most nursing homes to withhold CPR from their residents.

The debate on proper policies regarding performing CPR in nursing homes continues and, like other treatments that tend to prolong the life of an already debilitated individual, it is difficult for the clinician to balance patient autonomy with supplying a treatment that is considered nonbeneficial.

Terminal Care

Terminal care is geared toward providing a protective, nurturing, and homelike environment in which there is a large involvement of the health care team in decision making for the patient. Since the elderly resident is dependent on the staff for personal hygiene, meals, and medication, the resident assumes a subservient role by trading his or her autonomy and dignity for the attentive care received.[3]

The older person's own home has a certain therapeutic value that is often not recognized. Home health care is, therefore, receiving new recognition. In this setting, individuals will be more likely to exercise their right to make decisions. There is, however, a danger of a patient becoming overconfident and having unrealistic views regarding his or her capacity to care for him- or herself, which the home care provider must be careful in assessing.[3]

Unlike an acute care setting, the treatment in a long-term care facility is routine and repetitive, making violations of the individual's autonomy more probable. Older people often may have the power to decide but are unable to carry out their personal decisions without the aid of the staff. Without this assistance their freedom to decide is useless and their autonomy infringed upon.[36]

Value systems are important to examine when considering the long-term care setting. An individual may be placed in a facility that does not share his or her values and goals or the patient's status may change while in the facility, making the setting no longer appropriate. It is important for the primary care physician to manage this and prevent or resolve ethical mismatches.[3] For example, the elderly resident in a nursing home may not share the enthusiasm of the physical therapist to participate in an exercise program.

Although nursing home residents vary in age, degree of function, and levels of cognition and interests, a common denominator is the difficulty in exercising choice. In order to enhance patient autonomy in long-term care facilities, increased staff, space, and resources are needed. Society is responsible for making the decision whether or not this should be a priority. The changes that do not require extra funds should of course be investigated first, and efforts should be made to find out the preferences of nursing home residents themselves.[37]

Hospice

The question of how society should deal with their dying population has always represented a void in the health care system that, in the past two decades, has been filled with the fast growth of the hospice. The growth of the hospice setting has received widespread support in the United States, sparking the interest of the health professional specializing in geriatrics, since approximately 66% of the patients in hospices are over 65.[38]

In the hospice, health care and service is provided for the patient and the family and is available at all times. Care is planned and provided by a medical inter-disciplinary team, as well as by using family and volunteers to provide physical, emotional, and spiritual care to the patient with an emphasis on palliative care. The hospice is sensitive to needs of the family who obviously experience stress with the patient's terminal illness and also provides follow up care after the patient dies.[38]

The focus of the hospice is to help the dying patient live the remaining time as fully as possible instead of concentrating on the disease process itself. The care is directed primarily at symptom and pain control to improve quality of life rather than disease control. There are major philosophical differences between hospices and the traditional health care setting, with hospice rules and regulations being extremely flexible to enhance the life of the dying patient.[39]

The physical therapist does play a palliative role in the hospice setting, using pain control modalities but more importantly, he or she functions as an educator for both the patient and the family. As in a home care setting, the physical therapist teaches the patient functional and safe tasks, and the family is present to learn as well. Each member of the hospice health care team, including the physical therapist, assumes the role of counselor, which demands good listening and communication skills. The involvement of the therapist is dependent on the resources available as well as the desires of the patient and family.[39]

Suicide

The suicide rate of older people is double that of any other age group. These rates are most likely underestimated, given that the probability of not reporting suicides is highest in the elderly population. Older people are also more likely to complete the task of suicide, use a more violent means, and have a greater male to female ratio than any other age group. Conwell and co-authors[40] found that older suicide victims had a lower incidence of psychopathy and were responding to physical illness and loss.

Ethical debate regarding suicide and the elderly leaves health care providers confused about what their response should be. One question is whether suicide in the elderly should be treated like suicide in any other age group with an attempt to prevent it or to respect the right of the older person to choose to die. Health professionals desiring to prevent suicide rarely view it as a rational act well-thought out by the individual but as a symptom of depression and mental dysfunction. It is equally important to discuss whether or not killing oneself for reasons of old age alone without the presence of terminal illness is ethically justified.[6]

Arguments against the concept of a justifiable suicide are dominated by the belief that killing one's self is a terrible act regardless of the circumstances. Clinicians concerned with suicide prevention may argue that the state of mind of the older person may be temporary and, though circumstances may be bad, they may get better in the future. However, elderly individuals who have deliberated about suicide over a long period of time are not experiencing a passing mental state and, unlike their younger counterparts, the future of an older person is more predictable and less bright.[6]

There is a great desire to promote both "death with dignity" and the right to choose one's own destiny; however, there is a concern that society, as well as the elderly, will view suicide as a solution to problems associated with aging. Taking this a step further, elderly people who do not choose suicide may be viewed as selfish for not committing the act in order to remove their presence as a burden to society.[6]

The issue of suicide and the elderly is complicated by desires to preserve patient autonomy, as well as the fear that making suicide acceptable in the elderly will contribute overall to the reprehensible attitude that the older person is a burden and should be removed. Perhaps these ethical issues will become clearer when the young and old are able to come to terms with their own aging process and mortality.

CASE STUDY 1

A childless, 78-year-old woman was admitted to the hospital on July 14, 1981 because of weight loss and fever. Her husband died in 1972 and after his death she became depressed, refused to eat, and lost weight. An ileostomy tube was inserted for feeding purposes. It was successful, and the patient gained weight. Psychological interviews revealed her to be well oriented but possibly slightly demented because of her simple answers, and she did not show interest or awareness of events happening around her. She lost the ability to ambulate and developed multiple contractures. She also developed anemia secondary to poor nutrition. On November 30, 1982, when she was transferred to another facility, she still had the ileostomy, which had not been used for feeding for some time. The patient often complained about the tube and stated she would like it removed. On or around April 27, 1983, the end of the "J tube" broke off and the remaining portion appeared to be "flush" with the surface of the skin. On April 28, 1983 the tube slipped inside, causing the physicians to maintain a close observation of her status. The physician believed the tube would pass through the rectum in the feces, which it did several days later. The patient then stated she thought she was going to die and appeared quite depressed. The ethical question in this case is: Should the tube have been removed at the request of the patient given the presumed competent state she was in.

CASE STUDY 2

A 95-year-old woman living at home independently with diabetes and congestive heart failure was hospitalized after developing gangrene of one foot. While hospitalized she refused amputation but consented to continue management of her other medical problems, including medication and localized treatment for her foot. She became unpopular with the hospital staff and other patients because of the foot's odor and the related infection control hazards. The house staff on her case expressed that she must be crazy since she refused life-sustaining treatment. The physician and a psychologist experienced in competency assessment evaluated the patient and determined that the patient's cognitive abilities were intact. The evaluation also concluded that the patient refused the surgery due to personal values of not wanting to continue life at her age without her foot even if death without intervention was imminent. Presentation of positive examples of life as an amputee did not change her position. In order to pacify the concern of the staff regarding infection and odor, the ward was visited frequently by in infection control specialist and the patient received whirlpool treatments of the foot. The patient died several weeks later with her wishes respected.[7]

CASE STUDY 3

An 83-year-old woman whose status postoperatively included a right CVA, was admitted into a nursing home directly from the hospital. At the time of admission, the patient was extremely dependent and could only ambulate short distances with the maximum assistance of two people. She refused to use an assistive device. A mental evaluation performed by the nursing home staff physician revealed the patient was not oriented to time or place but was aware of her medical condition and recognized her daughter who visited her frequently. The physician and the patient's daughter agreed it was important to continue the physical therapy that was initiated in the hospital in order to promote restoration of function as well as independence. When the transporter arrived to take the patient to her first physical therapy session, the patient verbally refused, but she was placed in the wheelchair by the transporter under the direction of the nurse in charge on the floor. In the physical therapy department, the patient expressed the desire to return to her room repetitively and reluctantly cooperated during the evaluation performed by the therapist. Even after a great deal of coaxing and encouragement the physical therapist was unable to convince the patient to ambulate with a walker or a quad cane. In spite of the patient's verbal refusals, she was brought to physical therapy daily where she ambulated short distances with the assistance of two people but refused to perform any other exercises.

CONCLUSION

The ethical treatment of patients is an important but underemphasized aspect of medical care. Given the current trend away from high cost, high technology health care, today's health professional must reevaluate the role ethical issues play in their attitudes toward providing the best care, especially for older patients. This chapter has addressed the therapist's attitude toward the older patient, and how these attitudes impact decision making in rehabilitation. In addition, the more controversial areas of medical ethics, such as allocation of resources, care giver stress, patient dignity and patient rights, informed consent, and death and dying issues were discussed. Finally, the chapter stressed that these issues not only play a critical role in the day-to-day care of patients, but have a long-term impact as well.

PEARLS

- The shift in modern medicine from a paternalistic role toward giving the patient more responsibility in decision making may be threatening to the aged who are more comfortable with traditional roles.

- The physical therapist should practice beneficence in medical decision making and not be a neutral party. They should encourage acceptance of an appropriate treatment, being careful not to coerce or deceive the patient.

- Ombudsman funded by Medicare are available to provide information regarding patient rights and protection in long-term care facilities.

- In informed consent, physical therapists are obliged to provide information in language a patient can understand regarding risks, benefits, and alternate treatment options, except when the therapist exercises therapeutic privilege (i.e., withdrawing information that the therapist feels will cause the patient direct harm as a result of knowledge).

- Advanced directions, such as a living will, are documented desires of medical management used to ward off unwarranted care and promote death with dignity.

- The American Geriatric Society opposes active euthanasia and feels that while lethal injections may be appropriate for a few patients suffering from unrelenting pain, there is too much at risk for abuse for frail, disabled, and economically disadvantaged elderly.

- Older people have double the suicide rate of any other age group.

REFERENCES

1. Spencer FC. The vital role in medicine of commitment to the patient. *Am Coll Surg Bull.* 1990; 75:7–19.
2. *Miranda* v. *Arizona*, 384 U.S. 436 (1966).
3. Talar GA, Waymack MH. Ethics and the elderly. *Primary Care.* 1989; 16;529–541.
4. Purtilo RB. Ethical considerations. In: Jackson OL, eds. *Therapeutic Considerations for the Elderly.* New York: Churchill Livingstone; 1987:173.
5. Harris J, Fiedler CM. Preadolescent attitudes toward the elderly: an analysis of race, gender, and contact variables. *Adolescence.* 1988; 23:335–340.
6 Lesnoff-Caravaglia G. *Values, Ethics and Aging.* New York: Human Sciences Press; 1985.
7. Goldstein MK. Ethical care of the elderly: pitfalls and principles. *Geriatrics.* 1989; 44:101–106.
8. Lynn J. Conflicts of interest in medical decision-making. *J Am Geriatr Soc.* 1988; 36:945–950.
9. Dubler NN. Legal issues. *Merck Manual.* Rahway, NJ: Merck, Sharp, and Dohme Research Laboratories; 1990: 1142–1161.
10. Coates R. Ethics and physicotherapy. *Aust Physiotherapy.* 1990; 36:84–87.
11. Kilner JF. Age criteria in medicine. *Arch Intern Med.* 1989; 149:2343–2346.
12. Barondess JA, Kalb P, Weil WB, et al. Clinical decision-making in catastrophic situations: The revelance of age. *J Am Ger Soc.* 1988; 36:919–937.
13. Daniels N. Why saying no to patients in the United States is so hard. *N Engl J Med.* 1986; 314:1380–1383.
14. Eddy DM. The individual vs society: is there a conflict? *JAMA.* 1991; 265:1446–1450.
15. Rabins PV, Fitting MD, Eastham J, et al. Emotional adaptation over time in care-givers for chronically ill elderly people. *Age and Ageing.* 1990; 19:185–190.
16. Szulc T. How we can help ourselves age with dignity. *Parade.* May 29 1988;4–7.
17. American Physical Therapy Association Code of Ethics. Alexandria, VA: American Physical Therapy Association.
18. Moon MA. Task force to protect rights of nursing home patients. *Intern Med News.* 1983; 16:23.
19. Appelbaum PS, Roth LH. Patients who refuse treatment in medical hospitals. *JAMA.* 1983; 215:1296–1301.
20. Coy JA. Autonomy-based informed consent: ethical implications for patient noncompliance. *Phys Ther.* 1989; 69:826–833.
21. Arras JD. The severely demented, minimally functional patient: an ethical analysis. *J Am Ger Soc.* 1988; 36:938–944.
22. Gunn AE. Mental impairment in the elderly: medical-legal assessment. *J Am Ger Soc.* 1977; 25:193–198.
23. Fitten LJ, Lusky RL, Hamann C. Assessing treatment decision-making capacity in elderly nursing home residents. *J Am Ger Soc.* 1990; 38:1097–1104.
24. Rendon DC, et al. The right to know, the right to be taught. *J Gerontol Nurs.* 1986; 12: 33–37.
25. Simm J. Informed consent: ethical implications for physiotherapy. *Physiotherapy.* 1986; 72:584–587.
26. Greco PJ, Schulman KA, Lavizzo-Mourey R, et al. The patient self-determination act and the future of advance directives. *Ann Intern Med.* 1991; 115:639–643.
27. Malloy DW, Clarnetle RM, Braun EA, et al. Decision making in the incompetent elderly: "the daughter from California syndrome." *J Am Ger Soc.* 1991; 39:396–399.
28. Annas GJ. The health care proxy and the living will. *N Engl J Med.* 1991; 324:1210–1213.
29. Rachels J. Active and passive euthanasia. *N Engl J Med.* 1975; 292:78–80.
30. AGS Public Policy Committee. Voluntary active euthanasia. *J Am Ger Soc.* 1991; 39:826.
31. Teno J, Lynn J. Voluntary active euthanasia: the individual case and public policy. *J Am Ger Soc.* 1991; 39:827–830.
32. Blackhall LJ. Must we always use CPR? *N Engl J Med.* 1987; 317:1281–1285.

33. Council on Ethical and Judicial Affairs, American Medical Association. Guidelines for the appropriate use of do-not-resuscitate orders. *JAMA*. 1991; 265:1868–1871.

34. Zimmerman JE, Knaus WA, Sharpe SM, et al. The use and implications of do not resuscitate orders in intensive care units. *JAMA*. 1986; 255:351–356.

35. Finucane TE, Boyer JT, Bulmash J, et al. The incidence of attempted CPR in nursing homes. *J Am Ger Soc*. 1991; 39:624–626.

36. Collopy BJ. Ethical dimensions of autonomy in long-term care. *Generations*. 1990; XIV: 9–12.

37. Kane RL, Kane RA. Long-term-care financing on personal autonomy. *Generations*. 1990; XIV:86–94.

38. Greer DS. Hospice: Lessons for geriatricians. *J Am Ger Soc*. 1983; 31:67–70.

39. Toot J. Physical therapy and hospice, concept and practice. *Phys Ther*. 1984; 64:665–671.

40. Conwell Y, Rotenber M, Caine ED. Completed suicide at age 50 and over. *J Am Ger Soc*. 1990; 38:640–644.

CHAPTER *17* SEVENTEEN

Education Services: Learning, Memory, and Intelligence

Elders of the tribe were once considered teachers and the founts of wisdom. Today, little respect is given to the experiences of a lifetime, and myths perpetuate the notion that learning abilities and memory capabilities decline with age. On the contrary, in our society, elderly individuals must learn new skills as new technology alters basic systems of communication, transportation, finance, and recreation on a nearly daily basis. As values change, societal rewards change, and new learning is required.

Learning means the acquisition of information or skills, and it is usually measured by looking for improvements in task performance. When someone improves his or her performance at a given intellectual or physical task, then he or she has learned, and studies of performance in elderly individuals indicate a decline with age. Clearly, there are a number of factors other than learning ability that affect performance. Some of these include physiological responses, physical health status, and motivation. In practice, it is extremely difficult to separate the components of performance in order to examine the influence of learning ability, although a number of studies have attempted to do so. Despite evidence that other factors contribute to the decline in task performance, most researchers still attribute part of this decline to a diminished ability to learn with age.

All age groups can learn. Older individuals just require more time. Tasks that involve manipulation of distinct and familiar symbols or objects, unambiguous responses, and low interference from prior learning are particularly conducive to good performance by older individuals.[1]

At various points in time, different approaches to the study of learning and memory have been dominant. In the 1960s the associative view of learning was most popular. In the 1970s theories on information processing were established as the mode for learning and memory, whereas today a growing emphasis in learning theories concerns a contextual approach.[2] It is important, therefore, to briefly review the research on learning and memory from each of these approaches.

Learning and memory are closely related concepts. People must learn before they can remember, and learning without memory has limited use. Learning is often assessed by memory tasks. "How much you have learned?" is translated to "How much do you remember?" Learning is defined as the acquisition of a new skill or information through practice and experience. Remembering is defined as the retrieval of information that has been stored in memory.[2]

The general learning/memory system involves three processes: acquisition, storage, and retrieval. Memory is often discussed in terms of information: How is information put into the system, how is it stored, and how is it retrieved? This is the approach of modern information processing theories, and in this view, learning is part of memory; that is, the acquisition, registration, or encoding phase.

When adding the dimension of age, there are many questions that arise. How do learning abilities change? How does memory change? Does it fade? Do old people forget new things and remember the past? How do societal demands affect learning and memory?

ASSOCIATIVE LEARNING

Based on the assumption that learning and memory involve the association of ideas or events that occur together in time, the associative learning theory involves a stimulus–response bond, and paired association is the most commonly employed mode for testing memory using this theory. The task is to learn an association between two commonly unrelated items, such as basket–therefore or orange–until. The subject is first presented with two unrelated words, and the subsequent task is to give a correct response to each stimulus word when it appears alone. The ability to recall a paired stimulus represents the contents of memory. There are several factors that appear to influence the amount of information that can be processed with increasing age, including the pace of learning and the environment in which learning occurs, which may be influenced by cautiousness, anxiety, and interference from previously learned information.

The pace of learning is the speed with which a task is performed and is one variable known to affect older learners more than younger ones. The pace of learning can be manipulated in two ways. The anticipation interval is the time allotted for a response. Older subjects perform poorly when this interval is short but do much better when they are given more time to respond.[3] Younger subjects also improve as the anticipation interval increases but less than older subjects do. If a method called "self-pacing" is permitted (i.e., if the learner is allowed as much time as he or she wants), older subjects improve in the number of correct responses they are capable of giving. The second element of pacing in paired associative learning is the time the pair of items is presented for study. This period is referred to as the study time or inspection interval. Increasing the study time also improves the performance of older learners, though old and young subjects have been shown to benefit equally from longer study times.[4] Again, if "self-pacing" is allowed, older subjects benefit more than younger subjects.

The ability to perform associative learning tasks may be affected by variables like cautiousness, anxiety, and interference. These factors are often associated with errors of omission (not responding) or errors of commission (responding incorrectly). Errors of omission occur most often in fast-paced, associative learning situations (rather than errors of commission). Errors of omission reflect a cautiousness or a reluctance to venture a response unless one is absolutely certain of its accuracy. It has been suggested by researchers that the poorer performance of older adults, as reflected in omission errors, is a function of their being more cautious.[2]

To overcome cautiousness, or to test this hypothesis, experimenters have requested or demanded responses be made, even if they are wrong. This failed to improve the learning rate of older subjects or to reduce the number of errors of omission.[5] However, in another test of the cautiousness hypothesis, a small monetary reward was given for each correct response, each incorrect response was rewarded but at a slightly lower value, and the absence of a response received no reward. In this situation, older learners significantly reduced the number of errors of omission,[6] which suggests that older learners could do better if they took a few more chances.

Another hypothesis regarding the poorer performance of the elderly on paired associative learning suggests that anxiety affects performance. Eisdorfer and associates[7] tested this theory by introducing a drug that blocked physiological arousal. This resulted in significantly fewer errors in older subjects on associative learning tasks compared to elders given an inactive drug.

A final hypothesis suggests that in some instances of associative learning, older adults are more susceptible to the effects of interference from prior learning. When one word is frequently associated with another word in everyday situations, such as dark–light and water–ocean, the pair is said to have high associative strength. When one word is infrequently associated with another, such as dark–fast and water–book, the pair has low associative strength. If the associative habits of older individuals are more established through a greater number of years of experience, it follows that age related differences should be least for high associative pairs. This appears to be the case. In a comprehensive study, Botwinick and Storandt[8] found no age related differences in performance on an easy list but marked age related differences in performance on moderate to high difficulty lists. The older adults appear to be more handicapped when learning and recall involve forming associations that are contrary, or in competition with, previously learned verbal associations.

Judging from studies of associative learning, the rate of learning slows gradually through the adult years. Only after the age of 65 does one's learning become demonstrably poorer than that of young adults. The nature of this age deficit remains unclear. Older subjects profit from a slower pace of learning much more than do young adults. Moreover, the older learner may become too anxious or cautious, or may encounter interference from previously learned associations.

HUMAN MEMORY

There are many myths about the effects of aging on memory. For example, people are supposed to forget things they have recently learned, but memories from the distant past are supposed to be clear and vivid, sometimes startlingly so.

Memory is closely related to both intelligence and learning, since remembering is part of the evidence of learning and learning is part of the measurement of intelligence. For example, if a person does not learn, that person has nothing to remember. Conversely, if the individual cannot remember, there is no sign of learning.[9]

There are essentially four types of memory. Short-term or immediate memory involves recall after very little delay (as little as 5 seconds up to 30 seconds). Recent memory involves recall after a brief period (from 1 hour to several days). Remote memory refers to recall of events that took place a long time ago but that have been referred to frequently throughout the course of a lifetime. Old memory refers to recall of events that occurred a long time in the past and that have not been thought of or rehearsed since.

Regardless of type, there are three stages of memory: registration (encoding), retention (storage), and recall (retrieval). Registration refers to the recording of learning or perceptions, and it is more commonly referred to as encoding. In concept, it is analogous to the recording of sound on a tape recorder. Retention refers to the ability to sustain registration over time. Recall is retrieval of material that has been registered and retained. Obviously in any type of memory a failure at any of these stages will result in no measurable memory.

It is commonly believed that all kinds of memory show a decline with advancing age; however, studies do not consistently support this idea. While it is true that there is an age related deficit in recall of various types, it is not clear whether this deficit results from declining memory or declining ability to learn in the first place. If one is interested only in whether or not there is a decline in the ability to reproduce previously exposed material with age regardless of what the basis for the decline may be, the evidence points to an age deficit in the performance of both immediate and delayed recall.[10]

There appears to be a greater loss with age in short-term and recent memory than in remote or old memory. Also, the decline with age in memory function is less for rote memory (i.e., material that has been memorized) than for logical memory (i.e., material requiring problem solving from past learning).[2]

People with higher intelligence are less susceptible to memory loss with increasing age than are their less intelligent counterparts, and some older people escape memory loss altogether.[11] This pattern suggests that the memory loss that is associated with age may not in fact be due to processes of sensecence. It suggests that perhaps memory losses are associated with disuse, and, in fact, people who exercise their memories tend to maintain both remote and recent memory.[2]

Any attempt to try to reverse or compensate for a decline in memory functions must obviously depend on some notion of why people forget. There are a number of theories of forgetting, and each has implications for various treatment solutions.

One biological theory proposed that memory is located in ribonucleic acid (RNA). This theory states that loss of memory is the result of loss of RNA with age due to the influence of certain enzymes. Studies of subjects with severe memory decline suggest that memory is improved by administering RNA either orally or by intravenous injection.[12] Cameron[12] has asserted that this procedure (RNA therapy) is the only method that has reversed memory deterioration in cases of organic brain syndromes, but scant follow-up research does not substantiate this claim.

Another proposed theory has to do with previously learned material interfering with new learning.[2] If the interference theory is accurate, then all that could be done to ward off memory decline would be periodic rehearsal. Faulty encoding could be at least partly countered by allowing plenty of time for learning, perception, or both to take place. Not much could be done about a decline in the ability to retain material that has been registered.

The information processing theory deals with the acquisition of learned material. Within this approach, learning is viewed as part of memory and is based in the acquisition phase.[13] Studies of memory encoding often overlap with studies of perception, for both involve initial processing. Memory psychologists distinguish three phases of memory: encoding, storage, and retrieval.

Learning is often called encoding. Just as information must be translated into the proper code (or "language") for a computer to process it further, information from the environment must be encoded for the human processing system to store, use, and later retrieve it.

Encoding is the learning or acquisition phase of memory, but storage is perhaps the phase most people think of as memory. It is the laying away of encoded information in "storehouses" for later use. The sensory store is conceptualized as a very brief way station for essentially unprocessed information from the environment.[14] In order for information to be recalled, it must be processed and transferred to later stores (short-term and long-term). Short-term stores are presumed to hold relatively small amounts of information for a slightly longer time than a sensory store (a phone number from directory assistance), commonly on the order of a few seconds, whereas the long-term store is seen as having a very large capacity for storing information that can be retained over long periods of time. Figure 17–1 provides a schematic representation of the memory system.[15]

The final phase of memory is retrieval, which is the finding of information when it is needed. The major age differences in memory performance are related to short-term and long-term store.[16] There do not appear to be significant age differences in sensory store, but there is evidence that some of the age differences in memory lie specifically in the retrieval phase. Older people may have the necessary information in storage, but they cannot get to it as easily as younger people.[17] One way to show that retrieval, rather than learning or storage difficulties, are involved is to compare two common methods of retrieval: recall and recognition. Recall is the remembrance of what has been learned or experienced, while recognition is the perception that an object or person has been encountered and learned before. What does it mean, then, when one can recognize material that one cannot recall? It means that the information was learned and stored, because it can be recognized as correct, but it also means that the individual could not retrieve it when asked for simple recall, though she or he can if presented with multiple choices. It means that the failure of recall was a failure in retrieval; that the search for the desired information in the storehouses of memory failed even though the information was there.

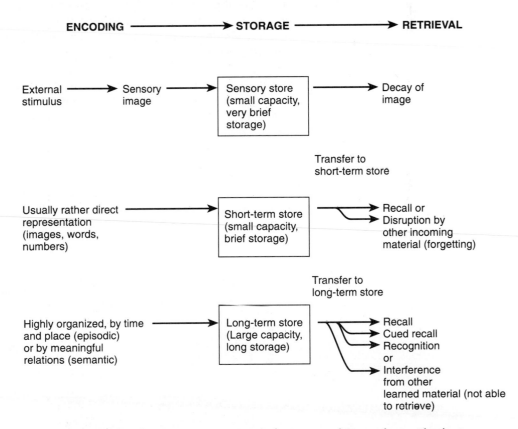

Figure 17–1. The memory system is a rough approximation of memory theories. This chart's primary purpose is to illustrate (1) the three phases of memory (encoding, storage, and retrieval) and (2) the three storage systems (sensory, short-term, and long-term). The additional material shows the differences in encoding, storage, and retrieval for the three stores. *(Reproduced with permission from Atkinson JW, Shiffrin RM. Human memory: a proposed system and its control processes. In: Spence KW, Spence JT, eds. The Psychology of Learning and Motivation. New York: Academic Press; 1968;2.)*

Research suggests that encoding and retrieval problems are the cause of the memory difficulties of older adults.[17] Some of these difficulties occur because older adults do not spontaneously use effective encoding and retrieval strategies. When instructed in these strategies, their performance improves.

The relationship of age to encoding has been cross-sectionally studied, and the findings indicate only a slight decline in encoding ability until age 65.[16] Are there age differences in encoding? Encoding, when viewed from the information processing theory, is the learning or acquisition phase. The earlier discussion suggests that encoding will be found to be less efficient in older subjects. In particular, a slower pace of learning leads to a more efficient encoding of the information.[18] If initial learning between young and old groups is compared, memory will be essentially the same, though elderly individuals need more repetition.[19] This implies that older subjects are less efficient in encoding the material and that they require more repetitions or better organization of the material to build an adequate code.

One of the best ways to encode information for later retrieval is to organize it.[20] Evidence suggests that many older subjects do not spontaneously organize information for later recall.[17] In one investigation, lists of words with clusters based on similarity in meaning (ocean/sea) or relatedness (piano/music) were used to test age related differences.[21] These natural ways to organize and encode the list of words were used by younger learners but rarely were used by older learners. If older subjects were instructed in the memory-enhancing advantages of organization, they improved their position relative to younger subjects.[22] This was true of subjects who were old and were found to have low intelligence in verbal ability.[23] An example of this type of study is one in which subjects were first given experience in sorting words into categories, which trains them in organizing words.[24] Later, given a similar list to learn, older subjects did better relative to younger subjects who did not have the prior training in sorting words into categories (Fig. 17–2).

Another way to encode information for later retrieval is to use what are commonly called mnemonic devices.[25] These techniques use verbal or visual associations to link pieces together that might not by themselves have clear relationships. A common verbal mnemonic is "i before e, except after c." An example of visual

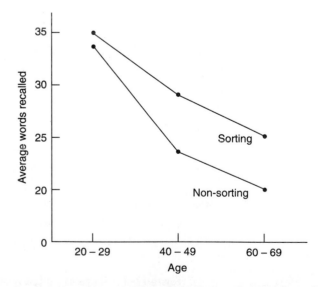

Figure 17–2. Average number of words learned as a function of age. Prior to learning, about half of the subjects carried out a sorting task designed to aid in organizing word lists; the rest of the subjects performed a task that did not involve sorting. *(Reproduced with permission from Hultsch D. Adult age differences in free classification and free recall. Devel Psych. 1971; 4:338–342. © 1971 by the American Psychological Association.)*

mnemonics might be "picturing" a shopping list (milk, mushrooms, and suntan lotion) by visually imagining a cow sunning on a mushroom.

In a study of the effectiveness of various types of encoding instructions,[26] younger and older adults were given pairs of unassociated words to learn. Three different groups were instructed to simply learn the pairs as best they could; to think of some property or characteristic common to both words, or to form a visual image of an interaction. To test retention, one word of a pair was given, and the subject was asked to recall the second word. Both age groups who were instructed to use imagery did better. Encoding was facilitated by the use of imagery and retrieval was facilitated by using cues to stimulate recall.

In another investigation,[27] individuals in their 60s and 70s were instructed in a venerable old memory trick called the "method of loci." This method involves imagining items to be remembered in various familiar locations. The older subjects who learned this trick remembered significantly more than those not instructed in this method.

Another way to examine age differences in the encoding phase of memory is to consider the "depth" at which information from the environment is processed. The depth-of-processing approach was first proposed in 1972 to explain why some tasks involve greater memory demands than others.[28] In general, deeper levels of processing involve processing words at a semantic level; that is, they involve examining the meaning of the word rather than superficial characteristics of the stimuli. The deeper the level, the more remembered. As with their apparent difficulties with organization and mediation, older subjects do not seem to process information as deeply as younger subjects. The data suggest that without direct and detailed instructions, older subjects process words in a list simply by thinking about their sounds (acoustic encoding), whereas younger subjects process them by thinking about their meaning (semantic encoding).[17,29]

Age differences in memory can be reduced or eliminated altogether if older adults are instructed in the use of encoding strategies and given additional time to complete memory tasks.[14] Age differences in encoding and the use of organizational strategies are most evident in "effortful" tasks; those that require constant attention or are novel or unfamiliar (for example, following a new recipe, driving an unfamiliar car, or driving to a familiar place by a different route). Automatized tasks require little attention or conscious awareness (such as routine household chores or playing a familiar tune on the piano).[30]

Several lines of evidence suggest that part of the age difference typically observed in studies of memory lies in the encoding phase of memory.[4,18] Older subjects do not spontaneously organize information as quickly or as effectively as younger ones. It appears that it is harder for older learners to form associations, and it takes them longer to do so. They use less effective verbal mediators when they mediate at all. Also, older adults do not seem to process information as deeply as younger adults; therefore, they store less information and consequently can retrieve less. This has been explained by researchers as a problem in motivation or anxiety, because older persons are either unwilling or unable to explore the lists at a deeper level. Another factor could be less education in elderly people and a different learning mode. In the early 1900s, "rote learning" was the emphasized mode for learning.

THE STORAGE PHASE OF MEMORY RELATED TO AGE

The second phase of memory, storage, involves retention or loss of information. Traditionally, studies of memory storage deal with capacity or "how much" information an individual can store. Another important consideration in the study of memory storage in addition to capacity is duration, or "how long" the information can remain in storage before it is lost or displaced and forgotten. The three storage systems defined earlier guide studies of retention and storage.[15] Sensory and short-term stores are viewed as limited capacity structures in that they ordinarily retain information for only brief periods of time. The long-term store is considered to have an almost unlimited capacity, and information is rarely lost from it.

Sensory memory is considered to be sense-specific, that is, the information is stored according to the sensory modality that receives it. Two types of sensory modalities are defined within this context of memory. The visual memory store is called iconic memory, and it is considered to be a fleeting memory based on visual information. Facsimiles of auditory stimuli are termed echoic memory. Many psychologists consider these brief facsimiles to be an initial stage of information processing. There is almost no information available on the effects of aging on echoic memory.[31] Iconic memory is often studied by presenting a stimulus (for example, a letter or letters) to a subject briefly and then presenting a second stimulus that interferes with or "masks" the first one. Iconic memory is assessed as the extent to which the initial stimulus is recalled after the mask.[32]

Since visual abilities decline with age, it might be expected that the declines in the sensory store be larger than they are. It is possible that age differences in sensory store make some stimuli more difficult for older people to attend to and remember. Speech comprehension is one likely candidate, but the minor deficits in sensory store that do occur probably do not contribute significantly to the more severe memory problems in long-term store experienced in the elderly.[16] This is because age differences in short-term memory, the next stage in the information processing system, appear to be small, and it is in short-term memory that information is prepared for long-term memory.

The short-term store is considered to be temporary and to have a limited capacity (i.e., six to nine items with acoustic encoding). The purpose of the short-term store is to "work on" the information so that it is in proper form for storing in the more permanent long-term store. As a result, the short-term memory store is sometimes called "working memory." The short-term store uses the encoding processes of organization, mediation, and depth of processing, which helps prepare or encode information for permanent storage in long-term store. There are age differences in the facility with which adults use these encoding processes, as has been previously discussed. If information is bumped out of short-term store before it is properly encoded, it probably will be lost forever.

While there are age differences in encoding in the short-term store, there do not appear to be any in the capacity of short-term store.[17,19,33] Studies of memory span (the ability to recall the longest string of items, such as numbers, letters, or words, that can be repeated after a single, brief presentation) show few age differences. An example would be hearing a phone number from directory assistance with no pen in hand. Lack of age differences in short-term storage is provided by a second line of evidence called the recency effect. Subjects typically do best on the first (primary effect) and the last few words given (recency effect). The only age difference found is the pace with which the lists are presented. Older learners need more time.[34] Old and young people do not differ in the capacity of the short-term store, but when encoding information into long-term store, the problems experienced by older adults may be a result of their tendency to use repetition rather than a more appropriate encoding strategy.

The long-term store is what people generally think of as memory. There may be large age differences in long-term memory, particularly when the material to be remembered exceeds the capacity of short-term store.[2] Since the probability of diseases that can affect brain tissue (i.e., cardiovascular) or brain functions (i.e., neurological) is much greater in old people, this sort of loss may be a factor in age differences in memory. Most of the discussion of age differences in long-term storage centers not on capacity or loss of information but rather on the ease or difficulty that people have when trying to locate information in this vast repository of facts and ideas. This is the issue of retrieval, the third phase of memory.

RETRIEVAL RELATED TO AGE

As with encoding, older adults also have more difficulty retrieving the information they have stored, because older people have more trouble getting the information into their long-term stores and more trouble getting it out. Difficulties in encoding and retrieval account for most of the overall age differences observed in memory experiments.[16]

The distinction between recall and recognition is key to studying the retrieval process of memory. Often elderly subjects can recognize words but cannot recall them. An example of this is that older subjects might not be able to recall BASKET, but can recognize it when asked, "Was BASKET on the list?" Studies show that age differences on recognition tests are small or nonexistent, whereas age differences found for recall of factual information are significant.[16,35] Recall and recognition may be affected by different encoding strategies,[36] and the use of efficient encoding strategies may be especially important for recall. In a comprehensive 21-year longitudinal study,[37] word recognition showed modest gains until age 60 and only moderate declines thereafter. In contrast, the word recall test showed marked age changes beginning in young adulthood and accelerating in old age.[37] The conclusion of this study was that older subjects have a lot of information in memory storage that they cannot get to in difficult retrieval tasks that involve recall. Older subjects benefit more than younger subjects when retrieval cues are improved; recognition tests provide more and better cues than recall tests. Cued recall (i.e., starts with . . . , or categories: animals, names, professions, vegetables, etc.) aided elderly individuals in better recall.[19]

The magnitude of age differences in recall and recognition may also be affected by the subjects' verbal ability. Several studies showed no differences between younger and older groups who had high verbal ability, but age differences were found between young and old low verbal ability groups.[38,39]

Recall of ancient memories is an interesting area in the study of memory and aging. Another of the myths of aging is that old people cannot remember recent events but can recall, with great clarity, events in the distant past.[40] In the nineteenth century, one theorist went so far as to formulate what has come to be known as Ribot's Law,[26] which states that information is forgotten in a sequence that is the reverse of the order in which it was acquired. As a general rule, memory for an event is greatest immediately following the event and then declines systematically; recognition memory declines less rapidly than recall. The literature on age differences in remote memory suggests that such differences are minimal. Even though remote memory holds up well in older adults, it is not superior to the recall of recent events.[40]

Remote memory is commonly evaluated by recall and recognition of public events (i.e., World War II or Kennedy's assassination). No age related differences in recall of recent events as compared to remote events has been found.[41] What is probably happening when people feel that ancient events are clearer in their mind is that a particularly sharp memory from the past is being compared with some vaguely encoded event of the last day or two.[40] Strong memory, called a "flashbulb memory," is evident when a remote event was of such personal significance that it has strong emotions associated with it or was thought about (rehearsed) many times.[42]

Young and middle-aged adults experience this strange reversal of memory strengths where remote memories are stronger than recent memories.[42] Old people encode recent events less well than younger adults, and it is possible that they rehearse ancient memories more often (reminiscing), but the reversal of memory strengths is a natural phenomenon that occurs at all ages and is incorrectly viewed as a sign of aging. The truth is that memory is a notoriously leaky repository in humans of all ages. The myth that old memories are set in mental concrete that has hardened to the extent that it will not accept new inputs is pure nonsense!

Atypical difficulties in encoding new events often result from temporary or permanent changes in brain function or changes in brain chemistry.[43] In humans, such changes can be induced in adults of all ages by prescription drugs or voluntary use of alcohol or drugs. These effects are usually transient. In elderly adults, and sometimes in younger adults, brain disease that results in a biochemical imbalance is often reflected in the inability to remember recent events (because they are not encoded and stored, although memory for less recent events in unimpaired).[44]

Everyday memories have been studied as a more relevant area of memory testing in older subjects.[45] The older subjects may have more difficulty in encoding word lists into memory and later retrieving them. They do not, however, seem to have difficulties remembering the time and place of the experiment, and they retrieve with ease information about income, education, or number of grandchildren, and they have no difficulty encoding the instructions for the experiment.[45] Elders may not spontaneously organize word lists for effective recall, but ask a 70-year-old fan of soap operas to recount the last 2 weeks of "The Young and the Restless" or "Days of Our Lives" and you are likely to observe a confident, highly organized, and accurate response.

Some memory researchers distinguish episodic memories, which concern specific events (episodes) that occurred at a specific time and place, from semantic memories, which concern general, context-free facts about the world, such as the meaning of words, rules of grammar and arithmetic, or personal beliefs. Episodic memory studies investigate the recall of activities that have already occurred. In contrast, prospective memory involves remembering something in the future (i.e., a dental appointment or turning off the oven when the cake is done). Though elders reported problems with forgetting prospective memory, most studies indicate they performed as well or better than younger subjects.[46] Time monitoring strategies, such as a calendar or a kitchen timer, were found to be important modalities for enhancing prospective memory for both young and older adults.

The contextual approach to learning and memory takes into account the subject's prior knowledge, level of verbal ability, motivation, and other factors. Contextual approach studies involve the interaction between the characteristics of the subject, the type of material used in the task, and memory performance.[47] These studies investigate the processing of information from prose passages that are common in everyday experience (i.e., newspapers or magazines). Age differences are not as common in text (prose) memory performance as they are in recall of lists. The presence or absence of age differences is a function of the contextual factors that mediate the subject's processing of text materials. Age differences have been found to be smaller when the text is well organized, when there is prior knowledge, and when the subject has above average verbal ability. Recalling "the gist" of a well-organized text passage proved to be as strong in the older subjects as in young adults.[48] The old may focus on the main idea, whereas the young may be more observant of detail. What appears to be inefficient processing in older people may actually reflect adaptive changes. As a result of life experiences or lower levels of energy, the old may focus on higher levels of meaning and devote less attention to detail.[48]

Self-reports of memory are included in the contextual approach to investigating learning and memory in older adults. It was found that at all ages learners may present a distorted picture of what actually occurred. When questioned however, older adults report more memory failures and are more likely to be upset when memory failure occurs.[49] Older adults reported that they forget names, routines, and objects more often than younger adults do. This self-reporting of memory problems was more common in unfamiliar situations or when the subjects were required to recall information they had not recently used.[45,46] External aids, such as visual cues, proved to be helpful tools in assisting with recall, particularly with regard to prospective memory.

Distortion of long-term memory has been found to occur in all age groups.[50] Theorists suggest that information is permanently stored once it has been placed in long-term memory; that information is not lost even when it cannot be retrieved. Research in which subjects witnessed a complex event (i.e., a crime or accident) and were subsequently given misleading information confirmed that the distortion of memory was consistent in all age groups. Provided with the initial event and a confounding, interfering piece of information both young and old subjects later recalled the event incorrectly. Distortions in memory are more likely when the interval between the event and the misinformation is long. Memories of violent events are more likely to be distorted and postevent information is more likely to be accepted if it is presented in an auxiliary clause than if it appears in a main clause of a sentence. Memory distortion is minimized if subjects are warned that the postevent message contains misinformation.[51]

Memory complaints, depression, and drug use are important variables to consider when assessing memory loss. The extent of memory problems is probably exaggerated with age, especially when posited against depression, drug use, or both.[52] Complaints of memory problems do not correlate with scores on objective tests of memory performance,[53-55] but significant correlations between depression and complaints of poor memory have been found.[52] There is a tendency for depressed persons to underestimate their abilities.

Drug side effects may also affect cognitive function in general and memory in particular. Drugs, such as tranquilizers, antidepressants, and sedatives, reinforce some of the cognitive slowing tendencies. Inappropriate dosages or the interaction of drugs (i.e., multiple drug use) can result in mental confusion and memory loss.[44]

There is also a potential for drugs to improve cognitive functioning and memory by improving neurotransmitter and neuroendocrine functioning.[16,43] No drug, to date, has been found that significantly improves memory function. To find a drug that improves memory function, the researcher must first target a specific cognitive process that a drug is supposed to influence. Also, problems resulting from metabolic variations often mask any significant changes in study groups of elderly.

PROBLEM SOLVING

Many of the learning and memory tasks described in previous sections involve relatively simple problems. Another type of cognitive activity, problem solving, is more complex and may involve aspects of learning and memory not previously discussed. Problem solving requires that a person assess the present state of a situation, define the desired state (or goal), and find a way to transform the present state to the desired state.[56]

The process of solving a problem has been broken down into four steps.[57] The first step is to understand the problem, which involves gathering information on the problem and identifying its important elements. The second step is to devise a plan, using past experience for guidance. The use of a relevant strategy would ensure that one devises an efficient plan. The third step is to carry out the plan, and the final step is to review what has been done (i.e., was the problem solved?).

There are many types of studies that address problem solving from a "laboratory" perspective (using prefabricated laboratory situations that do not necessarily duplicate problems encountered in real life). One such mode of testing is termed concept attainment. In concept attainment tasks, items in a set are divided into two subsets in accordance with some characteristic or rule. The subject demonstrates mastery of the rule by distinguishing the items that reflect the rule from those that do not. An example of this would be "choose the red circle; do not choose the green circle." Another example is presenting meal content lists with the rule that certain food types may induce illness and having the subjects identify those meals that would make them ill following consumption. A number of studies of this type, in which performance of younger and older adults were compared, found that the old solved fewer problems than the young.[58-60] Some of the difficulties encountered were that older subjects failed to ignore irrelevant information and tended to fixate on useless hunches.[60] Although elderly people do not spontaneously employ effective strategies, several training studies have found that their performance could be improved with brief training procedures.[61,62]

"Twenty questions" is another means of testing problem-solving abilities. In this type of task, the subject is presented with an array of pictures or words, only one of which is the correct choice. The task is to determine the correct choice by asking less than 20 questions that can be answered with a "yes" or "no." The most efficient strategy is to ask questions that are constraint-seeking (i.e., "Is it a vegetable?"), each of which eliminates a set of possible answers. Asking questions that refer to only one item is inefficient. Again, the elderly tend to do poorer on these tasks than younger groups,[63] but their performance improved significantly after training in the use of constraint-seeking questions.

Piagetian theory has been applied to problem-solving measurement as well. Piagetian theory assumes that concrete operational abilities (i.e., the ability to think logically about concrete or tangible problems), such as classification and conservation (the recognition that the amount of matter does not change when it is rearranged), develop during middle childhood and that formal operational abilities (i.e., the ability to think logically about hypothetical situations or problems) are achieved in adolescence. Do these abilities decline in old age? One hypothesis suggests that operational abilities decline in reverse of the order in which they develop.[64,65] In other words, formal operational thought would decline before conservation. Studies of the elderly's performance on various Piagetian tasks have yielded mixed results. Some show that the elderly do poorer than younger people[66]; others find no age differences in formal operational tasks.[67] Success is positively correlated with higher levels of education and higher intelligence scores. Training has been shown to improve the elderly's performance as well.

In summary, these studies suggest that there are age differences in problem-solving abilities and that the elderly do less well on a number of types of tasks. Several explanations have been offered. It may be that problem-solving ability is a function of educational level, fluid intelligence, or both, rather than aging per se. These factors, in turn, may reflect cohort differences. Additionally, brief educational training has been shown to improve all the types of problem solving discussed here,[68] which suggests that the elderly possess the competence to perform the tasks but do not spontaneously employ the necessary strategies. Even after training, the elderly may not transfer the use of these strategies to the problems encountered in real life.

INTELLIGENCE

When considering intelligence, a potential and an actual ability are implied. In practice, however, measured ability is always dealt with. Thus, conceptually intelligence, as it is studied by psychologists, has three aspects: potential intelligence, actual intelligence, and measured intelligence. This discussion will center around age changes in measured intelligence.

Measured intelligence is actual mental ability (i.e., measured performance of basic cognitive abilities) defined in terms of responses to items on a test. Yet no matter how extensive or well-prepared a test is, there is always a margin of error in its measurement of actual mental ability. The most frequently used test in studies of adult intelligence and age related changes is the Wechsler Adult Intelligence Scale (WAIS).

Intelligence quotient (IQ) is a test score that is compared with the normal or average score of 100. When the WAIS is used for adults aged 20 to 75 years and over, there is an age factor built into the determination of what is normal. In Figure 17–3, the heavy black line indicates the mean raw scores on the WAIS by age. Note that measured performance peaks about age 25, and declines thereafter, particularly after age 65. In scoring measured performance a handicap or advantage is built into the WAIS IQ score to control for age. There could be a 40 point difference between the score at age 25 and the score at age 75, and yet the IQ score would be the same. The importance of this is that the most frequently used test of mental ability incorporates an assumption that a 40 point drop in score from age 25 to 75 is normal.

In practical terms, however, the average decline with age in WAIS scores masks a large amount of individual variation. Any given older person might have an extremely high IQ even when compared to the young. In fact, the correlation between age and IQ is not particularly high, only around –0.40. This means that if the odds against predicting the IQ score were 10 to 1, then knowledge of age would reduce these odds to 6 to 1, not a particularly stunning reduction.

Intelligence testing does not measure a single ability; it measures a set of abilities. Broadly, the WAIS yields separate scores for verbal and performance IQs. The WAIS includes subtests measuring information, vocabulary, comprehension, arithmetic, similarities, digit span, picture completion, object assembly, block design, picture arrangement, and digit symbol tasks.[10] Elderly subjects do best on the information subtest and worst on the digit symbol subtest. The subtests can be broken into two sets; one set dealing with verbal ability and the other dealing with performance ability, and older people consistently do better on the verbal tests than they do on the performance tests. Subtest patterns on the WAIS indicate that stored information and verbal abilities are sustained in old age at a much higher level than are psychomotor, perceptual, and integrative skills.[69] Of relevance here is that most of the performance subtests are timed while many of the verbal subtests are not. Timed tests may be influenced by the individual's reaction time, which is subject to an age related decline (see Chapter 3).

There are a number of factors that influence age changes in IQ. Perhaps the most important is the individual's initial level of functioning. People with scores in

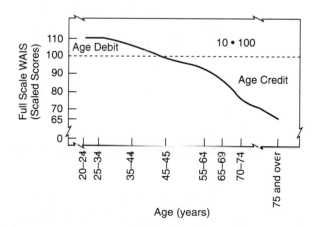

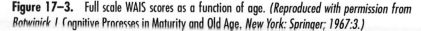

Figure 17–3. Full scale WAIS scores as a function of age. *(Reproduced with permission from Botwinick J. Cognitive Processes in Maturity and Old Age. New York: Springer; 1967:3.)*

the 95th percentile (i.e., with scores high enough that 95% of all scores fall below theirs), show a leveling off in vocabulary scores between the ages of 20 and 30. Thereafter, these individuals' scores showed a plateau or a slight rise with advancing age.[70] On the other hand, people in the 25th percentile show a marked decline in vocabulary scores after the age of 30. This suggests that those with a stronger verbal base to begin with continue to acquire verbal intelligence as the years progress, and those with a weaker verbal foundation initially show a progressive decline in ability as the years go by.

Performance on an intelligence test is closely related to such factors as motivation, anxiety, and cooperation. An environment producing anxiety or a poorly motivated or uncooperative individual will prevent accurate measurement of what that individual is actually capable of accomplishing intellectually.

Another factor that has great influence on the performance on an intelligence test is the level of education: the higher the educational level, the higher the test scores. It is difficult to determine whether intelligence or education comes first, but they are highly correlated.

IQ is also affected by the health status of the individual being tested. Suboptimal levels of health have been shown to have a negative influence on performance on IQ tests. In fact, it has been hypothesized that rapid declines in IQ after the age of 65 could very likely be the result of poor health. For example, arteriosclerosis has been correlated to markedly decreased scores.

Most studies of intelligence and age compare test scores of people of different ages using a cross-sectional study model and assume that the only variable is age. This assumption is obviously difficult to defend. Older people have lived through a different era and developed a different body of "symbols" than younger people. Life experience is likely to be a strong influencing variable. The studies discussed measured age differences as opposed to age changes in intelligence. The most accurate study design in the examination of age changes in intelligence would be a longitudinal study following the individual through life with periodic measurements of intelligence. Such studies have been conducted and have shown the same patterns of changes already noted except that the declines observed in the overall scores were much smaller. This would suggest that at least part of what appears to be the decline in the intelligence of older people is actually a change in skills that are being emphasized by the culture.

Memory is also a factor influencing older individual's performance on intelligence tests. Studies have shown that short-term memory tends to lose efficiency with advancing age, as previously discussed. Since perceptive and integrative skills depend heavily on short-term memory, and vocabulary and information skills depend mainly on long-term memory, these findings may account for much of the observed difference in IQ test performances between older and younger individuals.

TEACHING STRATEGIES FOR THE ELDERLY

Life is an educational process. Some education occurs in formal settings, such as schools, but most learning occurs informally through everyday experiences. It has been shown that adults of all ages benefit from education and that formal educational experiences can assist the older adult to prepare for career changes and retirement. Learning environments are also useful in compensating for deficits in sensory input, memory, and physical changes that may occur with aging.

Though the research previously reviewed indicates that older adults may have more difficulty in the acquisition or encoding of information and in retrieving stored information, these age differences have been found to be quite minimal. Clearly, adults of all ages, in the absence of pathology, have no difficulty learning.[71]

Most of the studies on memory training involves encoding information into long-term store and focuses on training older learners in encoding strategies. Older adult learners do not automatically employ encoding strategies,[72] although when instructed in their use, elderly learners use these techniques effectively.

Face-name recall (i.e., remembering people's names) is one of the most common memory problems. Yesavage,[73] in a series of studies, examined the effectiveness of imagery in face-name recall. Elderly subjects were taught to form associations using visual imagery,[73,74] and those subjects who learned this technique were found to have significantly improved face-name recall. In a subsequent study, pretraining in muscle relaxation techniques reduced performance anxiety and significantly improved learning in the same subjects using imagery.[74] These imagery studies used elderly subjects living in the community, which raises the question, "Can similar procedures in memory training be used to improve functioning of elderly individuals with dementia?" So far, the evidence is not very encouraging. In a study examining the effectiveness of visual imagery training among subjects with cognitive declines, subjects improved somewhat in tests given immediately following the training, however, there was no latency or long-term retention, and these improvements were not maintained.[75] However, with intensive memory training in subjects with retrograde and anterograde amnesia and head injury patients, Wilson and Moffat[76] found some improvement in both immediate and latent recall.

It appears that memory performance of healthy elderly people can be improved through memory training. Whether or not this improvement is maintained over time has not been well documented. It is also not evident that elderly people spontaneously employ these training strategies in everyday situations. Rehearsal of encoding strategies is effective in keeping information in short-term memory, but for encoding information into long-term memory, organizational strategies, mnemonics, and imagery are more useful. Likewise, in prospective memory (i.e., remembering an appointment), using time monitoring strategies, like calendars or timing devices, have been shown to be particularly effective. Most of the research on memory focuses on the use of internal memory aids (encoding strategies). As most people, young or old, generally use external aids, such as making lists, it would be helpful for future research to examine external strategies for improving memory in the elderly.

The elderly do just as well as younger people on recognition tasks but have more difficulty with verbatim recall.[37] They also are adept at retaining the gist of a text but have difficulty remembering the details. These findings are important when developing a means of assessing learning in the elderly. For example, multiple choice or true/false items may be more effective procedures, since both involve recognition memory. Short answer or fill-in-the-blank questions, on the other hand, would be difficult because they require recall of specific information. Providing sufficient time for recall is also important.

When teaching the elderly, it must be keep in mind that there may be some loss of vision or hearing. Compensation for these losses could facilitate the processing of the information. Aids like larger print, avoidance of rapid speaking, seating the hearing impaired near the speaker to facilitate lip reading, and repetition of the main points are helpful in assisting the elderly in learning tasks and retaining information. The capacity to pay attention may decline with age,[18] and repetition ensures that the learner may grasp a point even if she or he was inattentive when it was first presented.

Many principles of learning amplify the information processing model of learning: People learn best in pleasant surroundings; they are most likely to repeat activities that they experience as pleasant; overlearning allows task performance to be accomplished automatically; and people are most likely to remember those tasks in which they have been actively involved (i.e., "doing" influences the depth of encoding and storage). In addition, if an individual "forgets" something they once knew, they relearn it faster than if they had never learned it before.[2]

TEACHING IN THE THERAPEUTIC SETTING

In the process of implementing treatment, allied health professionals consistently function in the role of "teacher." It is important for them to be knowledgeable not only about the content of the information they are conveying, but even more importantly, about the capability of the elderly individual for learning. Therapists must understand the developmental changes that occur in older persons that ultimately affect their learning capabilities and adapt instructional sessions to enhance the learning process.

Documented changes in sensory function can limit or distort reception, perception, monitoring, feedback, and transmission of incoming stimuli. A general slowing of the neural processes seems to occur with age, as demonstrated by decreased conduction over multisynaptic pathways. There is also a progressive, age related change in response to cutaneous, proprioceptive, vestibular, and other stimuli.[77] There are reported visual declines in acuity, accommodation, field luminance factors, color sensitivity, perception of ambiguous figures and illusions, figural aftereffects, serial learning, figure ground organization, closure, spatial abilities, and visual memory.[78] Some of these variables have been considered in the IQ and memory research reviewed, though not comprehensibly by any one study. If all of these factors are not considered, then these sensory variables may be confounding with cognitive variables.

Aging changes also occur in the outer ear, the inner ear, and central auditory processing that are reflected in a decreased ability to inhibit background noise and other irrelevant signals and a decreased auditory acuity and perception of high-frequency sounds. The older person's ability to hear and understand speech in less than ideal listening environments is particularly affected.[79] Attentional deficits further compromise the accuracy of input and registration of stimuli. Inaccuracies in the first stage of learning (input and registration) affect the subsequent stages of information processing. Stimuli that is not adequately registered cannot be effectively encoded or retrieved.

A marked slowing in the learning ability in the elderly is reported whether a simple motor movement or a complex cognitive process is involved. Older adults benefit from having longer periods of time for inspection and response. Self-paced learning leads to the best performance.[80] The elderly tend to make more errors of omission than errors of commission.[81] Concrete information is learned more accurately and efficiently than abstract information,[82] and concept learning is also better when information is conveyed in concrete (as opposed to abstract) language.[81] When the opportunity to practice psychomotor tasks is given, learning and performance improve, regardless of the difficulty of the task.[83] When unlimited numbers of trials are given for the mastery of a task, the elderly can recall information as effectively as younger persons; however, more trials are required by elderly to attain this goal.[81] Elderly who are given verbal feedback concerning their performance improve significantly on subsequent related problems. As a general rule, they perform best when instructions are given in a supportive manner.[81] These factors that influence older adult learning all need to be considered if learning is to be accomplished in the therapeutic setting.

In considering the age related changes in learning, it becomes clear that health care professionals who interact with the elderly must be particularly sensitive to learner needs and be diligent in structuring teaching settings to maximize and individualize learning. For example, some people are auditory learners, and some are visual learners, while others need kinesthetic input and learn by doing. Some tasks are better taught by demonstration and some by verbal instruction.

The learning environment determines and influences the educational experience. An environment that is conducive to learning promotes the process, and as a general rule, an environment that is familiar to the learner is the preferred environment for learning new skills. Familiar settings induce a sense of security in which pertinent new information can be attended to. Learning in the natural environment (i.e., the home or work environment) eliminates the need for the client to transfer or generalize information to a home or work setting. In unfamiliar settings, the learner is more likely to be attracted by, and responsive to, novel environmental stimuli. When unfamiliar treatment environments must be used, they should be structured to simulate the natural environment whenever possible and to diminish the number of competing stimuli. Once a new skill is learned, practice in a variety of environments will assist in generalizing its use.

Environments and procedures that are orderly and organized enhance the learner's ability to process information in an orderly and organized fashion. A cluttered or busy environment creates irrelevant, distracting stimuli in the learning environment and impedes the learning process.

Physical and psychological comfort are also important to consider in the treatment setting. Noise levels, color schemes, adequate lighting, ventilation, and comfortable room temperature should all be considered. Glossy, highly waxed floors and work surfaces that distort and reflect light should be avoided. Comfortable chairs and proper table heights are recommended. Background noises (i.e., computers, air conditioners, running water, and other appliances) should be eliminated so that they will not interfere with foreground sound perception. Most kitchen and bathroom settings compromise hearing: The lack of carpeting, drapes, and padded furniture impose additional noise and reverberating sounds.

The persona of the therapist is also an important source of psychological comfort for the elderly learner. A calm, patient, unhurried, interested, knowledgeable, and assured health care provider can decrease situational stress and promote a climate of acceptance and reassurance. Conveying verbally and nonverbally that the elderly individual is a valued person with valuable ideas to contribute and that experimentation and failure are important processes in learning new skills enhances the environment. Positive reinforcement for good efforts, as well as good performance, is crucial in facilitating the learning process in an elderly person.

Teaching methods and techniques in the therapeutic setting include all those behaviors employed by instructors to communicate particular pieces of information to the learners. Variables that influence learning include the organization of material, the rate of presentation, the choice of task, the mode of presentation, and covert strategies.[81]

Organization of Information

New information needs to be presented in a highly organized fashion. Visual displays should be simple configurations that explicitly demonstrate a few salient points. Verbal instructions and directions must emphasize the most important information in a simple manner. Written instructions need to be clear, have section headings, be written in large print, and emphasize the major points. Only information relevant to the task at hand should be presented. Differences and similarities between new and old tasks need to be identified. Whole-part-whole learning is a recommended strategy with the elderly. With this technique the entire task and anticipated goal are introduced, then the parts are identified, and each is related to the preceding steps and to the whole. For instance, the person whose end goal is independent meal preparation has to accomplish many component steps in the process of reaching that goal. It is important for the individual to understand the importance of each step (e.g., mobilizing joints and strengthening particular muscle groups or increasing fine motor coordination and endurance) and how each step relates to the end objective.

Rate of Presentation

Information should be presented at a rate compatible with the learner's ability to comprehend and respond. Generally, this rate will correspond with the complexity of concepts and tasks being taught. Simple, concrete tasks require less time to learn. When instructing the elderly, directions should be presented slowly and ample time for practice provided. If fatigue or confusion occur, the instructional sessions should be kept short.

Task Choice

It is important that the choice of task be directed toward attainment of a pre-established, desirable goal. The task should allow the learner to express and fulfill their own personal needs (e.g., creativity, socialization, mastery). Tasks that interest the learner should be selected, if possible. A preliminary development of an interest inventory will identify what is important to the individual learner. In other words, activities chosen need to be relevant and meaningful to the learner, and the purpose for learning each task needs to be clear. Self-care tasks seem to have the greatest relevance for most elderly individuals. Goals, such as transfer training, eating, and dressing, are concrete and usually are experienced as meaningful. Practice of self-care tasks in a familiar environment is best for obtaining follow through of the learned tasks. Activities, such as mat exercises or fine hand coordination exercises, may not seem relevant to the older learner. In these cases, it is important to relate the activities to the established treatment goals. Explain and demonstrate the mobility and strengthening components of mat activities as they relate to functional goals. This will help in making the activities more concrete and necessary for accomplishing the end goal.

Tasks should be sufficiently challenging but easy enough to assure successful experiences. Building on past successes will promote advancing toward the treatment goals. A knowledgeable, enthusiastic therapist can also help to motivate learners to engage in the necessary tasks to be learned.

Presentation of Information

Instructions for the older learner need to be concrete, simple, clear, and one step at a time. The learner should be given the opportunity to practice each step before subsequent steps are introduced. Demonstrations, which are carefully planned, are also helpful modes of education. With a good demonstration, the learner is given the opportunity to initiate the exact movement until each step has been completed. It is also advised that demonstrations be done in the same position as the learner will be in when they are doing the task. For demonstration to be effective in influencing the learner, it requires skillful observation and visual memorization of the teacher's movements, followed by a transfer of the complex visual information to an opposite orientation. This can be frustrating for the older learner.

To compensate for a hearing loss, the instructor needs to be within 10 feet of the listener, use a low-pitched speaking voice with a moderate volume (shouting distorts sound for those with hearing losses), and position themselves so that the listener can see their mouth. Since a lot of information is communicated by facial expression, gestures and body language are important facilitators for conveying information. Verbal and nonverbal language needs to be congruent, because understanding is enhanced when nonconfusing visual stimuli accompany auditory information.

To compensate for some of the changes in vision with aging use a large, bold print on a solid background for printed material. The use of a visual aid, such as a magnifying glass, may be helpful when large print is not available. Lighting is also important. Too much light can create glare, and too little light will diminish the older learner's ability to see anything.

Motor learning may be enhanced by physically guiding the learner's extremities through the desired patterns of movement. It is preferable for the teacher to stand behind the learner so that the learner can concentrate on the sensation of movement. Movements should be repeated several times without any alterations. The learner is eventually weaned from guided patterning and asked to perform the movement without the teacher's tactile, proprioceptive, and motoric assistance.

Covert Strategies

Older adults tend not to spontaneously use organized methods or ploys to enhance learning and memory, as was previously discussed. They do, however, benefit from instructions in memory strategies. The use of memory strategies is a means of compensating for real or anticipated deficits in memory.

It is important to optimize overall health status by implementing the concept of "independence." The more one can do for oneself, the more one is capable of doing independently. The more that is done for an aged individual, the less capable he or she becomes of functioning on an optimal independent level and the more likely is the progression of a disability. The advancing stages of disabilities increase the individual's vulnerability to illness, emotional stress, and injury. Aged persons' subjective appraisal of their health status influences how they react to their symptoms, how vulnerable they consider themselves, and when they decide they can or cannot accomplish an activity. Often an aged person's self-appraisal of her or his health is a good predictor of a rehabilitation clinician's evaluation of health and functional status, but such assessments may also differ in many ways. In older persons, perceptions of their health may be determined in large part by their level of psychological well-being and by whether or not they continue in rewarding roles and activities.[84]

As an aged individual's perception of their health status is an important motivator in compliance with a rehabilitation program, it is important to discuss this further. One notable study showed that even when age, sex, and health status (as evaluated by physicians) were controlled for, perceived health and mortality from heart disease were strongly related.[85] Those who rated their health as poor were two to three times as likely to die as those who rated their health as excellent. A Canadian longitudinal study of persons over 65 produced similar results.[86] Over 3 years, the mortality of those who described their health as poor at the beginning of the study was about three times the mortality of those who initially described their health as good, regardless of their actual (or measured) health status.

Despite this awareness among older persons of their actual state of health, the aged are known to fail to report serious symptoms and wait longer than younger persons to seek help. It is with this in mind that rehabilitation professionals need to listen carefully to their aged clients. It appears that, contrary to the popular view that older individuals are somewhat hypochondriacal, the aged generally deserve serious attention when they bring complaints to their care givers. Their perceived level of health will greatly impact the outcomes of functional goals in the geriatric rehabilitation setting whether it be acute, rehabilitative, home, or chronic care.

Rosillo and Fagel[87] found that improvement in rehabilitation tasks correlated well with the patient's own appraisal of her or his potential for recovery but not well with others' appraisals. Stoedefalke[88] reports that positive reinforcement (frequent positive feedback) for older persons in rehabilitation greatly improved their performance and feelings of success. This indicates that aged persons can improve in their physical functioning when modifications in therapeutic interventions provide more frequent feedback. Some research indicates that older persons with chronic illness have low initial aspirations with regard to their ability to perform various tasks.[89] As situations in which they succeeded or failed occurred, their aspirations changed to more closely reflect their abilities. Older persons may have different beliefs about their abilities as compared to younger persons.[90] When subjects were given an unsolvable problem, younger subjects ascribed their failure to not trying hard enough, while older subjects ascribed their failure to inability. On subsequent tests, younger individuals tried harder, and older subjects gave up. These age differences indicate a variation in the perceived locus-of-control. This holds extreme importance in the rehabilitation potential of an aged person. If the cause of failure is seen as an immutable characteristic by the person, then little effort in the future can be expected.

Aged individuals may have a higher anxiety level in rehabilitation situations because they fear failure or are afraid of "looking bad" to their family or therapist. Eisdorfer found that if anxiety is high enough, then the behavior is redirected toward reducing the anxiety rather than accomplishing the task.[91] Weinberg[92] found that subjects set their own goals for task achievement even if they are directed to adopt the therapist's goals. In another study, Mento, Steel, and Karren[93] reported that the best performance at difficult tasks (as many rehabilitation tasks are) occurs when the aged person sets a very specific goal, such as walking 10 feet with a walker. If the person simply tries to do better, then performance is not improved as much.

These are important motivational components to keep in mind when working with an aged client, because the therapeutic approach of the clinician may perhaps have the greatest impact on the successful functional outcomes in a geriatric rehabilitation setting.

CONCLUSION

The process of aging may inexorably bring with it changes that interfere with learning, especially in the presence of pathology. An elderly individual's competence may decline, and environmental influences may also be a prominent impediment to learning. Therefore, if the elderly are to gain maximum benefit from therapeutic interactions that are educational in nature, therapists must give much thought and attention to the environments in which they teach older adults, as well as to the methods they rely upon to convey information.

PEARLS

- Learning is defined as the acquisition of a new skill or information through practice and experience, whereas remembering is the retrieval of information that has been stored in memory.

- Encoding and retrieval problems are the cause of memory difficulties in older adults, and instruction in organizing, slower pacing, and verbal and visual associations can improve performance.

- Sensory and short-term stores of memory are limited in capacity, whereas long-term store has an unlimited storage capacity.

- Problem-solving ability appears to decline with age and may be due to education level and fluid intelligence. Training can improve older people's problem-solving ability, however, they may not transfer these strategies to problems encountered in real life.

- Memory performance of healthy elderly can be improved through memory training.

- Orderly environments enhance an older person's ability to process information, whereas a cluttered, busy environment creates distracting stimuli and impedes learning.

- Variables that positively influence learning for the older person are

  1. Highly organized presentation of information.

  2. Appropriate rate of presentation of information (i.e., simple tasks quickly, more complex slowly).

3. Choosing meaningful tasks.

4. Clean, simple, concrete, step-by-step information presentation.

5. Use of memory strategies.

REFERENCES

1. Gardner DL, Greenwell SC, Costich JF. Effective teaching of the older adult. *Top Ger Rehab.* 1991; 6(3):1–14.
2. Merriam SB, Cafferella RS. *Learning in Adulthood.* San Francisco: Jossey-Bass; 1991.
3. Arenberg D, Robertson-Tchabo EA. Learning and aging. In: Birren JE, Schaie KW, eds. *Handbook of the Psychology of Aging.* New York: Van Nostrand Reinhold; 1977.
4. Canestrari RE. Age changes in acquisition. In: Talland GA, ed. *Human Aging and Behavior.* New York: Academic Press; 1968.
5. Taub HA. Paired associates learning as a function of age, rate and instructions. *J Genetic Psych.* 1967; 111:41–46.
6. Leech S, Witte KL. Paired-associate learning in elderly adults as related to pacing and incentive conditions. *Dev Psych.* 1971; 5:174–180.
7. Eisdorfer D, Nowlin J, Wilkie F. Improvement of learning in the aged by modification of autonomic nervous system activity. *Science.* 1970; 170:1327–1329.
8. Botwinick J, Storandt M. *Memory, Related Functions and Age.* Springfield, Ill: Charles C Thomas; 1974.
9. Fisher J, Pierce RC. Dimensions of intellectual functioning in the aged. *J Geron.* 1967; 22:166–173.
10. Botwinick J. *Cognitive Processes in Maturity and Old Age.* New York: Springer; 1967.
11. Ryan EB. Beliefs about memory changes across the adult life span. *J Geron.* 1992; 47(1):41–47.
12. Cameron DE. Ribonucleic acid in psychiatric therapy. In: Maserman JH, ed. *Current Psychiatric Therapies.* New York: Grune and Stratton; 1964.
13. Craik FIM, Trehub S, eds. *Aging and Cognitive Processes.* New York: Plenum; 1982.
14. Hoyer WJ, Plude DJ. Attentional and perceptual processes in the study of cognitive aging. In: Poon L, ed. *Aging in the 1980's.* Washington, DC: American Psychological Association; 1980.
15. Atkinson JW, Shiffen RM. Human memory: a proposed system and its control processes. In: Spence KW, Spence JT, eds. *The Psychology of Learning and Motivation.* New York: Academic Press; 1968; 2.
16. Poon L. Differences in human memory with aging: nature, causes, and clinical implications. In: Birren JE, Schaie KW, eds. *Handbook of the Psychology of Aging.* 2nd ed. New York: Van Nostrand Reinhold; 1985.
17. Craik FIM, Rabinowitz JC. Age differences in the acquisition and use of verbal information. In: Long J, Baddeley A, eds. *Attention and Performance.* Hillsdale, NJ: Erlbaum; 1984;X.
18. Craik FIM, Byrd M. Aging and cognitive deficits: the role of attentional resources. In: Craik FIM, Trehub S, eds. *Aging and Cognitive Processes.* New York: Plenum; 1982.
19. Craik FIM. Age differences in human memory. In: Birren JE, Schaie KW, eds. *Handbook of the Psychology of Aging.* New York: Van Nostrand Reinhold; 1977.
20. Kausler DH. *Experimental Psychology and Human Aging.* New York: Wiley; 1982.
21. Denney NW. Classification abilities of the elderly. *J Geron.* 1974; 29:309–314.
22. Schmitt FA, Murphy MD, Sanders RE. Training older adult free recall rehearsal strategies. *J Geron.* 1981; 36:329–337.
23. Botwinick J. *Aging and Behavior.* 2nd ed. New York: Springer; 1978.
24. Hultsch D. Adult age differences in free classification and free recall. *Dev Psych.* 1971; 4:338–342.
25. Hartley JT, Harker JO, Walsh DA. Contemporary issues and new directions in adult development of learning and memory. In: Poon L, ed. *Aging in the 1980's.* Washington, DC: American Psychological Association; 1980.
26. Rabinowitz JC, Craik FIM, Ackerman BP. A processing resource account of age differences in recall. *Canadian J Psych.* 1982; 36:325–344.

27. Robertson-Tchabo EA, Hausman CP, Arenberg DA. A classic mnemonic for old learners: a trip that works. *Ed Geron.* 1976; 1:215–226.

28. Craik FIM, Lockhart RS. Levels of processing: a framework for memory research. *J Verbal Learning and Verbal Behavior.* 1972; 11:671–684.

29. Treat N, Reese H. Age, imagery, and pacing in paired associate learning. *Dev Psych.* 1976; 12:119–124.

30. Shiffrin RM, Schneider W. Controlled and automatic human information processing: II. perceptual learning, automatic attending and a general theory. *Psych Rev.* 1977; 84:127–190.

31. Crowder RG. Echoic memory and the study of aging memory systems. In: Poon LW, Fozard JL, Cermak LS, Arenberg D, Thompson LW, eds. *New Directions in Memory and Aging: Proceedings of the George A Talland Memorial Conference.* Hillsdale, NJ: Erlbaum; 1980.

32. Cerella J, Poon L, Fozard J. Age and iconic read-out. *J Geron.* 1982; 37:197–202.

33. Fozard JL. A time for remembering. In: Poon L, ed. *Aging in the 1980's.* Washington, DC: American Psychological Association; 1980.

34. Poon L, Fozard J. Speed of retrieval from long-term memory in relation to age, familiarity and datedness of information. *J Geron.* 1980; 5:711–717.

35. Schonfield D, Robertson EA. Memory storage and aging. *Canadian J Psych.* 1966; 20:228–236.

36. Smith A. Age differences in encoding, storage, and retrieval. In: Poon LW, Fozard JL, Cermak LS, Arenberg D, Thompson LW, eds. *New Directions in Memory and Aging: Proceedings of the George A Talland Memorial Conference.* Hillsdale, NJ: Erlbaum; 1980.

37. Schaie KW. Cognitive development in aging. In: Obler LK, Alpert M, eds. *Language and Communication in the Elderly.* Lexington, Mass: Heath; 1980.

38. Bowles NE, Poon L. An analysis of the effect of aging on memory. *J Geron.* 1982; 37:212–219.

39. Cavanaugh J. Effects of presentation format on adult's retention of television programs. *Exp Aging Res.* 1984; 10:51–54.

40. Erbert JT. Remote memory and age: a review. *Exp Aging Res.* 1981; 1:189–199.

41. Poon L, Fozard J, Paulshock D, Thomas J. A questionnaire assessment of age differences in retention of recent and remote events. *Exp Aging Res.* 1979; 5:401–411.

42. Brown R, Kulick J. Flashbulb memories. *Cognition.* 1977; 5:73–99.

43. Marsh GR. Introduction to psychopharmacological issues. In: Poon L, ed. *Aging in the 1980's,* Washington, DC: American Psychological Association; 1980.

44. Butler RN, Lewis MI. *Aging and Mental Health.* 3rd ed. St. Louis, Mo: Mosby; 1982.

45. West RL. Practical memory mnemonics for the aged: preliminary thoughts. In: Poon L, Rubin D, Wilson B, eds. *Everyday Cognition and Memory.* Hillsdale, NJ: Erlbaum; 1986.

46. Poon L, Schaffer G. *Prospective Memory in Young and Elderly Adults.* Paper presented at the meeting of the American Psychological Association; Washington, DC: August, 1982.

47. Hultsch D, Dixon R. Memory for text materials in adulthood. In: Baltes PB, Brim OG, eds. *Life-Span Development and Behavior.* New York: Academic Press; 1984;6.

48. Labouvie-Vief G, Schnell D. Learning and memory in later life. In: Wolman BB, ed. *Handbook of Developmental Psychology.* Englewood Cliffs, NJ: Prentice-Hall; 1982.

49. Cavanaugh J, Grady J, Permutter M. Forgetting and use of memory aids in 20 to 70 year olds' everyday life. *Int J Aging Hum Dev.* 1983; 17:113–122.

50. Loftus E. Misfortunes of memory. *Philosophical Trans Royal Society London.* 1983; 302:413–421.

51. Loftus E, Fienberg S, Tanur J. Cognitive psychology meets the national survey. *Am Psych.* 1985; 40:175–180.

52. Zarit SH. *Aging and Mental Disorders.* New York: Free Press; 1980.

53. Kahn RL. The mental health system and the future aged. *Gerontologist.* 1975; 15:24–31.

54. Perlmutter M. What is memory aging the aging of? *Dev Psych.* 1978; 14:330–345.

55. Thompson L. Testing and mnemonic strategies. In: Poon LW, Fozard JL, Cermak LS, Arenberg D, Thompson LW, eds. *New Directions in Memory and Aging: Proceedings of the George A Talland Memorial Conference.* Hillsdale, NJ: Erlbaum; 1980.

56. Reese HW, Rodeheaver D. Problem solving and complex decision making. In: Birren JE, Schaie KW, eds. *Handbook of the Psychology of Aging.* 2nd ed. New York: Van Nostrand Reinhold; 1985.

57. Polya G. *How to Solve It: A New Aspect of Mathematical Method.* 2nd ed. Princeton, NJ: Princeton University Press; 1971.

58. Crovitz E. Reversing a learning deficit in the aged. *J Geron.* 1966; 21:236–238.
59. Offenbach SI. A developmental study of hypothesis testing and cue selection strategies. *Dev Psych.* 1974; 10:484–490.
60. Hartley AA. Adult age differences in deductive reasoning processes. *J Geron.* 1981; 36:700–706.
61. Sanders JA, Sterns HL, Smith M, Sanders RE. Modification of concept identification performance in older adults. *Dev Psych.* 1975; 11:824–829.
62. Sanders RE, Sanders JA, Mayes GJ, Sielski KA. Enhancement of conjunctive concept attainment in older adults. *Dev Psych.* 1976; 12:485–486.
63. Denney NW. Task demands and problem-solving strategies in middle-age and older adults. *J Geron.* 1980; 35:559–564.
64. Papalia D, Bielby D. Cognitive functioning in middle and old age adults: a review of research based on Piaget's theory. *Hum Dev.* 1974; 17:424–443.
65. Muhs PJ, Hooper FH, Papalia-Finlay DE. An initial analysis of cognitive functioning across the life-span. *Int J Aging Hum Dev.* 1980; 10:311–333.
66. Rubin KH. *Decentration Skills in Institutionalized and Noninstitutionalized Elderly.* Proceedings of 81st Annual Convention, American Psychological Association. 1973; 8(Part 2):759–760.
67. Papalia-Finley DE, Blackburn J, Davis E, et al. Training cognitive functioning in the elderly—Inability to replicate previous findings. *Int J Aging Hum Dev.* 1980; 12:111–117.
68. Willis SL. Towards an educational psychology of the older adult learner: intellectual and cognitive bases. In: Birren JE, Schaie KW, eds. *Handbook of the Psychology of Aging* 2nd ed. New York: Van Nostrand Reinhold; 1985.
69. Hulicka IM. Age changes and age differences in memory functioning. *Gerontologist.* 1967; 7(2, part II):46–54.
70. Jones HE. Intelligence and problem-solving. In: Birren JE, ed. *Handbook of Aging and the Individual.* Chicago: University of Chicago Press; 1959:700–738.
71. Poon L, Rubin D, Wilson B. *Everyday Cognition and Memory.* Hillsdale, NJ: Erlbaum; 1986.
72. Poon L, Walsh-Sweeney L, Fozard J. Memory skill training for the elderly: salient issues on the use of imagery mnemonics. In: Poon L, ed. *New Directions in Memory and Aging: Proceedings of the George A Talland Memorial Conference.* Hillsdale, NJ: Erlbaum; 1980.
73. Yesavage JA. Imagery pretraining and memory training in the elderly. *Gerontology.* 1983; 29:271–275.
74. Yesavage JA, Rose T. The effects of a face-name mnemonic in young, middle aged, and elderly adults. *Exp Aging Res.* 1984; 10:55–57.
75. Zarit SH, Zarit J, Reever K. Memory training or severe memory loss: effects of senile dementia. *Gerontologist.* 1982; 22:373–377.
76. Wilson B, Moffat N. *Clinical Management of Memory Problems.* Rockville, Md: Aspen; 1984.
77. Kenney RA. *Physiology of Aging.* Chicago: Year Book Medical Publishers, Inc.; 1982.
78. Cristarella MC. Visual functions of the elderly. *Am J Occup Ther.* 1987; 31:432–440.
79. Gladstone VS. Hearing loss in the elderly. *Phys & Occup Ther Ger.* 1992; 2:5–20.
80. Feldman HS, Lopez MA. *Developmental Psychology for the Health Care Professions: Adulthood and Aging.* Boulder, Co: Westview Press; 1982;2.
81. Okun MA. Implications of geropsychological research for the instruction of older adults. *Adult Education.* 1987; 27:139–155.
82. Rabbitt P. Changes in problem solving ability in old age. In: Birren JE, Schaie KW, eds. *Handbook of the Psychology of Aging.* New York: Van Nostrand Reinhold Co.; 1987; 606–625.
83. Botwinick J. *Aging and Behavior.* 3rd ed. New York: Springer; 1983.
84. Siegler IC, Costa PT Jr. Health behavior relationships. In: Birren JE, Schaie KW, eds. *Handbook of the Psychology of Aging.* 2nd ed. New York: Van Nostrand Reinhold; 1985.
85. Kaplan E. *Psychological Factors and Ischemic Heart Disease Mortality: A Focal Role for Perceived Health.* Paper presented at the annual meeting of the American Psychological Association; Washington, DC: 1982.
86. Mossey JM, Shapiro E. Self-rated health: a predictor of mortality among the elderly. *Am J Pub Health.* 1982; 72:800–808.
87. Rosillo RA, Fagel ML. Correlation of psychologic variables and progress in physical therapy: I. degree of disability and denial of illness. *Arch Phys Med Rehabil.* 1970; 51:227.
88. Stoedefalke KG. Motivating and sustaining the older adult in an exercise program. *Top Ger Rehab.* 1985; 1:78.

89. Nader IM. Level of aspiration and performance of chronic psychiatric patients on a simple motor task. *Percept Mot Skills.* 1985; 60:767.
90. Prohaska T, Pontiam IA, Teitleman J. Age differences in attributions to causality: implications for intellection assessment. *Exp Aging Res.* 1984; 10:111.
91. Eisdorfer L. Arousal and performance: experiments in verbal learning and a tentative theory. In: Talland GA, ed. *Human Aging and Behavior.* New York: Academic Press; 1968.
92. Weinberg R, Bruya L, Jackson A. The effects of goal proximity and goal specificity on endurance performance. *J Soc Psychol.* 1985; 7:296.
93. Mento A, Steele RP, Karren RJ. A metaanalytic study of the effects of goal setting on task performance: 1966–1984. *Organ Behav Hum Decis Process.* 1987; 39:52.

Administration of Geriatric Services

As the role of the geriatric rehabilitation therapist continues to evolve, the development of excellent clinical skills and the ability to interpret research in the literature has become more important to the geriatric physical therapist. In addition, as the nation's health care system is revised, nursing homes, hospitals, rehabilitation centers, outpatient clinics, and home health agencies will be looking for therapists with good administrative skills to provide administrative advisement and supervision for professional, as well as adjunct staff.

It is imperative, therefore, that physical therapists become aware of all aspects of administration. A greater understanding of administrative services will facilitate communication not only within the discipline but also with other disciplines, including nursing and social work.

This chapter has two goals: first, to familiarize therapists with administrative terms and concepts, and second, to serve as a reference for therapist working in a rehabilitation facility or a physical therapy department.

DESCRIPTION OF ADMINISTRATION

Administration is an extremely complex term. It involves not only paperwork for developing a policy and procedure manual, finance, and budgeting, but also developing guidelines for effectively managing and motivating people. For the purposes of this chapter, administration will be divided into five areas:

1. Finance and budgeting.
2. Policies and procedures.
3. Legal concerns.
4. Employee relations.
5. Marketing.

The needs of administration vary by position. For example, if the therapist is a staff therapist, his or her administrative needs may be minimal. This therapist may be asked to fill out documentation forms, send in billing slips, and play a very limited role in managing employees. On the other hand, if a therapist is in charge of an entire department, he or she may need to develop personnel information, such as employee handbooks, billing procedures, documentation procedures, or finance and budget procedures, as well as equipment use forms and marketing strategies. Therefore, the best approach to acquiring an understanding of administrative needs is to gain an understanding of the information in each of the five major areas listed.

FINANCING AND BUDGETING

Financing and budgeting can be defined as a monetary sketch of the needs and plans of a department in any setting. If a therapist works in an outpatient facility, for example, items that must be budgeted are rental of space, equipment, staff time, and ancillary personnel (such as receptionists or aides), as well as laundry and other line items. Based on the number of patients that will be seen, the income, and the costs, the therapist must establish a workable formula for the amount of money dispersed versus the amount of incoming money.

A realistic budget is essential to the financial well-being of a physical therapy business. No matter how effective the treatment and how dedicated the staff, the hard reality is that if income does not exceed expenditures, the business will fail. Descriptions of the nuances of finance and budget can be gleaned from any elementary course in business, but the difficult part is applying the practices to an actual business.

Figure 18–1 is a notational example of a budget for a medium-sized (gross annual income between $500,000 and $1,000,000), physical therapy business, adapting data from an actual practice in a large metropolitan area. While the specifics are dependent on a wide range of variables, the rough order of magnitude of the percentages spent on various services should be a useful guide.

Figure 18–1 illustrates several points. First and foremost, a profit *must* be made to ensure the long-term viability of the practice. Next, the income comes from services delivered, and expenses should only be made for those items that contribute to earning that income. Finally, there are controllable and noncontrollable expenses. Time and effort should be spent on the controllable expenses, such as salary, postage, and so on, without agonizing over those expenses that cannot be controlled (i.e., taxes or repairs).

Budgets should also be living documents. No matter how well planned a budget is actual income and expenses will vary, and the budget should be modified accordingly during the year.

The financial health of the business should be checked at least once a month. This is a useful time period, since it coincides with the normal cycle of bank statements, as well as payments by insurers and other health care agencies.

In a nursing home setting, therapists who are planning and working in a department will use a similar type of budget and have similar types of concerns. Figures 18–2A and 18–2B give examples of a financial report and budget for a nursing home.

Sample Budget for a Medium Sized Outpatient Physical Therapy Practice.

INCOME

Fees & Services	$745,000
Sales - Equipment	5,000
Total Income	$750,000

EXPENSES

Direct Expenses

Salaries: Owners/officers	$200,000
Salaries: Other employess	230,000
Medical supplies	30,000
Payroll taxes	30,000
Total Direct Expenses	490,000
Gross Profit (Loss)	260,000

Operating Expenses

Accounting	9,000
Advertising	2,000
Annual Report	100
Bank service charges	100
Business meals	4,000
Cleaning	1,000
Contributions	2,000
Data processing	1,000
State income tax (@10%)	5,000
Credit card discount	4,000
Delivery expenses	400
Depreciation	15,000
Dues and subscriptions	1,000
Entertainment	3,000
Education and seminars	2,000
Gifts	2,000
Insurance	24,000
Interest expenses	1,000
Legal fees	4,000
Licenses and permits	500
Miscellaneous expenses	1,200
Office expenses	3,000
Office supplies	6,000
Parking	2,000
Postage	3,000
Printing and stationery	5,000
Publications and books	1,000
Rent	84,000
Repairs and maintenance	2,000
Taxes, personal property	1,500
Tax, sales	200
Telephone	7,000
Travel	5,000
Temporary Help	5,000
Utilities	3,000
Total Operating Expenses	210,000
Income before taxes	50,000
Federal income tax	7,500
NET INCOME	$42,500

Figure 18–1.

Sample SNF Rehab Budget: Small Unit

	Physical Therapy	Occupational Therapy	Speech Therapy	Total Therapy
Charges	157,000	154,000	28,000	339,000
Expenses	84,000	88,000	14,000	186,000
Overhead	71,000	52,000	8,000	131,000
Gross Margin	2,000	14,000	6,000	22,000
Nonbill	3,000	2,000	2,000	7,000
Adjust to Cost	2,000	14,000	6,000	22,000
Net Loss	(3,000)	(2,000)	(2,000)	(7,000)

ASSUMPTIONS/NOTES

1. 134 bed facility

2. Medicare average daily census = 7.5 beds or 5.7% of total census

3. Therapy unit staffing

	FTEs
Physical therapist	1.00
Physical therapy aide	1.00
Occupational therapist	1.00
Certified occupational therapy assistant	1.00
Speech language pathologist	0.25
Director of rehab (MD)	0.05

4. Square footage

	SQ. FEET
Physical therapy	644
Occupational therapy	50
Speech therapy	0
Total facility	23,677

5. Facility general & administrative expenses = $490,000/year

6. Rehab services payor mix:

	Mix (%)
Medicare - Part A	60
Medicare - Part B	37
Private/other	2
Welfare	1

7. Loss is due to nonbillable services to welfare patients and services under all-inclusive insurance contracts (where services are covered in the per-diem rate).

Figure 18–2A. *(Reprinted with permission from Kurtz H, Medical and Rehabilitation Specialist.)*

Sample SNF Rehab Budget: Large Unit

	Physical Therapy	Occupational Therapy	Speech Therapy	Total Therapy
Charges	802,000	268,000	258,000	1,328,000
Expenses	490,000	102,000	66,000	658,000
Overhead	254,000	58,000	32,000	344,000
Gross Margin	58,000	108,000	160,000	326,000
Nonbill	45,000	50,000	46,000	141,000
Adjust to Cost	55,000	87,000	181,000	273,000
Net Loss	(42,000)	(29,000)	(17,000)	(88,000)

ASSUMPTIONS/NOTES

1. 118 bed facility

2. Medicare average daily census = 15.5 beds or 14% of total census

3. Therapy unit staffing

	FTEs
Physical therapist	5.75
Physical therapist assistant	4.00
Physical therapy Aide	1.16
Occupational therapist	2.16
Certified occupational therapy assistant	1.00
Occupational therapy assistant	1.00
Speech language pathologist	1.58
Director of rehab (MD)	0.25

4. Square footage

	SQ. FEET
Physical therapy	2,071
Occupational therapy	496
Speech therapy	134
Total facility	32,584

5. Facility general & administrative expenses = $480,000/year

6. Rehab services payor mix:

	Mix (%)
Medicare - Part A	81
Medicare - Part B	8
Private/other	11
Welfare	0

7. Loss is due to nonbillable services to welfare patients and services under all-inclusive insurance contracts (where services are covered in the per-diem rate).

Figure 18–2B. *(Reprinted with permission from Kurtz H, Medical and Rehabilitation Specialist.)*

ORGANIZING AND PLANNING FOR PERSONNEL, EQUIPMENT, AND SUPPLIES

Equipment and supplies can be broken up into the equipment and supplies needed by the department versus the equipment and supplies needed for the patient. With respect to departmental equipment, physical therapists specializing in geriatrics must assess whether or not their equipment will provide a return on investment.

For example, if one were to purchase an expensive piece of exercise equipment, would this in fact provide enough revenue to justify the expense? If for example, the piece of equipment is $10,000, the therapist must assess in what way this $10,000 will be returned to the facility. If a therapist could put a patient on this piece of equipment for 10 minutes, this would free the therapist up to work with another patient. Doing this approximately eight times during the day would free up 80 minutes. Over the course of the year, this amounts to approximately 350 hours. A piece of equipment that supplies this magnitude of free time for a therapist, plus the effects of the machine (i.e., strengthening, motivation, and endurance training) will recoup its cost in year (an excellent pay back rate).

When writing requests for equipment or in looking for equipment for self-purchase, the therapist should keep in mind these variables: need, advantages, disadvantages, and cost. Therapists, for example, can purchase parallel bars, and these bars provide needed standing support for gait, balance, and posture work. The advantage of parallel bars is that there is a well-documented history of use in the clinical setting. The main disadvantages are that they are expensive and space-consuming. Access to a sturdy railing might be an alternative. In this type of setting, the railing also can be used for gait training.

A department can be sparse, with hooks on the wall for attachment of exercise bands to be used in progressive resistance exercises, or it can be more high technology, with isokinetic equipment and high-tech balance machines. However, this level of sophistication is not always necessary. Table 18–1 presents a listing of the minimum equipment necessary for a nursing home, as well as a more comprehensive listing for a high-tech facility.

Another important category of equipment and supplies is durable medical

TABLE 18–1. MINIMAL AND MAXIMAL EQUIPMENT LISTS FOR PT DEPARTMENTS

Basic Equipment Needs	Maximum Equipment Needs
Exercise mat	List A plus
Treatment table (plinth)	Cybex
Mirror(s)	Kinetron
Stairs	UBE
Complete set cuff weights: 1/2 to 10 lbs	Fitron
Parallel bars or sturdy railings	Balance Master
Restorator or bike	KAT
Hot Pack (Hydrocollator)	Tekdyne
Wall pulleys	Pro-Stretch
Assortment of ambulation aids: Walkers, pick-up, 2 wheel, 4 wheel canes, single point, quad, hemi crutches	Complete Theraband Line
	Zelex
Additional Recommended Equipment	Hip Machine
Multi-mode electrical stimulator	
Ultrasound	
Tilt table	
Whirlpool	

TABLE 18–2. SAMPLE POLICY AND PROCEDURE FOR EQUIPMENT PURCHASE OR RENTAL

Short-term rental may be appropriate if there is an *occasional* need for the equipment. If the facility routinely uses the equipment on patients, it would be considered part of the departmental costs and would not be billable as a medical supply. All equipment must be ordered by the patient's physician and billed under Part A Medicare Claims.

Examples of billable rental equipment:
1. *CPM (constant passive motion) machines:* Used for total joint replacements.
2. *Reclining wheelchairs:* Used for patients allowed only minimal hip flexion.
3. TENS units.
4. Bucks traction unit for lower extremity fractures.

equipment. To administer efficiently what a facility needs of this type of equipment, therapists must develop policies and procedures to monitor rental, purchase, and resale of the equipment. Therapists in the administrative setting must develop procedures for purchase or rental of equipment for patient use based on the type of equipment that the patient needs.

Table 18–2 provides a sample of procedural record dispersement of medical supplies in a nursing home facility. This policy and procedure can be modified slightly to be used in an outpatient and hospital setting as well.

DEVELOPING GOALS, PHILOSOPHY, AND ORGANIZATIONAL PLANS

Before developing an outpatient or nursing home department, therapists should carefully review their expected goals and plan accordingly. What is the mission statement of the department? In other words, what are the goals and what kind of plan is one going to use to attain these goals in this setting? In an existing setting, the organizational goals and plans should be reviewed periodically to see that they correspond to the current structure of the practice.

Organizational Goals

Reviewing an organization's goals and objectives will provide the therapist with an idea of the direction in which the practice is or should be moving. Is the practice providing standard care to a small community, moving toward high-quality care in the current area, or expanding into a larger area or both? Therapists must determine if these goals agree with their own goals for the future. Does the therapist want to stay in a small practice, working a regular schedule, and doing the best possible job with available resources? Or is the therapist trying to expand the practice, get involved in a larger company, or both? In trying to focus on these issues is important to clarify the individual therapist's goals as they relate to the organizational goals of the practice.

Table 18–3 provides a sample mission statement and philosophy statement. The therapist in a supervisory role should use the type of guidelines suggested in Table 18–3 to develop their own personal philosophy, taking into consideration not only current goals but expected goals for the next 5 to 10 years.

Organizational Plan

The organizational plan is a visual chart of the administrative hierarchy of the department, facility, or entire company. It is a charting of the various employees' positions in relation to others (Fig. 18–3). This can be done on a small scale (e.g., one to two person department) or on a larger scale (e.g., a company of 1000).

This can be very useful for getting an idea of how a company's hierarchy operates, how a person fits into the practice, or how a setting will change if a new

---

TABLE 18–3. SAMPLE MISSION STATEMENT AND PHILOSOPHY STATEMENT

Mission Statement

Our mission is to provide the highest quality rehabilitation services that:

• Meet and maximize each resident's individual needs.
• Promote the quality of life of each resident entrusted to our care.
• Use highly trained rehabilitation professionals.
• Integrate an interdisciplinary approach toward the rehabilitative potential of each resident.

Philosophy of Resident Care

Our goal in rehabilitation services is to provide the highest quality of service to each individual resident who needs assistance in returning to his or her maximal functional abilities.

The rehabilitation therapist at the facility plays a vital role in the operation of the skilled nursing facility, not only by being involved with the residents currently receiving therapy, but also by providing input for all residents in the facility through staff education and consultation, attendance at key meetings within the facility, routine therapy programs, and involvement in RNA programs.

Each resident has some potential for rehabilitation, however small. It is the responsibility of the health care team to evaluate the medical, physical, and psychosocial needs of each resident. From this assessment, a health care plan is designed that encourages maximum functional independence and above all promotes the well-being and quality of life of each resident.

Reprinted with permission from Therapy Management Innovations, Inc.

person is hired. For example, an administrator can simply add the new employee to the chart in various places to see how it affects the chain of command.

LEGAL CONSTRAINTS

Legal ramifications are extremely important for therapists in both administrative and practicing capacities. Therapists must be certain that they have taken

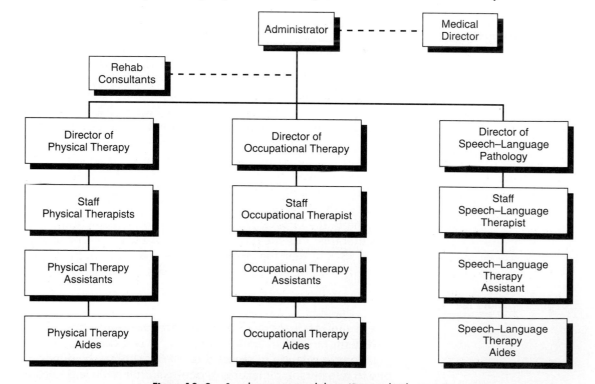

Figure 18–3. Sample organizational chart. *(Reprinted with permission from Therapy Management Innovations, Inc.)*

adequate measures to provide an optimal and legally safe environment for their patients.

A major concern of therapists is being sued for malpractice or negligence. The remainder of this section provides information to assist in understanding the legal climate and prepares the geriatric therapist for some common scenarios that may occur.

The malpractice scenario is as follows: the plaintiff, who is the person suing, tries to provide evidence that, through a failure to meet accepted standards, a patient has been injured. The defendant, or the person being sued, tries to show that quality care was given. Therefore, it is imperative that the therapist constantly complies with regulations and safety practices. The safety practices of the clinic should be outlined in the policy and procedure manual, and the therapist must constantly document that safety measures are in place. Legal documentation, separate from the documentation used for the purposes of reimbursement, is therefore essential.

When sued, a health professional must be able to show that they provided care equal to or exceeded by the national, as well as the local, standard. If called to appear in court, local practitioners who can attest to local practices, or national experts who can testify on the differences between local and national standards, may be useful.

If a patient receives minimal or nonspecific harm because of treatment, a suit would be improper. Therapists can only be sued because actual harm resulted from treatment. For example, if a patient states that the therapist did not diagnose a particular problem, but the therapist did not prevent the patient from obtaining an adequate diagnosis, there is no fault. However, if, because of an inadequately maintained piece of equipment, a patient is injured, the therapist is at fault.

Additionally, liability for injury must be based on proximate cause. That is, the therapist's wrongful conduct must have actually caused the problem. For example, if the therapist walks the patient through a puddle of water, and the patient slips and falls, injuring the coccyx, that is considered proximate cause and the therapist may be sued for unsafe practice and negligence.

For the therapist in a supervisory capacity, as well as in a clinical capacity, it is advisable to use a systematic approach in writing notes, to ensure the therapist is legally covered. The best system for this is the FACT System,[1] which stands for *factual, accurate, complete,* and *timely.* The FACT System states that therapists should write down *factual* comments, what they see, hear, smell, and feel, not what they suppose or assume. They should be *accurate:* never document for someone else and never ask other therapists to document them. Be *complete.* Do not leave any blank spaces, because the attorney will allude to the possibility that space was left to be filled in at a later date.

Finally, be *timely.* Try to write your notes on time. If a late entry is necessary, do not write it in the margins; note that it was a late entry. If a late entry follows other entries and it is dated, it will look as though it was filled in after the fact in a methodical fashion. This reflects a better organized chart compared to squeezing notes in the margins. Do not erase errors, run a line through them and initial the correction. Table 18–4 provides additional dos and don'ts to help in legal documentation.

Finally, from an administrative advisory standpoint, therapists should keep in mind a risk management program to avoid legal complications. To develop an effective risk management program, take the following five steps: (1) identify the potential risks; (2) measure potential risks; (3) select the best technique to control the risks; (4) implement the best technique chosen; and (5) evaluate the technique chosen.

For example, if a potential risk is water spilling from a Hubbard tank, the therapist needs to assess if it is just a minimal amount of water leaking out. If it stays in the Hubbard tank area and does not move to a patient traffic area, there may not be a significant risk. If, however, the drip results in a large puddle, and the patients

TABLE 18–4. DOS AND DONT'S FOR LEGAL DOCUMENTATION

1. Do put in patient's behavior.
2. Don't get personal.
3. Do use quotes.
4. Don't advertise incident reports.
5. Don't use charts to settle disputes.
6. Do be neat and legible.
7. Don't try to keep secrets.

walk in it, then some measure needs to be taken to keep the environment safe. To drain the excess water, a pump may need to be installed in the floor, or a therapist or aide should be assigned the task of water control and clean up in the hydrotherapy unit. If either measure is used, it should be monitored to see if it is, in fact, solving the problem. If it is, it should be continued; if not, the risk assessment/management should be repeated until the situation is rectified. Some additional red flags that may indicate the liabilities of a law suit and of which therapists should be aware are listed in Table 18–5.[2]

Another area of legal concern for physical therapists is the malfunction or misuse of equipment. Unlike other specialties in medicine, equipment can play a large role in the legal ramifications of physical therapy department. Therefore, therapists should be particularly aware of the following areas.

All equipment should be checked and calibrated annually or more periodically, if deemed necessary. The current certification should be clearly displayed on each piece of equipment as well as the last time that the equipment was checked. Finally, the procedure for the checking of equipment should be listed in the policy and procedure manual (see Appendix A).

Even simple equipment may pose a problem. For example, thermometers used in hot pack warmers, paraffin machines, and whirlpools may become dysfunctional. Temperature in these pieces of equipment should be checked monthly with a second thermometer to see if, in fact, they are correct. Hot pack covers showing bald spots and other warning signs should be replaced immediately.

Safety regulations should be posted on all pieces of equipment that require sophisticated techniques (e.g., Cybex equipment or balance machines). All timers

TABLE 18–5. RED FLAGS FLAGS FOR POSSIBLE LITIGATION

1. A patient refuses or leaves treatment.
2. Patient has cardiac arrest during treatment.
3. Patient sees doctor at completion of treatment.
4. Patient goes to hospital within 72 hours.
5. Patient burned during treatment.
6. Patient isn't properly prepared or equipment fails.
7. Patient falls during visit.
8. Patient not informed of his or her condition or complications.
9. Postoperative pain is greater than expected.
10. Patient not encouraged to call doctor if they have a problem.
11. Patient wait longer than 15 minutes.
12. Patient uncomfortable about sexual questions.
13. Patient given unclear instructions.
14. Therapist unfriendly or discourteous.
15. Patient feels therapist didn't spend enough time with them.

TABLE 18–6. HINTS FOR EXPERT WITNESSES

1. Be sure you understand the question.
2. Answer directly and simply. Don't volunteer information.
3. Do not guess. Don't be too proud to admit the limits of your expertise.
4. Take time to think before you answer
5. Do your homework.
6. Speak clearly. Say yes or no, don't just shake your head.
7. Always complete your answer. Don't let the opposing counsel cut you off.
8. Be polite but firm, not cocky.
9. Stop instantly when the judge interrupts you.
10. Never lose your temper or argue with the attorney.
11. When in court, talk directly to the members of the jury and explain your answers in lay person's terms.
12. Dress professionally and conservatively.

and call bells should be checked daily, and foot stools should be eliminated if they have worn pads. Wheelchairs and stretchers should be checked to make certain that locks, straps, and belts are in proper working order.

The best idea for assessing safety is to have someone examine the department weekly, as though he or she were an insurance or safety inspector or a skeptical patient keeping an eye out for hazards.

The final step of any legal administrative program is being prepared to go to court or to be deposed. Table 18–6 presents some useful hints for being an outstanding expert witness, being deposed, or being cross-examined.

The following is a list of the most frequent reasons why therapists are sued, according to the APTA Risk Management Manual[2]:

1. Failure to perform a physical therapy diagnosis.
2. Failure to refer.
3. Failure to properly treat.
4. Failure to monitor the patient.
5. Failure to maintain equipment or equipment failure.
6. Failure to follow doctor's orders.

Improper practice by the therapist may lead to patient injury. Some common causes for patient injury are

1. Being improperly treated with heat or electric equipment.
2. Incorrectly performing exercises with various types of equipment.
3. Improper manipulation.
4. A slip and fall accident.
5. Improper range of motion testing.

PERSONNEL MANAGEMENT: EMPLOYEE RELATIONS

Personnel management encompasses policies and procedures for employee orientation, benefits and other programs. Providing proper supervision is another important part of personnel management. Many books have been written on how to successfully supervise employees. One of the easiest and most succinct books on supervision is *The One Minute Manager*.[3] The text, which takes about 1 minute to read, states that it takes 1 minute to acknowledge an employee's positive attributes and only 1 minute to reprimand them when necessary.

A good supervisor is one that is aware of employee needs and acknowledges good as well as inadequate performances. In addition, a good supervisor gives immediate feedback to the employee frequently.[4]

Employee orientation, quality assurance, inservices, and meeting attendance and orientations for aides are all areas that will require policy development as well as managerial expertise. Providing detailed information on this subject is beyond the scope of this text, but some guidelines for supervisors are provided in Appendix A. These guidelines can be used by supervisors to assist in hiring, training, and managing employees.

MARKETING

The final area to be covered in this chapter is marketing. Marketing is often a foreign concept for rehabilitation professionals. Frequently, marketing is thought of as selling, which it is not. Marketing is the process of identifying services to be offered and then, promoting, pricing, and distributing these services to the patients.[4]

For example, before opening a physical therapy department that will provide geriatric care in the Los Angeles suburbs, it is imperative to research the composition of the population in the area to see if it will support the practice. This background information can be developed by reviewing Chamber of Commerce data, performing interviews with citizens, conducting random sampling by telephone or a mail survey, and general information gathering. Once a need has been identified, decisions can be made on pricing and promoting the service.

It is not easy to open a practice. Studies of demographics, compensation, and other factors must be thoroughly examined before a new practice can be opened. It is essential to develop a fair scheme for charging, to prepare a schedule that meets the needs of the community, to establish the most centrally located site for the services, and to make sure that the site is accessible to all clients.

The next step is to promote the service. Let people know that the service is available, show how it differs from other services in the area, and try to expose people to information about the clinic. This can be done in a number of ways, ranging from sending out letters or making telephone calls to preparing seminars or just advertising by word of mouth.

Targeting marketing efforts is very important. In many areas, therapists are dependent on physicians for referrals. Thus, marketing may need to be targeted at physicians. In other areas, targeting patients who may want physical therapy but cannot get physician orders may be the best approach.

Marketing can be divided into two categories: external and internal. External marketing has already been described and it involves letting people from the outside know about the practice's services. Internal marketing focuses on the inner workings of the facility and how the efficiency and high quality of the services provided encourages patients to return or refer others to the clinic. Good questions to assess internal marketing efforts are: (1) Is the staff courteous? (2) Is a visit to the clinic a pleasant experience? (3) Are patients provided with information about the facility? (4) Does the staff know what the goals of the clinic are and act with these in mind?

Internal marketing strategies are discussed widely in the literature and although providing more detail is beyond the scope of this section, additional references are available.[5-8] Table 18–7 provides a simple and succinct marketing strategy handout for therapists, discusses professional level marketing and community level marketing, and gives examples of how to implement these strategies.

TABLE 18–7. MARKETING STRATEGY

Rehabilitation departments frequently succeed or fail due to their ability to plan and implement ongoing marketing programs to showcase rehabilitation services. Marketing concepts must be kept in mind at all times and not only during low volume periods. The following is an example of marketing techniques that each therapist is encouraged to develop relative to their facility and specialized programs.

Marketing falls into three general categories:
1. Community
2. Professional
3. Facility

1. Community Level
   A. Volunteer to an organization, such as Spinal Cord Club, MS, MD.
   B. Advertise facility based community service programs, such as "Caring for the Stroke Patient at Home." Could be for families in the facility as well as on a local public level.
      Organize a posture screening in a mall or senior center.
      Teach a special exercise class at a retirement center.
      Develop educational activities for osteoporosis month (May).
   C. Presentations to Special Interest Groups
      Service clubs.
      Geriatric groups.

2. Professional Level
   A. Doctor visits
      Initial introduction to new physicians.
      Introduce new programs or equipment in the physical therapy department.
      Discuss continuing education course.
      When getting started, you may want to discuss postop protocols (i.e., for THR, TKR to determine general approach to weight bearing, exercise).
      Accompany patients on follow-up physician visits.
      Send typed discharge summaries frequently.
   B. Acute Care Physical Therapy Visits
      Introduce yourself to all staff.
      If new to area, may ask for informatio on local APTA chapter, TENS distributors, recommendations on good medical supply companies.
      Tour the facility.
      Ask for input on Skilled Nursing Facility (SNF) Physical Therapy needs in the community.
   C. Discharge planners
      Administrator, director of nursing, and physical therapist make a good team to visit hospital discharge planners.
      Leave brochures and business cards when available.
      Send discharge planners typed discharge summaries on those patients they referred to you as soon as possible.
      Develop and introduce new programs.
   D. Enterostomal therapist
      Excellent contact person for wound care referral.
      Ask them to provide inservices to your facility.
   E. Attend local continuing educational courses, especially those sponsored by your referring hospitals.
   F. Attend APTA local chapter meetings

3. Facility Level
   A. Admission Meetings: Attendance by the Physical Therapist is mandatory.
   B. Inservices to Nursing Staff
      Four per year are required, however, you are encouraged to provide them as deemed necessary in cooperation with director of nursing and staff development director.
      Consult with certified nurse assistant classes to teach certain portions of the class, such as bodymechanics, range of motion, positioning, and the rehabilitation team approach.
      Periodic departmental head inservices.
      Assist in coordination of other inservices with occupational and speech therapy.
   C. Rehabilitation Conferences: Used to teach rehabilitation approach to nursing staff.
   D. Consult with activities director to help coordinate an exercise class.

CONCLUSION

As stated previously, it is imperative that therapists not only understand the clinical aspects of geriatric rehabilitation but the administrative aspects as well. Most of the information on administration is not directly available in rehabilitation texts, and the therapist may need to consult other sources to find some information. The best sources are business publications and seminars. A mixture of good clinical and administrative skills can provide therapists with a very rewarding practice.

PEARLS

- The components of administration are finance and budgeting, policies and procedures, legal concerns, employee relations, and marketing.

- Budgeting is defined as providing a monetary sketch of the department or clinic, and a realistic budget is essential to the financial well-being of the business.

- Need, advantages, disadvantages, and cost are all important considerations when purchasing equipment.

- An organizational plan is a visual chart of the administrative hierarchy.

- The plaintiff has a case if they can show actual harm resulted from an action, or if the therapist practiced below local or national standards.

- Equipment should be calibrated annually, and more sophisticated equipment should have precautions and directions posted.

- Marketing is identifying services to be offered and promoting, pricing, and distributing these services to the patients.

REFERENCES

1. Bergeson S. More about charting with a jury in mind. *Nursing.* April 1988; 50–58.
2. American Physical Therapy Association. *Risk Management.* Alexandria, VA: APTA; 1990.
3. Blanchard K, Spencer J. *The One Minute Manager.* New York; Berkeley Books; 1982.
4. Solomon R. *Clinical Practice Management.* Gaithersburg, Md: Aspen Publishers; 1991.
5. Kotler P, Clarke R. *Marketing for Health Care Organizations.* Englewood Cliffs, NJ: Prentice-Hall; 1987:244.
6. Husted S, Varble D, Lowry J. *Principles of Modern Marketing.* Needham Heights, Mass: Allyn and Bacon; 237.
7. Scott J, Warshaw M, Taylor J. *Introduction to Marketing Management.* 5th ed. Homewood, Ill: Irwin; 1985; 11–12.
8. *Journal of Health Care Marketing.* American Marketing Association, 250 S. Wacker Dr., Chicago, Ill, 60606; *Journal of Medical Practice Management.* Williams and Wilkins, 428 E. Preston St., Baltimore, 21202.

Appendix A. Guidelines for Hiring, Training, and Managing Employees

Orientation of Therapy Aides

Orientation and Training
Checklist: PT Aide

Physical Therapy Aide
Work Performance
Evaluation Checklist

Committee Meetings

Daily Stand-up Meeting

Rehabilitation Meeting

Resident Care
Planning Conference

Utilization Review

Department Head Meeting

Resident Care Policy Review

Quality Assurance
and Assessment

Orientation of Therapy Aides

Policy

All new OT, PT, SLP aides will be oriented in a timely manner by the director of physical therapy or a designee (i.e., other staff therapists). Upon satisfactory completion of orientation and skills assessment, the aide will be assessed at 3 months, 1 year, and yearly thereafter.

Purpose

To assure competent skills in both direct and indirect patient care activities.

Scope

Orientation procedure must be followed on all new therapy aides.

Guidelines

1. Orientation process will vary depending on employee's prior work experience and will be at the discretion of the supervising therapist.
2. The therapy aide will be trained in the use of selective therapy modalities and procedures as deemed appropriate by the supervising therapist. All modalities that may be performed by the aide will be documented on work performance evaluation checklist by the trainer.
3. When responsibilities are added to the tasks performed by therapy aides, these are documented on the work performance evaluation checklist to indicate training has been done.
4. Orientation checklists will be completed on each new therapy aide.
5. Work performance evaluation checklists are updated on an ongoing basis and maintained, and a copy is kept in the aide's personnel file.

Figure 18A–1. *(Reprinted with permission from Therapy Management Innovations, Inc.)*

Orientation and Training Checklist: PT Aide

General Orientation to Facility

- [ ] Mission/Philosophy Statements
- [ ] Introductions
    Facility Staff
    Rehab Staff
- [ ] Tour
- [ ] Supplies & Equipment
    List supplies or equipment issued (i.e., dep't. key, gait belt, etc.)
- [ ] Body Mechanics Instruction

Roles

- [ ] PT Aide Job Description
- [ ] Supervision Requirements
- [ ] Interdisciplinary Team Approach (common goals, communication, etc.)
- [ ] PT Role
- [ ] Other Rehab Roles
- [ ] Other Facility Staff
- [ ] Consultants
- [ ] Nursing/Rehab Integration of Services

Clinical Information

- [ ] Effects of Aging (i.e., systems, multiple dx., myths v. facts, etc.)
- [ ] Common Diagnoses/Problems/Precautions
- [ ] CVA
- [ ] Upper extremity fracture
- [ ] Hip fracture
- [ ] Hip replacement
- [ ] Knee replacement
- [ ] Fracture of spine
- [ ] Arthritis
- [ ] Progressive neurological conditions
- [ ] Head injury
- [ ] Cardiac
- [ ] COPD
- [ ] Amputation
- [ ] Wounds
- [ ] Medical conditions
- [ ] Functional Levels Defined
- [ ] Identifying Change of Condition (functional)
- [ ] Reporting Patient Information what, to whom, when, written, verbal
- [ ] Family Interactions

Treatment Modalities/Procedures

- [ ] Bed Mobility Training (Consider: hemiplegia, UE or LE fracture, hip, replacement, fracture of spine)

- [ ] Transfer Training/Use of Gait Belt (Consider: hemiplegia, LE fracture or joint replacement, amputee)
- [ ] Ambulation Activities/Use of Gait Belt (Consider: hemiplegia, LE fracture, or joint replacement)
    - ■ Types of gait
    - ■ Precautions
    - ■ Safely assisting
    - ■ Equipment—types, adjustments
- [ ] Balance Activities
    - ■ Sitting
    - ■ Standing
- [ ] Positioning (Consider: hemiplegia, UE or LE fracture, UE or LE fracture, LE joint replacement, wounds)
    - ■ Bed
    - ■ Wheelchair
- [ ] Wheelchair Mobility Training
    - ■ Safe transport of patients
    - ■ W/C adjustments
    - ■ Brakes, footpedals, leg rests
    - ■ Propulsion

Therapeutic Exercise

- [ ] Passive ROM
- [ ] Self ROM
- [ ] Active/assisted
- [ ] Active
- [ ] Resistive use of equipment (i.e., pulleys, weights, rickshaw, thera-band, etc.)
- [ ] Group

Other Procedures

- [ ] Whirlpool (Incl. routine use, cleaning, culturing per procedure)
- [ ] Hot Packs
- [ ] Cold Packs
- [ ] Contrast Bath
- [ ] Paraffin

Physiological Monitoring

- [ ] Pulse, Rate, and Rhythm
- [ ] Respirations, Rate, SOB

Use of Specialized Equipment

- [ ] Tilt Table
- [ ] Mechanical Lift
- [ ] CPM

Continued

545

───────────────── *Continued from previous page* ─────────────────

☐ Parallel Bars
☐ Specialized Exercise Equipment

Documentation (if applicable)

☐ Medical Record Format
☐ Patient Subjective & Objective Information
   (pt. comments & treatment given)
☐ Acceptable Abbreviations
☐ Functional Levels
☐ Co-signature by PT

Clerical Support

☐ Telephone Protocol

☐ Copying
☐ Faxing
☐ Ordering Supplies/Equipment (therapeutic and
   office needs)
☐ Scheduling
☐ Therapy Logs (for billing)
☐ Cleaning and Maintenance of Treatment Area

Other

☐ Reporting Incidents/Unusual Occurrences
☐ CPR
☐ Fire Safety Procedures
☐ Infection Control
☐ Disaster Procedures

Figure 18A–2. *(Reprinted with permission from Therapy Management Innovations, Inc.)*

PHYSICAL THERAPY AIDE WORK PERFORMANCE EVALUATION CHECKLIST

Procedure/Modality	INITIAL ASSESSMENT			3-MONTH			YEARLY		
	Date	PT Initials	AIDE Initials	Date	PT Initials	AIDE Initials	Date	PT Initials	AIDE Initials

Figure 18A–3. *(Reprinted with permission from Therapy Management Innovations, Inc.)*

Committee Meetings

Policy

To improve communication between Rehabilitation Services and the facility, each therapy service is requested to share information at specific committee meetings. This information should be given to the committee coordinator prior to its commencement if the therapist is unable to attend.

The following committee meetings are required, as appropriate, in your facility:

- Admissions.
- Rehabilitation.
- Resident Care Planning Conference.
- Quality Assurance.
- Use Review.
- Department Head Meeting.
- Patient Care Policy Review.
- Corporate/Regional Rehab Meeting.
- Quality Assurance and Assessment.

Procedure

1. Obtain the dates and times of these meetings from your administrator.
2. Schedule meetings accordingly.

Figure 18A–4. *(Reprinted with permission from Therapy Management Innovations, Inc.)*

Daily Stand-Up Meeting

Meeting name: This meeting may be known by different facilities; it may be called the Admissions or Stand-up or Census Meeting.

Purpose: To provide coordinated interdisciplinary communication regarding patient inquiries, admissions, discharges, and room transfers.

Frequency: Every day, for approximately 15 minutes.

Members: Administrator, director of nursing, admissions coordinator, physical therapist, occupational therapist, speech-language pathologist, medical records, bookkeeper and appropriate department heads.

Items Discussed:

- Inquiries pending, level of care/payor status.
- New admissions.
- Discharges.
- Room transfers.
- Patient's change of condition.
- Special programs/activities for the day.

Figure 18A–5. *(Reprinted with permission from Therapy Management Innovations, Inc.)*

Rehabilitation Meeting

Purpose: To provide an opportunity for interdisciplinary team members to discuss a patient's plan of treatment.

Frequency: Weekly.

Members: Administrator of nursing, charge nurse, RNA, physical therapist, occupational therapist, speech-language pathologist, social services, and discharge planner. Dietary services and CNA should attend as appropriate.

Items Discussed:

- Interdisciplinary goals.
- Patient's progress.
- Equipment needs.
- Discharge planning.
- Family teaching.

Documentation: Minutes of each meeting should be kept. These should include date of the meeting, members present, patients reviewed, and necessary follow-up. A notebook containing rehabilitation meeting minutes can be kept in the rehabilitation department and used as a reference for each minute.

Figure 18A–6. *(Reprinted with permission from Therapy Management Innovations, Inc.)*

Resident Care Planning Conference

Purpose: To provide the highest quality of care planning through use of a coordinated interdisciplinary approach.

Frequency: Twice weekly or as needed per facility census.

Members: Director of nursing, dietary, social services, activities, physical therapist, occupational therapist, and speech-language pathologist, RNA and CNA staff as needed.

Items Discussed:

- Interdisciplinary problems, goals, and treatment approaches are discussed and listed on the patient care plan.
- New admissions are discussed within 7 days of admit.
- Residents are discussed with updates and deletions recorded at least quarterly.
- Appropriateness of care plan entries.
- Changes in condition.

Figure 18A–7. *(Reprinted with permission from Therapy Management Innovations, Inc.)*

Utilization Review

Purpose: To maintain a medical committee to determine Medicare coverage and to appropriately use facility services.

Members: Two or more physicians, including medical director, administrator, director of nursing, medical records, social services, physical therapist, occupational therapist, and speech-language pathologist.

Committee Functions: In order to promote the highest quality of resident care, the committee is responsible for conducting medical care evaluation studies, extended duration reviews, and consideration of any other cases brought to its attention. The committee will also review discharge plans for individual residents.

Rehabilitation Involvement: The rehabilitation team has an important role to play in the decision made by the utilization review committee. A list of patients should be reviewed prior to the meeting in order for the therapist to give an accurate update on the patient's therapy progress and expected duration of treatment. If a therapist is unable to attend, their patients should be discussed with the director of nursing to ensure their treatment plans are taken into consideration by the committee.

Figure 18A–8. *(Reprinted with permission from Therapy Management Innovations, Inc.)*

Department Head Meeting

Purpose: To facilitate open communication and sharing of information between key personnel. Each department head is responsible to share appropriate information with his or her staff.

Frequency: Scheduled as needed by the administrator; may be weekly or daily.

Members: Administrator, director of nursing, rehabilitation services, dietary, social services, activities, housekeeping/laundry, maintenance.

Items Discussed:

- Department update.
- Changes in policies and procedures.
- Corporate updates.
- Facility activities.
- Department head and consultant schedules.
- Community education.

Figure 18A–9. *(Reprinted with permission from Therapy Management Innovations, Inc.)*

Resident Care Policy Review

Purpose: To review and revise the Resident Care Policy Manual.

Frequency: At least yearly, usually prior to survey. It may be scheduled more frequently, as needed.

Members: Administrator, director of nursing, rehabilitation services, social services activities, dietary, housekeeping/laundry, maintenance.

Items Discussed:

- Review policies and procedures for accuracy.
- Delete nonexistent policies.
- Update and revise appropriate policies.
- Include new policies and procedures, as appropriate.

The Rehabilitation Policy and Procedure Manual should be reviewed and revised yearly. This may be completed during this meeting. Once completed, the manual is signed and dated.

Figure 18A–10. *(Reprinted with permission from Therapy Management Innovations, Inc.)*

Quality Assurance and Assessment

Purpose: To provide a systematic and ongoing self-evaluation process geared toward identifying and resolving problems, targeting areas for program improvement and development, and enhancement of overall resident care and quality of life.

Frequency: Monthly.

Members: Administrator, medical director, director of nurses, and at least three other staff members from various departments, such as social service, activities, dietary, rehabilitation, or housekeeping.

Items Discussed:

- Identification of areas to be studied.
- Format for data collection and communication of finding.
- Establishment of CQI studies, including time frames, responsibilities, data collection, tools, and reporting mechanism.

Figure 18A–11. *(Reprinted with permission from Therapy Management Innovations, Inc.)*

CHAPTER *19* NINETEEN

Consultation

The consultant role is not new to physical therapy, because physical therapists serve as consultants to other health care team members in daily treatment delivery. The physical therapist's role as a consultant is, however, new in the realm of geriatrics. Most literature on the subject of the consultant in geriatrics has only been published in the last 15 years.

The general literature on geriatric consultation states several reasons for its development. These reasons include patient care, professional education, public relations screening, and quality assurance. In the medical literature, the major reasons for requesting geriatric consultation were medical management (25%), discharge planning (18%), evaluation and management of dementia (17%), and failure to thrive (15%).[1] According to another study, the major reasons for requesting consultation were geriatric evaluation (28%), assessing rehabilitation potential (27%), and mental status evaluation (3%).[2]

Several benefits of geriatric consultation have been enumerated in the literature. These benefits are

1. Decreased length of hospitalization.[3]
2. Increased use of rehabilitation services.[3]
3. Improved patient care.[4]
4. Decreased use of expensive health care resources.[5]
5. Increased identification of new diagnoses.[6]
6. Provides a source of education.[7]

The negative aspects of geriatric consultation are

1. Conflicts may arise among the disciplines when there is a "turf" battle over the overall management of the patient.
2. Geriatric consultation can be time consuming.
3. This type of consultation can also be costly.[7]

The final introductory point on geriatric consultation is efficacy. The general literature reveals no definitive conclusions as to the efficacy of consultation. The literature is fraught with complications about the type of patient classically referred to a medical geriatric consultant. The frailer patients are more frequently referred and are more difficult to manage. Secondly, the recommendations of the consultant are often only partially followed.[8,9] Even with the controversy in geriatric consultation, the potential benefit to the older person in different treatment settings outweighs the negative aspects cited.

IDENTIFYING THE PHYSICAL THERAPY CONSULTANT'S ROLE

Settings

The variety of settings available to the physical therapy consultant in geriatrics is only limited by the therapist's imagination, but the major areas of consultation are nursing homes, home care, senior centers, hospitals, rehabilitation centers, and outpatient clinics.

Nursing Homes

In the nursing home a physical therapist can work as a staff therapist and receive a regular salary with all the benefits he or she can contract. Contract basis in the nursing home can take many forms, the most common of which are the hourly, per patient, or direct bill. In the hourly arrangement, the therapist charges the nursing home for any hours spent in the facility with the majority of time being spent in direct patient care. In addition, the therapist may set up restorative programs, provide in-service education, conduct screenings, and assist in quality assurance. The therapist is simply reimbursed on a time spent basis.

The per patient arrangement reimburses the therapist based on how many patients are seen. This can be a flat figure per patient or be based on a percentage of charges. The percentage method can be further broken down into the percentage of charges billed and the percentage of charges received. It is obvious that it is more advantageous to the therapist to contract on a percentage billed basis, while the nursing home would prefer to use the percentage received. The pros of the first situation are that the therapist does not have to wait for the money and is not dependent on the nursing home's filing ability. In addition, the therapist does not risk a denied claim. The therapist who contracts on a percentage basis has several options in providing nonpatient care services: They can be included as part of the package on a gratis basis, the therapist can be reimbursed on a hourly basis for any time spent in presentation and preparation, or a flat fee can be assessed on a weekly, monthly, or yearly basis for these extra services.

The final, most common method of consulting in a nursing home with direct patient care as the major emphasis is direct billing of the patient. In this situation the therapist offers to treat any appropriate patients and to bill the respective insurance company. This form of consultation is riskier and more inundated with paperwork than the previously mentioned methods; however, it can prove to be the most lucrative. (For specific information on inpatient and outpatient contracting see Appendix D.)

Home Care

Consultation in home care is identical to the situations already described when the consultant subcontracts with an agency. In this situation the therapist can be salaried, hourly, or per patient. In an even more independent situation, a therapist can hang up a shingle and treat patients in the home. The therapist will direct bill the patient and the insurance company. To treat Medicare home patients the independent therapist must have a certified office. (See Appendix A for Criteria for a Certified Office.)

Senior Centers

Senior centers and retirement homes provide a creative way of consulating in the geriatric realm, and therapists can serve in several capacities. For example, they can conduct environmental assessments, develop and teach exercise classes, or provide screening programs. The financial arrangements for these types of programs can be quite varied. The consultant can offer the facility a menu of these activities with a cost per activity charge. Another alternative is an hourly arrangement to provide whatever services are needed. The consultant can also directly charge the participants. For example, a consultant may charge each exercise class participant $5 per session, or $20 for four sessions. The consultant may want to provide some of the services for free as a public relations effort for future programs.

Hospitals, Rehabilitation Centers, and Outpatient Clinics

Hospital consulting is a new area of physical therapy, therefore, the physical therapist seeking hospital privileges is a relatively new and controversial topic. (See Appendix A for practice privileges from the state of California and criteria for certified office, as well as for information on performance standards for independent practitioners.)

The consultant in the hospital, rehabilitation center, and outpatient clinic can always contract to provide direct patient care on an hourly, per patient, or direct bill basis. He or she can also act to provide special assessment for older patients, which may take the form of a screening, such as an osteoporosis, balance, or foot evaluation. The consultant may also be called in to provide expert advice on how to improve the outcomes of therapy or to perform specific functional assessment specific for older persons (see Chapter 6 for functional assessment tools). In addition to providing these services in the hospital, rehabilitation and outpatient settings, the consultant can provide continuing education and screening programs to the public, as well as quality assurance expertise. The financial arrangement for this could take the form of an hourly contract, fee for service, or flat fee contract.

In all of these settings the geriatric consultant may be asked to design a program where none has existed previously. This will require the consultant to create policy and procedure manuals, employee handbooks, and billing procedures and forms. In the author's opinion the best approach to this type of arrangement is to develop an hourly contract. A flat fee contract can also be used, however, this does not give the consultant the freedom to spend time on unforeseen complications that may arise in the process of designing a program.

Identifying Consultant Activities

Screening Programs

Screening programs are one of the major activities of the geriatric consultant. They can be conducted in any of the settings listed as well as in a public setting (i.e., shopping malls). (Appendix B has examples of screening programs for the community.)

Direct Patient Care

Physical therapists can provide part-time or full-time direct patient care as another type of activity, and it can be very creative. In many situations the physical therapist conducts the evaluations and discharges, and the physical therapy assistant provides the hands-on treatment under the supervision of the physical therapist. Some therapists set up classes for providing care to similar patients in the hospital, nursing home, or community setting. The options for care in this setting are limitless. Nevertheless, the important components of this type of consulting are appropriate evaluation, progressive treatment strategies, and comprehensive discharge. Through this process the therapist must provide appropriate documentation.

Consulting on OBRA

In the nursing home setting, additional consultative roles are constantly developing. In 1989 and 1990, for example, the US government took action on some previous legislation that directly impacted the physical therapist. The scenario with a consultative view of an approach to the problem follows.

The Omnibus Reconciliation Act (OBRA) of 1987 and the Federal Nursing Home Amendment are two of the most influential pieces of legislation affecting long-term care. Even though OBRA was published in 1987, the guidelines for the implementation of this legislation are still being written. One portion of these guidelines that will affect physical and occupational therapy dramatically is the "Interpretive Guidelines on Physical Restraints: Implemented October 1, 1990."

A quote from these guidelines illustrates the importance of physical and occupational therapists with regard to interpreting the legislation and administering the guidelines: "A facility must have evidence of consultation with appropriate health professionals, such as occupational or physical therapists in the use of less restrictive supportive devices, *prior to* using physical restraints as defined in this guideline for such purposes."

The four major types of patients who are candidates for physical restraints are

- The cognitively impaired wanderer.
- The aggressive patient.
- Patients who interfere with medical treatment.
- The unsteady patient.

The physical and occupational therapist will be most effective in assessing the necessity for restraining devices for the fourth group because of the clear benefits associated with aiding these patients to maintain their quality of life. For this group, the guidelines call for several major areas of assessment. The first major area of assessment is the risk of falls or a decline in functional status if physical restraints are not applied. The next area of assessment is the risk of falls or decline in function if physical restraints are applied. The third and fourth areas of concern are to use less restrictive measures and the application of restraints. The final area to be assessed is the facility's ability to provide the least restrictive environment.

To tie or not to tie is a difficult question. Understaffed nursing homes are fearful of guidelines that may cause an increase in the responsibilities of overburdened and underpaid staff. In addition, the possibility of increased legal pressure has been a source of apprehension regarding nonadherence to the guidelines. The proponents of untying the elderly, however, are advocating unassailable issues in the area of quality of life that must be considered in a comparison of risks and benefits.

Physical and occupational therapists can be extremely important players in allaying the fears of staff in this area, as well as in helping to ensure that the least restrictive and most freedom enhancing environment for older persons is established. Figure 19–1 is a Physical Restraint Form,[10] which is self-explanatory. Questions 1–16 on the Physical Restraint Consultation Form address the area of risk of falls both intrinsic and extrinsically. The next areas of concern, possible less restrictive measures and application of restraints, respectively, are addressed by the questions under #17 in the Physical Restraint Consultation (PRC) form. The third area of the assessment form is the risk of falls or decline in function if physical restraints are applied. The same tools already noted will answer this concern, as well as question #18 on the PRC form. The final area of assessment is the facility's ability to provide the least restrictive environment. This is addressed in question #19.[10]

Physical Restraint Consultation Form

1. Name _____ Date _____

2. Current medical problems _____

3. Medications _____

4. History of falls _____

    Frequency _____

    Time of day _____

    Position _____

    Activity _____

5. Balance with eyes open _____

6. Balance with eyes closed _____ (see Chapter 6)

7. Get up and go _____ (see Chapters 11, 12, and 13)

8. Vertebral artery syndrome _____

9. Blood pressure change with position change _____

10. Flexibility _____

11. Strength _____

12. Posture _____

13. Gait (eyes open) _____ (eyes closed) _____

14. Tandem walk _____

15. Psychological _____

16. Environment

    Noise level _____

    Chairs _____ Stable _____ Locked _____

    Beds _____ Low _____ Locked _____

    Lighting _____ Adequate _____ Glare _____

    Toilet _____ Raised _____ Handrails _____

    Colors _____ Raised _____ Safe _____

17. Recommendations

A. Physical Restraints Y _____ N _____ (If yes, state time, placement, precautions, and suggestions) _____

B. Does the resident need devices for alignment, proper body position, or prevention of contractures? Y _____ N _____ (If yes, specify) _____

C. Does resident need to be in nonrestrained area of constant observation? _____

D. Other suggestions (P.T., O.T., exercise class, or assistive devices). Specify _____

18. Has the use or will the use of physical restraints cause:

A. Chronic constipation or incontinence _____

B. Pressure sores _____

C. Loss of muscle tone _____

D. Loss of independent mobility _____

E. Increased agitation _____

F. Loss of balance _____

G. Symptoms of withdrawal or depression _____

H. Reduced social contact _____

19. Is the least restrictive restraint being used? Y _____ N _____ If no, why not _____

20. When should the resident be reevaluated for use of physical restraints? _____

Figure 19 1. *(Reprinted with permission from Lewis C: How to handle upcoming guidelines PT Bull. June 27, 1990;18–19.)*

Quality Assurance and Chart Review

Physical therapists can also act in a consultative capacity to provide quality assurance and chart review assistance. To provide this type of service the therapist should consult several references in this area. References 11–17 are particularly useful for information on quality assurance. Several groups exist across the country that provide this type of service. However, if it can be done in-house or locally for less money and inconvenience, then the therapist is providing a worthwhile consultant service.

THE CONSULTATION PROCESS

To execute a successful consultation program a methodical and reproducible process should be followed. The steps in this process are

1. Needs assessment.
2. Query.
3. Proposal.
4. Negotiation.
5. Implementation.
6. Evaluation.

A needs assessment can be conducted simply or through a very sophisticated process. In its simplest form, a needs assessment is conducted either by asking people if they think a program would be beneficial or by observing the site. Increasing in sophistication, a needs assessment would be a random phone survey, a written survey to a specific audience, or tapping the data from a community or facility survey.

The query portion of the process entails asking detailed questions to assist in the design of the program. For example, if a posture screening program is to be developed, questions about the time of day, acceptable waiting time, price, expectations, and people and facilities available would be useful (Fig. 19–2).

A proposal can also be simple or sophisticated. A simple proposal would be a telephone call to the general manager of a community mall, with a discussion that included information on the therapist's background. If space is available, the therapist should ask what the appropriate times are, about the available manpower, and about additional expense requirements. This can be followed up by a letter restating the terms. A formal proposal is given in Appendix C.

The negotiation step of the consultation process entails discussing the therapist's needs with the facility contracted with. In this process, the therapist must come into the meeting with both an optimal situation and the minimal ac-

---

Sample Query

Your group has expressed an interest in a low back exercise class. To design the class to meet your needs, please take a few moments to fill out the questions below.

1. What time of day is good for you?
2. Is five dollars per class acceptable?
3. What do you expect from this class?
4. How often would you like to come to the class?

Figure 19–2.

ceptable situation. Begin the negotiation by describing the optimal situation, then ask the negotiatee about their optimal scenario. If the two match, both will be very happy. If the responses are completely opposite, then ask what their minimal acceptable situation is. If this situation is vastly different than the minimal criteria the therapist has established prior to this meeting, then he or she should graciously leave.

The implementation of the consulting process can be divided into four phases: long-term planning, short-term planning, execution, and continuation. Long-term planning begins from the moment the negotiations end and the contract is signed and lasts until the day before the project begins. Activities to be accomplished during this phase are the design or completion of any administrative forms. For example, if a therapist consults to provide an exercise class, in the long-term phase he or she will need to develop medical releases and get them filled out before the class begins (Fig. 19–3). Participant evaluation forms will be needed as well as handouts and contracts, and the class will need to be advertised (see Appendix C). The final aspect of the long-term implementation is preparing the exercise class. In preparing for the first class, an introduction must be designed for the therapist and a way of meeting the class's participants must also be designed. Then a format for the class must be developed. Finally, the class should be practiced several times so the therapist is comfortable teaching it.

In the short-term phase of implementation (1 to 2 days before the class) areas to plan for are environmental and advertising. Environmentally, check the room one more time before the class. Is there enough room? Is the temperature correct?

Implementation Phase

	EXERCISE CLASSES	SETTING UP	PHYSICAL THERAPY DEPT.
Long-term	Medical releases Evaluation forms Contracts with individual Handouts Sign-in sheet Advertise		
Short-term	Check space Get equipment Get music Appropriate clothes Advertise		
Execution	Check water Check temperature Check music Check handouts Check lights		
Continuation	New handouts Reevalulate forms New equipment/music Advertise		

Figure 19–3A.

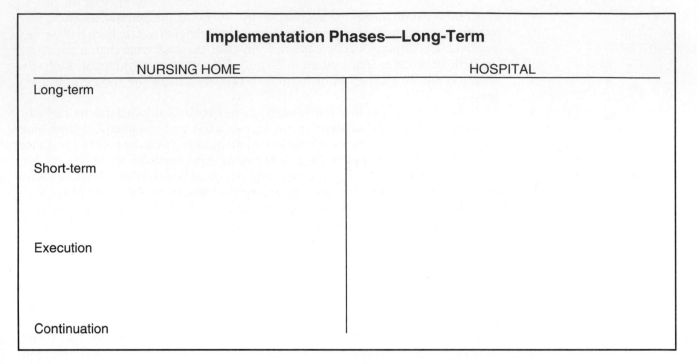

Figure 19–3B.

Is the music system appropriate and do the tapes work on the equipment? Do you have tapes and do you feel comfortable working the equipment? The therapist is also part of the environment. What are you going to wear? There are several considerations here. First, you need to look professional, and yet you need to move around to teach an exercise class. Tailored slacks and a professional blouse will work. Second, the colors should be in the optimal appreciation range for the older person, that is the reds, oranges, and golds. See Chapter 12 for more information on colors.

The final aspect of the short-term implementation phase is intense advertising. In the last 24 to 48 hours, advertisements can be repeated for one more time. Flyers can be used to catch the participant's attention.

The execution phase is teaching the class. Do a last minute check of the environment. Check to be sure the temperature and lighting are correct and that water is close by. Check to be sure the handouts are ready and that the music is working. At the last minute, check to be sure you are relaxed and comfortable.

The continuation phase is composed of what it takes to continue the consulting activity. In the preceding example, the continuation phase is relatively simple, but in a contracted physical therapy department, it can be much more difficult. For example, in the department setting the consultant is frequently confronted with patient load fluctuations and staff shortages. These types of problems constantly plague these settings and should be planned for in the continuation. Returning to the example of the continuation phase in the exercise classes, activities to enhance this phase are developing new handouts, programs, equipment usage, musical background, and continuing advertisement. In addition, frequent reevaluations of the class participants, using the initial evaluation to show progress can help to motivate individuals to continue in an exercise program.

The final phase of the consultant process is the evaluation phase, which can be accomplished simply or in a more sophisticated fashion. In the simplest form, evaluation can be done by asking the recipients if they like the services. This can be done by spontaneous feedback or by a formal questionnaire (Fig. 19–4).

In the hospital or nursing home setting, the recipients of the service are not the only consumers. Nurses and referring doctors should also receive questionnaires

Patient Satisfaction Survey

The following is a survey that Crescent City Physical Therapy sends to patients within 30 days of their discharge date. What we hope to accomplish is to determine if we are meeting your needs and expectations. Crescent City Physical Therapy cares about what you think. We want to offer you the highest quality of patient care. So, please take a brief moment and complete this short survey, and return it in the stamped, self-addressed envelope. Thank You!!

1. The treatment you received from your physical therapist was?

    ☐ Excellent   ☐ Average   ☐ Poor   ☐ No response

2. The treatment you received from your physical therapy aid was?

    ☐ Excellent   ☐ Average   ☐ Poor   ☐ No response

3. The service you received from the front desk when you first set up an appointment was?

    ☐ Excellent   ☐ Average   ☐ Poor   ☐ No response

4. The service you received at the front desk when checking in for your appointment was?

    ☐ Excellent   ☐ Average   ☐ Poor   ☐ No response

5. The service you received at the front desk when setting up a return appointment was?

    ☐ Excellent   ☐ Average   ☐ Poor   ☐ No response

6. The manner or promptness in which billing the responsible party (insurance company, attorney, workman's compensation, or private pay) was?

    ☐ Excellent   ☐ Average   ☐ Poor   ☐ No response

7. Was the manner in which statements were sent easily understood?

    ☐ Excellent   ☐ Average   ☐ Poor   ☐ No response

8. The manner in which the Crescent City Physical Therapy office handled your telephone calls was?
    ☐ Excellent   ☐ Average   ☐ Poor   ☐ No response

Figure 19–4.   *(Reprinted with permission from Crescent City Physical Therapy & Sports Rehabilitations Services, Inc.)*

on the services. Evaluations can be done periodically or at set intervals (i.e., every 6 months), and the can also be used to assess outcomes.

Outcomes can be broken down into two broad categories. The first is patient or recipient outcomes. In the example of the exercise class, the participant outcome can be easily assessed by comparing initial and follow-up data. The same is true for direct service consulting. Patient initial evaluation and subsequent evaluation comparison can show outcomes. (See Chapter 20 for statistical analysis.) The second outcome variable of overall institutional benefits is much more elusive and difficult to assess. The simplest way of assessing this variable is to choose one outcome. For example, in the direct service area, you may want to compare the number of falls prior to implementation of your physical therapy program and after.

CONCLUSION

The possibilities of consulting in the realm of geriatrics are limitless, because the consultant has the luxury of designing unique programs in a variety of settings. Through this the physical therapist can contribute worthwhile information to the rehabilitation process.

PEARLS

- The primary reasons for consultation services in geriatrics are patient care, professional education, public relations, screening, and quality assurance.

- The benefits of geriatric consultation are

  1. Decreased length of hospitalization and use of expensive health care resources.

  2. Increased use of rehabilitative services and identification of new diagnoses.

  3. Improved patient care.

  4. Greater access to educational resources.

- Physical therapists may serve as consultants in nursing homes, senior centers, hospitals, and rehabilitation centers, as well as home care. The consultant's role will change in each setting.

- The four major types of patients who are candidates for restraints are

  1. Cognitively impaired wanderers.

  2. Aggressive patients.

  3. Patients who interfere with medical treatment.

  4. Unsteady patients.

- The steps in a successful consultation process are needs assessment, query, proposal, negotiation, implementation, and evaluation.

- The most important phase of the consultation process is the evaluation or outcome phase. The step can be as simple as checking patient satisfaction or as sophisticated as statistical analysis of postprogram scores.

REFERENCES

1. Duthie EH, Gambert SR. Geriatrics consultation implication for teaching and clinical care. *Gerontol Geriatric Education.* 1983;4:59.
2. Burley L, Currie C, Smith R, et al. Contribution from geriatric medicine within acute medical wards. *Br Med J.* 1979;2:90.
3. Hogan DB, Fox RA, Badley BWD, et al. Effects of a geriatric consultation service on management of patients in an acute care hospital. *Can Med Assoc J.* 1987;136:713.
4. Allen C, Becker P, McVey L, et al. A randomized controlled clinical trial of a geriatric consultation team. *JAMA.* 1986;255:2617.
5. Barker WH, Williams TF, Zimmer JG, et al. Geriatric consultation team. *J Am Ger Soc.* 1985;33:422.
6. Lichtenstein H, Winograd CH. Geriatric consultation: a functional approach. *J Am Ger Soc.* 1984;32:356.
7. Lee T, Pappus EM, Goldman L. Impact of inter-physician communication on the effectiveness of medical consultation. *Am J Med.* 1983;74:105.
8. Katz P, Dube D, Calkins E, et al. Use of a structured functional assessment format in a geriatric consultation service. *J Am Ger Soc.* 1985;33:681.
9. Campion EW, Jette A, Beckman B. An interdisciplinary geriatric consultation service: a controlled trial. *J Am Ger Soc.* 1983;31:792.
10. Lewis C. How to handle upcoming guidelines. *PT Bull.* June 27, 1990;18–19.
11. Borden LP. Patient education and the quality assurance process. *QRB.* 1985;11(4):123–127.
12. Chauhan L, Hutchings D, LePoer K. Quality assurance manual in PT services. *Clin Manage in Phys Ther.* September/October 1986;6(5):28–31.
13. Ellingham CT, Deschler MJ. Quality control circles. *Clin Manage in Phys Ther.* 1985;5(5):42–43.
14. Gaynor L. Quality assurance quarterly screening review. *Clin Manage in Phys Ther.* September/October 1985;5(5):38–41.
15. Glendinning M. Quality assurance in physiotherapy. *Austin Clin Rev.* November 1981;(3):22.
16. Goode DH, Jamieson HD, Warrington DM. Quality assurance in physiotherapy. *Laser NZ J Physiother.* April 1984;12(1):27–28.
17. Quality Assurance. *Hosp Peer Rev.* March 1980;5(3):29–40.
18. Lewis C, Campanelli L. *Health Promotion and Exercise for Older Persons.* Rockville, Md: Aspen Publishers; 1990.

Appendix A. Practice Guidelines

Performance Standards in Long-Term Care Facilities

Practice Privileges for Physical Therapists

Medicare Regulations—

Conditions for Coverage

Outpatient Physical Therapy Services furnished by Physical Therapists in Independent Practice

Performance Standards for Registered Physical Therapists in Long-Term Care Facilities

The purpose of these standards shall be to ensure that Physical Therapy services rendered in Long-Term Care facilities shall subscribe to Standards of Practice as established by the American Physical Therapy Association.

I. Admissions

    The Registered Physical Therapist shall advise and/or participate in the Admissions Process to ensure:

    A. That sufficient information is available at the time of admission review including a comprehensive summary of previous physical therapy received by the patient;

    B. That restorative services and equipment available in the facility are appropriate to meet the needs of patients being considered for admission;

    C. That a record review of every patient admitted to the facility is accomplished to determine the need for physical therapy evaluation services, or maintenance care.

II. Direct Services

    A. The Registered Physical Therapist shall provide direct service to any patient upon referral by the physician.

    B. The therapist shall conduct a:

        1. physical therapy evaluation and in consultation with the patient, the physician and other members of the patient care team develop a goal and treatment plan or recommend to the physician that no treatment or maintenance care only is indicated;

        2. provide skilled physical therapy services directly or direct the services performed by the qualified PT assistant;

        3. maintain progress notes at designated intervals in the clinical record indicating:

            a. progress toward goals;

            b. changes in status or new problems;

            c. re-evaluations.

    C. The RPT will periodically reassess goals and review and revise the patient care plan accordingly.

    D. Contact the patients physician as required or indicated.

    E. Maintenance programs may be planned by the RPT and carried out by the patient, nursing staff or family members.

        1. The therapist should ensure that the maintenance program is clearly understood by the personnel designated to carry out the plan.

        2. The therapist should re-evaluate patients on maintenance routines periodically but not less than every 60 days.

    F. Discharge Planning:

        1. The RPT shall assist in implementing an appropriate discharge plan for those individuals transferring to another facility or returning home.

        2. Activities of the therapist may include but not be limited to:

            a. developing PT discharge summary;

            b. discharge home;

                1. home visit to assess architectural barriers and recommend modifications

                2. establish home physical therapy program (copy in chart) that is understood by patient and family

            c. discharge to another facility;

                1. provide a physical therapy summary (including treatment given and patient status on discharge).

III. Indirect Services

    A. The Registered Physical Therapist shall provide consultation regarding the rehabilitation needs of patients in the facility by any of the following:

        1. Participation in Multi-Disciplinary Patient Care meetings or conferences to:

            a. assist in identifying patient problems;

            b. state short and long term goals and recommend how these objectives can be reached;

            c. review patient's progress and reassess appropriateness of the direct services or maintenance program as part of the total patient care plan.

    B. The Registered Physical Therapist shall participate in formal and informal in-service training.

        1. provide in-service training to other long term care facility staff;

Continued

Continued from previous page

2. attend relevant in-service training programs provided in the facility.

C. Attends UR committee meetings or other conferences at the request of administration.

D. Submit a written summary of indirect services provided in accordance with facility policy.

IV. Physical Therapy Audit

The Registered Physical Therapist should be encouraged to participate in and/or develop peer review activities as recommended by the Massachusetts Chapter APTA; these activities may include: Physical Therapy Audit, Department structure review, process review, outside review by persons designated by Massachusetts Chapter APTA.

V. Policies and Procedures

The RPT shall have appropriate input into development of parts of policy and procedure manual pertaining to Physical Therapy.

Figure 19A–1. *(Reprinted with permission from Massachusetts APTA Chapter Newsletter, June 15, 1979;4(5):4.)*

Practice Privileges for Physical Therapists: Model Policy and Procedure

Application: Physical Therapists seeking full or limited practice privileges, physical therapy department director, medical staff committee on interdisciplinary practice.

Policy: A physical therapist holding a current license as required by California law to practice physical therapy is eligible for practice privileges in this hospital only if he or she meets the following qualifications:

1. Is a registered physical therapist licensed by the Board of Medical Quality Assurance to practice in the State of California.
2. Adequately documents experience, background, training, demonstrated ability, experience, judgment, and physical and mental health status to demonstrate qualification to exercise practice privileges within the hospital, and that any patient treated will receive that professional level of quality and efficiency of care established by the hospital.
3. Is determined, on the basis of documented references, to adhere strictly to the accepted ethics of the physical therapy profession; to work cooperatively with others in the hospital setting; and to assist the hospital in fulfilling its obligations related to patient care, within the areas of his or her professional competence and credentials.

Purpose: This policy establishes a mechanism for reviewing credentials and granting practice privileges to physical therapists who practice outside the employment of the hospital.

Definitions

1. *Physical Therapists with Practice Privileges:* A physical therapist, eligible for practice privileges by meeting the qualifications set forth under this policy, who chooses to practice outside the employment of the hospital. He or she shall meet the eligibility requirements for employment by the hospital should both parties wish to pursue this arrangement.
2. *Full Practice Privileges:* Includes all areas of practice as defined by the Physical Therapy Practice Act, State of California, as they pertain to the scope of physical therapy services provided in the hospital and defined in hospital department policies and procedures.
3. *Limited Practice Privileges:* Limited to specified areas of practice or patient population, such as but not restricted to, electromyography, cardiac rehabilitation, or neonatal intensive care.

Procedures

1. Granting of Practice Privileges: A physical therapist seeking practice privileges at this hospital must apply and qualify for such privileges. Applications for initial granting of practice privileges and subsequent renewal there of shall be submitted and processed in a parallel manner to that provided in the Medical Staff Bylaws for other practitioners.

   a. A completed Allied Health Professional application with pertinent support documentation is to be submitted to the Medical Staff Office.

   b. Upon written verification of required information, the application is forwarded to the Director of Physical Therapy for review and recommendations. Input from the physical therapy department's Medical Director is obtained as needed. The Application is then forwarded to the medical Staff Committee on Interdisciplinary Practice (CIP), or similar appropriate committee.

   c. While considering applications for practice privileges in physical therapy, the Director of Physical Therapy, or his or her designee, shall be present at CIP meetings. The CIP shall review and recommend approval or denial of the application, then forward it to the Medical Executive Committee.

   d. The Medical Executive Committee's recommendation is then presented to the Board of Trustees for final approval.

   e. The applicant shall be notified in writing as to the approval or denial of his or her request for practice privileges. Individuals whose applications have been denied may have the decision reconsidered by requesting a personal appearance at a regularly scheduled meeting of the CIP.

   f. The CIP reviews the status of all physical therapists with practice privileges biannually and recommends reappointment or denial of continued privileges.

   g. The President of the Medical Staff may grant temporary practice privileges for individual physical therapists.

   h. Assignment: Each physical therapist who is qualified for initial granting of practice privileges shall be assigned to a clinical department appropriate to his or her professional training, and shall be subject to the policies and procedures of that department.

   i. Monitoring requirement: Except as otherwise recommended by the Medical Executive Committee and approved by the Board of Trustees, each physical therapist initially granted practice privileges shall complete a period of monitoring. Monitoring may include direct observation of the therapist's performance and chart review. Each initial appointee shall be assigned a monitor(s) for evaluation of his or her performance. The purpose of the monitoring requirement

Continued

———— *Continued from previous page* ————

is to determine the appointee's eligibility to exercise the practice privileges initially recommended. An initial appointee shall remain subject to monitoring until a favorable recommendation for his or her removal from monitoring is received in writing from his or her Monitor and approved by the CIP, the Medical Executive Committee, and the Board of Trustees.

Term of Monitoring Period: The term of monitoring for initial appointment or modification of privileges shall extend for a minimum period of 6 months and for a minimum number of cases determined by the CIP with input from various Clinical Service Committees as requested.

2. Prerogatives: the prerogatives that may be extended to a physical therapist with practice privileges shall be defined in hospital/departmental policies and procedures. Such prerogatives may include

   a. Provision of specified patient care services consistent with Physical Therapy Department/Hospital policies and procedures; consistent with the practice privileges granted, being full or limited; and within the scope of the physical therapist's licensure or specialized certification, if applicable.

   b. Service on medical staff, department, and hospital committees.

   c. Attendance at the meetings of the department where assigned, and attendance at hospital education programs in his or her special area of practice or at those programs deemed mandatory by the Hospital.

3. Responsibilities: Each physical therapist with practice privileges shall

   a. Meet those responsibilities required by Medical Staff Rules and Regulations, and if not so specified, meet those responsibilities specified in the Medical Staff Bylaws, Section on Membership as generally applicable to the practice of physical therapy.

   b. Retain appropriate responsibility within his or her area of professional competence for the care and supervision of each patient in the Hospital for whom he or she is providing services.

   c. Participate as appropriate in patient care quality review, evaluation, and monitoring activities required of physical therapists; in supervising initial appointees of his or her profession, and in discharging such other functions as may be required from time to time.

   d. Maintain his or her professional competence by pursuing professional development opportunities, which would include, but are not limited to, formal education, seminars, conferences, workshops, self-study, and advanced clinical residencies.

   e. Abide by the Medical Staff Bylaws and Rules and Regulations as they pertain to physical therapists, and all other physical therapy practice standards, departmental policies, and procedures.

   f. Prepare and complete in a timely fashion, the medical and other required records for all patients for which he or she provides services in the hospital.

   g. Abide by the lawful ethical principles of the profession of physical therapy.

   h. Abide by the laws of the State of California, including the California Physical Therapy Act, and the California Business and Professional Code, Section 654.2 (disclosure of ownership interest in a service to which referrals are made).

   i. Work cooperatively with other physical therapists, both institutionally based and those with practice privileges, as well as medical staff members, nurses, and other hospital personnel.

   j. Assist in providing continuing education programs for the physical therapy staff, physicians, nurses, and other hospital personnel.

Figure 19A–2.   *(Reprinted with permission from California Chapter APTA.)*

Medicare Regulations—Conditions for Coverage: Outpatient Physical Therapy Services Furnished By Physical Therapists in Independent Practice

[¶20,698A]

§ 405.1730. Conditions for Coverage—Services Furnished by Physical Therapists in Independent Practice—General.

(a) In order to be covered under the program of health insurance for the aged and disabled as a supplier of outpatient physical therapy services, a physical therapist in independent practice must meet State licensure and requirements set forth in section 1861(p)(4) of the Act, 42 U.S.C. 1395x(p)(4), and other requirements established pursuant to this provision. This section of the law states specific requirements which must be met by such suppliers and authorizes the Secretary of Health, Education, and Welfare to prescribe by regulation other requirements relating to the health and safety of beneficiaries as may be found necessary.

(b) Section 1861(p) provides in pertinent part as follows:

"(p) The term 'outpatient physical therapy services' means physical therapy services furnished by a provider of services, a clinic, rehabilitation agency, or a public health agency, or by others under an arrangement with, and under the supervision of, such provider, clinic, rehabilitation agency, or public health agency to an individual as an outpatient—

* * *

"The term 'outpatient physical therapy services' also includes physical therapy services furnished an individual by a physical therapist (in his office or in such individual's home) who meets licensing and other standards prescribed by the Secretary in regulations, otherwise than under an arrangement with and under the supervision of a provider of services, clinic, rehabilitation agency, or public health agency, if the furnishing of such services meets such conditions relating to health and safety as the Secretary may find necessary"

¶ 20,698A   Reg. § 405.1730

(c) The requirements included in the statute and the additional health and safety requirements prescribed by the Secretary are set forth in the Conditions for Coverage for Outpatient Physical Therapy Services Furnished by Physical Therapists in Independent Practice (see § § 405.1732–405.1737).

.01 Source

As adopted 41 F.R. 20863 (May 21, 1976, effective June 21, 1976); recodified from 20 CFR 405.1730 at 42 F.R. 52826 (Sept. 30, 1977).

[¶20,698B]

§ 405.1731. Definitions Relating to Physical Therapists in Independent Practice

As used in § § 405.1731–405.1737, the following definitions apply:

(a) *Physical therapist.* A person who is licensed as a physical therapist by the State in which he is practicing if the State licenses physical therapists, and—

(1) Has graduated from a physical therapy curriculum approved by the American Physical Therapy Association, or by the Council on Medical Education and Hospitals of the American Medical Association, or jointly by the Council on Medical Education of the American Medical Association and the American Physical Therapy Association, or

(2) prior to January 1, 1966:

(i) Was admitted to membership by the American Physical Therapy Association: or

(ii) Was admitted to registration by the American Registry of Physical Therapists; or

Continued

Continued from previous page

(iii) Has graduated from a physical therapy curriculum in a 4-year college or university approved by a State department of education; or

(3) Has 2 years of appropriate experience as a physical therapist and has achieved a satisfactory grade on a proficiency examination approved by the Secretary except that such determinations of proficiency shall not apply with respect to persons initially licensed by a State after December 31, 1977, or seeking qualifications as a physical therapist after such date; or

(4)(i) Was licensed or registered prior to January 1, 1966; and

(ii) Prior to January 1, 1970, had 15 years of full-time experience in the treatment of illness or injury through the practice of physical therapy in which services were rendered under the order and direction of attending and referring doctors of medicine or osteopathy; or

(5) If trained outside the United States:

(i) Was graduated since 1928 from a physical therapy curriculum approved in the country in which the curriculum was located and in which there is a member organization of the World Confederation for Physical Therapy;

(ii) Meets the requirements for membership in a member organization of the World Confederation for Physical Therapy;

(iii) Has 1 year of experience under the supervision of an active member of the American Physical Therapy Association: and

(iv) Has successfully completed a qualifying examination as prescribed by the American Physical Therapy Association.

(b) *Physical therapist in independent practice:* A person who is licensed as a physical therapist by the State in which he is practicing, meets one of the qualification requirements in paragraph (a) of this section, and furnishes services under the circumstances described in § 405.232(e)(2)(ii).

(c) *Supervision:* The presence, at all times, of a qualified physical therapist when physical therapy services are rendered in the physical therapist's office or in the patient's place of residence.

(d) *Physician.* A person who is—

(1) A doctor of medicine or osteopathy legally authorized to practice medicine and surgery by the State in which he or she performs these functions or actions; or

(2) A doctor of podiatric medicine, but only with respect to the functions which he or she is legally authorized to perform by the State in which he or she performs them.

.01 Source

As adopted, 41 F.R. 20863 (May 21, 1976, effective June 21, 1976); recodified from 20 CFR 405.1731 at 42 F.R. 52826 (Sept. 30, 1977); amended at 53 F.R. 12010 (Apr. 12, 1988, effective May 12, 1988).

[¶ 20,698C]

§ 405.1732. Condition for Coverage—Compliance with Federal, State, and Local Laws

The physical therapist in independent practice and staff, if any, are in compliance with all applicable Federal, State, and local laws and regulations.

(a) *Standard: Licensure of facility.* If any State in which State or applicable local law provides for the licensing of the facility of a physical therapist, such facility is:

(1) Licensed pursuant to such law; or

(2) If not subject to licensure, is approved (by the agency of such State or locality responsible for licensing) as meeting the standards established for such licensing.

Medicare and Medicaid Guide

(b) *Standard: Licensure or registration of personnel.* The physical therapist in independent practice and staff, if any, are licensed or registered in accordance with applicable laws.

Continued

Continued from previous page

.01 Source:

As adopted, 41 F.R. 20863 (May 21, 1976, effective June 21, 1976); recodified from 20 CFR 405.1732 at 42 F.R. 52826 (Sept. 30, 1977).

[¶ 20,698D]

§ 405.1733. Condition for Coverage—Physician's Direction and Plan of Care

Patients in need of outpatient physical therapy services are accepted for treatment by the physical therapist in independent practice only on the order of a physician who indicates anticipated goals and is responsible for the general medical direction of such services as part of the total care of the patient. For each patient, there is a written plan of care established and periodically reviewed by the physician.

(a) *Standard: Medical findings and physician's orders.* The following is made available to the physical therapist, prior to or at the time of initiation of treatment:

(1) The patient's significant past history,

(2) Diagnosis(es),

(3) Physician's orders,

(4) Rehabilitation goals and potential for their achievement,

(5) Contraindications, if any,

(6) The extent to which the patient is aware of the diagnosis(es) and prognosis, and

(7) Where appropriate, the summary of treatment provided and results achieved during previous periods of physical therapy services or institutionalization.

(b) *Standard: Plan of care.* For each patient there is a written plan of care established by the physician or by the physical therapist who furnishes the services, which indicates anticipated goals and specifies the type, amount, frequency, and duration of physical therapy services. The plan of care and results of treatment are reviewed at least once every 30 days by the attending or other physician and the indicated action is taken.

(c) *Standard: General medical direction.* Patients are seen by a physician at least once every 30 days. General medical direction at appropriate intervals is evident from the clinical record.

(d) *Standard: Notification of physician.* The attending physician is promptly notified of any changes in the patient's condition. If changes are required in the plan of care, such changes are approved by such physician and noted in the clinical record.

Reg. § 405.1733   ¶ 20,698D

(e) *Standard: Indexes.* Clinical records are indexed at least according to name of patient to facilitate acquisition of statistical clinical information and retrieval of records for administrative action.

.01 Source

As adopted, 41 F.R. 20863 (May 21, 1976, effective June 21, 1976); recodified from 20 CFR 405.1736 at 42 F.R. 52826 (Sept. 30, 1977).

[¶ 20,698H]

§ 405.1737. Condition for Coverage—Physical Environment

The physical environment of the office and/or facility of the physical therapist in independent practice affords a functional, sanitary, safe, and comfortable surrounding for patients, personnel, and the public.

(a) *Standard: Building construction.* The construction of the building housing the physical therapy office meets all applicable State and local building, fire, and safety codes.

(b) *Standard: Maintenance of the physical therapy office and equipment.* There is established a written preventive-maintenance program to ensure that equipment is operative and that the physical therapy

Continued

——— *Continued from previous page* ———

office is clean and orderly. All essential mechanical, electrical, and patient-care equipment is maintained in safe operating condition, and is properly calibrated.

(c) *Standard: Other environmental considerations.* The building housing the physical therapy office is accessible to, and functional for, patients, personnel, and the public. Written effective procedures in aseptic techniques are followed by all personnel and such procedures are reviewed annually, and when necessary, revised.

(d) *Standard: Emergency procedures.* The physical therapist is aware of the possibility of the occurrence of fire and other non-medical emergencies and has documented: (1) A means of providing for safe patient egress from the physical therapy office and the building housing the office, such means being demonstrated by fire exit signs, etc., and (2) Other such provisions necessary to ensure the safety of patients.

.01 Source

As adopted, 41 F.R. 20863 (May 21, 1976, effective June 21, 1976); recodified from 20 CFR 405.1737 at 42 F.R. 52826 (Sept. 30, 1977).

.01 Source

As adopted, 41 F.R. 20863 (May 21, 1976, effective June 21, 1976); recodified from 20 CFR 405.1733 at 42 F.R. 52826 (Sept. 30, 1977); amended at 53 F.R. 12010 (Apr. 12, 1988, effective May 12, 1988).

[¶ 20,698E]

§ 405.1734. Condition for Coverage—Physical Therapy Services

The physical therapist in independent practice provides an adequate program of physical therapy services and has the facilities and equipment necessary to carry out the services offered.

(a) *Standard: Adequate program.* The physical therapist will be considered to have an adequate physical therapy program when services can be provided, utilizing therapeutic exercise and the modalities of heat, cold, water, and electricity; patient evaluations are conducted; and tests and measurements of strength, balance, endurance, range of motion, and activities of daily living are administered.

(b) *Standard: Supervision of physical therapy services.* Physical therapy services are provided by, or under supervision of, a qualified physical therapist.

.01 Source

As adopted, 41 F.R. 20863 (May 21, 1976, effective June 21, 1976); recodified from 20 CFR 405.1734 at 42 F.R. 52826 (Sept. 30, 1977).

[¶ 20,698F]

§ 405.1735. Condition for Coverage—Coordination of Services with Other Organizations, Agencies, or Individuals

The physical therapy services provided by the physical therapist in independent practice are coordinated with the health and medical services provided to the patient by organizations, agencies, or individuals.

(a) *Standard: Exchange of clinical records and reports.* When a patient is receiving or has recently received health and medical services from providers, organizations, physicians, or others that are related to and that may involve the physical therapy program, the physical therapist shall, on a regular basis, exchange with such providers, organizations, physicians, or others in accordance with § 405.1736(a) documented information which has a bearing on the patient's health and welfare so as to ensure that services effectively complement one another.

.01 Source

As adopted, 41 F.R. 20863 (May 21, 1976, effective June 21, 1976); recodified from 20 CFR 405.1735 at 42 F.R. 52826 (Sept. 30, 1977).

——— *Continued* ———

Continued from previous page

¶ 20,698E   Reg. § 405.1734

[¶ 20,698G]

§ 405.1736. Condition for Coverage—Clinical Records

The physical therapist in independent practice maintains clinical records on all patients in accordance with accepted professional standards and practices. The clinical records are completely and accurately documented, readily accessible, and systematically organized to facilitate retrieving and compiling information.

(a) *Standard: Protection of clinical record information.* Clinical record information is recognized as confidential and is safeguarded against loss, destruction, or unauthorized use. Written procedures govern use and removal of records and include conditions for release of information. A patient's written consent is required for release of information not authorized by law.

(b) *Standard: Content. The clinical record information.* Clinical record in-record contains sufficient information to identify the patient clearly, to justify the diagnosis(es) and treatment, and to document the results accurately. All clinical records contain the following general categories of data:

(1) Documented evidence of the assessment of the needs of the patient, of an appropriate plan of care, and of the care and services provided,

(2) Identification data and consent forms,

(3) Medical history,

(4) Report of physical examination(s), if any,

(5) Observations and progress notes,

(6) Reports of treatments and clinical findings, and

(7) Discharge summary including final diagnosis(es) and prognosis.

(c) *Standard: Completion of records and centralization of reports.* Current clinical records and those of discharged patients are completed promptly. All clinical information pertaining to a patient is centralized in the patient's clinical record.

(d) *Standard: Retention and preservation.* Clinical records are retained for a period of time not less than:

(1) That determined by the respective State statute or the statute of limitations in the State, or

(2) In the absence of a State statute: (i) 5 years after the date of discharge or, (ii) in the case of a minor, 3 years after the patient becomes of age under State law, or 5 years after the date of discharge, whichever is longer.

Figure 19A–3. *(Reprinted with permission from Commerce Clearing House, Inc., 1988.)*

Appendix B.   Screening and Prevention

Foot Care Demonstration Project   Institutional Screening

Foot Care Demonstration Project for Frail, Low-Income Elderly

This project is designed to demonstrate the development, use, and efficacy of a foot care program for low income, frail elders. The focus of the program is several-fold:

1. Preventative education.
2. Screening for identification and treatment of foot disorders before disabling complications occur.
3. Remediation of foot disorders through appropriate home care, education, orthotics, shoes, exercise, or both.
4. Follow-up care for individuals who receive orthoses, shoes, podiatric care, exercise programs, or educational instruction.

The objectives of this program are to improve mobility, function, and quality of life for elders through:

1. Improving foot function.
2. Reducing the incidence of painful feet.
3. Preventing foot dysfunction from producing loss of mobility and independence.

The hypotheses of this demonstration project are that:

1. There is a correlation between foot pain and level of function.
2. There is a significant difference in function with those clients with foot pain/deformity and those without.
3. Specific interventions will result in a decrease of soft tissue abnormalities and pain and an increase in function.

The Foot Care Demonstration Project is carried out by a team, including a physical therapist, podiatrist, orthotist/podiatrist, and social worker. Foot screening, preventive education, intervention and follow-up care is provided to approximately 400 low income, frail elderly individuals in 14 communities located within central Massachusetts.

A data base has been developed describing foot dysfunction, pain, functional ability, and socioeconomic characteristics within the population served. Success of the education and intervention programs will be determined by comparing pain, function, and foot deformity prior to and following 1 year in the Foot Care Program for each client.

This Foot Care Demonstration Project is an outgrowth of a foot care clinic that had been started through Cushing Hospital in January 1986. The Demonstration Project serves to measure the short-term (1 to 2 years) efficacy of this type of intervention in reducing disability, loss of mobility, or hospitalization of elders as a consequence of foot disorders. It will also serve as a basis for a longitudinal study of foot deformities among low income elderly.

Figure 19B–1.

A Screening Mechanism to Identify Potential Physical Therapy Geriatric Clients in Institutional Settings

Frequently, for a variety of reasons, patients are not referred to physical therapy. In many instances, there is an inadequate understanding of the physical therapy services available as well as a lack of appreciation for the benefits available to the patient and institution through physical therapy programs.

Informational programs and materials identifying physical therapy services and the skills of physical therapy practitioners are frequently presented to health care practitioners and the community. However, frequently physical therapists do not identify the improved quality of life and cost effectiveness of their services, such as reducing the amount of care and services needed by clients and the prevention of complications as well as further disability.

No formal follow-up was conducted following the program. However, surveys reported using the suggested criteria during survey sessions and found them to be helpful. In Mississippi, state certifying licensure groups were aware of many individuals perceived to need additional service but were unaware of the specific types of patient problems that physical therapists could offer assistance with in the nursing home setting. Furthermore, many of the surveyors felt that more residents should be receiving physical therapy but without guidelines to follow it was difficult to make recommendations with any certainty. However, surveyors had no guidelines for effectively identifying potential patients. So, agency personnel approached a physical therapist requesting an inservice for surveyors. The topic for the meeting was to be "identifying nursing home residents who might benefit from physical therapy services."

The therapist planning the workshop developed the following objectives for the session: (a) describe the professional qualifications and skills of physical therapists; (b) identify quality of life and cost effective outcomes produced through physical therapy; (c) describe problems and diagnoses that frequently require a physical therapy referral and (d) develop an easy mechanism to identify potential physical therapy patients.

To summarize the 2 hour program and provide the participants with a practical, easy to use mechanism for patient identification, a short check list was developed. The surveyors were told that if a patient needed assistance with two or more of the problems listed, had a condition in the diagnostic category, and met onset criteria, a referral for physical therapy evaluation was probably indicated. In addition, they were alerted to check for information on any previous rehabilitation services.

1. Diagnostic Categories: The individual has one or more of the conditions listed:
   a. cerebral vascular accident (i.e., stroke)
   b. fractures
   c. impaired cognitive function or organic brain syndrome (i.e., Alzheimer's)
   d. arthritis
   e. amputation
   f. chronic lung disease
   g. Parkinson's disease
   h. general dehabilitation
   i. cardiovascular problems
   j. postsurgery
   k. cardiovascular disease

2. Onset Criteria: The patient has physical problems:
   a. a recent decrease in mobility skills or activities of daily living
   b. the onset of disease or disability occurred less than 6 months ago

3. Physical Problems: The patient has problems, such as:
   a. muscle weakness in one or both upper and lower extremitiesm
   b. very limited physical endurance

Continued

Continued from previous page

  c. range of motion limitations

  d. diminished sensory function

  e. coordination/balance difficulties

  f. posture

4. Equipment problems: The patient needs assistance with:

  a. self-care activities or using adaptive equipment

  b. learning skills (e.g., one handed skills, wheelchair mobility, ambulation)

  c. adaptive equipment procurement and maintenance

5. Activities of Daily Living Problems: The patient needs to develop and/or practice:

  a. self-care skills

  b. daily living activities

  c. ambulation activities

  d. mobility skills

6. Mental Status Problems: The patient has had a change in:

  a. mental alertness since admission

  b. socialization is limited

7. Previous Rehabilitation Services

  a. what, when, where, response, and discharge status

No formal follow-up was conducted following the program. However, surveys reported using the suggested criteria during survey sessions and found them to be helpful.

Figure 19B–2. *(Reproduced with permission from Greenwald MF. A Screening Mechanism to Identify Potential Physical Therapy Geriatric Clients in Institutional Settings. Geritopics. Winter 1991;14(1):26.)*

Appendix C.   Marketing Protocols

Introductory Letter

Introduction Phone call

Sample Visit

Topic List for Classes

Sample Contract

Sample Letter to Class Members

Sample Flyer

Participant Consent Form

Medical Release Form

Physical Activity Profile

Medical History Form

Sample Class Invitation

Sample Class Outline

Perfect Posture Handout

Introductory Letter

Ms. Ann Jones
Mill Vill Retirement Home
South Pond, WY 12345

Dear Ms. Jones:

My name is Carole Smith, and I am interested in talking to you about setting up some very special exercise classes. My background is in physical therapy, and I have worked for more than 10 years with older people. I would like to share some of my expertise with the members of Mill Vill Retirement Home before they need the individualized services of a physical therapist.

My classes are special because they are on different subjects, such as arthritis, back pain, and neck stiffness, to name just a few.

I have enclosed my resumé as well as a list of topics for the exercise group. Please review the information at your leisure. In the meantime, if you have any questions, I can be reached at 555–1212.

I plan to call you to set up a meeting in a week. Thank you for your time.

Sincerely,

Carole Smith, PT

Figure 19C–1. *(Reprinted with permission from Lewis C. Health Promotion and Exercise for Older Adults. Gaithersburg, Md: Aspen Publishers Inc.; 1990.)*

Introductory Phone Call

Hello, Ms. Jones. My name is Carole Smith. I wrote to you about a week ago about the possibility of my conducting an exercise class. I was wondering if you would like to get together and discuss this. What is a good time for you? Good, I look forward to seeing you then.

Figure 19C–2. *(Reprinted with permission from Lewis C. Health Promotion and Exercise for Older Adults. Gaithersburg, Md: Aspen Publishers, Inc.; 1990.)*

Sample Visit

Hi, Ms. Jones. I'm Carole Smith. [Make small talk here; discuss the weather, how nice the facility is.] Did you have a chance to look over the material I sent you? [If not, have an extra copy to give her, and discuss the topics.] Do you think this program would be a welcome addition at Mill Vill? Are you interested? I would like to start doing the class on a weekly basis and see how well it is received. My fee is $100 per class. Is that agreeable to you? Good. I have a contract that I brought to protect both of us. If you will sign it, I can begin in 3 weeks. In the meantime, I have a letter to your residents to introduce me and get their ideas. If you could pass these out, I will be back in a week to get the responses. Then, 1 week before class, I will come around with flyers announcing the class.

Figure 19C–3. *(Reprinted with permission from Lewis C. Health Promotion and Exercise for Older Adults. Gaithersburg, Md: Aspen Publishers, Inc.; 1990.)*

Topic List for Classes

- Fancy footwork
- Lavish legs
- Knowledgeable knees
- Happy hips
- Better backs
- Nice necks
- Supple Shoulders
- Agile arms
- Wonderful wrists
- Hardy hands and flexible fingers
- Improving balance
- Realizing relaxation
- Abatable arthritis
- Preventing Parkinson's problems

- Opposing osteoporosis
- Perfect posture
- Getting stronger
- Better breathing
- Stopping stroke
- Ways to walk
- Facts on flexibility
- Correcting coordination
- Understanding aerobics
- All about Alzheimer's disease
- Achieving perfect body weight
- Exercising facial muscles
- Hidden exercises

Figure 19C–4. *(Reprinted with permission from Lewis C. Health Promotion and Exercise for Older Adults. Gaithersburg, MD: Aspen Publishers, Inc.; 1990.)*

Sample Contract

I, _____ contract with _____

_____ to provide a _____ exercise/discussion
(frequency)
class on various topics.

I agree to bring handouts and cassette tapes. _____ agrees to provide <u>chairs, stereo,</u>

<u>and batons</u> as well as $100.00 (one hundred dollars) per class to be paid within 2 weeks of the class.

This contract can be terminated with 30 days' notice by either party.

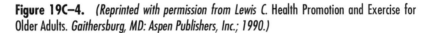

_____   _____
Date   Signature

_____   _____
Date   Signature

Note: An attorney can suggest additions and variations of this sample agreement and should be consulted regarding the full implications of any contractual commitments.

Figure 19C–5. *(Reprinted with permission from Lewis C. Health Promotion and Exercise for Older Adults. Gaithersburg, Md: Aspen Publishers, Inc.; 1990.)*

Sample Letter to Potential Class Members

Dear Mill Vill Residents:

Allow me to introduce myself. My name is Carole Smith and I am a physical therapist with 10 years' experience. My specialty is the bone and muscle problems of older people.

On Monday, June 18, from 11:00 to 12:00, I will be leading an exercise class and a brief discussion of osteoporosis. I will be returning to conduct other discussions as well and would like you to help me determine which ones would be of interest to you. Please check those of interest and add any others. Thank you in advance for your help.

See you in exercise class soon!

Sincerely,

Carole Smith, PT

Please fill out and return to the front desk.

TOPICS

☐ Arthritis	☐ Increasing Flexibility
☐ Posture	☐ Getting Stronger
☐ Neck Pain	☐ Aerobics—Pros and Cons
☐ Relieving Back Pain	☐ Stress Management
☐ Fixing Shoulder Problems	☐ Walking Programs
☐ All about Knees	☐ Exercises for You
☐ Feet Work	☐ Helping Hands
☐ Improving Balance	☐ Better Breathing
☐ Correct Coordination	☐ Hidden Exercises
☐ Walking Better	☐ _____

Figure 19C–6. *(Reprinted with permission from Lewis C. Health Promotion and Exercise for Older Adults. Gaithersburg, Md: Aspen Publishers, Inc.; 1990.)*

Sample Flyer

OSTEOPOROSIS CLASS

11:00–12:00

Monday, June 18th
in the
Dining Room

MEET

Carole Smith, Physical Therapist

LISTEN, LEARN, & EXERCISE

for Osteoporosis

and

HAVE FUN DOING IT!

Figure 19C–7. *(Reprinted with permission from Lewis C. Health Promotion and Exercise for Older Adults. Gaithersburg, Md: Aspen Publishers, Inc.; 1990.)*

Participant Consent Form

I understand that the purpose of this (project or program) is to enhance my health-fitness status.

I verify that my participation is fully voluntary, and no coercion of any sort has been used to obtain my participation.

I understand that I may withdraw from the (project or program) without prejudice or malice at any time during the involved period or session.

I have been informed of the procedures and methods that will be used in the (project or program) and understand what will be necessary for me as a participant.

I understand that my participation will remain anonymous unless expressed name permission is given by me.

Signed: _____

Date: _____

Figure 19C–8. *(Reprinted with permission from Lewis C. Health Promotion and Exercise for Older Adults. Gaithersburg, Md: Aspen Publishers, Inc.; 1990.)*

Medical Release Form

_____ has my permission to participate in a physical exercise program to be given at _____ . I understand that this course consists of gentle stretching and strengthening programs of a mild exercise performance level. I have listed below any problems that the health professional leading this class should be aware of and that may affect this patient's performance in the class.

Name of Physician _____

Diagnosis _____

Limitation _____

Areas To Emphasize _____

Medications _____
_____

Figure 19C–9. _(Reprinted with permission from Lewis C. Health Promotion and Exercise for Older Adults. Gaithersburg, Md: Aspen Publishers, Inc.; 1990.)_

Physical Activity Profile

Name: _____

Date: _____

We would like to know more about you in order to improve our fitness program and meet your individual needs. Please fill in the following:

1. What was/is the nature of your employment (e.g., manufacturing, sales, teacher)? _____
_____
Year of retirement, if applicable: _____

2. How would you rate the physical activity you perform/performed at work? (Check one)

_____ little (sitting, typing, driving, talking)
_____ moderate (standing, walking, bending, reaching)
_____ active (light physical work, climbing stairs)
_____ very active (moderate and physical work, lifting)

3. My physical activity during the "working hours" of the day has:
_____ stayed the same   _____ decreased   _____ increased

4. What physical and recreational activities are you presently involved in (e.g., dancing, swimming, walking, bowling)? _____
_____ How often? _____

5. My goal(s) for joining a fitness program is:

_____ to lose body fat   _____ to stay active
_____ because my doctor advised me to   _____ because I am concerned
                                                            about my health (e.g.,
                                                            blood pressure, arthritis,
                                                            bad back)

6. Check the activity you participate in and place the appropriate category next to the activity:

1 if total time spent is less than 15 minutes (3 times/day)

2 if total time spent is at least 20 minutes (3 times/week)

3 if activity is sustained for more than 20 minutes (3 times/week)

_____ walking   _____ swimming   _____ golf
_____ jogging   _____ dancing   _____ other _____

Figure 19C–10. *(Reprinted with permission from Lewis C. Health Promotion and Exercise for Older Adults. Gaithersburg, Md: Aspen Publishers, Inc.: 1990.)*

Medical History Form

Name: _____ Date: _____

1. Have you any medical complaints at present (i.e., lower back pain, arthritis, neck pain, hypertension, diabetes, cardiovascular problems, etc.)? _____
   _____

2. What major illnesses required hospitalization (give dates)? _____
   _____

3. Smoking status (circle one):
   a. never smoked   b. smoke now   c. smoked in past, not now

4. History of cardiovascular disease:
   NO   YES   Personal, if so, what _____
   _____
   NO   YES   Family history, if so, what _____
   _____
   NO   YES   Other _____
   NO   YES   Other _____

5. (Muscular history) Present or previous injury?
   a. NO   b. YES
   c. If yes, specify: _____

6. (Bone-joint history) present or previous bone or joint disease?
   a. NO   b. YES
   c. If yes, specify: _____

7. Check off each of the following ailments that apply to you:
   _____ Frequent dizziness   Hernia _____   Diabetes _____
   _____ Physical impairments, if any, specify: _____
   _____

8. On the average, how many times do you visit your physician each year?
   _____

9. How many times do you take medication each day? What types of medications are they? _____
   _____

10. Do you have any limitations not mentioned previously that will place limitations on complete participation in the fitness program? _____

Figure 19C–11. *(Reprinted with permission from Lewis C. Health Promotion and Exercise for Older Adults. Gaithersburg, Md: Aspen Publishers, Inc.; 1990.)*

Sample Class Invitation

Posture tells people a lot about you. Good posture also helps your body function better.

Posture exercises are easy to learn so join us to find out about . . .

PERFECT POSTURE

at:

_____

on:

_____

in:

_____

Taught by: _____

LISTEN, LEARN, AND EXERCISE!

PERFECT POSTURE

Figure 19C–12. *(Reprinted with permission from Lewis C. Health Promotion and Exercise for Older Adults. Gaithersburg, Md: Aspen Publishers, Inc.; 1990.)*

Sample Class Outline

PERFECT POSTURE

Lecture/Discussion

Posture tells people a lot about you. Posture affects how you look, obviously; standing with your head in a very forward position makes you look sort of unhappy and depressed, while standing in a very chin-tucked, upright position makes you much more attractive. Good posture can also enhance your musculoskeletal and your cardiopulmonary functioning. For example, try this: stick your head way forward as far as you can (*demonstrate*), take a deep breath, and blow it out. Now, sit back in your chair, pull your head up as high as you can, and take a nice deep breath. Notice that you can take a much bigger breath when you head is back in the chin-tuck position. So, posture is extremely important not only for physical attractiveness, but also for physical functioning.

Good posture can be looked at from either the side or the front. From the side, if you have good posture, you can draw a straight line from your ear, through your shoulder, knee, and ankle. Take a look at my posture. Then stand up, and take a quick look at the posture of the other members of the class (*go around to all the participants, giving quick little hints to people if they have a forward head, rounded shoulders, or bend in their knees; try to be positive, but try to give good useful feedback*).

You can assess posture from the front or the back, too. People often have asymmetries. One shoulder may be higher; one hip may be higher. Such as asymmetry may cause problems. There may be a tightness or soreness in the higher shoulder. A higher hip may cause tightness in the back area as well. So again, stand up, and let me take a look at your posture (*again, go around the room and give individual feedback*).

Good posture is also needed when you are sitting down. For this, you need to support yourself with the back of a chair, behind your low back, and behind your upper back area. So let's all sit back with good posture (*watch the participants, and give feedback to them*).

Try and become aware of your posture, and know when your posture is good. Do not take posture for granted. You really need to work on posture all the time. Put dots around your house or apartment, and every time you see a dot think to yourself that you need to tuck your chin in or pull your shoulders back. I will give you a hand-out before you leave today with some other reminders (*Figure 19C–14; read aloud and discuss, if desired.*) Now we are going to go on to posture exercises.

Exercises

1. Deep breaths. Do three times.
2. Turtle. Push head forward in an exaggerated motion, then pull back. Do three times.
3. Chin tucks. Do three times.
4. Head motions. Do three times each.
   (a) Forward
   (b) Backward
   (c) Side to side
   (d) Over each shoulder
5. Shoulder shrugs. Do three times.
6. Shoulder circles. Do three times.
7. Shoulder backs. Pull your shoulder blades back. Do three times.
8. Arm reaches up. Reach as high as you can to the sky. Do three times.
9. Arm reaches back. Reach as far backward as possible. Do three times.
10. Side tilts. Do three times.
11. Pelvic tucks. Do three times.
12. Gluteal sets. Tighten your buttock muscles as tight as you can. Do three times.
13. Knee ups. Bend your knees up to the ceiling. Alternate knees. Do three times.
14. Knee outs. Let your knees flop outward. Do three times.
15. Knee twists. Turn your knees inward. Do three times.
16. Ankle bends. Do three times.
17. Ankle circles. Do three times.
18. Toe curls. Do five times.
19. Spine lengtheners. As you take a deep breath, imagine your spine extending from your hips to the top of your head. Do three times.
20. Body extenders. Gently pull your spine into extension. Do three times.

Figure 19C–13. *(Reprinted with permission from Lewis C. Health Promotion and Exercise for Older Adults. Gaithersburg, Md: Aspen Publishers, Inc.; 1990.)*

Perfect Posture Handout

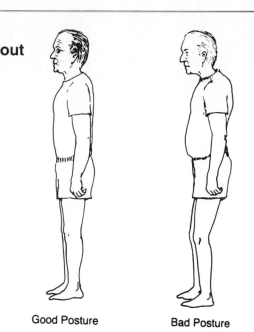

Good Posture   Bad Posture

Dos

1. Tuck in your chin.
2. Pull your shoulders back as much as you can.
3. Try to keep your ear over your shoulders, over your hips, over your ankles.
4. When sitting, support your back and legs as much as possible.
5. Think lengthening.
6. Try to sleep in a position that optimizes good posture and flexibility of muscles.
7. Be aware of your posture as much as possible.

Don'ts

1. Do not sit in one position too long.
2. Do not stand in one position too long.

Exercises

1. Deep breaths: Do three times.
2. Turtle: Do three times.
3. Chin tucks: Do three times.
4. Head motions: Do three times each.
   a. Forward
   b. Backward
   c. Side to side
   d. Over each shoulder
5. Shoulder shrugs: Do three times.
6. Shoulder circles: Do three times.
7. Shoulder backs: Do three times.
8. Arm reaches up: Do three times.
9. Arm reaches back: Do three times.
10. Side tilts: Do three times.
11. Pelvic tucks: Do three times.
12. Gluteal sets: Do three times.
13. Knee ups: Do three times.
14. Knee outs: Do three times.
15. Knee twists: Do three times.
16. Ankle bends: Do three times.
17. Ankle circles: Do three times.
18. Toe curls: Do five times.
19. Spine lengtheners: Do three times.
20. Body extenders: Do three times.

Figure 19C–14. *(Reprinted with permission from Lewis C. Health Promotion and Exercise for Older Adults. Gaithersburg, Md: Aspen Publishers, Inc.; 1990.)*

Appendix D. Guide to Consultation

A Guide for Contracting Out Inpatient and Outpatient Physical Therapy

Consulting Service for Hospital and Nursing Home Physical Therapy Departments

HOSPITALS' RFP GUIDE: CONTRACTING OUT INPATIENT AND OUTPATIENT PHYSICAL THERAPY

by Jerome B. Connolly, PT

Member of the Executive Committee of the American Physical Therapy Association & Past Chairman of the Montana Board of Physical Therapy Examiners

SCORING SCALE: Rank each proposal on the criteria below and total section scores on the heavy line in front of the section heading.
0 = Not Available
1 = Would Try
2 = Limited Experience
3 = Experienced
4 = Expert

Introduction

With physical therapists and other health professionals in short supply, more hospitals are turning to experienced physical therapists with entrepreneurial skills to manage, market, and maintain high quality, productive departments. Included here are the key factors to consider when contracting for physical therapy services.

1. CONTROL

_____ 1.1 The contract stipulates that ultimate control remain with the hospital. The physical therapy services must comply with existing hospital policy.

_____ 1.2 The physical therapy department policy and procedure manual development and maintenance is the responsibility of the physical therapy (PT) contractor, but is subject to the approval of the hospital governing board and administrator.

2. INCOME

_____ 2.1 The hospital should be able to derive attractive income from the PT services

_____ 2.2 while simultaneously divesting itself of the profit-eating expenses of personnel recruitment, retention, benefits, turnover, sick leave, vacation coverage,

_____ 2.3 equipment acquisition, and

_____ 2.4 continuing professional education Moreover, a long-term commitment to a contract PT service develops a more consistent service, greater market share,

more respect and recognition in the community and a more satisfied medical staff

3. EXPERIENCE

_____ 3.1 Experience in PT evaluation and treatment,

_____ 3.2 practice management,

_____ 3.3 marketing, and promotion are at the top of the list when it comes to selecting the contractor. Experienced PTs with proven track records who can develop programs based on need and drawing from their own experience in such programs are essential for success of this kind of arrangement. The physical therapy contractor must be able to relate professionally to referring physicians, earn respect, and develop rapport.

4. QUALITY

Physical therapy patient care should be of the highest quality with an emphasis placed on

_____ 4.1 comprehensive, objective patient evaluation,

_____ 4.2 thorough treatment planning and implementation,

_____ 4.3 demonstration of progress through reevaluation measures, and

_____ 4.4 prompt, complete documentation from intake to discharge. Cooperative interdisciplinary approaches are to be used as appropriate and

_____ 4.5 timely communication with all necessary parties is essential.

5. INFORMATION NETWORKS

_____ 5.1 Physical therapists who are active in their state and national professional association matters (*The American Physical Therapy Association*) have at their disposal the most recent information in the field.

_____ 5.2 They also develop nationwide networks that prove valuable. Physical therapists who have a high profile in the APTA can more easily attract and recruit qualified and dedicated professionals.

_____ 5.3 Experience on a State Board of Physical Therapy Examiners is highly desirable.

Developed by First Physical Therapy, PC, Billings, MT.

— **Continued** —

— Continued from previous page —

6. Personnel
_____ 6.1 Recruitment and retention of qualified dedicated, professional, and support staff
_____ 6.2 Payroll, benefits,
_____ 6.3 performance evaluations,
_____ 6.4 staff motivation, communication, and
_____ 6.5 professional development (continuing education).
_____ 6.6 Scheduling of staff including providing adequate relief for vacation, sick, and professional development leave.

7. Equipment
_____ 7.1 While maintenance of the hospital's existing equipment in optimal functional condition should remain the responsibility of the hospital,
_____ 7.2 any new equipment acquired should be acquired and maintained by the contractor.
_____ 7.3 New equipment should be acquired promptly as needed to remain competitive and progressive.

8. Contract Development
_____ 8.1 Development of the contract language should be accomplished by the PT contractor and be subject to approval of the hospital administrator, governing board, and attorneys. This puts the bulk of the legal expenses in drafting the contract on the contractor rather than the hospital.

9. Administration
_____ 9.1 Recruitment and retention of qualified staff.
_____ 9.2 Staffing department for existing and developing need.
_____ 9.3 Scheduling patients on a prompt and timely basis.
_____ 9.3 Fiscal analysis and reporting to hospital administrator.
_____ 9.4 Submission of complete month-end reports to hospital administration.
_____ 9.5 Oversight of complete, timely, and accurate PT documentation.
_____ 9.6 Arrange and comply with fiscal relationship established with hospital (_rent, fee for service, percentage of revenue, etc._).

10. Marketing
_____ 10.1 Determination of existing, emerging, and future needs.
_____ 10.2 Planning to meet identified needs.

_____ 10.3 Assessing satisfaction of referral source.
_____ 10.4 Development of a market-driven service.
_____ 10.5 Program and protocol development. Secure necessary approval of programs and protocols developed.

11. Strategic Planning
_____ 11.1 Creation of a mission statement for the service consistent with that of the hospital.
_____ 11.2 Development of an environmental statement as it affects the provision of physical therapy in the area.
_____ 11.3 Development of 1 year specific objectives supplemented by an action plan to accomplish the objectives.
_____ 11.4 Development of a 3 to 5 year long-range plan to include new market niches.
_____ 11.5 Development of an ongoing action plan, regular activities essential to the ongoing operation of a progressive physical therapy service.

12. Physician Relations
The contractor should be able to successfully establish and maintain a strong rapport with the medical staff.
_____ 12.1 Evidence of this capability should be demonstrable.
_____ 12.2 Physician references should be provided.

13. Quality Assurance
_____ 13.1 Through chart and program review and
_____ 13.2 in-house professional development sessions, high quality standards are promoted and achieved. Cooperation with other hospital departments is essential to this.

14. Risk Management and Professional Liability
_____ 14.1 Through an organized and concerted awareness program the professional and support staff should be sensitized to the latest malpractice trends and risks confronting physical therapy. This is the responsibility of the PT contractor in addition to
_____ 14.2 providing proof of insurance at $1 million/$3 million levels and naming the hospital as an additional insured.

— Continued —

Continued from previous page

15. Community Involvement
The physical therapist contractor and staff should have a commitment to the community.
_____ 15.1 Periodic talks, presentations,
_____ 15.2 events,
_____ 15.3 articles, and the like are all part of the quality service that demonstrates the hospital's commitment to the community in terms of prevention and wellness as well as treatment. This is also an effective component of marketing the hospital's PT services and programs.

16. Injury Prevention Programs
The PT contractor should be willing to participate in the hospital's employee orientation program as well as showing a commitment to employee health and
_____ 16.1 well-being by providing back and sports injury prevention programs.
_____ 16.2 Similar programs should be offered to the community and to local and regional business and industry.

17. Program Development
Through frequent and close interaction with the medical staff and consumers the PT contractor should develop
_____ 17.1 programs and services to meet the needs as identified, and
_____ 17.2 should demonstrate the ability to successfully sell and implement these programs.

18. Professional Development and Continuing Education
A significant emphasis should be placed on the continuing professional development of the staff. This should be demonstrated by the contractor through
_____ 18.1 in-house as well as
_____ 18.2 external, formal programs that keep the professionals current in the field.
_____ 18.3 The emphasis must be provided by the PT contractor by whom the cost is borne and the example set.

TOTAL

For more information about contracting for physical therapy services, call Jerry Connolly at First Physical Therapy.

Figure 19D–1A.

SCORING GUIDE

Interpreting the scores and comparing them must of course take into account the size and type of your facility.

After assigning a point rating of 0–4 to each factor (i.e., factor 2.2 received a "3"), add all of the factors up for each section to give an overall score for that area (i.e., Risk Management scored a "7"). Then add all the section scores together for an overall ranking of the proposal. If you use all of the sections, which we recommend, there are 236 points possible on the 59 questions. A minimum threshold score should be no lower than 130. If the potential contractor scores in that range, proceed with caution as their inadequacies and inexperience could well negate most of the benefits of contracting physical therapy services outside the staff. A "C+" score or 2.5 avg. would be 150 points. If some of these sections are deemed by you to be areas already handled elsewhere in the hospital or infeasible for your operation, eliminate the section(s) from the scoring.

If you would like further assistance in this area, First Physical Therapy can develop your facilities' RFP, distribute it, screen and score applicants, and even develop and negotiate the contract for the selected Physical Therapy provider. Simply call us to discuss the possibilities.

Figure 19D–1B.

Consulting Services Offered by First Physical Therapy for Hospital & Nursing Home Physical Therapy Departments

Whether you are starting, upgrading, fine-tuning, or just evaluating your physical therapy service, First Physical Therapy's wealth of experience in a variety of physical therapy settings and arrangements can assist you in identifying and achieving your goals for your physical therapy services.

Do You Face These Now Common Problems in Physical Therapy Departments?

1. High Staff Turnover
   - Continuous recruiting efforts that result in uneven compensation packages that sap morale.
   - Recent graduates forced into management roles.
   - Difficulty in maintaining the high quality standards that the hospital or nursing home stands for.
   - Staffing unresponsive to physicians' demands and needs.
   - The high cost of traveling PTs/locum tenems (*avg. $320/day,* $83–91,500/yr).
2. Loss of faith in the department by physicians.
3. Underperforming profit center.
4. Inability of the department to contribute fully to the hospital's overall mission.
5. Inattentiveness to equipment maintenance.
6. Loss of continuity and an inability to develop a proactive, market-driven department.
7. A department that is not as responsive as desired to physician demand.

Our Professional Experience

The principals of First Physical Therapy have cumulative experience in excess of 50 years. This has been earned in a multitude of settings, including hospitals, long-term care facilities, home care, outpatient centers, school systems, industry, work-hardening, wellness programs, health clubs, and others. Moreover, the firm currently operates three outpatient clinics and provides physical therapy as a contractor to five nursing homes and hospitals in Montana.

How can First Physical Therapy directly help your hospital or nursing home?

1. Assessment and planning of your physical plant.
2. Identification of local market needs.
3. Determination of local market size for supporting PT services.
4. Competitor analysis.
5. Differentiation of your services from competitors.
6. Other market research.
7. Analysis of current operations' practices and effectiveness.
8. Staff performance assessment.
9. Environmental statement development.
10. Strategic planning.
11. Professional development of current staff.
12. Recruitment strategies.
13. Contract review or development.
14. Equipment needs and use assessment.
15. Physician relations enhancement.
16. Risk management and professional liability analysis.
17. Injury prevention and wellness consulting.
18. Productivity analysis
19. Environmental analysis and forecasting.
20. Marketing and public relations assistance.
21. Department oversight or management.
22. Reimbursement analysis-cash flow.

Continued

─── *Continued from previous page* ───

Examples of Program and Protocol Development of Particular Interest to Hospitals

- Industrial physical therapy.
- Temporomandibular joint (TMJ) protocols
- Sports physical therapy.
- Injury prevention programs.
- Risk management.
- Quality assurance.
- Documentation for optimal reimbursement.
- Customer service practices.
- Dealing with managed care/PT-managed care.
- Work-hardening programs.

Nonbillable time
PHASE I:
Information Gathering
Preliminary Assessment
Scope of Services Defined
Time/Expense Estimate

Billable time
PHASE II:
Assignment Definition
Methodology Selection
Goal & Results Targeted

PHASE III:
Work Plan & Timeline
Implementation
Analyze Findings
Draw Conclusions

PHASE IV:
Report of Findings & Documentation
Formal Presentation

PHASE V:
Oversee Implementation of Recommendations
Conduct Training
Evaluate Outcome
Followup as Appropriate

WHY USE A CONSULTANT WITH YOUR CURRENT PHYSICAL THERAPY DEPARTMENT?

Experience: With over half a century in cumulative PT experience there is little we haven't seen. We offer specialized service management from the perspective of these many years of experience.

Efficiency: Because we are specialized and extensively involved in the profession of physical therapy we have resources at our disposal that allow us to perform an assignment better, faster, and more thoroughly than clients can on their own.

Concentration: We can focus on accomplishing a critical assignment quickly, our clients are free to operate the ongoing services without diversions.

─── *Continued* ───

────── *Continued from previous page* ──────

Confidentiality: We are an independent physical therapist-owned private firm. We do not reveal the identity or purpose of our clients except when permitted to do so. We will not reveal critical information without prior approval.

Objectivity: We can offer a fresh viewpoint, unencumbered by hierarchical pressure, traditions, bias, or conflict of interest. If we are unable to help, we will refer the client to other appropriate resources.

Client Relationships and Billing

Work is carried out in a manner that best satisfies the client. This can be accomplished on an hourly basis or on a retainer for a stipulated period or even as a single project assignment. Itemized billing of time, materials, and expenses will be provided on a monthly basis. Invoices are due payable within 10 days of receipt.

There is no charge for Phase I consulting services. The plan developed is converted to contractual language by FPT and is subject to the approval of the hospital administrator or governing board before implementation.

To discuss your specific needs, contact Lorin Wright or Jerry Connolly at First Physical Therapy.

Figure 19D–2.

CHAPTER **20** TWENTY

Scientific Inquiry and Research

Competency in the area of geriatric physical therapy would not be complete without an understanding of research. Research is critical in providing good physical therapy care because of the necessity to interpret current methods and to look to the future for more efficacious means of providing care.

This chapter will discuss methods of evaluating research in general and will examine problems with rehabilitation and aging research in particular. It will also discuss measurement issues often encountered in psychological research, and it will talk about clinical research and provide several different means of assisting clinicians in designing clinical research. The final part of the chapter is designed to show how to do research and how to get clinicians to use research in daily practice.

HOW TO ANALYZE RESEARCH ARTICLES

Research articles contain several general elements. Most articles start off with an abstract, which is a concise paragraph preceding the research article whose main purpose is to summarize the remaining body of the article (e.g., introduction, methods, results, conclusions, and relevance of the article to the clinician).[1] Frequently, an abstract can be read to save time and to note results. However, if a clinician is interested in delving deeper into the topic and wants to evaluate the conclusions reached by the researcher, the entire article should be examined.

The next part of the research article is the introduction, which contains several elements:

1. The problem statement.
2. The literature reviewed.
3. The purpose of the study.
4. The type of study.
5. The expected results.
6. The research question (null hypothesis).[1]

The most important aspect of the introduction is clarity. Did the author clearly state the purpose, type of study, expected results, and research question? The literature reviewed must be complete and exhaustive, and it should note any gaps in the literature that have been identified.[1]

The method section provides the reader with specifics as to how the study was conducted. This section should describe the subjects in detail as to their characteristics in regard to age, sex, and diagnosis, and it should describe sample size and the method of selection of the sample. Any instrument used in the study should be described in terms of validity and reliability and the procedures used should be described in detail so that the reader could replicate the study.

The next section of the article is data analysis, which should provide in detail the method of data analysis and applicability to this particular study. In the description of data analysis p-values must be presented. The results section should clearly describe the results generated from this study and define their practical and statistical significance.

The discussion section provides more interpretive information as compared to the results and methods section. In this part, the author is defining in greater detail accepted or rejected results of the hypothesis and any weakness in the experimental design. Here the author can further discuss any relevant literature that may apply to the study results. The author's opinions on how these relate to the research finding can be stated. The conclusion section briefly states the results that should flow logically from the remainder of the article. Table 20–1 outlines these guidelines for evaluating research articles and can help a clinician by providing more information on evaluating research.

PROBLEMS WITH REHABILITATION RESEARCH

Before discussing the problems of aging research, it is imperative to look at the difficulties that might be encountered in the area of rehabilitation research. Cicely Partridge[2] did an excellent job of describing research guidelines for physical therapists, and her text developed stages of the research project.[2] Figure 20–1 provides an example of her checklist for following the various stages of research, and this can be very helpful to the therapist starting off. In addition, she cites many obstacles that may occur in the rehabilitation setting, making it more difficult for physical therapists to achieve research. These are[1]

1. Finding an appropriate question in the research environment.
2. Finding a population that can tolerate research in various rehabilitation techniques.
3. Finding literature to support the research hypothesis.
4. The physical therapist's knowledge of the research process.
5. Availability of funding, and financing facilities.
6. Time to conduct research.
7. Cost of research.

TABLE 20–1. GUIDELINES FOR EVALUATING A RESEARCH ARTICLE

Introduction

Is problem clearly stated?
Is literature review complete?
Do authors identify a gap in the literature?
Is purpose clearly stated?
Is expectation or hypothesis identified, if indicated?

Methods

Are subjects well described?
How was sample selected?
How large is the sample?
Is a control group used?
Is the instrumentation well described?
Are measuring instruments valid and reliable?
Is the procedure well described?
Could you replicate the study?
Does the design have internal validity?
Is data analysis well described?
What questions are addressed by each test?
Is the analysis appropriate to the question and to the data?
What p-value was used, if indicated?

Results

Are results presented clearly?
Are results statistically significant?
Are results practically significant?

Discussion

Clarifies if hypothesis was accepted or rejected or if results were as expected?
Do authors identify weaknesses in the experimental design?
Is further literature cited to expand on unexpected findings?
Are results applied to clinical practice?
Are suggestions for further study presented?

Conclusions

Are results restated briefly?
Do conclusions follow logically from the results?

Reprinted with permission from Domholdt E, Malone T. Evaluating research literature: the educated clinician. Phys Ther. April 1965; 65(4):487–491.

8. Cooperation of the patients to undergo the rigors of the rehabilitation process as well as the study.
9. Availability of subjects that meet specific criteria for the research project.
10. Familiarity with coding and statistically analyzing data.
11. Ethics.
     Is it ethical to withhold treatment from various subjects for the sake of research?
     Is it ethical to go through patients' records?
     What are the ethical limits of informing patients of the results of the research?
     Is it ethical to withhold the new therapy from the control group and cause the possible loss of therapeutic benefit?

Research guidelines: A handbook for therapists

	Yes	No	Not applicable
1. Asking questions, developing ideas			
Reading the literature			
Defining the research question			
Statement of objectives for the study, or producing a hypothesis for testing			
2. Deciding on appropriate research design			
Organization and approaches to field work			
Writing the research proposal			
Applying to grant-awarding bodies			
Ethical committees or other bodies concerned with the use of human subjects			
3. Considering methods of collecting information			
Preparing forms and questionnaires			
Considering analysis of data			
Consulting a statistician			
4. Collection of information			
Pilot work			
Main study			
5. Analysis of results			
Writing the report			
Presentation of oral and written papers			

Figure 20–1. *(Reprinted with permission from Partridge C, Barnitt R. Research Guidelines: A Handbook for Therapists. Rockville, MD: Aspen; 1986.)*

Is it ethical to withhold the standard therapy from the experimental group, again with possible loss of therapeutic benefit?
Is it ethical to ask the experimental group to receive a new, unproven therapy, which may have side effects as yet unknown?[3]

PROBLEMS WITH AGING RESEARCH

The problems with aging research are quite numerous, ranging from sampling and subject recruitment to cross-sectional design. In the area of sampling, the article by Wayne[4] showed that people in cross-sectional samples tended to have longer nursing home stays, as well as less social support and more behavioral and functional problems than persons in the admissions sample, who tended to have shorter stays and more acute medical problems. Therefore, looking at a cross-sectional sample could skew the results of research findings. When conducting research in a nursing home, it is imperative to look at the samples chosen to control for the particular and cultural problems already listed.[4]

In the area of subject recruitment, several variables must be considered for the elderly. For example, older persons experience decreased mobility. Therefore, a study requiring mobility, such as the ability to drive a car or use public transportation to get to the test site, may eliminate participants from the study. To generalize the abilities of the subject's recruited is also difficult. For example, the majority of the elderly do not live in nursing homes: Therefore, to assume that they are a representative sample of all older people would be erroneous. In addition, when recruiting subjects from various settings, you may disrupt the normal functioning of that person's day and, therefore, make it difficult to generalize the results of the study.[5]

Gerontological research has been painfully aware of the effects of variability in subjects of aging research. Nelson and Dannifer,[6] however, present compelling information to the geriatric researcher to attend to the diversity and analyze the homogeneity of variance on control for aging research methodology. Their work showed an increase in variability with age up to 65%, which was more pronounced in longitudinal versus cross-sectional studies.[6]

Andrews[7] makes a very strong point for controlling cultural variables in aging research and points out that attitudinal, religious, social, and behavioral influences can affect many outcome measures commonly explored by rehabilitation researchers and cites numerous examples, one of which is nutrition.[7] A person's religious background, for example, can strongly influence a person's nutritional intake. This may affect rehabilitation variables, such as the desire to walk, independence, or assistance from others. These attitudinal, religious, and social variables should be controlled for when doing rehabilitation research to be sure to check for the effects of the study.[7]

In aging research, methodology can significantly impact research outcomes. Research designs can vary from cross-sectional to longitudinal. In cross-sectional research, all variables are measured at one point in time. Longitudinal research looks at an extended period of time and variables are measured over it. The benefits of cross-sectional studies are the short-term commitment and minimal financial implications. However, the ability to attribute differences between groups to variables of age is very difficult, and this particular study design does not take into consideration other confounding variables. For example, cohort differences can influence demographic variables. People who lived during the Depression developed a specific sense for understanding how to function in the economy when the availability of money is lowered. Therefore, as a group they have a new understanding of functioning. This shared experience is a cohort effect, which is difficult to figure out when using cross-sectional studies.[8]

Longitudinal studies, on the other hand, take a much longer amount of time and can be impractical in terms of time and money involved. In a longitudinal study, for example, a therapist may choose to examine patients at age 20 to check for arthritis of the knee and follow them until they reach 90. This requires 70 years of study and is, therefore, impractical. Another problem with longitudinal studies in the area of aging research is the discrimination of socialization. How, for example, can a therapist determine if the variables are actually age or activity level related? Has a patient's medication or periods of rest affected the outcome or is it the aging process?[8]

Dr Schale[9] proposes a cross-sectional and time-sequential analysis to differentiate the presence of cohort and age differences. He also suggests that this type of research can minimize problems of longitudinal methodologies. His method is called the cohort sequential method[9] and it controls for historical events by following two or more cohorts over different age and time ranges. For example, he may follow a 20-year-old group, a 50-year-old group, and a 70-year-old group for 10 years to look at the effects of arthritis of the knee. He believes this method will cut the time involved in doing aging research and will control the cohort differences. It will, however, give some longitudinal perspective as to the aging research.[9]

Another problem with aging research can result from the use of the survey used. It is well known that some older persons have problems with vision, hearing, and mentation that may affect the extent to which they are able to respond to the survey instrument. The older person may also be more fearful of test-taking, and, therefore, it may be more difficult to obtain informed consent from older populations.[10]

Finally, the degree to which physical or mental impairments affects the older population may require special explanations for research participation.[10]

MEASUREMENT ISSUES

Reliability

In reviewing and conducting research, it is imperative that therapists are aware of measurement issues in research. The first area is reliability, which is essentially the internal consistency of a measurement tool. For example, if quadricep strength is measured by one therapist and then another therapist measures quadricep strength of an older person, are the two measures similar? For example, if the first therapist rates the quadriceps as 3/5 or fair and the other therapist rates the quadriceps as 5/5, there is no interrater reliability, which means there is a discrepancy between the two therapists' measures. Interrater reliability is, therefore, consistency between examiners. Interrater reliability means that if a therapist rates the quadriceps as 3/5 of an older person at one point in time and, 2 months later, assuming that there was no change in the quadricep strength, the therapist again rates the quadriceps as 3/5 of the same older person. Interrater reliability is consistency within an individual's measurements over time. These principles must be met or the measures themselves will be incorrect. Although reliability is important, it is not the only measurement issue to consider when evaluating measurement tools.

Validity

There are numerous types of validity. Validity assesses whether or not the scale measures what it is designed to measure, and there are six different types of validity:[11]

1. Concurrent validity correlates your test with other test variables. For example, manual muscle testing may be correlated with mechanical tests. You may develop a balance assessment tool that you want to correlate with standard and accepted balance assessment tools.
2. Content validity examines the components of the tool. Content validity examines each item of a test as to its representativeness of the entire sample. For example, if you want to look at balance and you have ten different questions related to balance, it looks at each one to see if, in fact, they individually relate to the final outcome of what you are trying to measure.
3. Predictive validity looks at the test's ability to predict outcomes. For example, on the Barthel Test, which has a predictive validity, a score of 50 would predict that a person is not independent, not ready for discharge and needs excessive help in personal care. Whereas if a person scores a 90, he or she could probably go home with a minimal amount of assistance.
4. Internal validity shows if the independent variable really caused the dependent variable.
5. External validity shows the extent to which findings can be generalized to other settings in the real world. For example, the results of a study testing muscle strengths on aging rats has external validity to a rat population but lacks external validity in humans.
6. Face validity is the easiest form of validity. It states that if you think its measuring what its supposed to measure then it is. For example, if you believe on a math test that your questions are math questions, therefore, you're measuring your students' ability to do math. If you are looking for the components of gait and you are doing a gait analysis on the face of it, you are measuring gait. Face validity is usually measured through professional judgment as to whether or not it is face valid.

The next major measurement issue is variables. Differentiating between independent and dependent variables is critical to understanding research design. Independent variables are those that the experimenter manipulates. Dependent variables are what the experimenter assesses as a result of the independent variable. For example, exercise classes to improve balance would be the independent variable, and balance outcomes as a result of the classes would be the dependent variable.

The final area of research is data analysis. The major components of descriptive statistical analyses are parametric and nonparametric statistics. Measures of central tendency and variance are parametric statistics. Measures of central tendencies can be subdivided into three categories[11]:

1. Mean or the average. To calculate the mean, the sum of all of the scores are added and then divided by the number of scores to produce the mean. For example, for the scores 1, 2, 4, 6, 8, 8, and 10, the mean is 5.57.
2. Median is the middle ranked score, the one that occurs exactly in the middle. For example, if the listed scores are 1, 2, 4, 6, 8, 8, and 10, the median would be 6.
3. Mode is the most frequently observed value in the data set. For example, with the above scores, 8 would be the model or most frequently observed value.

Variability

The concept of variability is also under the category of descriptive statistics. Variability has two types of measures:

1. Range, which essentially describes the highest to the lowest score. This can be very important if you are trying to talk about the person's response to an exercise program. For the data set given earlier, the range is 9.
2. Standard deviation is another measure of variability that looks at the distribution from the highest to lowest scores by calculating the square root of the variance.

A normal distribution curve, or bell curve, has a line representing the mean at its center (Fig. 20–2). To either side of the line, up to the dotted line, is the standard deviation. One standard deviation above or below the mean represents 34% of the sample. If it is on both sides it is 68%. To go two standard deviations would encompass almost the entire population or 95%.[11]

Data Analysis

The descriptive statistics already mentioned are considered parametric statistics (i.e., mean, median, variance, and standard deviation). Chi square is nonparametric.

Statistical analysis used for these parametric statistics can be at the nominal or ordinal level. A quick review of nominal, ordinal, interval, and ratio data may be helpful. When looking at numbers and measurements, they can be placed into a hierarchy, which ranges from nominal to ratio. Nominal numbers essentially de-

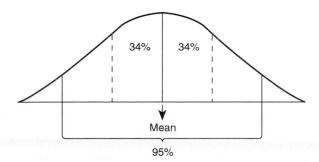

Figure 20–2. Normal distribution curve.

scribe categories. Something is nominal if it is naming something, such as the months of the year. Strong, weak, young, and old are examples of nominal level data. Nominal level information provides the reader with some descriptive information, but it has no hierarchial value.

Ordinal information has a hierarchial value and uses numbers to order objects with respect to some characteristic. For example, scales of stronger to weaker or faster to slower provide ordinal information. The numbers all represent values relative to each other.

The next level is interval. Interval data can be thought of as integers; it describes, provides a hierarchy, and ascribes a numerical difference. Examples of interval level measure are manual muscle tests, number of feet ambulated, and number of repetitions.

Finally, the highest level of measurement is ratio level data. Ratio level information has all three characterizations, as previously noted, with 0 as a reference point. Examples of ratio data are fractions, goniometric measurements, and timed scores.

To use parametric statistics appropriately you must have either interval or ratio level data. To use parametric statistics, you need to make statistical assump-

TABLE 20–2. PARAMETRIC STATISTICS

Test	General Use	Specific Example	
		Source	Application
t Test	Compare two independent groups	Ikeda ER, et al. *Phys Ther.* 1991;71:473–481.	Compared *joint movements* during rising from a chair in young versus elderly adults
		Schwartz RS, et al. *J Gerontol.* 1990;45:M181–M185.	Compared *distribution of body fat* in young versus elderly men
Paired *t* Test	Compare two groups of data where each value in group A is linked in some way to a value in group B	Blanke DJ, Hageman PA. *Phys Ther.* 1989;69:144–148.	Compared *gait characteristics* between young and elderly men who were matched by leg length
ANOVA	Compare multiple groups or treatments	Einkauf DK, et al. *Phys Ther.* 1987;67:370–375.	Compared *spinal mobility* in six groups of *women* who were grouped according to age
		Mossey JM, et al. *J Gerontol.* 1990;45:M163–M168.	Compared recovery from *hip fracture* in four groups of elderly who were grouped according to type of depressive symptoms
ANCOVA	Used to control initial differences when comparing various groups	Panton LB, et al. *J Gerontol.* 1990;145:M26–M31.	Studied *effects of aerobic and resistance training on reaction time* in elderly men; used ANCOVA to control for differences in pretraining reaction time in each group
Factorial ANOVA	Compare effects of two or more independent variables	Nelson RM, et al. *Phys Ther.* 1984;64:29–34.	Compared *differences in motor unit activity* based on age and percentage of maximal voluntary contraction strength
Repeated Measures ANOVA	Compare measurements taken under different conditions or on different occasions in a particular group or groups	Vandervoort AA, et al. *J Gerontol.* 1990;45:B125–B128.	Measured quad/ham torque in young and elderly females at different *isokinetic speeds and different contraction types:* concentric versus eccentric (combined repeated measures with factorial design)
Correlation	Determines the degree of association between two variables	Bohannon RW. *Topics Geriatric Rehabil.* 1990;6:51–58.	Determined relationship between *functional independence* and specific variables (age, gender, number of PT sessions, and so on) in patients recovering from hip fracture
Regression	Generally tries to see how well certain variables are able to predict another variable	Magaziner J, et al. *J Gerontol.* 1990;45:M101–M107.	Examined ability of several factors to *predict functional recovery* 1 year after hip fracture

Permission to reprint from Ciccone C. Lecture notes from Geriatrics, An Advanced Tutorial, *San Francisco: February 1992.*

tions about your data (e.g., normality or homogeneity of variance), whereas in nonparametric statistics, fewer assumptions need to be made. Nonparametric statistics make no assumptions about the form of the underlying distribution except that it be continuous. Chi square is nonparametric. Table 20–2 is a chart of parametric statistics that shows their use and application.

When reviewing and conducting geriatric research, it is imperative to examine the most appropriate use of statistical measures.

CONDUCTING CLINICAL REHABILITATION RESEARCH IN AGING

Once the therapist understands how to analyze the problems with aging research and rehabilitation, he or she can begin to pursue various forms of clinical research. One of the most interesting approaches has been developed by Rothstein and Ecternach and is called the "Hypothesis Oriented ALGORITHM (HOAC Model) for Clinicians."[13] This method is presented as a means to assist physical therapists in clinical decision making and patient management. Figure 20–3 illustrates the process by which the therapist can collect information and assess the efficacy of their efforts. The stages are

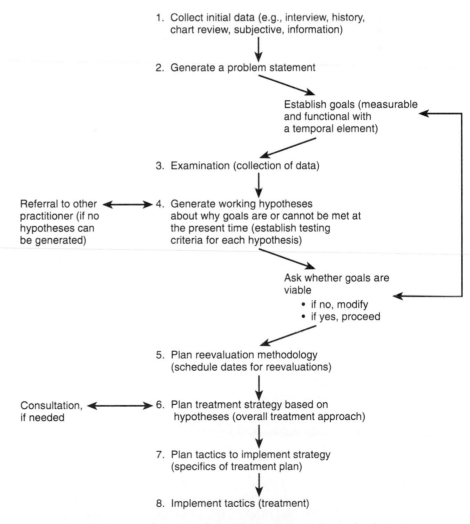

1. Collect initial data (e.g., interview, history, chart review, subjective, information)

2. Generate a problem statement

Establish goals (measurable and functional with a temporal element)

3. Examination (collection of data)

Referral to other practitioner (if no hypotheses can be generated)

4. Generate working hypotheses about why goals are or cannot be met at the present time (establish testing criteria for each hypothesis)

Ask whether goals are viable
- if no, modify
- if yes, proceed

5. Plan reevaluation methodology (schedule dates for reevaluations)

Consultation, if needed

6. Plan treatment strategy based on hypotheses (overall treatment approach)

7. Plan tactics to implement strategy (specifics of treatment plan)

8. Implement tactics (treatment)

Figure 20–3. Hypothesis-oriented algorithm for clinicians. *(Reprinted with permission from Rothstein J, Echternach J. Hypothesis-oriented algorithm for clinicians—a method for evaluation & treatment planning. Phys Ther. 1986;66(9):1388–1394.)*

1. Initial data collection: The therapist, through interview, chart review, or subject information, gathers information from the patient.
2. Problem statement: The therapist generates a question to explore.
3. Examination and collection of the data: The therapist conducts the study (e.g., collects data).
4. Working hypothesis: The therapist generates a working hypothesis about why the goals were met or not met and reassesses whether or not the goals were appropriate.
5. Reevaluation: The therapist then does a reevaluation of the methodology.
6. Future strategies: The therapist plans future treatment strategies based on the overall hypothesis.
7. Tactic for implementation: The therapist develops a tactic to implement the strategies.
8. Final implementation: The therapist finally implements this specific treatment protocol.

This is an initial way of using a research design for the evaluation and treatment of an individual patient or a group of patients.

Single Subject Design

Another interesting research methodology that can easily be used in the geriatric rehabilitation setting is the single subject design. This particular type of design is defined as a detailed documentation summary of the characteristics, diagnosis, problem, treatment, and response of one patient. In this study design, the patient will be viewed prior to any intervention, then the intervention will be introduced and then withdrawn. When intervention is applied, any changes in patient status will be noted and carryover from this particular status will also be noted after termination of the intervention.

This is an easy way of making an analysis of a particular treatment intervention. For example, let's take one Parkinson patient who has a difficult time getting out of a chair. The therapist records over several weeks the difficulties of the patient getting out of a chair and the time spent by the patient sitting in the chair. The therapist then applies education and the use of flexion activities to get the patient out of the chair. The therapist then records what happens when the patient, throughout the day, tries to get up out of the chair (i.e., a noted increase in the number of times the patient gets up and walks around is documented). The intervention of the flexion activities is withdrawn, and an effect is observed (i.e., number of times the patient gets out of the chair). This type of study has some difficulties for generalization in that there is only one patient being observed.[14,15]

Woolery[15] describes several ways of interpreting the data from single subject research design. Woolery discusses visual analysis of the graph data that relies on visual interpretation of the changes and another strategy of the use of statistical procedures, such as trend estimation, Rn statistic, and time series analysis all of which can provide valuable information in the single subject design.[15]

Qualitative Research

Another important area of research is qualitative research. Shepard provides an excellent description of this in the *Journal of the American Physical Therapy Association*,[16] where she discusses case studies, descriptive research, and quasi-experimental research as examples of both qualitative and quantitative methods for looking at the effects of rehabilitation. The case study method presents one case study and describes a patient, and it may have both quantitative and qualitative research methods. However, the qualitative aspect tends to be highlighted. In the area of descriptive research, she describes this as a way the clinician describes a certain patient population and then discusses relevant physical therapy clinical problems and how the current literature addresses those problems. It is a description of what actually occurs in the clinical setting.

In quasi-experimental research, the therapist conducts the actual research. The treatment techniques do not have to be as controlled as the level of laboratory studies, because it would be almost impossible to do this in the clinical setting. Variables, such as group support, mood swings, and family conflict are common in human research and are not an issue in rat sample studies. Therefore, the majority of research done in the clinical setting is of a qualitative nature.

Gail Jensen in the *Journal of the American Physical Therapy Association*[17] presents an outline guide designed for conceptual framework and qualitative research (Table 20–3) that provides an excellent framework for the therapist to understand qualitative research and to implement it in the clinical setting.

Finally, Table 20–4 examines ways to address potential threats to internal validity in qualitative research, which is the biggest threat to conducting qualitative research. Frequently, the therapist will be questioned as to the scientific basis for this research and will have to face these various problems.

Ethnography

Another method of research that may be employed by physical therapists in a geriatric setting is ethnography. This is a qualitative form of scientific research and is used to discover and describe human behavior through the perspective of the person studied. Table 20–5 lists the steps in the ethnography methodology.[18]

In addition, Table 20–6 lists the unique aspects of ethnography.[18] Ethnography has both pros and cons. The positive side of ethnography is that it is a very flexible process for data collection. It's a good tool for measuring behavior, which is fre-

TABLE 20–3. GUIDELINES FOR CONDUCTING QUALITATIVE RESEARCH

Questions	Suggestions
1. Is the description rich?	Provide sufficient detail so the account of observations comes to life. The goal is to capture what you observed. Avoid using abstract or passive words. For example, instead of stating the patient appeared to be in pain, describe what you saw so someone could infer the patient was in pain.
2. Is there concrete detail that portrays what actually happened?	Reconstruction of dialogue is important. Strive to record the subject's own words when possible. Nonverbal expressions should also be noted.
3. Is confidentiality maintained?	Usually, the researcher is dealing with a small number of subjects, and confidentiality is a critical factor. The researcher also relies on building trust and rapport with subjects to collect valid information.
4. Is the material presented pertinent to the research topic?	Once immersed in the research setting, it is easy to get off track and gather data that are not relevant. An initial, yet dynamic, conceptual framework can help guide your data collection.
5. Are multiple perspectives presented?	The researcher must continually look for data that might disconfirm preliminary insights. Field notes should reflect collection of supporting and disconfirming evidence. This evidence can in turn be used to revise the conceptual framework.
6. Has the researcher kept an account of his or her behaviors during the data collection?	Because the researcher is the data-collection instrument, it is important to keep track of behaviors, assumptions, or whatever else might affect the construction of field notes.

Reprinted with permission from Jensen G. Qualitative methods in physical therapy research: A form of disciplined inquiry. Phys Ther. June 1989;69(6):492–500.

TABLE 20–4. WAYS TO ADDRESS POTENTIAL THREATS TO INTERNAL VALIDITY IN QUALITATIVE RESEARCH

Threat	Recommendation
History	Qualitative researchers assume that history affects the nature of the data, because phenomena rarely remain constant. When process and change are the focus of the research, then the researcher must establish which baseline data remain stable over time and which data change. This process can be accomplished through the use of replication and time-sampling strategies.
Observer effects	Sufficient residence in the field and corroboration from multiple informants can reduce these effects. Participant reaction and confirmation, documented throughout the research process, will also help guard against observer effects.
Selection-regression	Qualitative researchers do not usually try to control selection and regression effects to isolate a treatment, but distortions in the data may occur by selection of participants. In complex field situations, an adequate inventory of groups, subgroups, events, or social scenes must be completed to ensure the findings are representative.
Mortality	Qualitative researchers assume that growth and attrition are normal processes in a natural setting and that what is important is the identification of their effects.
Spurious conclusions	Elimination of rival explanation in qualitative research requires effective and efficient data-collection systems and the use of corroborating sources of data. Negative confirming or disconfirming evidence is sought throughout the research process.

Reprinted with permission from Shepard K. Qualitative & quantitative research in clinical practice. Phys. Ther. *December 1987;67(12):1891–1894.*

TABLE 20–5. STEPS IN ETHNOGRAPHIC METHODOLOGY

The steps used in ethnographic methodology are presented in a sequential format, but in practice many of these steps occur simultaneously or concurrently, rather than in a fixed, sequential manner.

1. Identify a topic to study.
2. Pose research questions related to the topic of study.
3. Identify initial methods and sources for data collection based on questions posed (e.g., persons to interview or observe).
4. Develop operational definitions initially or as the need arises during the study.
5. Collect initial data by observations or interviews. Begin analysis of data as they are collected from initial observations or interviews. Preliminary concepts should emerge from the data.
6. Analyze data as they are collected and form tentative concepts that explain them.
7. Collect more data. For example, conduct additional observations, interview persons previously observed, or observe persons initially interviewed.
8. Continue to analyze all accumulated data and refine tentative concepts that explain the data.
9. Continue to collect and analyze data concurrently until the concepts established can explain all of the data collected. If tentative concepts do not explain (fit) the data, they should be modified until they do fit the data.
10. Analyze concepts to establish explanations of the interrelationships of two or more concepts. This analysis results in forming tentative hypotheses or propositions.
11. Formulate hypotheses into substantive theory that describes and explains phenomena that occur. The hypotheses also may serve as the basis for subsequent experimental or quasi-experimental design research.

Although the phases of ethnographic inquiry differ from those of quantitative scientific inquiry, the process for collecting and analyzing data is systematic and rigorous.

Reprinted with permission from Schmoll BJ. Ethnographic inquiry in clinical settings. Phys. Ther. *December 1987;67(12):1895–1897.*

TABLE 20–6. UNIQUE ASPECTS OF ETHNOGRAPHY

Ethnography is distinguished from quantitative research by the following characteristics:

1. The study is guided by general questions related to a topic rather than by preestablished hypotheses.
2. A review of the literature is treated as a data source that may be subjected to constant comparative analysis rather than serving as a basis for the generation of hypotheses.
3. The direct contact with the groups under study by observations or interviews, or both, is essential. Other forms of data, such as progress reports, surveys, medical records, quality assurance reports, and a review of the literature, may be used in combination with observations and interviews.
4. Variables are regarded as data.
5. Multiple phases of the inquiry occur simultaneously rather than in a fixed, sequential manner.
6. Ethnography begins with a broad general area for study that increasingly becomes focused more narrowly as the study proceeds.

Reprinted with permission from Schmoll BJ. Ethnographic inquiry in clinical settings. Phys. Ther. December 1987;67(12):1895–1897.

quently what is being measured and it enables the therapist to develop a theory about a fluid mix of behaviors in the clinical setting. The limitations of ethnography are that it is limited strictly to human interactions that impact human behavior and the lack of control variables and statistical analysis make the data inappropriate for quantitative statistical hypothesis testing. In addition, it requires meticulous documentation. Nevertheless, it may be an appropriate modality in the rehabilitation environment.

ENCOURAGING THE USE OF RESEARCH

The final component of this chapter is how to use research and how to encourage the use of research. According to Bohannon and LeVeau[19] the literature suggests that research information is not routinely used by human service professionals. What are some of the major factors that keep these health professionals from using research?

1. Frequently clinicians view scientists as different from themselves, and they question the type of research that is being conducted.
2. The communication of research findings is so overwhelming it may discourage its use by the professional.
3. The use of jargon in research that is not commonly used in the clinic may preclude its use.
4. The results may be too tentative, inconclusive, and not studied thoroughly enough.
5. The research may be delayed in its publication and of interest to only a few of the clinicians available.
6. Frequently people who are active clinically do not have the time to read new information, and they may not be using this type of information.
7. Clinicians tend to prefer practice articles over research articles because of the vast amount of information available and, when faced with time constraints, may frequently choose to read the clinical versus the research article.
8. Frequently clinicians, even if they do understand the report, may not be able to implement the findings, and they may resist implementing the various findings because they may go against what they have been taught previously.[19]

Consent Form for Human Subjects

Description

Subject's Name (Please print): _____

Project Title: _____

_____

Project Director/Researcher's Name: _____

_____

Describe the nature of the research project and what will be required of the participants:

Certification

I fully understand the program or activity in which I am being asked to participate and the procedures that will be performed. I have had an adequate chance to ask questions and understand that I may ask additional questions any time while the study is in progress.

I understand that I am participating in this activity of my own free will, and I am free to withdraw my consent and discontinue my participation at any time while the study is in progress.

This is to certify that I agree to participate in this program or activity under the direction of the researcher named above.

_____   _____
Date   Signature of Subject (or other
                                     authorized person, such as a
                                     child's parent or guardian)

                                     _____
                                     Witness (if necessary)

Figure 20–4.

These strategies could be used to increase the use of research information:

1. Prepare students to be consumers of research. Teachers, clinicians, and clinical affiliates should use research when talking to students and make it available so they can frequently refer to various articles. Encourage students to do research projects and to work on research projects. In addition, role models in the area of research are necessary in the various academic institutions.

2. Prepare physical therapists to be consumers of research by exposing them to research articles versus clinical tracts that may extrapolate the research information. Have those students go to the library and investigate original research. In addition, make research information available by providing annotated bibliographies, notebooks of current research, and highlight clinicians who have used research. Have a research member on board on a clinical staff.[19]

ETHICAL ISSUES AND RESEARCH

Before concluding the chapter on research, special mention must be made about ethical considerations. Prior to conducting any study using human subjects, therapists must have these subjects sign a consent form. Figure 20–4 is a sample consent form for research and can be modified as needed for various studies. Please note that at any time a subject has the right to withdraw from a study and that this must be clearly identified in the consent form.

CONCLUSION

Geriatric research is similar to research in the entire rehabilitation realm with a few exceptions. This chapter points out that the older population is slightly more difficult to study. Certain study methodologies might be better for obtaining information, and suggestions were given for different types of research tools that could be used in the rehabilitation environment. The future of geriatric rehabilitation truly is in the area of research. Understanding the differences in aging research, and the various ways of conducting aging research, may help to improve that future.

PEARLS

- A research article is composed of an abstract, introduction, method, data analysis, results, discussion, and conclusion sections.

- The introduction contains: (1) the statement of the problem, (2) the literature reviewed, (3) the purpose of the study, (4) the type of study, (5) the expected results, and (6) the research question.

- The major problems in aging research are sampling, subject recruitment, and design constraints.

- Understanding measurement issues, such as reliability, validity, and data analysis, are essential for therapists to properly interpret aging research reports.

- A method suggested for clinicians to assist therapists in a clinical decision making is the Hypothesis Oriented Algorithm for Clinicians (HOAC).

- An interesting research methodology that may be used to study the aged is ethnography (i.e., a qualitative form of research used to describe and discover human behavior from the perspective of the person studied).

REFERENCES

1. Domholdt E, Malone T. Evaluating research literature: the educated clinician. *Phys Ther.* April 1965; 65(4):487–491.
2. Partridge C, Barnitt R. *Research Guidelines: A Handbook for Therapists.* Rockville, Md: Aspen Publishers, Inc.; 1986.
3. Sim J. Methodology and morality in physiotherapy research. *Physiotherapy.* April 1989; 75(4):237–243.
4. Wayne S, Rhyne RL, Thompson RF, et al. Sampling issues in nursing home research. *J Am Ger Soc.* March 1991; 39(3):308–311.
5. Kelly P, Kroemer K. Anthropometry of the elderly: status and recommendations. *Human Factors.* October 1990; 32(5):571–595.
6. Nelson E, Dannefer D. Aged heterogeneity: fact or fiction? the fate of diversity in gerontological research. *Gerontologist.* 1992; 32(1):17–23.
7. Andrews G. Cross-cultural studies—an important development in aging research. *J Am Ger Soc.* May 1989; 37(5):483–485.
8. Schunk C. Research and the elderly. In: Lewis CB (ed.). *Aging: Health Care's Challenge.* Philadelphia: F.A. Davis; 1985.
9. Schale KW. Quasi-experimental research designs in the psychology of aging. In: Britton SE, Schale KW, eds. *Handbook of the Psychology of Aging.* New York: Van Nostrand Rheinhold; 1985:39.
10. Rayman I, Bloom S. Survey research as a tool for studying problems in the elderly. In: Kent B, Butler RN (eds.). *Aging: Human Aging Research—Concepts & Techniques,* Vol. 34. New York: Raven Press; 1988; 34:51–76.
11. Mattson D. *Statistics Difficult Concepts: Understandable Explanations.* Oak Park, Ill: Bolzchazy-Carducco Publishers, Inc.; 1986.
12. Ciccione C. Lecture notes from *Geriatrics: An Advanced Tutorial,* San Francisco, Calif.: February 1992.
13. Rothstein J, Echternach J. Hypothesis-oriented algorithm for clinicians—a method for evaluation & treatment planning. *Phys Ther.* September 1986; 66(9):1388–1394.
14. Connolly B, et al. Single-case research: when is it valid? *Phys Ther.* November 1983; 63(11):1767–1768.
15. Woolery M, Harris S. Interpreting results of single-subject research designs. *Phys Ther.* April 1982; 62(4):445–452.
16. Shepard K. Qualitative & quantitative research in clinical practice. *Phys Ther.* December 1987; 67(12):1891–1894.
17. Jensen G. Qualitative methods in physical therapy research: a form of disciplined inquiry. *Phys Ther.* June 1989; 69(6):492–500.
18. Schmoll B. Ethnographic inquiry in clinical settings. *Phys Ther.* December 1987; 67(12):1895–1897.
19. Bohannon R, LeVeau B. Clinicians' use of research findings. *Phys Ther.* January 1986; 66(1):45–50.

CHAPTER *21* TWENTY-ONE

Aging Network Resources

Helpful Organizations	Heart Disease
General Information	High Blood Pressure
Women's Health Issues	Alcoholism
Nutrition and Physical Fitness	Data Base Resources
Medications	Long-Term Care Issues
Accident Prevention	Housing Options
Osteoporosis	Financial Planning
Osteoarthritis	Care Giving
Urinary Incontinence	Widowhood
Cognitive Changes	Political Issues
Diabetes	Legal Issues
Cancer	Educational/Career Issues

The goal of this chapter is to give a meaningful sampling of the available resources for the elderly so that the reader can create his or her own network. The wonderful thing about the resources selected for this chapter is that they are bound to lead to others. A definitive list of resources would itself fill a large book and would encompass organizations and services that operate locally as well as nationally.

HELPFUL ORGANIZATIONS

General Information

Diseases and disabilities that afflict enough people have their own organizations like the American Lung Association, the American Cancer Society, and the American Heart Association. There are more than 200 of these repositories of general information, all user-friendly. Most of the organizations will send free booklets about their diseases, and they are excellent sources of patient educational materials.

Some national organizations are listed in the local yellow pages, or a printed listing of private and public sources can be ordered for $17.25 postpaid by writing to: Resource Information Guide, P.O. Box 990297, Redding, CA. 96099.

The National Health Information Center [1–800–336–4797] can also refer interested persons to the appropriate organizations. Don't be shy—the center receives calls for every disease imaginable, and its staff is armed with 1100 phone numbers. For less well-known illnesses, the National Organization for Rare Disorders, created by Abbey Meyers after she discovered how hard it was to get information on Tourette's syndrome (which her three children have), is another excellent source for information. This organization supplies the public with the kind of information to which she wishes she had had easier access. There is information available on 950 diseases. The pamphlets and informational materials cover symptoms and therapies for patient education, as well as current research reviews for the clinician. The first request is free; subsequent reports cost $3.25 each [1–203–746–6518].

Hot Lines

Hot lines have been created and are another excellent source of information. A prostate hot line, for instance, offers advice on treatments [1–800–543–9632]. The Y-ME National Organization for Breast Cancer offers information and support to women with breast cancer [1–800–221–2141 or 1–708–799–8228]. The Centers for Disease Control and Prevention offers information on risk factors for just about any disease and operates an AIDS hot line [1–800–432–AIDS].

For a list of some 100 hot lines call the National Health Information Center (telephone number in previous paragraph). For $1 they will send a roster of toll-free health information numbers. Some operate from nine to five, others are on call 24 hours. The National Health Information Clearinghouse (P.O. Box 1133, Washington, DC 20013; 1–800–336–4797 or 1–703–522–2590) will help locate resources pertaining to health information; specific questions about health are referred to appropriate experts or federal agencies.

Support Groups

Support Groups are another excellent source of information. While most people think such groups are merely sources of emotional support, they also provide a powerful function of information exchanges. For example, a patient developed a problem with such frequent urination that she could not leave the house. Her doctor told her there was no treatment for urinary incontinence, but he referred her to a self-help group for people who shared this affliction. From the group, she learned about a drug that offered relief, not yet approved in the United States, but available in Europe and Mexico. Armed with this information, she returned to her doctor, who obtained the drug for her through an experimental program. The drug was effective in resolving her urinary incontinence, and her functional level of activity has returned to a desirable balance.

The American Self-Help Clearinghouse at St Clares Riverside Medical Center in Denville, New Jersey, tracks more than 700 groups and publishes the *Self-Help Source-Book*, available for $10 [1–201–625–7101]. They will also provide numbers for clearing houses in 19 states: California, Connecticut, Illinois, Iowa, Kansas, Massachusetts, Michigan, Missouri, Nebraska, New Jersey, New York, North Carolina, Ohio, Oregon, Pennsylvania, South Carolina, Tennessee, Texas, and the District of Columbia. These regional clearinghouses can give information on specific local support groups. The National Self-Help Clearinghouse will also send a list of support group information. Just send a self-addressed stamped envelope (SASE) to: 25 West 43rd St., New York, NY 10036 [1–212–840–7606].

Patient and Professional Education

For patient and professional educational materials on just about any disease, disability, or social problem afflicting the elderly the US Department of Health and Human Services and the National Institute on Aging, which is a division of this agency, are excellent sources. To obtain a comprehensive listing of *all* available publications from these two institutions write to: Department of Health and Human Services, Public Health Service, Agency for Health Care Policy and Research, Executive Office Center, 2101 East Jefferson Street, Suite 501, Rockville, MD 20852 and NIA Information Center, 2209 Distribution Circle, Silver Spring, MD 20910. In addition, the Robert Wood Foundation, Consumer Information Center, Pueblo, CO 81009 and the American Association of Retired Persons, 1909 K Street, N.W., Washington, DC 20049 [1–202–872–4700] will provide numerous materials on issues related to aging and disease/disability.

Women's Health Issues

For women's illnesses, the National Women's Health Network provides information and referrals on 75 topics [1–202–347–1140]. The National Institute on Aging has a wonderful publication, called Health Resources for Older Women, that is free of charge and can be obtained by writing to: NIA Information Center, 2209 Distribution Circle, Silver Spring, MD 20910 and asking for NIH Publication No. 87–2899. This publication provides resources on age changes and health promotion, such as menopause, nutrition and physical fitness, skin changes, use of medicines, and accident prevention. In addition, common disorders such as osteoporosis, osteoarthritis, urinary incontinence, and cognitive changes are discussed and available resources are presented. Educational material is available on housing options, financial planning, care giving, and widowhood as well. The NIA also has an excellent and comprehensive booklet entitled: Who? What? Where?: Resources for Women's Health and Aging that includes resource information on all of these areas in women's health, in addition to materials and resources on Alzheimer's disease and other cognitive changes, depression, heart disease, and current research related to women and aging (NIH Publication No. 91–323, 1992).

The Center for Climacteric Studies (University of Florida, 901 N.W. 8th Avenue, Suite B1, Gainesville, FL 32601; 1–904–392–3184) was established to promote research, public education, and clinical service in areas related to women's health issues. HERS (Hysterectomy Education Resources, 422 Bryn Mawr Avenue, Bala Cynwyd, PA 19004; 1–215–667–7757) is also an excellent source of educational materials on menopause and OB-GYN surgical procedures. This organization publishes a quarterly newsletter that is a valuable update mechanism for research oriented toward women's health problems related to menopause. The American College of Obstetricians and Gynecologists (600 Maryland Avenue, S.W., Suite 300 East, Washington, DC 20024; 1–202–638–4680) offers patient education pamphlets entitled The Menopause Years, Estrogen Use, and Preventing Osteoporosis.

The National Women's Health Network (224 Seventh Street, S.E., Washington, DC 20024; 1–202–223–6886) is an organization that serves as a clearinghouse for information on women's health issues. It also publishes a newsletter on health and lobbying efforts.

Nutrition and Physical Fitness

Guidelines on specific nutritional requirements of older people are scarce. Current RDAs divide the adult population into only two age groups: those aged 23 to 50 and those over age 50. Relatively little research has been done to define the impact of age related physiological changes on human nutritional requirements. However, the few studies that have been done indicate that aging may affect the need for certain nutrients, vitamins, and minerals. For example, the ability of the body to absorb calcium and vitamin D declines substantially with age, possibly increasing older people's susceptibility to osteoporosis and risk of bone fractures.

With age the need for calories declines while the requirements for protein, minerals, and vitamins remains the same. Also, many people decrease their physical activity somewhat as they grow older, and this also reduces the need for calories. Good health depends on staying physically active. Current evidence from research shows exercise strengthens the heart and lungs, lowers blood pressure, reduces the risk of diabetes, reduces the level of certain fats in the blood, and strengthens bone. Thus, maintaining a regular fitness program is important. Exercise can safeguard health, help control weight, and contribute to a better mental outlook.

The American Dietetic Association (430 North Michigan Avenue, Chicago, IL 60611; 1–312–280–5000) is interested in improving the dietary habits of all people and works to advance the science of dietetics and nutrition, as well as to promote education in these areas. The American Physical Therapy Association (1111 North Fairfax Street, Alexandria, VA 22314–9902; 1–800–999–2782) can provide valuable information on exercise specific to the aging population. In addition, the President's Council on Physical Fitness and Sports (450 5th Street, N.W., Suite 7103, Washington, DC 20001; 1–202–272–3421) is mandated by an executive order signed by the president for the purpose of explaining to the public the importance of physical fitness. The council trains professionals to run health and fitness demonstration programs for the elderly and provides brochures, films, and speakers.

Medications

Drugs often affect the body differently as an individual increases in age, probably because of normal changes in the body's metabolism. Such changes can affect the length of time a drug remains in the body and the amount of the drug absorbed by body tissues. There are precautions that can be taken to reduce the risks associated with drug use (for example, taking the exact dosage prescribed and having a pharmacist or physician monitor the use of multiple drugs to avoid adverse reactions).

The AARP Pharmacy Service (P.O. Box NIA, 1 Prince Street, Alexandria, VA 22314; 1–703–684–9244) provides information on common prescription drugs, side effects, and cost differences between brand name and generic drugs. It has published a series of leaflets called Medication Information Leaflets for Seniors (MILS), which discuss 350 prescription drugs. For copies write to the Pharmacy Service, specifying the drugs you are interested in. The service also operates 12 pharmacies throughout the country for members of AARP.

Another excellent source of information on drugs, the American Pharmaceutical Association (2215 Constitution Avenue, N.W., Washington, DC 20037; 1–202–628–4410), is composed of practicing pharmacists, manufacturers, researchers, and publishers of pharmaceutical literature, promotes public health by establishing satisfactory drug standards. For answers to questions regarding drug approval, drug reactions, and other issues concerning new or approved medications, the Food and Drug Administration (Division of Regulatory Affairs, Center for Drugs and Biologics, 5600 Fisher Lane, Rockville, MD 20857; 1–301–295–8012) is a good resource for information.

Accident Prevention

Accidental injuries become more frequent and serious in later life. Several factors make people in this age group prone to accidents: poorer eyesight and hearing can decrease awareness of hazards; arthritis, neurological diseases, and impaired coordination and balance can affect steadiness; illness, use of medicines or alcohol, and preoccupation with personal problems can cause drowsiness or distraction. Falling is the most common cause of fatal injury in the aged. Each year it causes hip fractures in about 210,000 older person, 20% of whom die within the first year after an injury. In addition, a fall can result in months of pain and confinement or the fear of falling again. For some older persons it leads to institutionalization. Older women have a greater chance of developing osteoporosis and in combination with a greater risk of falls this increases the chances of fracture.

Automobile accidents are the second most common cause of accidents among older persons. Many of these accidents could be prevented, however, by limiting the distance traveled and the number of hours on the road, by using extra caution driving in evening rush hour and in winter weather, and by staying on familiar roads. The American Association of Retired Persons (AARP) (55 Alive/Mature Driving Program, Traffic and Driver Safety Program, 601 E Street, N.W., Washington, DC; 1–202–434–2277 or 1–800–434–2277) offers an 8-hour classroom, driver education refresher course for persons age 50 or older, taught by instructors who are 50 or older. In some states, a certificate of completion entitles the driver to a discount on automobile insurance. In addition, the American Automobile Association (AAA), offers the Mature Operator Program, an 8-hour classroom course for persons age 55 and over to enhance driving knowledge and awareness of new techniques and information about safe driving.

It is also especially important for older people to avoid prolonged exposure to extreme heat or cold. Accidental hypothermia (e.g., an abnormally low body temperature) can be avoided by wearing several layers of clothing and keeping the head covered. When older people live alone, they should arrange to have someone check on them daily when temperatures are very low. Overexposure to heat or to the sun can result in hyperthermia (heat stroke), a serious and potentially fatal condition. Older people, especially those with chronic diseases, can avoid hyperthermia by remaining in shady areas outside or in cool rooms during hot weather.

The National Safety Council (444 North Michigan Avenue, Chicago, IL 60611; 1–312–527–4800) is a nonprofit public service organization whose goal is to prevent accidents and improve the health of all Americans. The National Institute on Aging has some excellent materials on home safety, accidental hypothermia, and prevention of injury to older adults.

Osteoporosis

Osteoporosis is sometimes called the "silent disease" because it has no symptoms during its early stages. Unfortunately, the condition is usually not recognized until it reaches an advanced stage when fractures occur, most often in the spine, wrists, and hips. Current recommendations to prevent osteoporosis involve engaging regularly in weight bearing exercise and consuming adequate amounts of calcium and vitamin D throughout life. The American Academy of Orthopaedic Surgeons (222 South Prospect Avenue, Park Ridge, IL 60068; 1–312–823–7186) is a professional association whose members are orthopaedic surgeons. The staff offers an educational brochure entitled *Osteoporosis*. The National Institute of Arthritis and Musculoskeletal and Skin Diseases (NIAMS) (Public Information Office, Building 31, Room B2B15, Bethesda, MD 20892; 1–301–496–8188), one of the National Institutes of Health, supports clinical research on such chronic disabling diseases as osteoporosis, arthritis, and other musculoskeletal and skin diseases. The National Institute on Aging (Public Information Office, Building 31, Room 5C35, Bethesda, MD 20892; 1–301–496–2947) supports biomedical, social, and behavioral research on the aging process and special problems common to older people. The National Osteoporosis Foundation (1625 Eye Street, N.W., Suite 1011, Washington, DC 20006; 1–202–223–2226) offers programs nationwide to educate professionals and the public about osteoporosis and related research.

Osteoarthritis

Osteoarthritis (OA), one of the most common forms of arthritis, is a degenerative joint disease that develops in a large number of people by the age of 65 years. Only half of those affected experience pain and loss of mobility as a result of OA. It is important to reduce symptoms and prevent the disability and handicaps that result from inactivity. The form of treatment recommended depends on how severe the disease is and which joints are affected. General approaches to treatment are to control pain with drugs, to protect the joints from stress through rest, and by exercising regularly to strengthen muscles supporting the joints. Surgery for joint replacement is often indicated in the more severe cases of OA.

The Arthritis Foundation (1314 Spring Street, N.W., Atlanta, GA 30309; 1–404–872–7100) is a nationwide program committed to examining the cause and cure for arthritis and to improving treatments for arthritic patients. Services offered include public information and education about arthritis, a variety of publications for patient education, referrals to specialists, and community activities, such as arthritis clinics and rehabilitation and home care programs. The National Institute of Arthritis and Musculoskeletal and Skin Diseases, as mentioned in the previous section, is also an excellent source of patient and professional informational materials and research.

Urinary Incontinence

Urinary incontinence is especially common in women over the age of 65 years. Because those affected often isolate themselves, incontinence can be both a medical and a social problem. Two common types of incontinence are urge incontinence, in which the individual is unable to hold urine long enough to make it to the bathroom, and stress incontinence, in which leakage occurs during physical exertion or when sneezing, coughing, or laughing. Stress incontinence is also found in younger women as a result of pelvic floor weakening following pregnancy. The treatment method most often used to relieve incontinence include exercises (Kegel exercises to strengthen the pelvic floor muscles), medications, and surgery.

The HIP (Help for Incontinent People) Organization (P.O. Box 544, Union, SC 29379; 1–803–585–8789) is a self-help and patient advocacy group that offers encouragement, information, and resource listings for incontinent individuals. It also publishes the Resource Guide for Continence Aids and Services and the quarterly newsletter The HIP Report. The Simon Foundation (P.O. Box 835X, Wilmette, IL 60091; 1–800–237–4666) is a nonprofit educational group and serves as a clearinghouse for information on incontinence. It also publishes a newsletter entitled *The Informer*. Continence Restored (785 Park Avenue, New York, NY 10021; 1–212–879–3131 or 407 Strawberry Hill Avenue, Stamford, CT 06902; 1–203–348–0601) is a newly developed self-help organization that provides a wealth of information and support through the assistance of medically trained leaders. The US Department of Health and Human Services has an excellent set of publications that serve as a quick reference for clinicians (AHCPR 92–0041), a more extensive booklet on clinical practice guidelines (AHCPR 92–0038), and a patient's guide (AHCPR 92–0040), all of which are very comprehensive and valuable as educational tools in treating urinary incontinence in both men and women.

Cognitive Changes

Mental decline is not a normal part of growing older. Symptoms of cognitive decline, such as memory loss, bizzare behavior, personality changes, confusion, and extreme combativeness, in an older person may indicate the presence of any number of conditions, some of which are reversible. Two forms of incurable mental impairment that occur in old age are Alzheimer's disease and multi-infarct dementia.

What may appear to be profound mental impairment often is a reversible condition that can be easily corrected. Common causes of reversible impairment are poor nutrition, adverse drug reactions, high fever, and minor head injuries. Emotional problems frequently cause a reversible condition as well. Anxiety, boredom, loneliness, and depression can all appear as mental impairment. Depression, in particular, is the most common cause of pseudodementia.

The Alzheimer's Disease and Related Disorders Association (70 East Lake Street, Chicago, IL 60601; 1–800–621–0379) serves as a clearinghouse for all aspects of Alzheimer's disease, including medical, psychosocial, research, legal, political, fundraising, and family services and support. The National Institute of Neurological and Communicative Disorders and Stroke (NINCDS) (Public Information Office, Building 31, Room 8A06, Bethesda, MD 20892; 1–301–496–5751), one of the National Institutes of Health, supports research on neurological and communicative disorders and on stroke. It offers an excellent booklet entitled *The Dementias*. Nursing home resources are listed in the "Housing Options" section of this chapter. The Alzheimer's Disease Education and Referral Center (ADEAR) (P.O. Box 8250, Silver Spring, MD 20907–8250; 1–301–495–3311), established by NIA, distributes information to health professionals, patients and their families, and the general public on Alzheimer's disease, current research activities, and available services.

Diabetes

The best source for information on diabetes is the American Diabetes Association (ADA) (Two Park Avenue, New York, NY 10016; 1–212–683–7444). Members of ADA include physicians, research scientists, and dietitians, as well as diabetics and their families. The association sponsors educational lectures, film presentations, and diabetes screening clinics.

Cancer

The Cancer Information Service of the National Cancer Institute (NCI) (9000 Rockville Pike, Building 31, Room 10A18, Bethesda, MD 20892; 1–800–4–CANCER). In this program, trained NCI staff answer questions and offer publications about various aspects of cancer prevention, detection, causes, and treatments.

Heart Disease

The American Heart Association (AHA) (7320 Greenville Avenue, Dallas, TX 75231; 1–214–373–6300) supports research, education, and community service programs with the objective of reducing premature death and disability from cardiovascular disease and stroke. Local chapters are found in many communities. In addition, the Mended Hearts, a subgroup of the AHA, provides information, encouragement, and services to heart disease patients and their families. The National Heart, Lung, and Blood Institute (NHLBI) (9000 Rockville Pike, Bethesda, MD 20892; 1–301–496–4236), one of the National Institutes of Health, provides leadership for a national program of research and education on causes, prevention, diagnosis, and treatment of diseases of the heart, blood vessels, blood, and lungs, and on the use of blood and the management of blood resources.

High Blood Pressure

The High Blood Pressure Information Center (120/80 National Institutes of Health, Bethesda, MD 20892) is operated by the National Heart, Lung, and Blood Institute and provides information relating to research on the causes, prevention, methods of diagnosis, and treatment of heart, blood vessel, and blood diseases.

Alcoholism

The best source of information on alcoholism in the elderly is the National Council on Alcoholism (12 West 21st Street, New York, NY 10010; 1–212–206–6770). This is a voluntary organization whose purpose is to educate the public about the disease of alcoholism and to promote programs for prevention.

DATA BASE RESOURCES

More than any other tool, the computer has diminished the gap between health care providers and patients. There are as many as 245 data bases or computerized indexes of information today. The most important index, and the one on which most searches are based is Medline, a data base of 3600 medical journals. With a personal computer, a modem, and a $30 software package (e.g., Grateful Med), a search can be conducted for in-depth articles on any medical subject. For the Grateful Med software: 1–800–638–8480; for a free demo disk and brochure: 1–301–496–6308.

A guide to other data bases, Directory of Online Healthcare Databases, is available for $38 [1–503–471–1627]. This is a far-reaching directory with data bases on specific diseases and specific treatments. Most major medical libraries subscribe to Medline, and a reference librarian is an excellent source of information and guidance in how to use the system. In addition, some libraries, hospitals, and HMOs have desktop terminals that provide information for the "nonscientific public." For the nearest center, call: 1–800–227–8431 and ask for marketing. MDX Health Digest contains 200 health-oriented publications [1–503–471–1627]. Both of these services rely mainly on secondary sources and will link the user to more specific informational centers, and both information and materials are usually free.

If you are already into computer technology or are eager to learn, you can scan all kinds of exchanges between people delving into various medical subjects via some 300 electronic "bulletin boards." You can also send out a message and await a reply. For a list of health-oriented computer bulletin boards, send $5 and a SASE to Black Bag BBS, 1 Ball Farm Way, Wilmington, DE 19808, or with a modem, dial: 1–302–994–3772.

An extension of the computer bulletin board is the online conference, a sort of electronic self-help group accessible from your living room. The American Self-Help Clearinghouse organized the first online conference for agoraphobics (people who are afraid of open or public places). They linked up without having to leave the house and chat via keyboards. This could also be a boon for elderly people in rural areas.

CompuServe, an online information service, hosts several groups (for a membership fee of around $40, plus a small monthly charge). There is, for instance, a diabetes forum. For general information call: 1–800–848–8199. For cancer patients, there are numerous data bases. Designed both for medical practitioners and the public, they are among the most complete and easy to use. Medline, for instance, offers a separate cancer data base called CANCERLIT.

A list of treatment centers, plus some 1500 experimental programs, is available through the National Cancer Institute's data base called Physician Data Query (PDQ). PDQ also has a directory of physicians and organizations that provide cancer care. Although it is designed for doctors, you can tap into PDQ by using the Grateful Med software. You can also call 1–800–4–CANCER and request a free PDQ search, and they will mail it to you free of charge. If you have a fax, try Cancer-Fax at 1–301–402–5874 and an automated voice will tell you how to obtain detailed prognosis and treatment summaries on 80 kinds of cancers. The information is updated every month, and you can request a version intended for either medical professionals or for the general public.

Data base resources are also available through data brokers to meet the needs of health care professionals. The four listed here rely heavily on Medline, tend to be consumer oriented, and are staffed by professionals. The Health Resource Inc., a commercial enterprise, will provide Medline searches, article summaries, book excerpts, and medical journal articles, as well as lists of self-help groups. They cover alternative and holistic interventions along with the more mainstream sources of help. A report of 50 to 150 pages costs from $175 up, a mini-report (20 to 25 pages) runs $85. There is a 30-day money-back guarantee if you are not satisfied [1–501–

329–5272]. The nonprofit Planetree Health Resource Center provides an in-depth packet on a particular illness for $100. They will do a PDQ search for $25 per topic or a Medline search for $35 per topic. Medline searches are included in the comprehensive package, as are book excerpts and magazine articles [1–415–923–3680]. The Medical Information Service of the Palo Alto Medical Foundation was founded as a nonprofit service for medical professionals. They also provide information for the general public. A standard search, including Medline, costs $89 [1–800–999–1999]. The Medical Data Exchange offers a search on its own consumer health data base, MDX Health Digest, at a cost of $25. A Medline search is $48. If you need a more exhaustive, customized search, it is $60 an hour. This company also began as a data source for health professionals but recently launched into searches for lay people. [1–503–471–1627].

LONG-TERM CARE ISSUES

Housing Options

In later years changing circumstances often create the need for a new living arrangement. Costly maintenance and utility bills, the desire to relocate closer to family or to live in a smaller home, or a need for regular nursing attention are just a few of the considerations older persons have regarding housing. Today, a wide variety of housing options are available, some of which include new types of living arrangements that have evolved only in recent years. Some people arrange for "in-home" services for special needs. These might include homemaker or home health aide services, home-delivered meals, and escort or transportation services. Others consider renting out a portion of their home. Additional options include moving to a smaller home, moving in with family members, moving to a group home where older people share one residence, or moving to a community designed especially for older people. Many types of housing offer support services, as in a continuing care community or a nursing home.

The American Association of Homes for the Aging (AAHA) (1129 20th Street, N.W., Washington, DC 20036; 1–202–296–5960) is a national organization whose members include nonprofit nursing homes, independent housing facilities, continuing care facilities, and homes for the aging. They provide an excellent brochure entitled *The Continuing Care Retirement Community: A Guidebook for Consumers*. The National Association of Home Care (519 C Street, N.E., Stanton Park, Washington, DC 20002; 1–202–547–7424) monitors federal and state activities affecting home care and focuses on issues relating to home health care. They publish a magazine bimonthly called the *Caring Magazine*. The National Citizen's Coalition for Nursing Home Reform (1424 16th Street, N.W., Room L2, Washington, DC 20036; 1–202–797–0657) serves as a voice enabling consumers to be heard on issues concerning the development of long-term care systems. The Nursing Home Information Service (National Council of Senior Citizens, National Senior Citizens Education and Research Center, 925 15th Street, N.W., Washington, DC 20005; 1–202–347–8800) is a referral center for consumers of long-term care services. They offer information on nursing homes and alternative community and health services, and information on how to select a nursing home.

Financial Planning

Many older people are able to enjoy their retirement years with enough money to meet their basic needs and enjoy some leisure activities. Others face poverty for the first time in old age. Retirement savings often must be used for expensive medical treatment; fixed incomes or savings that many older persons depend on can be eroded by high inflation rates, and with a longer life expectancy, many older people simply outlive their assets.

Women are at a particularly high risk for becoming impoverished. Women generally earn lower salaries than men, and this further limits retirement benefits. Benefits are calculated on average lifetime earnings, so time spent at home to rear children reduces both pension and Social Security income in later life. Women are also more likely to work part-time and for employers who do not offer pension benefits, such as service businesses. Moreover, though Social Security is intended to supplement other forms of retirement income, for 60% of women over age 65 it is the only source of support. Another problem is that a large group of older women do not receive the benefits they are eligible for, either because they do not know about them or how to get them, or because they are too proud to accept this assistance. Others, especially those for whom English is a second language, may not understand the complicated paperwork necessary to initiate payments. Thus, only half of the elderly persons eligible for Supplemental Security Income actually receive benefits.

The Social Security Administration (SSA) (Office of Public Inquiries, 6401 Security Boulevard, Baltimore, MD 21235; 1–301–594–1234) is a federal agency that provides information about Social Security coverage, earnings records, claims eligibility, and adjustments. They also have information about Medicare and Medicaid programs. The Supplemental Security Income program is also administered by the SSA, and provides supplemental payments to older persons who already receive public assistance. Social Security branch offices are located throughout the country and are listed in local telephone directories. The Women's Equity Action League (1250 Eye Street, N.W., Suite 305, Washington, DC 20005; 1–202–898–1588) is a national organization whose members are dedicated to securing legal and economic rights for women by monitoring the implementation and enforcement of equal opportunity laws, conducting research, publishing reports, lobbying, and supporting lawsuits.

Care Giving

Care giving is the job of helping a relative or friend with meals, shopping, and other daily activities. A recent survey of care givers for elderly persons showed this role is most often taken on by women, usually wives or daughters. Care giving is also a policy issue growing in importance today since the number of people over age 85 (i.e., those in greatest need of daily help) is increasing rapidly and is expected to more than double within the next 15 years. With this rapid growth in the frail elderly population, a declining birth rate, and more women participating in the labor force, a wider diversity of groups are taking on responsibility for shouldering the tasks of care giving. Many groups are developing new ways of enabling families to share in partnership with other types of support systems, although the nature of such partnerships and the proper division of responsibility remain complex issues and are subject to much debate.

The Administration on Aging (AoA) (Office of Human Development DHHS, 330 Independence Avenue, S.W., Washington, DC 20201; 1–202–245–0724 [general information]; 1–202–245–0641 [publications]) is a federal agency and provides information about social services, nutrition, education, senior centers, and other programs for older Americans. It also offers A Directory of State and Regional Agencies on Aging, which lists local Area Agencies on Aging. These agencies are helpful in finding local services to answer a specific need. An organization called the Children of Aging Parents (2761 Trenton Road, Levittown, PA 19056; 1–215–945–6900) provides a variety of services, including starter packages for those interested in becoming care givers, a "matching" service for people starting a support group, workshops for the general community, and printed material. They also distribute a monthly newsletter.

Widowhood

The average age of widowhood for women in the United States is 56, which means half of all women over age 65 are living as widows. The average age of widowerhood for men is 72. This high rate of widowhood occurs because women tend to marry men older than themselves and because life expectancy from birth is 7 years longer for women than for men. Widowhood is often the end of a relationship that lasted most of a lifetime; it can cause profound grief. Thus recovery is often painful and takes time. The period of most intense grief can last from a few months to a year or more. During this time, it is normal for the widowed person to feel despair or depression, irritability, and even anger toward the person who died. After this grieving process, the individual is usually able to increase her or his range of independence and find new friends and activities to enrich life, although most people need special help with the social and psychological problems associated with being widowed.

Loneliness also commonly arises during this period. It sometimes takes an extra effort to find social activities and friends, but many resources are available on which to draw. Also, by offering their skills, many elderly individuals make new friendships through a variety of affiliations: with religious or civic organizations, voluntary activities, and other commitments. Women who find themselves alone as a result of widowhood may need to develop new skills for a changing role. For example, some must learn to manage financial matters for the first time, such as paying bills, balancing a checkbook, and handling insurance benefits.

To help both widows and widowers, a growing number of national and local organizations provide social and other types of support. ACTION (806 Connecticut Avenue, N.W., Washington, DC 20525; 1–800–424–8580) is a federal agency that administers domestic and international volunteer programs including the Peace Corps, Retired Senior Volunteer Program, Foster Grandparent Program, Senior Companion Project, and others. The Displaced Homemaker Network (1411 K Street, N.W., Washington, DC 20005; 1–202–628–6767) is an agency that fosters the development of programs across the United States with services to help displaced homemakers; these include individual counseling, support groups, employment/training seminars, vocational testing, and a "job club." The Widowed Persons Service is a part of AARP (American Association of Retired Persons, 1909 K Street, N.W., Washington, DC 20049; 1–202–872–4700). This is an outreach program for newly widowed persons. A service of the AARP, it provides group sessions, publication about legal matters, volunteer opportunities, and other services.

POLITICAL ISSUES

The Grey Panthers (3635 Chestnut Street, Philadelphia, PA 19104; 1–215–382–3300) is a coalition of activists who work to promote the concerns of the aged through newsletters and publications aimed at fighting various types of abuse and age discrimination. The National Coalition on Older Women's Issues (NCOWI) (2401 Virginia Avenue, N.W., Washington, DC 20037; 1–202–466–7837) is a nationwide network made up of member organizations and individuals concerned with improving the status of older women. Its focus is on the areas of employment, retirement income, and the health and well-being of women. NCOWI offers a list of organizations called Midlife and Older Women: A Resource Directory. The cost is $4.

The National Council on the Aging (NCOA) (600 Maryland Avenue, S.W., West Wing 100, Washington, DC 20024; 1–202–479–1200), in conjunction with other organizations, helps to promote concerns of interest to older persons. NCOA conducts seminars on wellness, offers a range of publications on public policy, advocacy, education, and career training, and functions as a resource for public education.

The National Organization for Women (425 13th Street, N.W., Washington, DC 20002; 1–202–347–2279) is an advocacy group that monitors local and national legislation affecting American women. Members participate in activities concerned with women's rights issues, such as economic protections for older women, participation in politics, recognition of the economic value of homemaking, and freedom from racial and educational discrimination. The Older Women's League (OWL) (1325 G Street, N.W., Lower Level B, Washington, DC 20005; 1–202–783–6686) has a national membership who are committed to helping meet various special needs of middle-aged and older women, especially in the areas of Social Security, pension rights, health insurance, and care giver support services. OWL uses volunteers to help with mailings, to maintain a referral resource file, and to answer letters from women writing in from across the country with questions.

LEGAL ISSUES

The Commission on Legal Problems of the Elderly (1800 M Street, N.W., Washington, DC 20036; 1–202–331–2297) is a commission that works to improve the quality and quantity of legal services for older citizens. It refers requests for services to appropriate agencies or groups. The National Senior Citizens Law Center (2025 M Street, N.W., Suite 400, Washington, DC 20036; 1–202–887–5280) is a public interest law firm with attorneys who specialize in areas of federal law having the greatest impact on the elderly poor. An excellent source of information on legal issues is the *American Civil Liberties Union Handbook* (Brown RN. *The Rights of Older Persons: A Basic Guide to the Legal Rights of Older Persons Under the Current Law*. Edwardsville, IL: Southern Illinois University Press; 1989). It covers every conceivable issue, from living wills to social security pensions, to patients' rights.

EDUCATIONAL/CAREER ISSUES

The American Association of University Women (2401 Virginia Avenue, N.W., Washington, DC 20037; 1–202–785–7700) is the largest national organization promoting the advancement of women in education and lifelong learning. For its members the AAUW holds monthly lectures and for the public it offers a variety of publications relating to education and career reentry. Elderhostel (80 Boylston Street, Suite 400, Boston, MA 02116; 1–617–426–7788) is a nonprofit educational program for adults age 60 and over. The program consists of 1-week courses taught in residence at various college campuses. The courses offer a range of liberal arts subjects presented at an introductory level. Free catalogues are available on request.

The National Commission on Working Women (1211 Connecticut Avenue, N.W., Suite 400, Washington, DC 20036; 1–202–332–1405) is a private organization that focuses on the concerns of women working in service industries, clerical occupations, retail stores, and factories.

INDEX